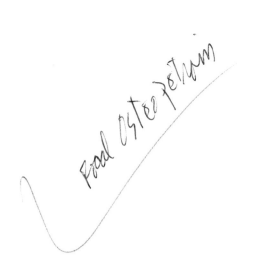

Food Osteopathy

D0759896

ORAL PATHOLOGY

ORAL PATHOLOGY
Clinical Pathologic Correlations

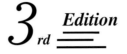

3rd *Edition*

Joseph A. Regezi, D.D.S., M.S.

Professor of Oral Pathology, School of Dentistry
Professor, Pathology, School of Medicine
University of California, San Francisco
San Francisco, California

James J. Sciubba, D.M.D., Ph.D.

Chairman, Department of Dental Medicine
Long Island Jewish Medical Center
New Hyde Park, New York
Professor, Department of Oral Biology and Pathology
School of Dental Medicine
State University of New York at Stony Brook
Stony Brook, New York

W.B. SAUNDERS COMPANY

A Division of Harcourt Brace & Company
Philadelphia   London   Toronto   Montreal   Sydney   Tokyo

W.B. SAUNDERS COMPANY
A Division of Harcourt Brace & Company

The Curtis Center
Independence Square West
Philadelphia, Pennsylvania 19106

Library of Congress Cataloging-in-Publication Data

Oral pathology: clinical pathologic correlations / Joseph A. Regezi, James J. Sciubba.—3rd ed.

p.   cm.

Includes bibliographical references and index.

ISBN 0–7216–7731–2

1. Mouth—Diseases.   2. Teeth—Diseases.   I. Sciubba, James J.   II. Title.
   [DNLM: 1. Tooth Diseases.   2. Mouth Diseases.   WU 140 R333o 1999]

RC815.R39 1999   617.5′22—dc21

DNLM/DLC   97-51667

ORAL PATHOLOGY: CLINICAL PATHOLOGIC CORRELATIONS, 3rd edition   ISBN 0–7216–7731–2

Printed in the United States of America.

Last digit is the print number: 9   8   7   6   5   4   3   2   1

Contributors

Ginat W. Mirowski, D.M.D., M.M.Sc., M.D.
Assistant Professor, Department of Oral
 Surgery, Medicine, and Pathology,
 Indiana University, School of Dentistry;
 Assistant Professor, Department of
 Dermatology, Indiana University, School
 of Medicine, Indianapolis, Indiana
Common Skin Lesions

Todd W. Rozycki, M.D.
Indiana University, School of Medicine,
 Indianapolis, Indiana
Common Skin Lesions

Jeffery C. B. Stewart, D.D.S., M.S.
Assistant Professor, Department of
 Pathology, University of Pennsylvania
 School of Dental Medicine, Philadelphia,
 Pennsylvania
Benign Nonodontogenic Tumors

Richard J. Zarbo, M.D., D.M.D.
Professor of Pathology, Case Western
 Reserve University School of Medicine,
 Cleveland, Ohio; Vice-Chairman,
 Anatomic Pathology, Henry Ford
 Hospital, Detroit, Michigan
*Malignant Nonodontogenic Neoplasms of the
Jaws*

Preface

The purpose of this book is to present current concepts of oral and maxillofacial pathology in a convenient and logical format. Its clinical orientation, as evidenced by disease classifications, descriptions, and photographs, should facilitate the identification and treatment of oral diseases. Microscopic correlations are also provided—an aspect that not only helps in the understanding of disease processes but also can provide an invaluable aid in clinical diagnosis and patient management. This text should help form a bridge between the didactic aspects of oral pathology and the practical clinical considerations.

This book is also designed to help enhance diagnostic skills through the use of differential diagnostic considerations. The development of a differential diagnosis is an effective academic teaching tool with considerable practical value in daily practice. An appreciation of the significance of all the possible diagnostic entities helps prevent needless delay or haste in treatment and helps eliminate the expense of unnecessary laboratory tests and consultations. Also, when a differential diagnosis is established, a more rational approach to biopsy and treatment can be followed.

Also presented in the text are contemporary theories on disease etiology and pathogenesis, current therapeutic regimens, and a brief up-to-date bibliography. When pertinent to etiology or diagnosis, immunohistochemical, immunofluorescent, and ultrastructural materials have been included. An additional distinctive feature of this book is the clinical overview found at the beginning.

How to Use This Book

The narrative or latter part of this book provides the body of information that is oral and maxillofacial pathology. It is the starting point for comprehensive study of this discipline. The overview or front section is essentially a distillation of the clinical aspects found in the main text and is designed to be used as a quick chairside and laboratory reference or as a rapid review. The two sections are keyed together through the page numbers listed after the various diseases in the overview so that detailed information is readily available at the readers' fingertips.

JOSEPH A. REGEZI
JAMES J. SCIUBBA

Acknowledgments

Although this book is the product of the authors, it would not have come to fruition without the direct and indirect support of many others. We are indebted to our oral pathology colleagues, fellow faculty members, biopsy contributors, and referring clinicians, who provided patients, tissue samples, and photographs that were the foundation of the illustrative material in this book. Appreciation is expressed to our colleagues, especially Drs. Amos Buchner, Richard Courtney, Troy Daniels, Mirdza Neiders, William Sprague, John Waterhouse, and Richard Wesley, who, following the publication of the first edition, helped us immeasurably with their constructive criticisms and comments. Gratitude is also expressed to Judith Fletcher and her capable staff at the W.B. Saunders Company for the production and marketing of this text.

We owe much to our own staffs, and to our mentors, Donald A. Kerr, John P. Waterhouse, and Leon Eisenbud, who as teachers and role models, significantly contributed to our professional and personal development. We are particularly indebted to our influential mentors/colleagues, John G. Batsakis and John T. Headington, for sharing their knowledge and providing exemplary professional character.

Our families are especially deserving of recognition. It is, unfortunately, from them that much of the time necessary to write this text was stolen. For their support and understanding, we are grateful.

Finally, acknowledgment must be accorded to the many fine students and residents we have come to know and love over the many years of our careers. It is the curious and motivated student who provides the stimulus and challenge that makes teaching rewarding work. It is the energy, the questions, and the new ideas from the student that will maintain the vitality of the profession.

JOSEPH A. REGEZI
JAMES J. SCIUBBA

NOTICE

Pathology is an ever-changing field. Standard safety precautions must be followed, but as new research and clinical experience broaden our knowledge, changes in treatment and drug therapy become necessary or appropriate. Readers are advised to check the product information currently provided by the manufacturer of each drug to be administered to verify the recommended dose, the method and duration of administration, and the contraindications. It is the responsibility of the treating physician, relying on experience and knowledge of the patient, to determine dosages and the best treatment for the patient. Neither the publisher nor the editor assumes any responsibility for any injury and/or damage to persons or property.

THE PUBLISHER

Contents

17

Clinical Overview*

*Photographs and text in Clinical Overview taken in modified form from Regezi J, Courtney R. *Clinical Oral Pathology.* University of Michigan, Ann Arbor, 1987. Reproduced by permission of the University of Michigan.

Vesiculo-Bullous Diseases

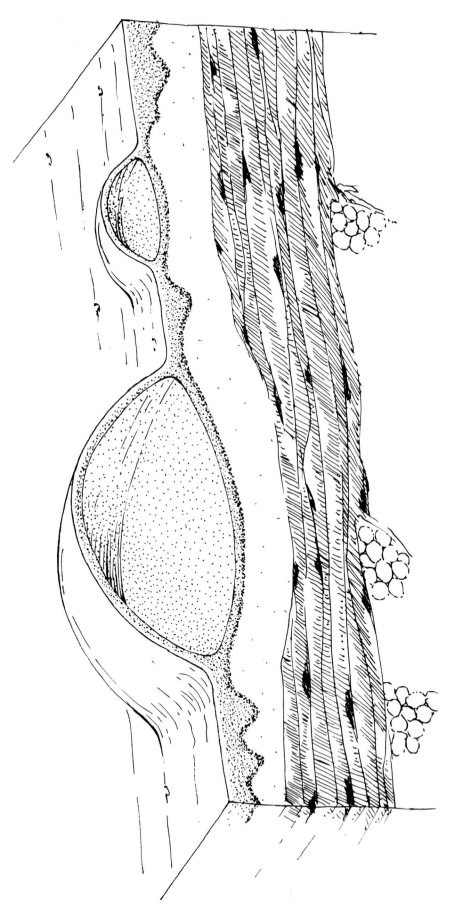

The presence or history of vesicles or bullae places an oral disease into a distinct and limited group of lesions. These generally include viral diseases and oral manifestations of dermatologic diseases. It is uncommon clinically to see bullae or vesicles, because most become ulcers in a matter of hours. The important question to ask of patients with oral ulcers, therefore, is whether or not the lesions were preceded by blisters. In patients with a positive history, the presence of systemic signs and symptoms would favor a viral etiology.

1

Vesiculo-Bullous Diseases

VIRAL DISEASES
Herpes Simplex Infections
Varicella-Zoster Infections
Hand-Foot-and-Mouth Disease
Herpangina
Measles (Rubeola)
CONDITIONS ASSOCIATED WITH IMMUNOLOGIC DEFECTS
Pemphigus Vulgaris
Cicatricial Pemphigoid
Bullous Pemphigoid
Dermatitis Herpetiformis
HEREDITARY DISEASES
Epidermolysis Bullosa

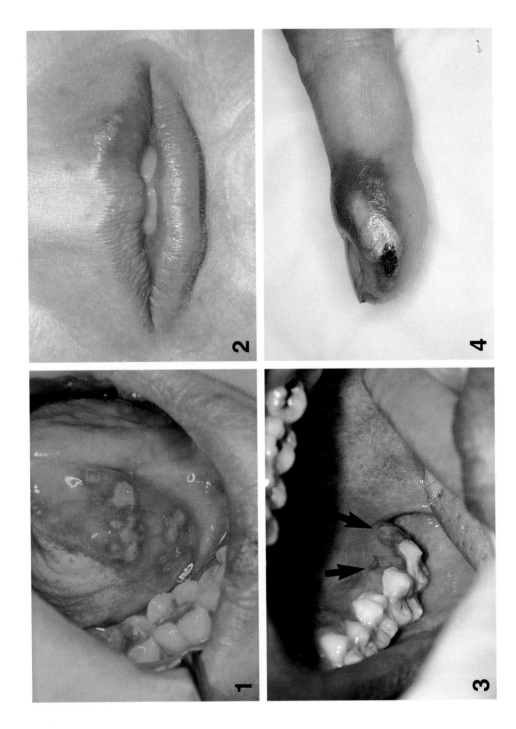

Vesiculo-Bullous Diseases

DISEASE	CLINICAL FEATURES	CAUSE	TREATMENT	SIGNIFICANCE
Herpes simplex infections Primary herpetic gingivostomatitis (Fig. 1) (p. 3)	Multiple painful oral ulcers preceded by vesicles; may have similar perioral and skin lesions; gingivitis usually present; usually affects children under 5 years; uncommon	Herpes simplex virus type I (occasionally type II)	Supportive; acyclovir occasionally useful	Self-limited, heals in about 2 weeks; reactivation of latent virus results in secondary infections; circulating antibodies provide only partial immunity
Secondary herpes simplex infection (Figs. 2–4) (pp. 3–4)	Multiple small ulcers preceded by vesicles; prodromal symptoms of tingling, burning, or pain; most common on lip, intraorally on palate and attached gingiva; called *herpetic whitlow* when occurs around fingernail; adults and young adults usually affected; very common	Herpes simplex virus—represents reactivation of virus and not reinfection; commonly precipitated by stress, sunlight, cold temperature, low resistance, and immunodeficiency	Symptomatic; the best virus-specific drug for oral herpes is acyclovir (especially systemic), but results are frequently disappointing	Self-limited; heals in 2 weeks without scar; lesions infectious during vesicular stage; patient must be cautioned against autoinoculation; herpes type I infections have not been convincingly linked to oral cancer; any site affected in AIDS patients
Varicella (pp. 7–10)	Painful pruritic vesicles and ulcers in all stages on trunk and face, few oral lesions; common childhood disease	Varicella-zoster virus	Supportive	Self-limited; recovery uneventful in several weeks
Herpes zoster (pp. 8–10)	Unilateral multiple ulcers preceded by vesicles distributed along a sensory nerve course; very painful; usually on trunk, head, and neck, rare intraorally; adults	Reactivation of varicella-zoster virus	Supportive; high-dose acyclovir, topical capsaicin for postherpetic pain	Self-limited, but may have a prolonged painful course; sometimes seen with lymphomas and immunodeficiency
Hand-foot-and-mouth disease (p. 10)	Painful ulcers preceded by vesicles on hands, feet, and oral mucosa; usually children; rare	Coxsackie virus	Supportive	Self-limited; recovery uneventful in about 2 weeks
Herpangina (pp. 11–12)	Multiple painful ulcers in posterior oral cavity and pharynx; lesions preceded by vesicles; children most commonly affected; seasonal occurrence; rare	Coxsackie virus	Supportive	Self-limited; recovery uneventful in less than a week
Measles (rubeola) (p. 12)	Oral Koplik's spots precede maculopapular skin rash; fever, malaise, plus other symptoms of systemic viral infection; children most commonly affected	Measles virus	Supportive	Self-limited; recovery uneventful in about 2 weeks

Vesiculo-Bullous Diseases

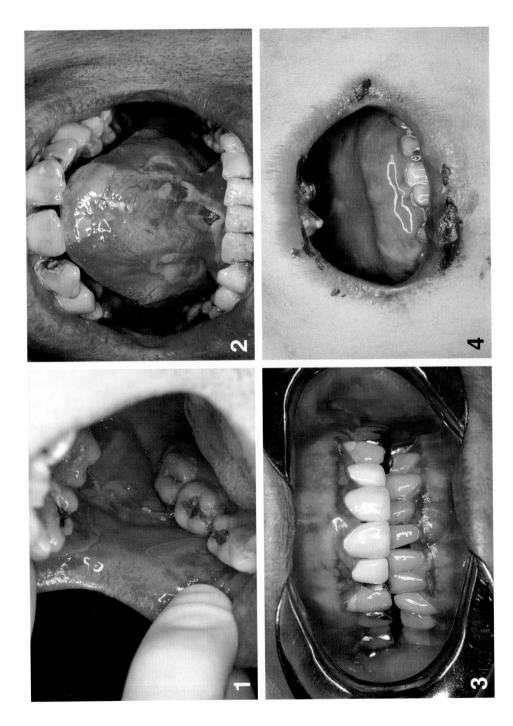

Vesiculo-Bullous Diseases *Continued*

DISEASE	CLINICAL FEATURES	CAUSE	TREATMENT	SIGNIFICANCE
Pemphigus vulgaris (Figs. 1 and 2) (pp. 13–18)	Multiple painful ulcers preceded by bullae; middle age; positive Nikolsky's sign; progressive disease, remissions or control with therapy; rare	Autoimmune; antibodies directed against desmosome-associated protein, desmoglein 3	Systemic steroids; occasionally immunosuppressive drugs for their steroid-sparing properties	May be fatal; significant morbidity from steroid therapy; oral lesions precede skin lesions in half the cases; prognosis improved if treated early
Cicatricial (mucous membrane) pemphigoid (Fig. 3) (pp. 18–22)	Multiple painful ulcers preceded by bullae; lesion may heal with scar; positive Nikolsky's sign; may affect mucous membranes of oral cavity, eyes, and genitals; when limited to attached gingiva only, may be called *desquamative gingivitis* or *gingivosis*; middle-aged or elderly women; uncommon; may be confused with lichen planus, chronic lupus of gingiva, and hypersensitivity	Autoimmune; antibodies directed against basement membrane antigens, laminin 5 and BP 180	Topical or systemic steroids	Protracted course; may cause significant debilitation if severe; ocular scarring may lead to symblepharon or blindness; death uncommon
Bullous pemphigoid (pp. 22–23)	Skin disease (trunk and extremities) with infrequent oral lesions; ulcers preceded by bullae; no scarring; elderly persons	Basement membrane autoantibodies are detected in tissue and serum	Systemic steroids/immunosuppressive drugs	Chronic course; remissions; uncommon
Dermatitis herpetiformis (pp. 23–25)	Skin disease with rare oral involvement; vesicles and pustules; exacerbations and remissions are typical; young and middle-aged adults	Unknown; IgA deposits in site of lesions; usually associated with gluten sensitivity	Dapsone	Chronic course that may require diet restriction or drug therapy
Epidermolysis bullosa (Fig. 4) (pp. 25–27)	Multiple ulcers preceded by bullae; positive Nikolsky's sign; inheritance pattern determines age of onset during childhood and severity; may heal with scar; primarily a skin disease, but oral lesions often present; rare	Hereditary, autosomal dominant or recessive	Steroids, reduction of trauma, antibiotics	Severe debilitating disease that may be fatal in recessive form; simple operative procedures may elicit bullae

Ulcerative Conditions

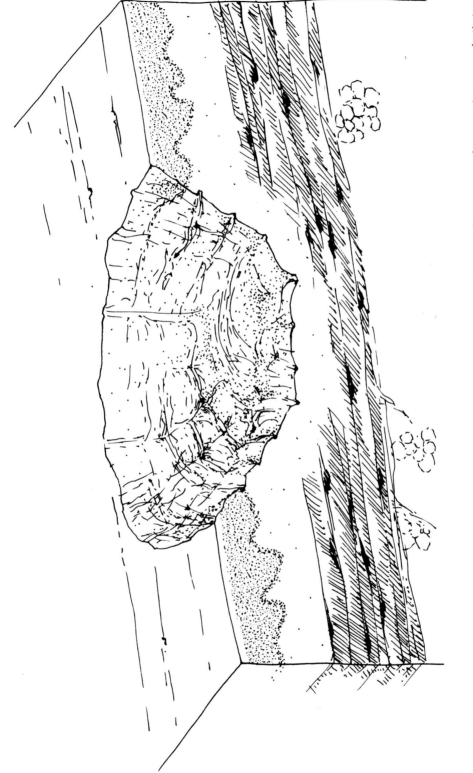

Ulcer is defined simply as loss of epithelium. Ulcerative lesions are commonly encountered in dental patients. Lesions range from reactive to neoplastic to oral manifestations of dermatologic disease.

2

Ulcerative Conditions

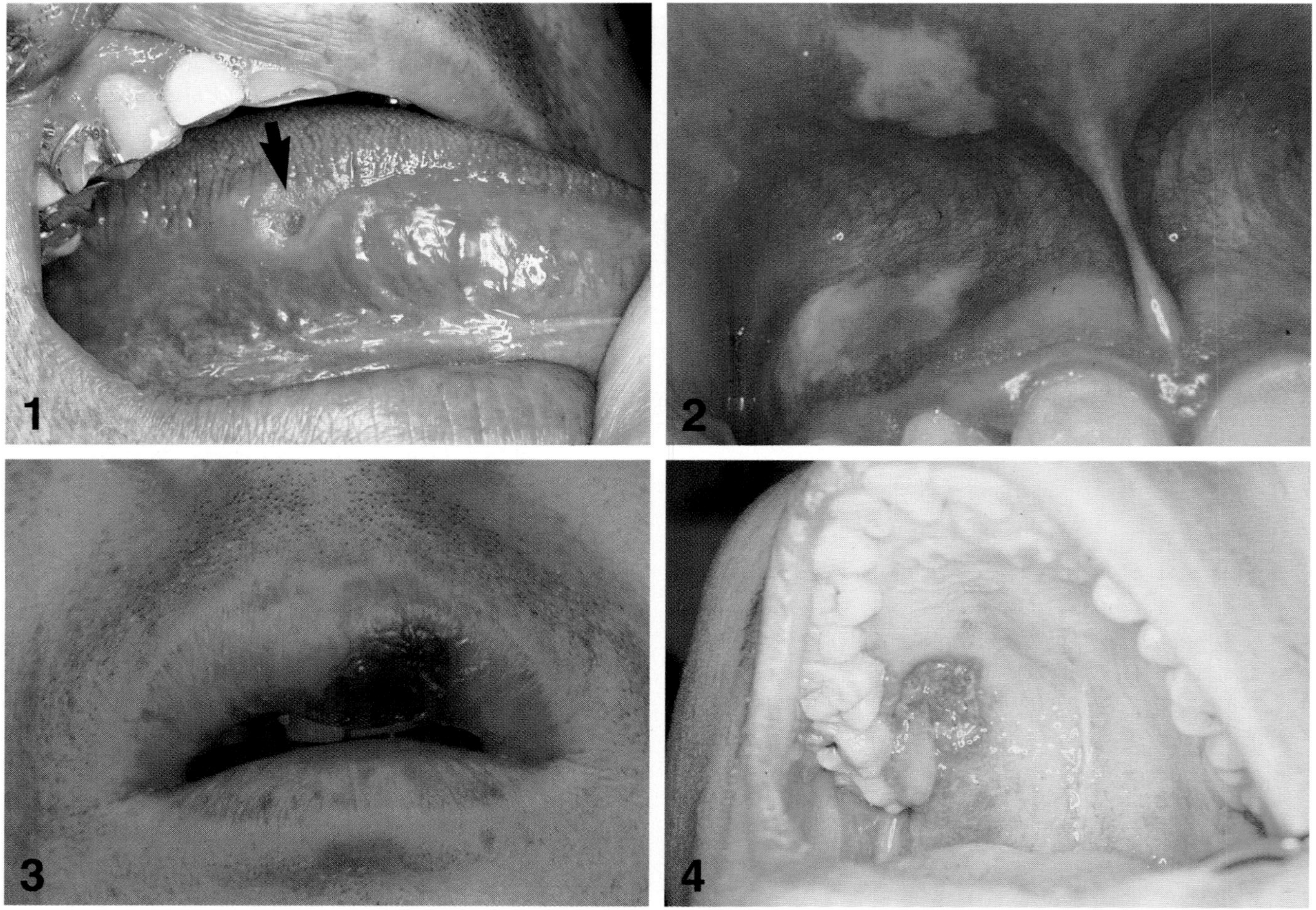
1
2
3
4

Ulcerative Conditions

DISEASE	CLINICAL FEATURES	CAUSE	TREATMENT	SIGNIFICANCE
Reactive lesions (Figs. 1 and 2) (pp. 30–35)	Painful ulcer covered by yellow fibrin membrane; diagnosis usually evident from appearance, when combined with history; common; traumatic factitional injuries are diagnostic challenge	Trauma, chemicals, heat, radiation	Symptomatic; remove causative agent if still active	Self-limited; heals in days to weeks; factitial injuries follow unpredictable course
Syphilis (Fig. 3) (pp. 35–38)	*Primary* (chancre)—single, indurated, nonpainful ulcer at site of spirochete entry, spontaneously heals in 4 to 6 weeks *secondary*—maculopapular rash on skin, ulcers covered by membrane (mucous patches) orally *tertiary*—gummas, cardiovascular and central nervous system lesions *congenital*—dental abnormalities (mulberry molars, notched incisors), deafness, interstitial keratitis (Hutchinson's triad)	Spirochete—*Treponema pallidum*	Penicillin	Primary and secondary forms are highly infectious; mimics other diseases clinically; if untreated, secondary form develops in 2 to 10 weeks; a minority of patients develop tertiary lesions; latency periods, in which there is no clinically apparent disease seen between primary and secondary and between secondary and tertiary stages
Gonorrhea (p. 38)	Typically genital lesions, with rare oral manifestations, painful erythema or ulcers, or both	*Neisseria gonorrhoeae*	Penicillin; alternate antibiotics may be required because of penicillin resistance	May be confused with many oral ulcerative diseases
Tuberculosis (Fig. 4) (pp. 38–40)	Indurated, chronic ulcer that may be painful—on any mucosal surface; differential includes oral cancer and chronic traumatic ulcer	*Mycobacterium tuberculosis*	Isoniazid, ethambutol, streptomycin, others	Lesions are infectious; oral lesions almost always secondary to lung lesions
Leprosy (pp. 40–41)	Skin disease, with rare oral nodules/ulcers	*Mycobacterium leprae*	Dapsone, rifampin, clofazimine	Rare in the United States but relatively common in Southeast Asia, India, South America
Actinomycosis (pp. 41–42)	Typically seen in mandible, with draining skin sinus	*Actinomyces israelii*	Long-term, high-dose penicillin	Infection follows entry through a surgical site, periodontal disease, or open root canal

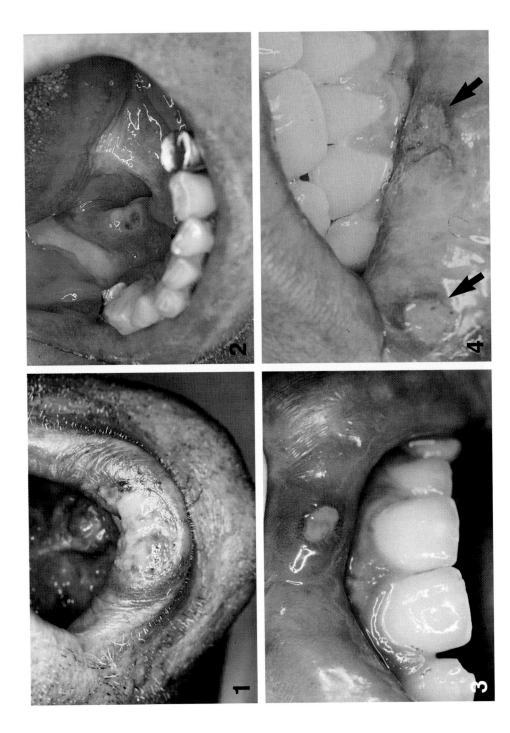

Ulcerative Conditions *Continued*

DISEASE	CLINICAL FEATURES	CAUSE	TREATMENT	SIGNIFICANCE
Noma (pp. 42–43)	Necrotic, nonhealing ulcer of gingiva or buccal mucosa; rare; affects children	Anaerobes in patient whose systemic health is compromised	Antibiotics and improve systemic health	Often associated with malnutrition; may result in severe tissue destruction
Deep fungal diseases (Fig. 1) (pp. 43–45)	Indurated, nonhealing, frequently painful, chronic ulcer, usually following implantation of organism from lung	*Histoplasma capsulatum, Coccidioides immitis*, others	Amphotericin B	Oral lesions are secondary to systemic lesions; some types are endemic
Subcutaneous fungal diseases (p. 45)	Nonspecific ulcers of skin and, rarely, mucosa	Usually *Sporothrix schenckii*	Iodides or ketoconazole	Sporotrichosis usually follows inoculation via thorny plants
Opportunistic fungal infections (pp. 45–46)	Occurs in compromised host; necrotic; nonhealing ulcer(s)	*Mucor, Rhizopus*, others	Amphotericin B plus treat underlying disease	Known collectively as *phycomycosis*; may mimic syphilis, midline granuloma, others; frequently fatal
Aphthous ulcers (Figs. 2–4) (pp. 46–53)	Recurrent, painful ulcers found on tongue, vestibular mucosa, floor of mouth, and faucial pillars; not found on skin, vermilion, attached gingiva, or hard palate; usually round or oval; ulcers not preceded by vesicles; *minor type*—usually solitary, less than 0.5 cm in diameter, common; *major type*—severe, heals in up to 6 weeks with scar (Fig. 4); *herpetiform type*—multiple, recurrent crops of ulcers	Unknown; probably an immune defect mediated by T cells; not caused by virus; precipitated by stress, trauma, other factors	Symptomatic; most remedies contain either steroid or tetracycline	Painful nuisance disease; rarely debilitating, except in major type; recurrences are the rule; more severe in patients with AIDS; may be seen in association with Behçet's syndrome and Crohn's disease
Behçet's syndrome (pp. 53–54)	Minor aphthae; eye lesions (uveitis, conjunctivitis); genital lesions (ulcers); arthritis occasionally seen	Probably an immune defect	Steroids, immunosuppressives	Biopsy and laboratory studies give nonspecific results; complications may be significant
Reiter's syndrome (p. 54)	Arthritis, urethritis, conjunctivitis or uveitis, oral ulcers; usually in white men in third decade	Unknown; ?immune response to bacterial antigen	Nonsteroidal antiinflammatory drugs	Duration of weeks to months; may be recurrent

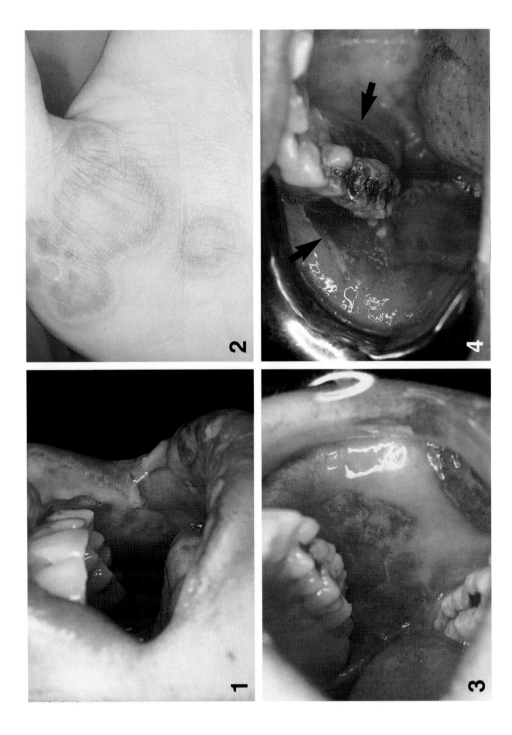

Ulcerative Conditions *Continued*

DISEASE	CLINICAL FEATURES	CAUSE	TREATMENT	SIGNIFICANCE
Erythema multiforme (Figs. 1 and 2) (pp. 54–57)	Sudden onset; painful widespread, superficial ulcers; usually self-limited; young adults; may also have target or iris lesions of skin; may be recurrent, especially in spring and fall; some cases become chronic; uncommon	Unknown; ?hypersensitivity; may follow drug ingestion or an infection such as herpes labialis or *Mycoplasma* pneumonia	Symptomatic; steroid usage controversial	Cause should be investigated; can be debilitating, especially in severe form, erythema multiforme major (Stevens-Johnson syndrome)
Lupus erythematosus (Fig. 3) (pp. 57–62)	Usually painful erythematous and ulcerative lesions on buccal mucosa, gingiva, and vermilion; white keratotic areas may surround lesions; chronic *discoid type*—generally affects skin and mucous membrane only; acute *systemic type*—skin lesions may be erythematous with scale (classic sign is butterfly rash across bridge of nose); also may have joint, kidney, and heart lesions; middle-aged women; uncommon	Immune defect; patient develops autoantibodies, especially antinuclear antibodies	Steroids, immunosuppressive drugs, others	*Discoid type* may cause discomfort and cosmetic problems; *systemic type* has guarded prognosis
Drug reactions (pp. 62–64)	May affect skin or mucosa; erythema, white lesions, vesicles, ulcers may be seen; history of recent drug ingestions is important	Potentially any drug via stimulation of immune system	Withdraw causative agent; antihistamines or corticosteroids	Reactions, such as anaphylaxis or angioedema, may require emergency care; highly variable clinical picture can make diagnosis difficult
Contact allergy (Fig. 4) (pp. 64–66)	Lesion occurs directly under foreign antigen; erythema, vesicles, ulcers may be seen	Potentially any foreign antigen that contacts skin or mucosa; cinnamon frequently cited	Eliminate offending material	Patch testing may be helpful for diagnosis; history is important
Wegener's granulomatosis (pp. 66–67)	Inflammatory lesions (necrotizing vasculitis) of lung, kidney, and upper airway; may affect gingiva when intraoral; rare	Unknown; ?immune defect, ?infection	Cyclophosphamide and prednisone	May become life threatening owing to tissue destruction in any of the three involved sites

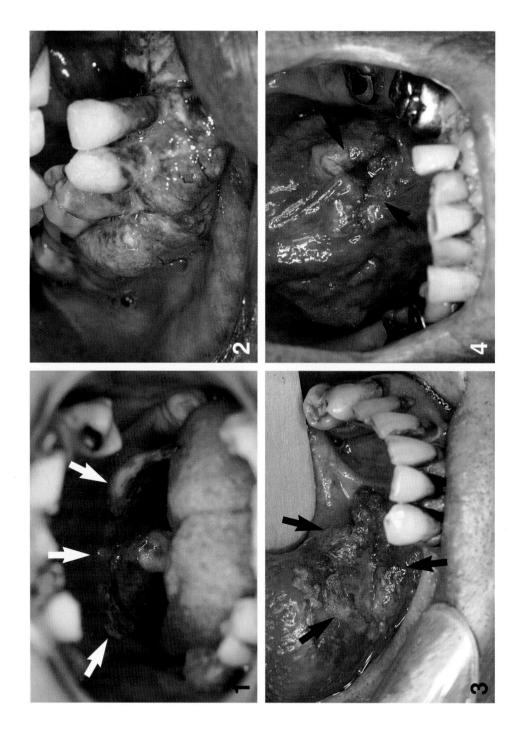

Ulcerative Conditions *Continued*

DISEASE	CLINICAL FEATURES	CAUSE	TREATMENT	SIGNIFICANCE
Midline granuloma (Fig. 1) (pp. 67–68)	Destructive, necrotic, nonhealing lesions of nose, palate, and sinuses; biopsy shows nonspecific inflammation; distinct from Wegener's granulomatosis; rare	Unknown; ?immune defect	Steroids, radiation	Poor; death may follow erosion into major blood vessels; may represent an occult lymphoma
Chronic granulomatous disease (pp. 68–69)	Recurrent infections in various organs; oral ulcers; males; rare	Genetic disease (X linked)	Antimicrobials	Altered neutrophil and macrophage function results in inability to kill bacteria and fungi
Cyclic neutropenia (p. 69)	Oral ulcers; infections; adenopathy; periodontal disease	Unknown	Supportive care	Rare blood dyscrasia
Squamous cell carcinoma (Figs. 2–4) (pp. 69–80)	Indurated, nonpainful ulcer with rolled margins; most commonly found on lateral tongue and floor of mouth; males affected twice as often as females; clinical appearance may also be as a white or red patch or mass	DNA alterations due to carcinogens such as tobacco, UV light, Epstein-Barr virus and human papillomavirus; alcohol and chronic irritation are co-carcinogens	Surgery or radiation	Overall 5-year survival rate is 45–50%; excellent prognosis if found in early stages, poor prognosis if metastasis to regional lymph nodes
Carcinoma of the maxillary sinus (pp. 80–81)	Patient may have symptoms of sinusitis or referred pain to teeth; may cause malocclusion or mobile teeth; may appear as ulcerative mass in palate or alveolus	Loss of genetic control of cell proliferation and invasion; carcinogens poorly understood	Surgery and/or radiation	Prognosis only fair; metastases are not uncommon

White Lesions

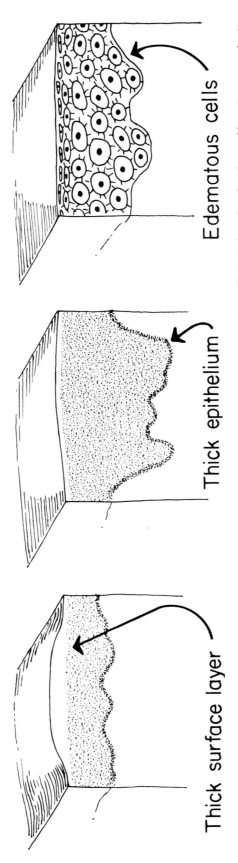

Thick surface layer

Thick epithelium

Edematous cells

Lesions generally appear white intraorally for one of several reasons (assuming that the lesion cannot be rubbed off). A thickened surface layer of keratin, an acanthotic (increase in thickness of the prickle cell layer) epithelium, and edematous epithelial cells all can produce clinically white lesions. Exudates and adherent surface debris may also appear white. With experience, the reason for a lesion's white appearance can often be determined clinically, but final proof rests on microscopic examination. This becomes especially important for idiopathic leukoplakia, because some of these lesions represent squamous cell carcinomas. The white lesions in the following list range from those that are genetically determined (genodermatoses) to those that are neoplastic.

3

White Lesions

HEREDITARY CONDITIONS
Leukoedema
White Sponge Nevus
Hereditary Benign Intraepithelial Dyskeratosis
Follicular Keratosis
REACTIVE LESIONS
Focal (Frictional) Hyperkeratosis
White Lesions Associated with Smokeless Tobacco
Nicotine Stomatitis
Solar Cheilitis
OTHER WHITE LESIONS
Idiopathic Leukoplakia
Hairy Leukoplakia
Hairy Tongue
Geographic Tongue
Lichen Planus
Dentifrice-Associated Slough
NONEPITHELIAL WHITE-YELLOW LESIONS
Candidiasis
Mucosal Burns
Submucous Fibrosis
Fordyce's Granules
Ectopic Lymphoid Tissue
Gingival Cysts
Parulis
Lipoma

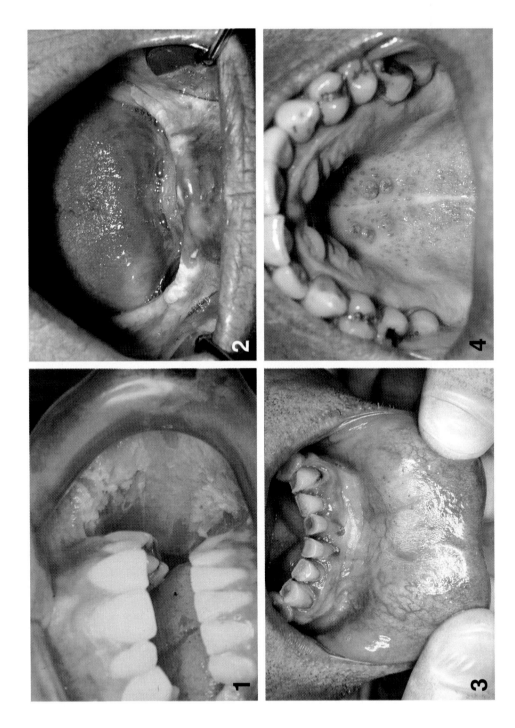

White Lesions

DISEASE	CLINICAL FEATURES	CAUSE	TREATMENT	SIGNIFICANCE
Leukoedema (pp. 83–84)	50% of whites and 90% of African-Americans affected; uniform opacification of buccal mucosa bilaterally	Unknown	None	Remains indefinitely; no ill effects
White sponge nevus (Fig. 1) (p. 84)	Asymptomatic, bilateral, dense, shaggy, white or gray, generalized opacification; primarily buccal mucosa affected, but other membranes may be involved; rare	Hereditary, autosomal dominant (Keratin 4 and/or 13)	None	Remains indefinitely; no ill effects
Hereditary benign intraepithelial dyskeratosis (pp. 84–85)	Asymptomatic, diffuse, shaggy, white lesions of buccal mucosa as well as other tissues; eye lesions—white plaques surrounded by inflamed conjunctiva; rare	Hereditary, autosomal dominant	None	Remains indefinitely
Follicular keratosis (pp. 86–87)	Keratotic papular lesions of skin and, infrequently, mucosa; lesions are numerous and asymptomatic	Genetic, autosomal dominant	Retinoids	Chronic course with occasional remissions
Focal (frictional) hyperkeratosis (Fig. 2) (pp. 87–88)	Asymptomatic white patch, commonly on edentulous ridge, buccal mucosa, and tongue; does not rub off; common	Chronic irritation	Remove irritant	May regress if cause eliminated
White lesions associated with smokeless tobacco (Fig. 3) (pp. 88–90)	Asymptomatic white folds surrounding area where tobacco is held; usually found in labial and buccal vestibules; common	Chronic irritation from snuff or chewing tobacco	Discontinue habit; biopsy suspicious areas	Increased risk for development of verrucous and squamous cell carcinoma after many years
Nicotine stomatitis (Fig. 4) (pp. 90–91)	Asymptomatic, generalized opacification of palate with red dots representing salivary gland orifices; common	Heat and smoke associated with combustion of tobacco	Discontinue smoking	Rarely develops into palatal cancer

White Lesions

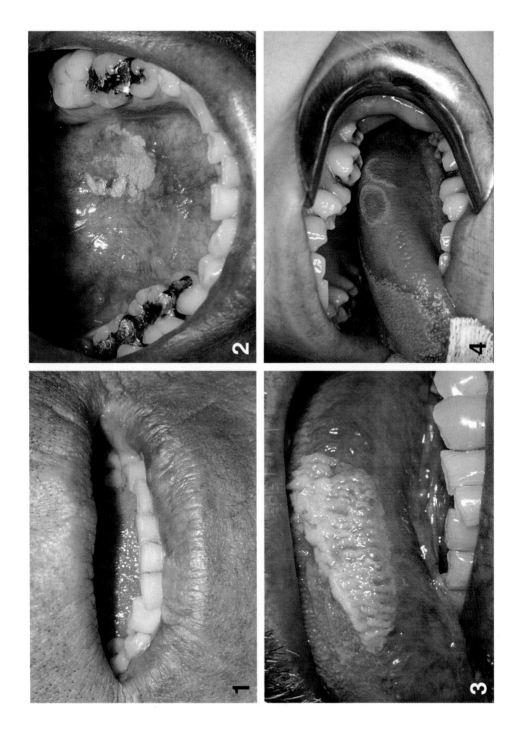

White Lesions *Continued*

DISEASE	CLINICAL FEATURES	CAUSE	TREATMENT	SIGNIFICANCE
Solar cheilitis (Fig. 1) (pp. 91–92)	Lower lip—atrophic epithelium, poor definition of vermilion-skin margin, focal zones of keratosis; common	UV light (especially UVB, 2900–3200 nm) and aging	Sunscreens (PABA) and sun blockers (zinc oxide, titanium dioxide), surgery in severe cases	May result in chronic ulceration of squamous cell carcinoma
Idiopathic leukoplakia (Fig. 2) (pp. 92–96)	Asymptomatic white patch; cannot be wiped off; males affected more than females	Unknown; may be related to tobacco and alcohol use	Biopsy, excision	May recur after excision; 5% are malignant, 5% become malignant
Hairy leukoplakia (Fig. 3) (pp. 96–99)	Filiform to flat patch on lateral tongue, often bilateral, occasionally on buccal mucosa; asymptomatic	Opportunistic Epstein-Barr virus infection	No specific treatment, evaluate for AIDS	Seen in 20% of HIV-infected patients; marked increase in AIDS; may occur in non–AIDS-affected immunosuppressed patients and rarely in immunocompetent patients
Hairy tongue (pp. 99–100)	Elongation of filiform papillae; asymptomatic	Unknown; may follow antibiotic or corticosteroid use	Improve oral hygiene; identify contributing factors	Benign process; may be cosmetically objectionable
Geographic tongue (Fig. 4) (pp. 100–101)	White annular lesions with atrophic red centers; pattern migrates over dorsum of tongue; varies in intensity and may spontaneously disappear; occasionally painful; common	Unknown	None; symptomatic treatment for painful lesions	Completely benign; spontaneous regression after months to years

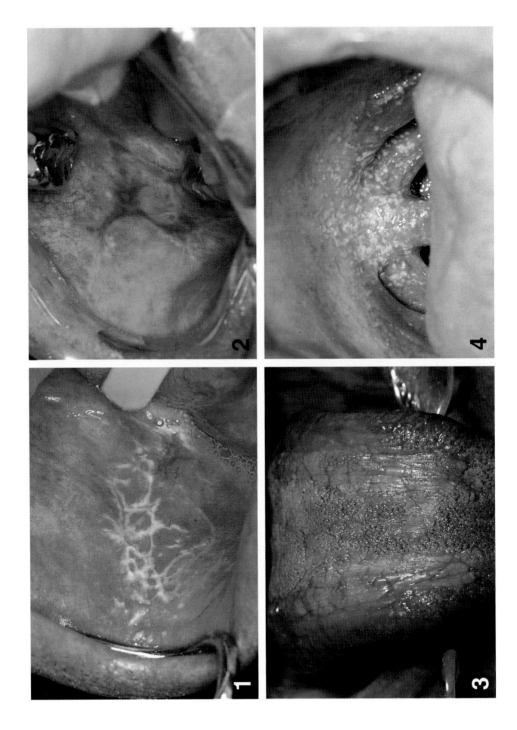

White Lesions *Continued*

DISEASE	CLINICAL FEATURES	CAUSE	TREATMENT	SIGNIFICANCE
Lichen planus (Figs. 1–3) (pp. 101–106)	Bilateral white striae (Wickham's); asymptomatic except when erosions are present (Fig. 2); skin lesions occasionally present and are purple pruritic papules; seen in middle age; buccal mucosa most commonly affected, with lesions occasionally on tongue, gingiva, and palate; forearm and lower leg most frequent skin areas; uncommon	Unknown; may be precipitated by stress; may be hyperimmune condition mediated by T cells	Topical or systemic steroids; retinoids may be helpful with or instead of steroids; follow-up examinations necessary	May regress after many years; treatment may only control disease; rare malignant transformation
Dentifrice-associated slough (p. 106)	Asymptomatic, slough of filmy parakeratotic cells	Mucosal reaction to components in toothpaste	Change brand of toothpaste	None
Candidiasis (Fig. 4) (pp. 107–113)	Painful elevated plaques (fungus) can be wiped off leaving eroded, bleeding surface; associated with poor hygiene, systemic antibiotics, systemic diseases, debilitation, reduced immune response; chronic infections may result in erythematous mucosa without obvious white colonies; common	Opportunistic fungus—*Candida albicans* and rarely other *Candida* species	Clotrimazole troches or nystatin suspension and treatment of predisposing disease	Usually disappears in 1 to 2 weeks after treatment; some chronic cases require long-term therapy

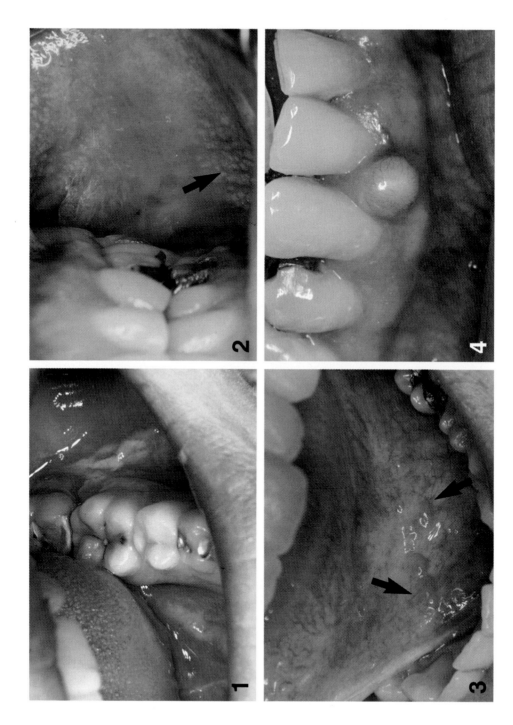

White Lesions *Continued*

DISEASE	CLINICAL FEATURES	CAUSE	TREATMENT	SIGNIFICANCE
Mucosal burns (Fig. 1) (pp. 113–114)	Painful white fibrin exudate covering superficial ulcer with erythematous ring; common	Chemicals (aspirin, phenol), heat, electrical burns	Remove cause; symptomatic therapy	Heals in days to weeks
Submucous fibrosis (pp. 114–115)	Areas of opacification with loss of elasticity; any oral region affected; rare	?Hypersensitivity to dietary constituents such as betel nut, capsaicin	None consistently effective	Irreversible; predisposes to oral cancer
Fordyce's granules (Fig. 2) (pp. 115–116)	Multiple asymptomatic, yellow, flat or elevated spots seen primarily in buccal mucosa and lips; seen in a majority of patients; many consider them to be a variation of normal	Developmental	None; lesions are diagnostic clinically and biopsy should not be performed	Ectopic sebaceous glands of no significance
Ectopic lymphoid tissue (Fig. 3) (p. 116)	Asymptomatic elevated yellow nodules less than 0.5 cm in diameter; usually found on tonsillar pillars, posterolateral tongue, and floor of mouth; covered by intact epithelium; common	Unknown	None	No significance; lesions remain indefinitely and are usually diagnostic clinically
Gingival cyst (Fig. 4) (pp. 117–118)	Small, usually white to yellow nodule; multiple in infants, solitary in adults; common in infants, rare in adults	Proliferation and cystification of dental lamina rests	None when in infants; excision when in adults	In infants, lesions spontaneously rupture or break; recurrence not expected in adults
Parulis (pp. 118–119)	Yellow-white gingival swelling due to submucosal pus	Periodontitis or tooth abscess	Treat periodontal pocket or nonvital tooth	Periodic drainage until primary cause is eliminated
Lipoma (p. 119)	Asymptomatic, slow-growing, well-circumscribed, yellow or yellow-white tumescence; rare benign neoplasm of fat; occurs in any area	Unknown	Excision	Seems to have limited growth potential intraorally; recurrence not expected after removal

Red-Blue Lesions

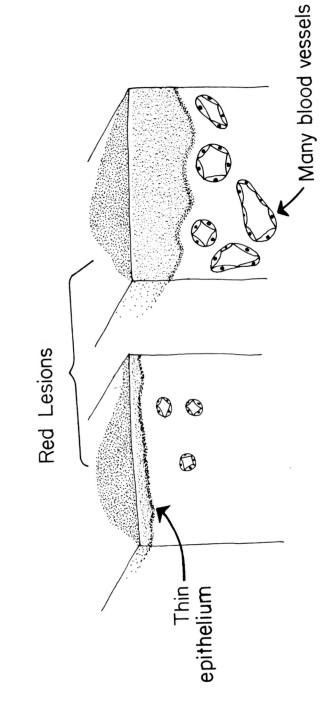

Red Lesions

Thin epithelium

Many blood vessels

Lesions may appear red either because of epithelial atrophy (allowing the submucosal vasculature to show, as in the tongue changes of pernicious anemia) or because of an actual increase in the number of submucosal blood vessels (hemangioma). They may also appear red because of extravasation of blood into soft tissues.

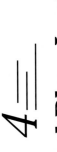

4
Red-Blue Lesions

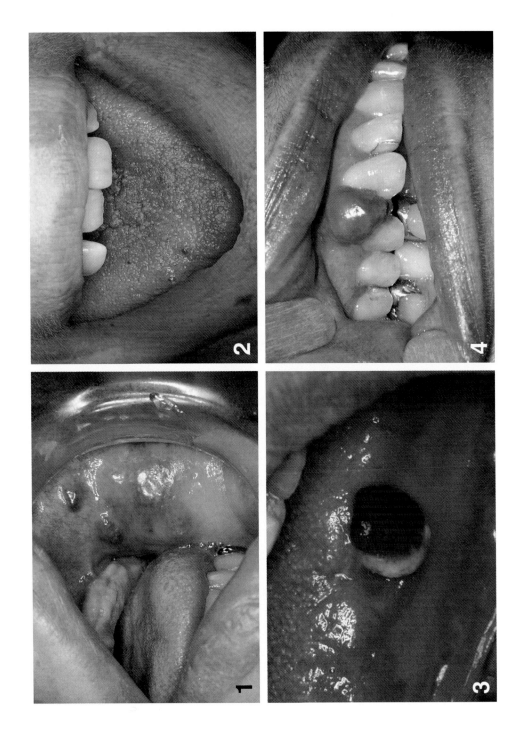

Red-Blue Lesions

DISEASE	CLINICAL FEATURES	CAUSE	TREATMENT	SIGNIFICANCE
Hemangioma (Figs. 1 and 2) (pp. 122–128)	Red or blue lesion that blanches when compressed; extent of lesion usually difficult to determine; skin, lips, tongue, and buccal mucosa most commonly affected; common on skin, uncommon in mucous membrane, rare in bone; part of Sturge-Weber syndrome (intracranial calcifications, seizures, mental retardation); telangiectasias (small focal dilations of terminal blood vessels) blanch when compressed; commonly found in sun-damaged skin, and seen with Rendu-Osler-Weber syndrome or hereditary hemorrhagic telangiectasia (HHT) (Fig. 2); venous varix is a form of vascular malformation seen on lower lip and ventral tongue	Some are benign congenital neoplasms, others are due to abnormal vessel morphogenesis (vascular malformation); *HHT*—autosomal dominant; *venous varix*—congenital or induced by UV light	Most congenital lesions involute without treatment; vascular malformations may require surgical removal; *HHT*—may be treated with surgery or cautery; *venous varix*—observe or surgical removal	May remain quiescent or gradually enlarge; hemorrhage may be a significant complication; often a cosmetic problem; *HHT*—epistaxis may be a problem
Pyogenic granuloma (Fig. 3) (pp. 128–130)	Asymptomatic red tumescence composed of granulation tissue; most commonly seen in gingiva; periodontal ligament origin; may be secondarily ulcerated; common	Trauma or chronic irritation; size modified by hormonal changes	Excision	Remains indefinitely; recurrence if incompletely excised; reduction in size if cause removed or after pregnancy
Peripheral giant cell granuloma (Fig. 4) (pp. 130–131)	Asymptomatic red tumescence of gingiva composed of fibroblasts and multinucleated giant cells; found mostly in adults in the former area of deciduous teeth; produces cup-shaped lucency when found in edentulous areas; uncommon	Trauma or chronic irritation	Excision	Remains indefinitely if untreated; a reactive lesion; clinical appearance similar to pyogenic granuloma

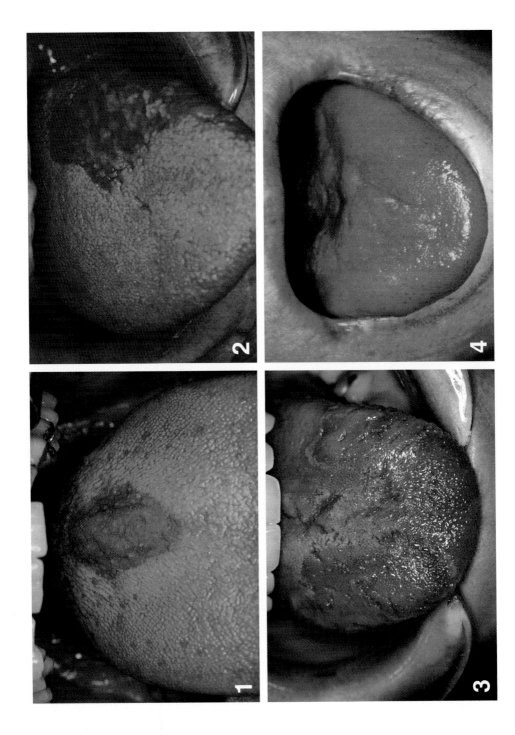

Red-Blue Lesions *Continued*

DISEASE	CLINICAL FEATURES	CAUSE	TREATMENT	SIGNIFICANCE
Median rhomboid glossitis (Fig. 1) (p. 131)	Red lobular elevation anterior to circumvallate papillae in midline	?Congenital versus chronic *Candida* infection	None	May support growth of *Candida albicans*
Erythroplakia (Fig. 2) (pp. 131–133)	Asymptomatic red velvety patch found usually in floor of mouth or retromolar area in adults; seen in older adults; red lesions may have foci or white hyperkeratosis (speckled erythroplakia)	Unknown	Excision	Most (90%) are *in situ* or invasive squamous cell carcinoma
Kaposi's sarcoma (pp. 132–135)	May be part of AIDS; usually on skin but may be oral, especially in palate; red to blue macules or nodules; rare, except in immunodeficiency	Endothelial cell proliferation related to cytokine/growth factor imbalance; HHV8 is part of etiology	Surgery, radiation, chemotherapy	Fair prognosis; poor when part of AIDS; incidence on the decline in AIDS patients
Geographic tongue (Fig. 3) (pp. 135–137)	White annular lesions with atrophic, red centers; white (keratotic) areas may be poorly developed, leaving red patches on dorsum of tongue; occasionally painful; common	Unknown	None; symptomatic treatment	Little significance except when painful; not premalignant
Psoriasis	Chronic skin disease with rare oral lesions; red skin lesions covered with silvery scales; oral lesions red to white patches	Unknown	Topical or systemic drugs; photochemotherapy	Must have skin lesions to confirm oral disease; exacerbations and remissions are typical
Vitamin B deficiency (Fig. 4) (p. 137)	Generalized redness of tongue due to atrophy of papillae; may be painful; may have an associated angular cheilitis; rare in USA	B complex deficiency	Vitamin B supplements	Remains until therapeutic levels of vitamin B are administered
Anemia (pernicious and iron deficiency) (pp. 137–139)	May result in generalized redness of tongue due to atrophy of papillae; may be painful; patients may have angular cheilitis; females more commonly affected than males; Plummer-Vinson syndrome—anemia (iron deficiency), mucosal atrophy, predisposition for oral cancer	Some forms acquired, some hereditary	Diagnosis and treatment of specific type of anemia	Some types may be life threatening; oral manifestations disappear with treatment; complication of oral cancer with Plummer-Vinson syndrome

Red-Blue Lesions

Red-Blue Lesions *Continued*

DISEASE	CLINICAL FEATURES	CAUSE	TREATMENT	SIGNIFICANCE
Burning mouth syndrome (pp. 139–141)	Wide range of oral complaints, usually without any visible tissue changes; especially middle-aged women; uncommon in males	Multifactorial—e.g., *Candida albicans*, vitamin B deficiency, anemias, xerostomia, idiopathic	Antifungal, steroid, vitamin B, iron; symptomatic; empathy and careful explanation required	May persist despite treatment
Scarlet fever (p. 141)	Pharyngitis, systemic symptoms, strawberry tongue	Group A streptococci	Penicillin	Complications of rheumatic fever and glomerulonephritis
Atrophic (erythematous) candidiasis (Fig. 1) (p. 141)	Painful, hyperemic palate under denture; angular cheilitis; red, painful mucosa	Chronic *C. albicans* infection; poor oral hygiene, ill-fitting denture are frequent predisposing factors	Nystatin, instruction on good oral hygiene, new denture	Discomfort may prevent wearing denture; not allergic or premalignant
Plasma cell gingivitis (p. 141)	Red, painful tongue; angular cheilitis; red gingiva	Allergic reactions to ?dietary antigen	Eliminate allergen	Gingival lesions similar to lupus, lichen planus, and pemphigoid lesions
Drug reactions and contact allergies (Fig. 2) (p. 142)	Red, vesicular, or ulcerative eruption	Hypersensitivity reaction to allergen	Identify and remove cause	Hypersensitivity reactions to drugs or HSV may produce erythema multiforme pattern clinically (Fig. 2)
Petechiae and ecchymoses Traumatic lesions (Fig. 3) (pp. 142–145)	Hemorrhagic spot (red, blue, purple, black) composed of extravasated blood in soft tissue; does not blanch with compression; may be seen anywhere in skin or mucous membranes after trauma; changes color as blood is degraded and resorbed	Follows traumatic insult such as that caused by tooth extraction-tooth bite, fellatio, chronic cough, vomiting	Observe	Resolves in days to weeks; no sequelae
Blood dyscrasias (Fig. 4) (pp. 142–145)	Hemorrhagic spots (small—petechiae, large—ecchymoses) on mucous membranes due to extravasated blood; may be spontaneous or follow minor trauma; spots do not blanch with compression; color varies with time; uncommon in general practice, but dental personnel may be first to observe	Lack of clotting factor, reduced numbers of platelets for various reasons, or lack of vessel integrity	Treatment of underlying blood disease	May be life threatening; must be investigated, diagnosed, and treated

Pigmentations of Oral and Perioral Tissues

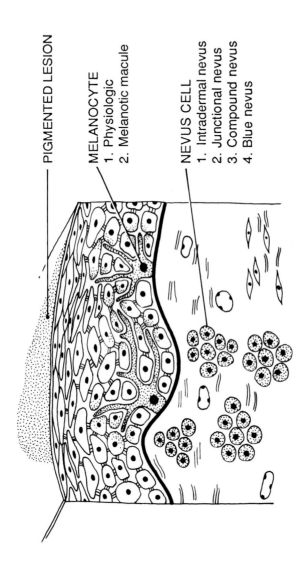

PIGMENTED LESION

MELANOCYTE
1. Physiologic
2. Melanotic macule

NEVUS CELL
1. Intradermal nevus
2. Junctional nevus
3. Compound nevus
4. Blue nevus

Pigmented lesions appear dark because of melanin production by either the melanocyte or its close relative, the nevus cell. Physiologic pigmentation, ephelides, and lentigines are due to melanocyte stimulation; the various types of nevi are due to pigment production by nevus cells.

5

Pigmentations of Oral and Perioral Tissues

Pigmentations of Oral and Perioral Tissues

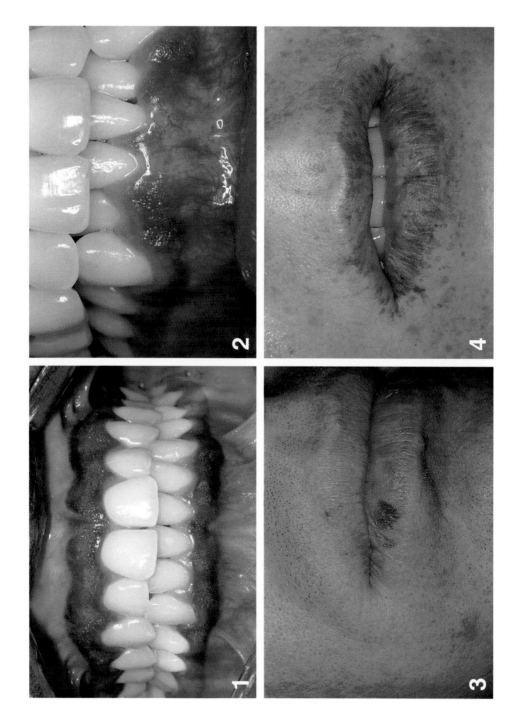

Pigmentations of Oral and Perioral Tissues

DISEASE	CLINICAL FEATURES	CAUSE	TREATMENT	SIGNIFICANCE
Physiologic pigmentation (Fig. 1) (pp. 146–147)	Symmetric distribution; does not change in intensity; does not alter surface morphology	Normal melanocyte activity	None	None
Smoking-associated melanosis (Fig. 2) (pp. 147–148)	Gingival pigmentation; especially women on birth control pills	Component in smoke stimulates melanocytes	Reversal after cessation of smoking	Cosmetic
Oral melanotic macule (Figs. 3 and 4) (p. 150)	Flat oral pigmentation less than 1 cm in diameter; lower lip, gingiva, buccal mucosa, palate usually affected; may represent oral ephelis, perioral lesions associated with Peutz-Jeghers syndrome (Fig. 4), Addison's disease, and postinflammatory pigmentation	Unknown; postinflammatory; trauma	Excision may be required to rule out melanoma	Remains indefinitely; no malignant potential

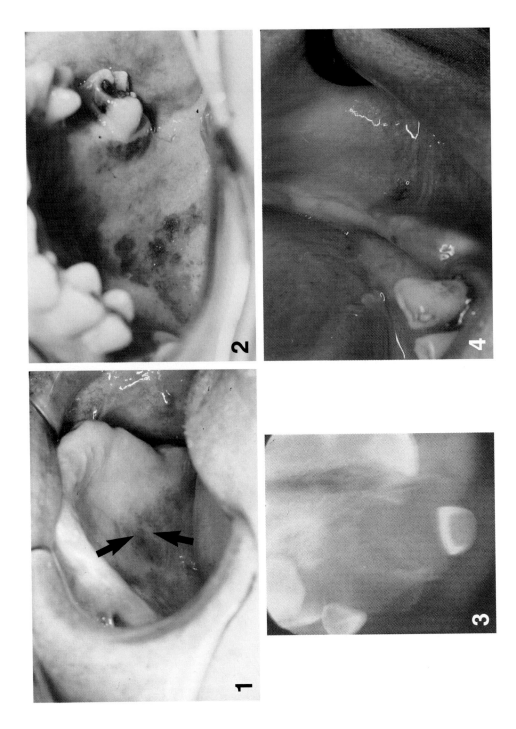

Pigmentations of Oral and Perioral Tissues *Continued*

DISEASE	CLINICAL FEATURES	CAUSE	TREATMENT	SIGNIFICANCE
Nevus (Fig. 1) (pp. 150–152)	Elevated pigmentations; often nonpigmented when intraoral; 15 per person on skin, uncommon orally; blue nevi seen in palate	Unknown, due to nests of nevus cells	Skin—excision of irritated or suspicious lesions to rule out melanoma; oral—excise all nevi to rule out melanoma	Remains indefinitely; cannot be separated from melanoma clinically
Melanoma (Fig. 2) (pp. 153–155)	Malignancy of pigmentary system; some have a radial growth phase of years duration (*in situ* type) before vertical growth phase, but invasive type has only vertical growth phase; oral melanomas may appear first as insignificant spot, especially on palate and gingiva; adults affected	UV light may be carcinogenic on skin; unknown for oral lesions	Wide surgical excision	Skin—65% 5-year survival; oral—20% 5-year survival; *in situ* melanomas have better prognosis than invasive melanomas; bad reputation because of unpredictable metastatic behavior
Neuroectodermal tumor of infancy (Fig. 3) (pp. 155–156)	Pigmented, radiolucent, benign neoplasm in maxilla of newborns; pigment is melanin; rare	Unknown; tumor cells of neural crest origin	Excision	Recurrence unlikely
Amalgam tattoo (Fig. 4) (pp. 156–157)	Asymptomatic gray-pigmented macule found in gingiva, tongue, palate, or buccal mucosa adjacent to amalgam restoration; may be seen radiographically if particles are large; no associated inflammation; common	Traumatic implantation of amalgam	Observe or excise if melanoma cannot be ruled out on clinical basis	Remains indefinitely and changes little; no ill effects
Heavy-metal pigmentation (pp. 157–158)	Dark line along marginal gingiva due to precipitation of metal; rare	Intoxication by metal vapors (lead, bismuth, arsenic, mercury) from occupational exposure	Treat systemic problem	Exposure may affect systemic health; gingiva pigmentation of cosmetic significance
Minocycline pigmentation (pp. 158–159)	Gray pigmentation of palate, skin, scars, bone, and, rarely, of formed teeth	Ingestion of minocycline	None	Must differentiate from melanoma; drug may cause intrinsic staining of teeth

Verrucal-Papillary Lesions

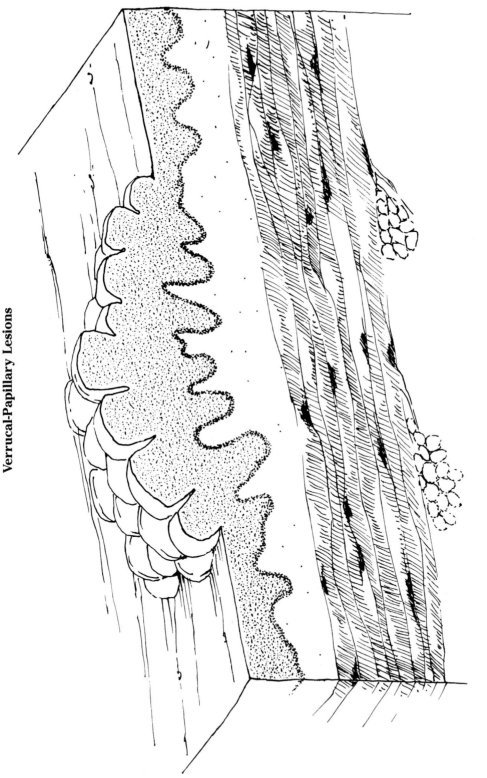

Lesions in this rather small group present as outgrowths from mucous membranes. They range from insignificant lesions of limited growth potential to verrucous carcinoma.

6

Verrucal-Papillary Lesions

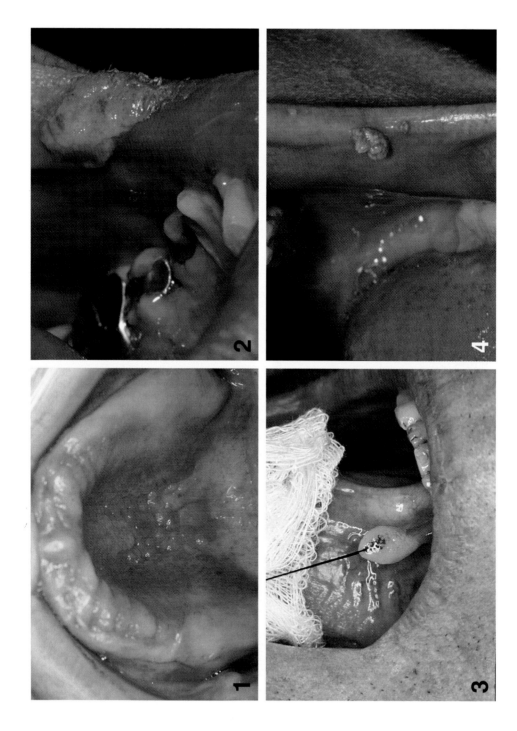

Verrucal-Papillary Lesions

DISEASE	CLINICAL FEATURES	CAUSE	TREATMENT	SIGNIFICANCE
Papillary hyperplasia (Fig. 1) (pp. 160–161)	Painless papillomatous "cobblestone" lesion of hard palate in denture wearers; usually red due to inflammation; common	Soft tissue reaction to ill-fitting denture and probable fungal overgrowth	Excision; construction of new denture	Lesion is not premalignant; may show significant regression if denture taken away from patient; antifungals may help
Condyloma latum (Fig. 2) (pp. 161–162)	Clinically similar to papillary hyperplasia; part of secondary syphilis	*Treponema pallidum*	Penicillin	Prognosis good with treatment
Squamous papilloma (Fig. 3) (pp. 162–164)	Painless exophytic granular to cauliflower-like lesions; predilection for tongue, floor of mouth, palate, uvula, lips, faucial pillars; generally solitary; soft texture; white or same color as surrounding tissue; young adults and adults; common	Most due to papillomavirus; some unknown	Excision	Lesion has no known malignant potential; recurrences rare
Oral verruca vulgaris (Fig. 4) (pp. 162–164)	Painless papillary lesion usually with white surface projections because of keratin production; may be regarded as a type of papilloma; children and young adults; common on skin, uncommon intraorally	Papillomavirus	Excision	Little significance; may be multiple and a cosmetic problem
Condyloma acuminatum (pp. 164–167)	Painless, pedunculated to sessile, exophytic, papillomatous lesion; adults; same color as or lighter than surrounding tissue; patient's sexual partner has similar lesions; rare in oral cavity	Papillomavirus	Excision	Oral lesions acquired through autoinoculation or sexual contact with infected partner; recurrences common

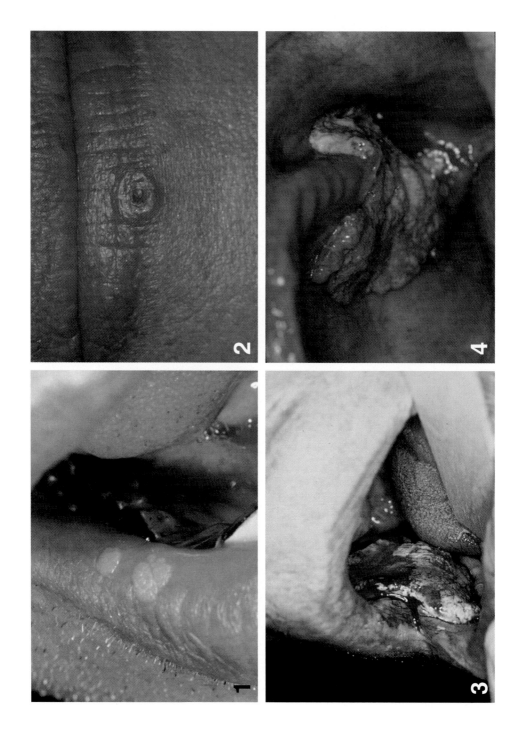

Verrucal-Papillary Lesions *Continued*

DISEASE	CLINICAL FEATURES	CAUSE	TREATMENT	SIGNIFICANCE
Focal epithelial hyperplasia (Fig. 1) (pp. 167–168)	Multiple soft nodules on lips, tongue, buccal mucosa; asymptomatic	Papillomavirus (HPV 13 and 32)	Excision	Little significance; may be included in differential diagnosis of mucosal nodules
Keratoacanthoma (Fig. 2) (pp. 168–170)	Well-circumscribed, firm, elevated lesion with central keratin plug; may cause pain; develops rapidly over 4 to 8 weeks and involutes in 6 to 8 weeks; found on sun-exposed skin and lips; rare intraorally; predilection for men	Unknown	Excision or observation	Difficult to differentiate clinically and microscopically from squamous cell carcinoma; may heal with scar
Verrucous carcinoma (Figs. 3 and 4) (pp. 170–171)	Broad-based, exophytic, indurated lesions; usually found in buccal mucosa or vestibule; men most frequently affected; uncommon	May be associated with use of tobacco, especially smokeless tobacco; HPV present in some lesions	Excision; radiation may have a role in therapy	Slow-growing malignancy; well differentiated, with better prognosis than usual squamous cell carcinoma; growth pattern is more expansile than invasive; metastasis uncommon
Pyostomatitis vegetans (pp. 171–173)	Multiple small pustules in oral mucosa; males more than females	Unknown	Topical preparations plus control of inflammatory bowel disease	May be associated with bowel disease such as ulcerative colitis or Crohn's disease
Verruciform xanthoma (p. 174)	Solitary, pebbly, elevated or depressed lesion occurring anywhere in oral mucous membrane; color ranges from white to red; rare	Unknown	Excision	Limited growth potential; does not recur

Submucosal Swellings (By Region)

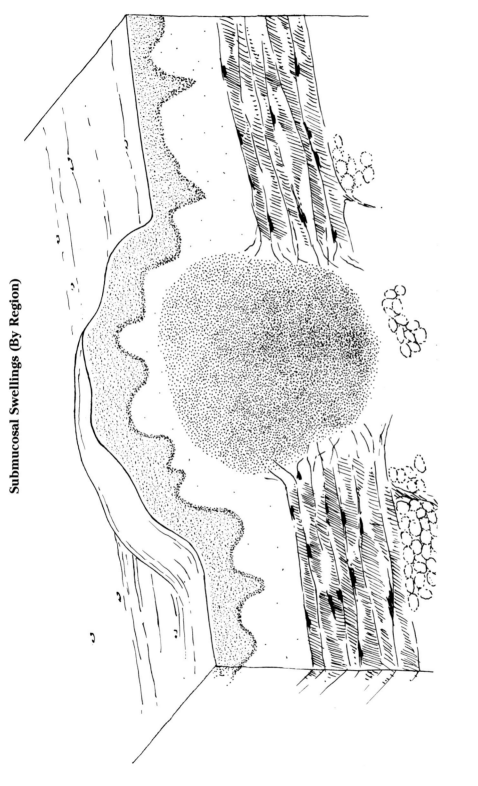

This group of lumps and bumps characteristically presents as asymptomatic swellings covered by normal, intact epithelium. A differential diagnosis is dependent on the region in which they are found. Many entities and disease subtypes not listed in this section are described in detail in Chapters 7, 8, and 9, on connective tissue, salivary gland, and lymphoid lesions, respectively.

O-48

7-9

Submucosal Swellings (By Region)

GINGIVAL SWELLINGS
Focal
Pyogenic Granuloma
Peripheral Giant Cell Granuloma
Peripheral Fibroma
Parulis
Exostosis
Gingival Cyst
Eruption Cyst
Congenital Epulis of the Newborn
Generalized Hyperplasia
Nonspecific Hyperplastic Gingivitis
Drug-Induced Hyperplasia
Hormone-Modified Hyperplasia
Leukemia-Induced Hyperplasia
Idiopathic (Genetically Influenced?) Fibrous Hyperplasia

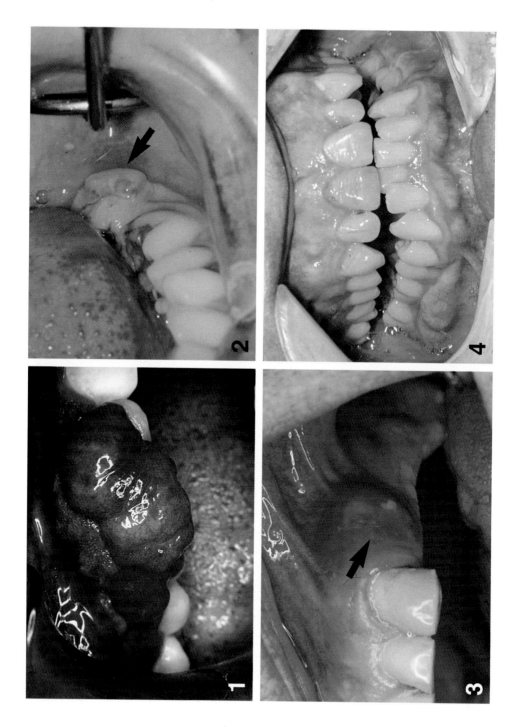

Gingival Swellings

DISEASE	CLINICAL FEATURES	CAUSE	TREATMENT	SIGNIFICANCE
Pyogenic granuloma (Fig. 1) (pp. 128–130)	Asymptomatic red tumescence found primarily on gingiva but may be found anywhere on skin or mucous membrane where trauma has occurred; common	Reaction to trauma or chronic irritation	Excision	May recur if incompletely excised; usually does not cause bone resorption
Peripheral giant cell granuloma (pp. 130–131)	Asymptomatic red tumescence of gingiva; cannot be clinically separated from pyogenic granuloma; uncommon	Reaction to trauma or chronic irritation	Excision	Completely benign behavior; unlike central counterpart; recurrence not anticipated
Peripheral fibroma (Fig. 2) (pp. 176–179)	Firm tumescence; color same as surrounding tissue; no symptoms; common; may be pedunculated or sessile	Reaction to trauma or chronic irritation	Excision	Represents overexuberant repair process with proliferation of scar; occasional recurrence seen with peripheral ossifying fibroma
Parulis (Fig. 3) (pp. 118–119)	Red tumescence (or yellow if pus filled) occurring usually on buccal gingiva of children and young adults; usually without symptoms	Sinus tract from periodontal or periapical abscess	Treatment of periodontal or periapical condition	Cyclic drainage occurs until underlying problem is eliminated
Exostosis (Fig. 4) (pp. 377–378)	Bony hard nodule(s) covered by intact mucosa found attached to buccal aspect of alveolar bone; asymptomatic; common; usually appears in adulthood	Unknown	None; may require removal for denture construction	No significance except in denture construction

Submucosal Swellings (By Region)

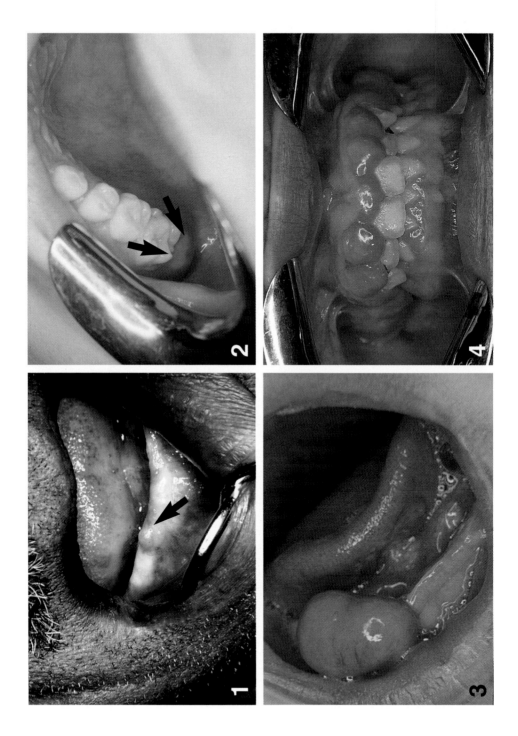

Gingival Swellings *Continued*

DISEASE	CLINICAL FEATURES	CAUSE	TREATMENT	SIGNIFICANCE
Gingival cyst (Fig. 1) (pp. 116–118)	Small, elevated, yellow to pink nodule(s); multiple in infants, solitary in adults; common in infants, rare in adults	Proliferation and cystification of dental lamina rests	None when in newborns; excision when in adults	Known as *Bohn's nodules* or *Epstein's pearls* in infants, lesions are unroofed during mastication; adult lesions do not occur
Eruption cyst (Fig. 2) (p. 296)	Bluish (fluid- or blood-filled) sac over the crown of an erupting tooth; uninflamed and asymptomatic; uncommon	Hemorrhage into follicular space between tooth crown and reduced enamel epithelium	None, tooth erupts through lesion	None, should not be confused with something else
Congenital epulis of the newborn (Fig. 3) (p. 200)	Firm pedunculated or sessile mass attached to gingiva in infants; same color as or lighter than surrounding tissue; rare	Unknown	Unknown	A benign neoplasm of granular cells similar to the granular cell tumor of the adult; does not recur
Generalized hyperplasia (Fig. 4) (pp. 179–183)	Firm, increased bulk of free and attached gingiva; usually asymptomatic; pseudopockets; nonspecific type common, others (drug induced, hormone modified, leukemia induced, genetically influenced) uncommon to rare	Local gingival irritants, plus systemic drugs (phenytoin [Dilantin], nifedipine, cyclosporine), hormone imbalance, leukemia, or hereditary factors	Improve oral hygiene, prophylaxis, gingivoplasty	Cosmetic as well as hygienic problem; causative factors should be eliminated if possible; improvement can be made by control of local factors

Submmucosal Swellings (By Region)

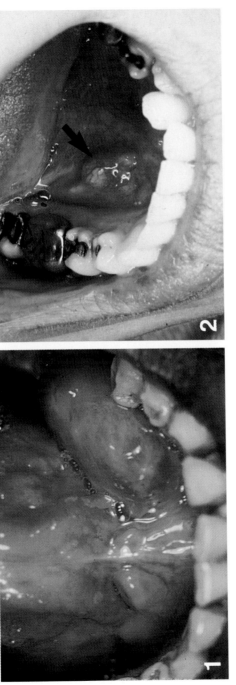

FLOOR OF MOUTH SWELLINGS
Mucus Retention Phenomenon (Ranula)
Dermoid Cyst
Lymphoepithelial Cyst
Salivary Gland Tumor
Mesenchymal Neoplasm

Floor of Mouth Swellings

DISEASE	CLINICAL FEATURES	CAUSE	TREATMENT	SIGNIFICANCE
Mucus retention phenomenon (ranula) (Fig. 1) (pp. 220–222)	Elevated, fluctuant, bluish-white mass in lateral floor of mouth; cyclic swelling often; usually painful; uncommon	Sialolith blockage of duct or traumatic severance of duct	Removal of stone or salivary gland extirpation	Most are due to sialoliths, some due to severance of duct with extravasation of mucin into soft tissues; recurrence not uncommon
Dermoid cyst (pp. 315–316)	Asymptomatic mass in floor of mouth (usually midline) covered by intact epithelium of normal color; young adults; feels doughy on palpation; rare	Proliferation of multipotential cells; stimulus unknown	Excision	Recurrence not expected; called *teratoma* when tissues from all three germ layers are present, and *dermoid* when secondary skin structures are dominant
Lymphoepithelial cyst (Fig. 2) (p. 315)	Asymptomatic nodules covered by intact epithelium less than 1 cm in diameter; any age; characteristically found on faucial pillars, floor of mouth, ventral and posterolateral tongue; yellowish-pink; uncommon within oral cavity, common in major salivary glands	Developmental defect	Excision	Ectopic lymphoid tissue of no significance; recurrence not expected
Salivary gland tumor (pp. 238–268)	Solitary, firm, asymptomatic mass usually covered by epithelium; malignant tumors may cause pain, paresthesia, or ulceration; young adults and adults; most frequent intraorally in palate, followed by tongue, upper lip, and buccal mucosa; uncommon	Unknown	Excision; may be extensive for some malignant tumors	Approximately half of minor salivary gland tumors are malignant; malignancies may metastasize to bones and lungs as well as regional lymph nodes; pleomorphic adenoma is most common benign neoplasm
Mesenchymal neoplasm (pp. 186–195)	Firm, asymptomatic tumescence covered by intact epithelium; may arise from any connective tissue cell	Unknown	Excision	Benign tumors not expected to recur; malignancies rare

Submucosal Swellings (By Region)

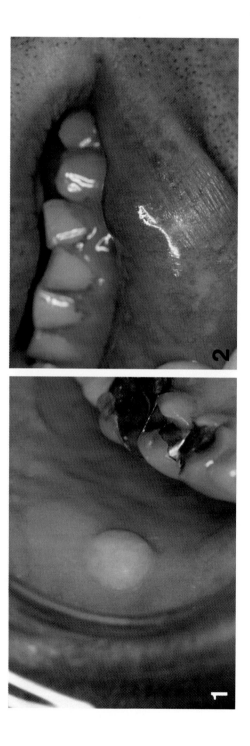

LIP AND BUCCAL MUCOSA SWELLINGS

Upper Lip
  Salivary Gland Tumor
  Mucus Retention Cyst
Lower Lip
  Traumatic Fibroma
  Mucus Extravasation Phenomenon (Mucocele)
Buccal Mucosa
  Traumatic Fibroma
  Mucus Extravasation Phenomenon
  Salivary Gland Tumor
  Mesenchymal Neoplasm

Lip and Buccal Mucosa Swellings

DISEASE	CLINICAL FEATURES	CAUSE	TREATMENT	SIGNIFICANCE
Salivary gland tumor			See Floor of Mouth Swellings	
Mucus retention cyst (pp. 219–220)	Solitary, usually asymptomatic, mobile, nontender; covered by intact epithelium; color same as surrounding tissue; adults over 50 years of age; common in palate, cheek, floor of mouth; uncommon in upper lip, rare in lower lip	Blockage of salivary gland excretory duct by sialolith	Excision	Recurrence not anticipated if associated gland removed; clinically indistinguishable from more significant salivary gland neoplasms
Traumatic fibroma (Fig. 1) (pp. 183–184)	Firm, asymptomatic nodule covered by epithelium unless secondarily traumatized; usually found along line of occlusion in buccal mucosa and lower lip; common	Reaction to trauma or chronic irritation	Excision	Represents hyperplastic scar; limited growth potential and no malignant transformation seen
Mucus extravasation phenomenon (Fig. 2) (pp. 217–219)	Bluish nodule (normal color if deep) usually covered by epithelium; may be slightly painful and have associated acute inflammatory reaction; most frequently seen in lower lip and buccal mucosa, rare in upper lip; adolescents and children; common	Traumatic severance of salivary gland excretory duct	Excision	Recurrence expected if contributing salivary gland not removed or if adjacent ducts are severed
Mesenchymal neoplasm			See Floor of Mouth Swellings	

Submucosal Swellings (By Region)

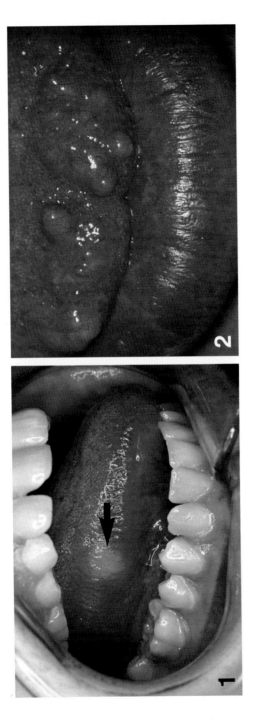

TONGUE SWELLINGS
Traumatic Fibroma
Pyogenic Granuloma
Granular Cell Tumor (Granular Cell Myoblastoma)
Neurofibroma
Salivary Gland Tumor
Lingual Thyroid

Tongue Swellings

DISEASE	CLINICAL FEATURES	CAUSE	TREATMENT	SIGNIFICANCE
Traumatic fibroma			See Lip and Buccal Mucosa Swellings	
Pyogenic granuloma			See Gingival Swellings	
Granular cell tumor (Fig. 1) (pp. 200–203)	Painless elevated tumescence covered by intact epithelium; color same as or lighter than surrounding tissue; strong predilection for dorsum of tongue but may be found anywhere; any age; uncommon	Unknown; cell of origin undetermined; Schwann cell; granularity due to cytoplasmic autophagosomes	Excision	Does not recur; of significance in that it must be differentiated from other lesions; no malignant potential
Neurofibroma/Palisaded encapsulated neuroma (pp. 204–209)	Soft, single or multiple, asymptomatic nodules covered by epithelium; same as or lighter than surrounding mucosa; most frequently seen on tongue, buccal mucosa, and vestibule but may be seen anywhere; any age; uncommon	Unknown; cell of origin is probably Schwann cell	Excision	Recurrence not expected; multiple neurofibromas should suggest von Recklinghausen's disease of nerve (neurofibromas with malignant potential; café au lait spots); palisaded encapsulated neuromas are not syndrome associated
Mucosal neuroma (Fig. 2) (pp. 208–209)	Multiple; lips, tongue, buccal mucosa; may be associated with MEN III syndrome	Unknown; MEN III syndrome is autosomal dominant	None	MEN III syndrome (pheochromocytoma, medullary carcinoma of the thyroid, and mucosal neuromas)
Salivary gland tumor			See Floor of Mouth Swellings	
Lingual thyroid (p. 316)	Nodular mass in base of tongue, may cause dysphagia; young adults; rare	Incomplete descent of thyroid anlage to neck	Excision only after demonstration of normal functioning thyroid tissue elsewhere	Lingual thyroid may be patient's only thyroid tissue

O-59

Submucosal Swellings (By Region)

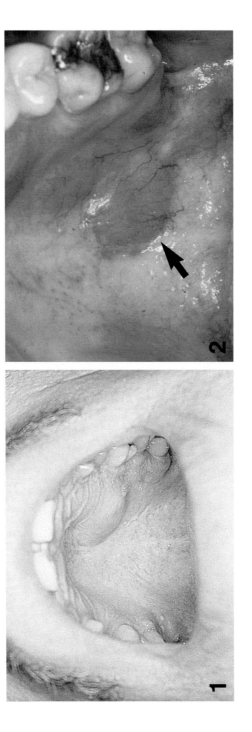

PALATAL SWELLINGS
Mucus Extravasation Phenomenon
Salivary Gland Tumor
Palatal Abscess from Periapical Lesion
Lymphoma
Torus
Neoplasm of Maxilla or Maxillary Sinus

Palatal Swellings

DISEASE	CLINICAL FEATURES	CAUSE	TREATMENT	SIGNIFICANCE
Mucus extravasation phenomenon			See Lip and Buccal Mucosa Swellings	
Salivary gland tumor (Fig. 1)			See Floor of Mouth Swellings	
Palatal abscess from periapical lesion	Painful, pus-filled, fluctuant tumescence of hard palate; color same as or redder than surrounding tissue; associated with nonvital tooth	Extension of periapical abscess through palatal bone	Incise and drain, treat nonvital tooth; antibiotics may be necessary	Pus may spread to other areas, seeking path of least resistance
Lymphoma (Fig. 2) (pp. 273–283)	Asymptomatic, spongy to firm tumescence of hard palate; rare in adults; relatively common in patients with AIDS	Unknown	Evaluation of other lymphoid organs for lymphoma; radiation/ chemotherapy; follow-up examinations	May represent primary lymphoma (non-Hodgkin's type); lymphoma work-up indicated; high-grade lesions seen in patients with AIDS
Torus (pp. 377–378)	Asymptomatic bony, hard swelling of hard palate (torus palatinus); bony, exophytic growths along lingual aspect of mandible (torus mandibularis); torpid growth; young adults and adults; affects up to 25% of population	Unknown	None; may be excised for prosthetic considerations	No significance; should not be confused with other palatal lesions
Neoplasm of maxilla or maxillary sinus	Palatal swelling with or without ulceration; pain or paresthesia; may cause loosening of teeth or malocclusion; denture may not fit; any age; rare	Unknown	Surgery or radiation	May represent benign or malignant jaw neoplasm or carcinoma of maxillary sinus; poor prognosis for malignant lesions

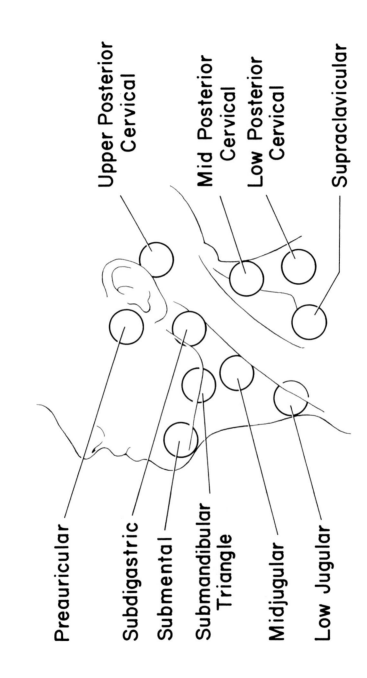

Preauricular

Subdigastric

Submental

Submandibular Triangle

Midjugular

Low Jugular

Upper Posterior Cervical

Mid Posterior Cervical

Low Posterior Cervical

Supraclavicular

NECK SWELLINGS
Lateral Neck
    Branchial Cyst
    Lymphadenitis—Nonspecific, Bacterial, Fungal
    Metastatic Carcinoma to Lymph Nodes
    Lymphoma
    Parotid Lesion—Neoplasm, Sjögren's Syndrome, Infection,
        Metabolic Disease
    Carotid Body Tumor (Paraganglioma, Chemodectoma)
    Epidermal Cyst
    Lymphangioma (Cystic Hygroma)
Midline
    Thyroglossal Tract Cyst
    Thyroid Gland Tumor
    Dermoid Cyst

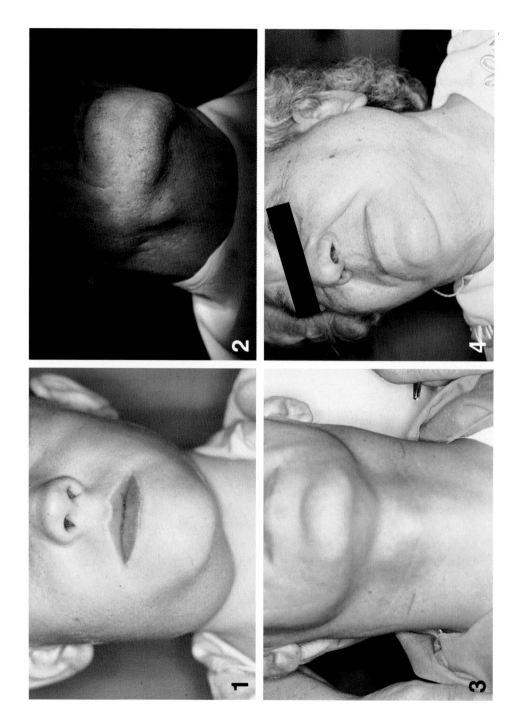

Neck Swellings

DISEASE	CLINICAL FEATURES	CAUSE	TREATMENT	SIGNIFICANCE
Branchial cyst (Fig. 1) (pp. 315–316)	Asymptomatic noninflamed swelling in lateral neck; soft or fluctuant; children and young adults; rare	Developmental, proliferation of epithelial remnants within lymph nodes	Excision	Clinical diagnostic problem
Lymphadenitis—nonspecific, bacterial, fungal	Single or multiple painful nodules (lymph nodes) in neck, especially submandibular and jugulodigastric areas; lesions are usually soft when acute and usually not fixed to surrounding tissue; nonspecific type common	Any oral inflammatory condition, especially dental abscess; oral tuberculosis, syphilis, or deep fungus may affect neck nodes	Treat specific cause	Neck disease often reflects in oral cavity
Metastatic carcinoma to lymph nodes (Fig. 2)	Usually single but may be multiple (rarely bilateral), indurated masses; fixed and nonpainful; most frequently affects submandibular and jugulodigastric nodes; adults; uncommon	Metastatic oral cancer; may occasionally come from nasopharynx lesion	Find primary lesion; surgery or radiation	Signifies advanced disease with poor prognosis
Lymphoma (Fig. 3) (pp. 273–283)	Single or bilateral swellings in lateral neck; indurated, asymptomatic, and often fixed; patient may have weight loss, night sweats, and fever; young adults and adults; uncommon	Unknown	Radiation and/or chemotherapy	After diagnostic biopsy, staging procedures are done; prognosis fair to excellent depending on stage and classification; relatively common in patients with AIDS
Parotid lesion (Fig. 4)	When tail of parotid affected, neck mass may occur; *neoplasm*—indurated, asymptomatic, single lump (Warthin's tumor—may be bilateral); *Sjögren's syndrome*—bilateral, diffuse, soft swelling plus sicca complex, affects primarily older women; *infection*—unilateral, diffuse, soft, painful mass	*Neoplasm*—unknown; *Sjögren's syndrome*—autoimmune; *infection*—viral, bacterial, or fungal; *metabolic disease*—diabetes, alcoholism	Treat cause	Requires diagnosis and treatment by experienced clinician
Carotid body tumor	Firm, movable mass in neck at carotid bifurcation; bruit and thrill may be apparent; adults; rare	Neoplastic transformation of carotid body (chemoreceptor) cells	Excision	Morbidity from surgery may be profound because of tumor attachment to carotid sheath

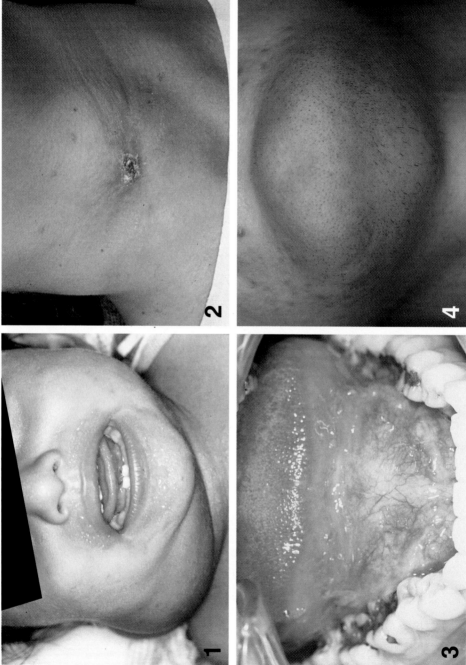

Neck Swellings *Continued*

DISEASE	CLINICAL FEATURES	CAUSE	TREATMENT	SIGNIFICANCE
Epidermal cyst	Elevated nodule in skin of neck (or face); usually uninflamed and asymptomatic; up to several centimeters in size; covered by epidermis and near skin surface; common	Epithelial rest proliferation	Excision	Recurrence not expected; more superficially located than other neck lesions discussed
Lymphangioma (Fig. 1) (pp. 196–197)	Spongy, diffuse, painless mass in dermis; may become large; lighter than surrounding tissue to red-blue; crepitance; children; rare	Developmental	Excision	May be disfiguring or cause respiratory distress
Thyroglossal tract cyst (Fig. 2) (pp. 316–321)	Midline swelling in neck above level of thyroid gland; may develop sinus tract (Fig. 2); most common developmental cyst of neck	Failure of complete descent of thyroid tissue from foramen caecum with subsequent cystification	Excision	Recurrence not uncommon because of tortuous course of cystic lesion
Thyroid gland tumor	Midline swelling in area of thyroid gland; firm, asymptomatic; uncommon	Unknown	Excision	Prognosis poor to excellent depending on stage and histologic type of tumor
Dermoid cyst (Figs. 3 and 4) (pp. 315–316)	Swelling in floor of mouth or midline of neck; young adults	Unknown	Excision	Recurrence not expected

10-15

Jaw Lesions

Jaw lesions can be classified in a number of ways. A common way is to separate them according to their general radiographic appearance of lucent, opaque, and mixed pattern. A disadvantage of this method is that an entity may have more than one radiographic pattern. Another is that most lesions in the jaws are radiolucent. The classification chosen for this section is division into the following groups:

Cysts of the oral region
Odontogenic tumors
Benign nonodontogenic tumors
Inflammatory jaw lesions
Malignant nonodontogenic neoplasms of the jaws
Metabolic and genetic jaw diseases

When considering a differential diagnosis, a step-by-step progression through the lesions in these groups provides a convenient and logical sequence of thought. Of considerable clinical importance is the combination of radiographic appearance, patient age, and location of the lesion. These three features considered together are very reliable signs for diagnosis of many jaw lesions and are emphasized in these tables.

Jaw Lesions

10

Cysts of the Oral Region

ODONTOGENIC CYSTS
Periapical (Radicular) Cyst
Dentigerous Cyst
Lateral Periodontal Cyst
Gingival Cyst of the Newborn
Odontogenic Keratocyst
Calcifying Odontogenic Cyst
Glandular Odontogenic Cyst
NONODONTOGENIC CYSTS
Globulomaxillary Lesion
Nasolabial Cyst
Median Mandibular Lesion
Nasopalatine Canal Cyst
PSEUDOCYSTS
Aneurysmal Bone Cyst
Traumatic (Simple) Bone Cyst
Static Bone Cyst
Focal Osteoporotic Bone Marrow Defect

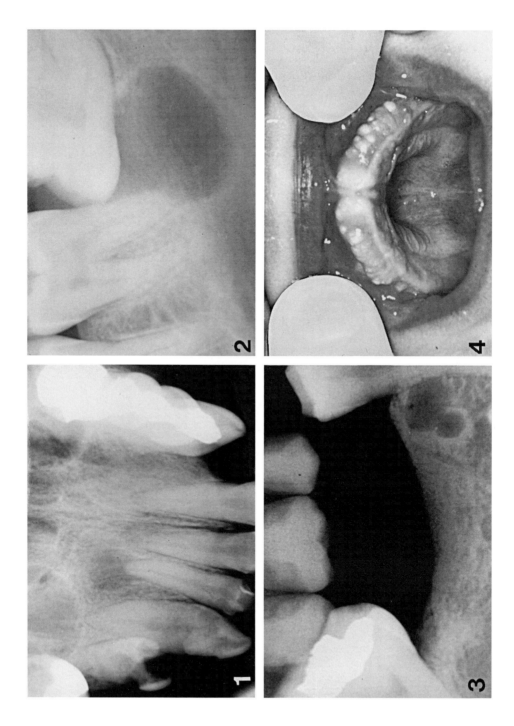

Cysts of the Oral Region

DISEASE	PATIENT AGE	LOCATION	RADIOGRAPHIC APPEARANCE	OTHER FEATURES
Periapical (radicular) cyst (Fig. 1) (pp. 288–291)	Any age; peaks in third through sixth decades	Apex of any nonvital erupted tooth, especially anterior maxilla	Well-defined lucency at apex of nonvital tooth	Cannot be distinguished radiographically from periapical granuloma; develops from inflammatory stimulation of rests of Malassez; incomplete enucleation results in *residual cyst*; chronic process and usually asymptomatic; common
Dentigerous cyst (Fig. 2) (pp. 291–296)	Young adults	Associated most commonly with impacted mandibular third molars and maxillary third molars and cuspids	Well-defined lucency around crown of impacted teeth	Complication of neoplastic transformation of cystic epithelium to ameloblastoma and, rarely, to squamous cell or mucoepidermoid carcinoma; some become very large, with rare possibility of pathologic fracture; common; *eruption cyst*—gingival tumescence developing as a dilatation of follicular space over crown of erupting tooth
Lateral periodontal cyst (Fig. 3) (pp. 296–299)	Adults	Lateral periodontal membrane, especially mandibular cuspid and premolar area	Well-defined lucency; usually unilocular but may be multilocular	Usually asymptomatic; associated tooth is vital; origin from rests of dental lamina; some keratocysts are found in a lateral root position; gingival cyst of the adult may be soft tissue counterpart
Gingival cyst of the newborn (Fig. 4) (pp. 299–300)	Newborn	Gingival soft tissues	Usually not apparent on radiograph	Newborns—common, multiple, no treatment; adult gingival cyst is rare, solitary, and treated by local excision

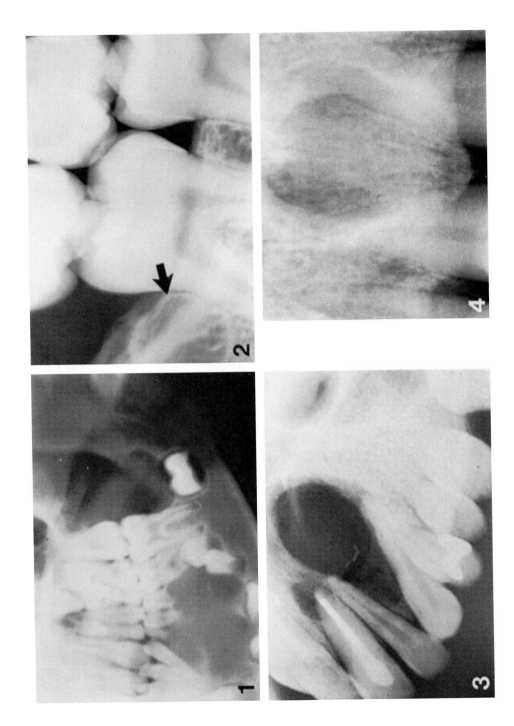

Cysts of the Oral Region *Continued*

DISEASE	PATIENT AGE	LOCATION	RADIOGRAPHIC APPEARANCE	OTHER FEATURES
Odontogenic keratocyst (Figs. 1 and 2) (pp. 300–304)	Any age, especially adults	Mandibular molar-ramus area favored; may be found in position of dentigerous, lateral root, periapical, or primordial cyst	Well-defined lucency; unilocular or multilocular	Recurrence rate of 5 to 62%; may have aggressive behavior; may be part of nevoid basal cell syndrome (keratocysts, skeletal anomalies, basal cell carcinomas); follow-up examination necessary; known as *primordial cyst* when found in place of tooth (Fig. 2)
Calcifying odontogenic cyst (pp. 304–305)	Any age	Maxilla favored; gingiva second most common site	Well-defined lucency, may have opaque foci	Origin and behavior are in dispute; ghost cell keratinization characteristic; may have aggressive behavior; rare
Glandular odontogenic cyst (p. 299)	Any age	Mandible favored	Well-defined lucency	Recurrence potential
Globulomaxillary lesion (Fig. 3) (pp. 305–306)	Any age	Between roots of maxillary cuspid and lateral incisor	Well-defined oval or pear-shaped lucency	Teeth are vital; asymptomatic; represents one of several different odontogenic cysts/tumors
Nasolabial cyst (pp. 306–307)	Adults	Soft tissue of upper lip, lateral to midline	No change	Origin likely from remnants of nasolacrimal duct; rare
Median mandibular lesion (pp. 307–308)	Any age	Midline mandible	Well-defined lucency	Teeth are vital; asymptomatic; represents one of several different odontogenic cysts/tumors
Nasopalatine canal cyst (Fig. 4) (pp. 308–309)	Any age	Nasopalatine canal or papilla	Well-defined midline maxillary lucency, may be oval or heart shaped	Teeth are vital; may be symptomatic if secondarily infected; may be difficult to differentiate from normal canal; common

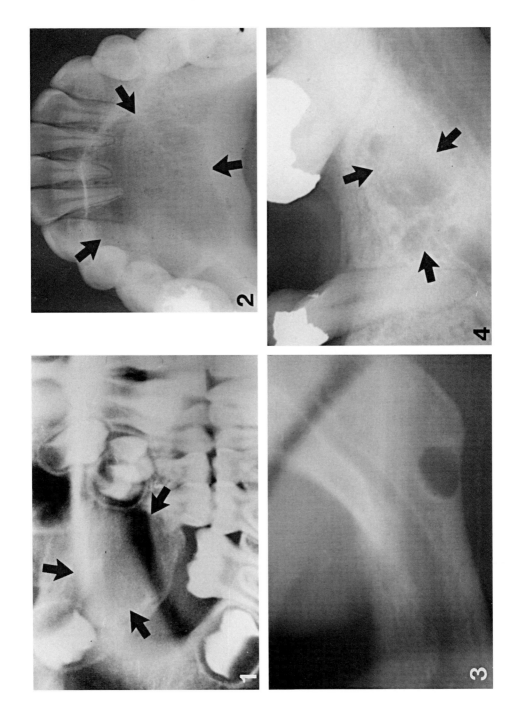

Cysts of the Oral Region *Continued*

DISEASE	PATIENT AGE	LOCATION	RADIOGRAPHIC APPEARANCE	OTHER FEATURES
Aneurysmal bone cyst (Fig. 1) (pp. 309–310)	Second decade favored	Either jaw; also long bones and vertebrae	Lucency, may be poorly defined; may have honeycomb or soap-bubble appearance	Represents vascular lesion in bone consisting of blood-filled sinusoids; blood wells up when lesion is entered; cause and pathogenesis unknown; rare; follow-up important
Traumatic (simple) bone cyst (Fig. 2) (pp. 310–313)	Second decade favored	Mandible favored	Well-defined lucency often extending between roots of teeth	Represents dead space in bone without epithelial lining; cause and pathogenesis unknown; uncommon in oral region; often part of florid osseous dysplasia
Static bone cyst (Fig. 3) (p. 313)	Developmental defect that should be apparent from childhood	Mandibular molar area below alveolar canal	Well-defined oval lucency, does not change with time	Represents lingual depression of mandible; filled with salivary gland or other soft tissue from floor of mouth; asymptomatic; an incidental finding that requires no biopsy or treatment; uncommon
Focal osteoporotic bone marrow defect (Fig. 4) (pp. 313–315)	Adults	Mandible favored	Lucency; often in edentulous areas	Contains hematopoietic marrow; probably represents unusual healing in bone; must be differentiated from other more significant lesions; uncommon

Jaw Lesions

11

Odontogenic Tumors

EPITHELIAL TUMORS
Ameloblastoma
Squamous Odontogenic Tumor
Calcifying Epithelial Odontogenic Tumor
Clear Cell Odontogenic Tumor (Carcinoma)
Adenomatoid Odontogenic Tumor
MESENCHYMAL TUMORS
Odontogenic Myxoma
Central Odontogenic Fibroma
Cementifying Fibroma
Cementoblastoma
Periapical Cemento-Osseous Dysplasia
MIXED (EPITHELIAL AND MESENCHYMAL) TUMORS
Odontoma
Ameloblastic Fibroma and Ameloblastic Fibro-Odontoma

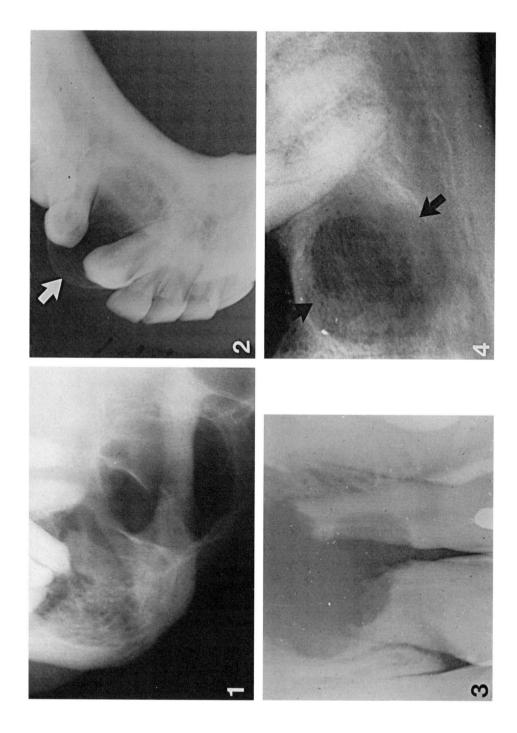

Odontogenic Tumors

DISEASE	PATIENT AGE	LOCATION	RADIOGRAPHIC APPEARANCE	OTHER FEATURES
Ameloblastoma (Fig. 1) (pp. 323–335)	Fourth and fifth decades	Mandibular molar-ramus area favored	Lucent; usually well circumscribed; unilocular or multilocular	May arise in wall of dentigerous cyst; may exhibit aggressive behavior; rarely metastasizes (usually to lung); recurrence rate low for unicystic type; usually asymptomatic; uncommon
Squamous odontogenic tumor (pp. 335–336)	Mean of 40 years; second through seventh decades	Alveolar process; anterior more than posterior	Lucency	Conservative therapy; few recurrences
Calcifying epithelial odontogenic tumor (pp. 336–339)	Mean around 40 years; second through tenth decades	Mandibular molar-ramus area favored	Lucent with or without opaque foci; usually well circumscribed; unilocular or multilocular	Behavior and prognosis are similar to those for ameloblastoma; rare
Clear cell odontogenic tumor (p. 339)	Seventh decade	Mandible, maxilla	Lucency	Rare
Adenomatoid odontogenic tumor (Fig. 2) (p. 339)	Second decade	Anterior jaws	Well-defined lucency, may have opaque foci	Usually associated with crown of impacted tooth; no symptoms; does not recur after enucleation; rare
Odontogenic myxoma (Fig. 3) (pp. 339–344)	Mean of about 30; ages 10 to 50	Any area of jaws	Lucent lesion, often multilocular or honeycombed; may be poorly defined peripherally	Tumors may exhibit aggressive behavior; no symptoms; uncommon; recurrence not uncommon
Central odontogenic fibroma (p. 344)	Any	Any area of jaws	Lucency, usually multilocular	Two microscopic subtypes exhibit same benign clinical behavior; differentiate from desmoplastic fibroma
Cementifying fibroma (Fig. 4) (pp. 344–346)	Fourth and fifth decades	Posterior mandible	Well-defined lucent lesion, may have opaque foci	Asymptomatic; grows by local expansion; recurrence unlikely; rare

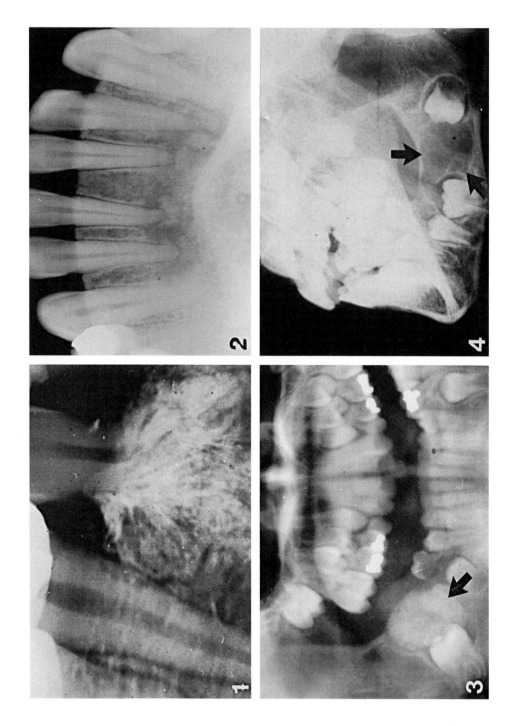

Odontogenic Tumors *Continued*

DISEASE	PATIENT AGE	LOCATION	RADIOGRAPHIC APPEARANCE	OTHER FEATURES
Cementoblastoma (Fig. 1) (pp. 347–348)	Second and third decades	Root of posterior teeth; mandible more than maxilla	Opaque lesion; attached to and replaces root; opaque spicules radiate from central area	May cause cortical expansion; tooth and lesion removed together; no symptoms; rare
Periapical cemento-osseous dysplasia (Fig. 2) (pp. 348–350)	Fifth decade	Mandible, especially apices of anterior teeth; usually more than one tooth affected	Starts as periapical lucencies that eventually become opaque in months to years	Regarded as a reactive lesion; always associated with vital teeth; requires no treatment; asymptomatic; common; rare variant known as *florid osseous dysplasia* represents severe form that may affect one to four quadrants and may have complications of chronic osteomyelitis and traumatic bone cysts
Odontoma (Fig. 3) (pp. 350–352)	Second decade	Anywhere, especially anterior mandible and maxilla	Opaque; *compound type*—tooth shapes apparent; *complex type*—uniform opaque mass	May block eruption of a permanent tooth; *complex type* rarely causes cortical expansion, no recurrence; *compound type* appears as many miniature teeth; *complex type* is conglomeration of enamel and dentin; probably represents hamartoma rather than neoplasm; common
Ameloblastic fibroma and ameloblastic fibro-odontoma (Fig. 4) (pp. 352–355)	First and second decades	Mandibular molar-ramus area	Well-defined lucency; may be multilocular and large; fibro-odontoma may have associated opaque mass representing an odontoma	Well encapsulated; recurrence not expected; no symptoms; if odontoma present, the lesion is called *ameloblastic fibro-odontoma*; rare

Jaw Lesions

12

Benign Nonodontogenic Tumors*

OSSIFYING FIBROMA
FIBROUS DYSPLASIA
OSTEOBLASTOMA
CHONDROMA
OSTEOMA
CENTRAL GIANT CELL GRANULOMA
HEMANGIOMA OF BONE
LANGERHANS CELL DISEASE (IDIOPATHIC HISTIOCYTOSIS)
TORI AND EXOSTOSES
CORONOID HYPERPLASIA

---

*Because of the similar microscopic appearance of a number of benign jaw lesions, they are frequently grouped together as fibro-osseous lesions. They are composed of a benign fibrous connective tissue stroma with various amounts of bone or cementum dispersed throughout. Vascularity ranges from slight to prominent in the various lesions. Diagnosis of fibro-osseous lesions depends on the correlation of clinical features, radiographic appearance, and microscopic findings.

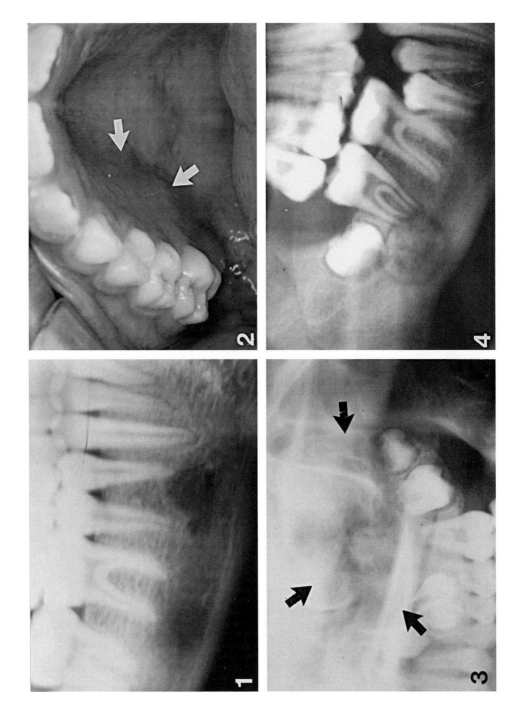

Benign Nonodontogenic Tumors

DISEASE	PATIENT AGE	LOCATION	RADIOGRAPHIC APPEARANCE	OTHER FEATURES
Ossifying fibroma (Fig. 1) (pp. 357–360)	Third and fourth decades	Body of mandible favored	Well-defined lucency, may have opaque foci	Slow growing and asymptomatic; may be indistinguishable from cementifying fibroma; does not recur; microscopy often similar to fibrous dysplasia; uncommon
Fibrous dysplasia (Figs. 2 and 3) (pp. 360–363)	First and second decades	Maxilla favored	Poorly defined radiographic mass; diffuse opacification often described as ground glass	Slow growing and asymptomatic; causes cortical expansion; may cease growing after puberty; a cosmetic problem treated by recontouring. Variants: *monostotic*—one bone affected; *polystotic*—more than one bone affected; *Albright's syndrome*—fibrous dysplasia plus café au lait macules and endocrine abnormalities (precocious puberty in females); *Jaffe-Lichtenstein syndrome*—multiple bone lesions of fibrous dysplasia and skin pigmentations; rare
Osteoblastoma (Fig. 4) (pp. 363–365)	Second decade	Either jaw	Well-defined, lucent to opaque lesion	Diagnostic feature of pain; microscopy often difficult, may be confused with osteosarcoma; recurrence not expected; rare
Chondroma (p. 366)	Any age	Any, especially anterior maxilla and posterior mandible	Relative lucency, may have opacities	May be difficult to separate microscopically from well-differentiated chondrosarcoma; rare

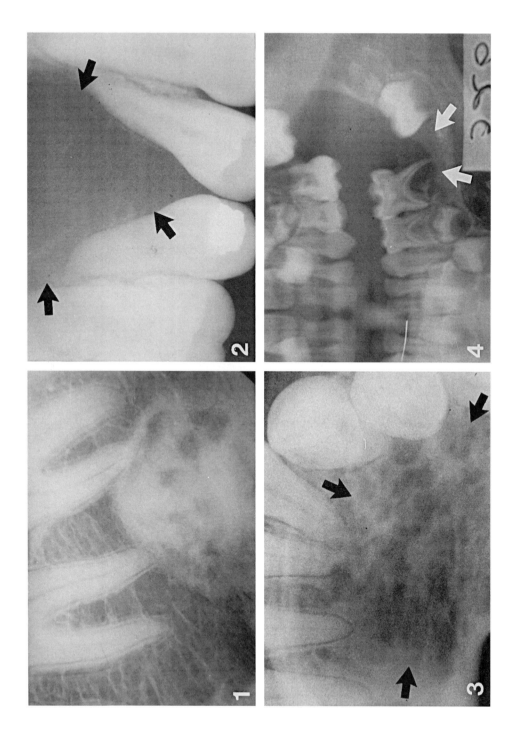

Benign Nonodontogenic Tumors *Continued*

DISEASE	PATIENT AGE	LOCATION	RADIOGRAPHIC APPEARANCE	OTHER FEATURES
Osteoma (Fig. 1) (pp. 366–368)	Any age	Either jaw	Well defined	Asymptomatic; may be part of Gardner's syndrome (osteomas, intestinal polyps, cysts and fibrous lesions of skin, supernumerary teeth); rare
Central giant cell granuloma (Fig. 2) (pp. 368–370)	Children and young adults	Either jaw	Usually well-defined lucency; may be multilocular or, less frequently, unilocular	May exhibit aggressive behavior; low recurrence rate; asymptomatic; uncommon; rule out hyperparathyroidism
Hemangioma of bone (Fig. 3) (pp. 371–372)	Young adults	Either jaw	Lucent lesion; may resemble honeycomb or be multilocular	Hemorrhage is significant complication with treatment; asymptomatic; rare
Langerhans cell disease (idiopathic histiocytosis) (Fig. 4) (pp. 372–376)	Children and young adults	Any bone	Single or multiple lucent lesions; some described as punched out; lesions around root apices sometimes described as resembling floating teeth	Three variants: *Letterer-Siwe syndrome (acute disseminated)*—organs and bone affected, infants, usually fatal; *Hand-Schüller-Christian syndrome (chronic disseminated)*—bone lesions, exophthalmos, diabetes insipidus and organ lesions, children, fair prognosis; *eosinophilic granuloma (chronic localized)*—bone lesions only, children and adults, good prognosis; surgery, radiation, or chemotherapy; cause unknown
Tori and exostoses (pp. 377–378)	Adults	Palate, lingual mandible, and buccal aspect of alveolar bone	May appear as opacity when large	Torus palatinus in 25% of population, torus mandibularis in 10%; cause unknown; little significance
Coronoid hyperplasia (p. 378)	Young adults	Coronoid process of mandible	Opaque enlargement	Cause unknown; may affect jaw function

Jaw Lesions

13

Inflammatory Jaw Lesions

ACUTE OSTEOMYELITIS
CHRONIC OSTEOMYELITIS
Focal Sclerosing Osteomyelitis (Condensing Osteitis)
Diffuse Sclerosing Osteomyelitis
Garré's Osteomyelitis (Chronic Osteomyelitis with
    Proliferative Periostitis)

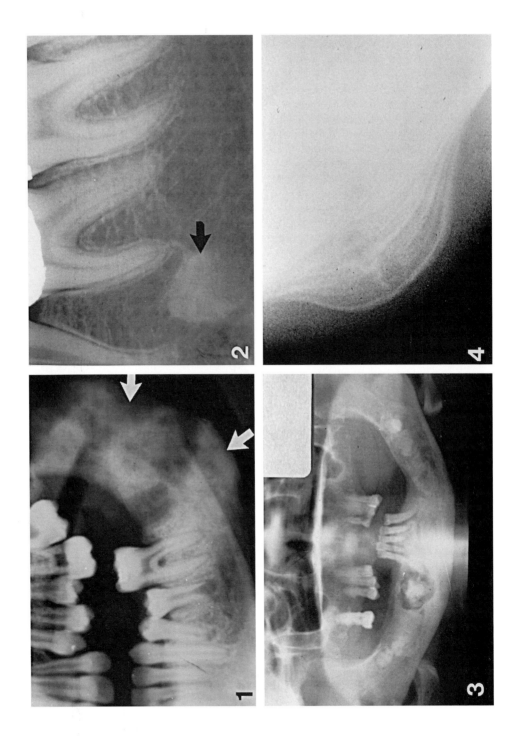

Inflammatory Jaw Lesions

DISEASE	PATIENT AGE	LOCATION	RADIOGRAPHIC APPEARANCE	OTHER FEATURES
Acute osteomyelitis (pp. 386–387)	Any age	Mandible favored	Little radiographic change early; after 1 to 2 weeks, a diffuse lucency appears	Pain or paresthesia may be present; pus producing if due to *Staphylococcus* infection; uncommon in severe form; most frequently caused by extension of periapical infection
Chronic osteomyelitis (pp. 387–390)	Any age	Mandible favored	Focal or diffuse; lucent with sclerotic foci described as a moth-eaten pattern (Fig. 1); *focal sclerotic type*—well-defined opacification (Fig. 2); *diffuse sclerotic type*—diffuse opacification (Fig. 3); *Garré's type*—onionskin periosteum (Fig. 4)	Usually asymptomatic but may be painful; most are related to chronic inflammation in bone of dental origin; many are not treated; nonvital teeth should be extracted or root canals filled; common; *Garré's type* is treated by extraction of offending tooth

Jaw Lesions

14

Malignant Nonodontogenic Neoplasms of the Jaws

OSTEOSARCOMA
Juxtacortical Osteosarcomas
Parosteal Osteosarcoma
Periosteal Osteosarcoma
CHONDROSARCOMA
Mesenchymal Chondrosarcoma
EWING'S SARCOMA
BURKITT'S LYMPHOMA
PLASMA CELL NEOPLASMS
Multiple Myeloma
Solitary Plasmacytoma of Bone
METASTATIC CARCINOMA

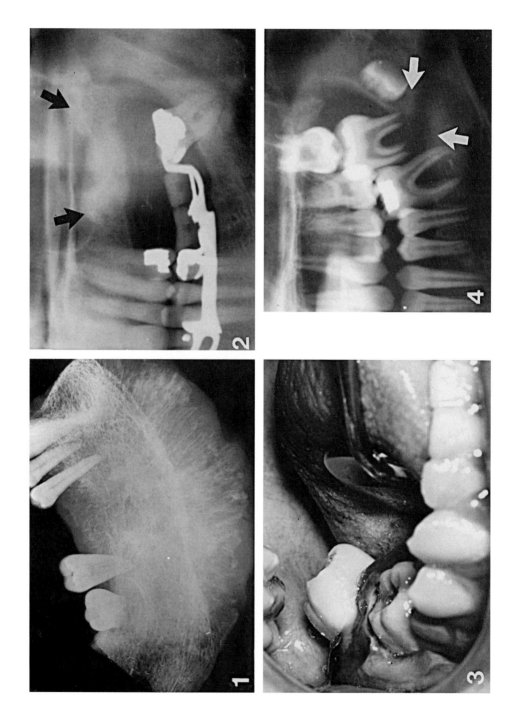

Malignant Nonodontogenic Neoplasms of the Jaws

DISEASE	PATIENT AGE	LOCATION	RADIOGRAPHIC APPEARANCE	OTHER FEATURES
Osteosarcoma (Figs. 1 and 2) (pp. 397–404)	Third and fourth decades	Mandible or maxilla; juxtacortical subtype (Fig. 2) arises from periosteum	Poorly defined lucency often with spicules of opaque material; sunburst pattern may be seen; juxtacortical lesion appears as radiodense mass on the periosteum	Swelling, pain, and paresthesia are diagnostic features; patients may have vertical mobility of teeth and uniformly widened periodontal ligament space; prognosis fair to poor, good prognosis for juxtacortical lesions
Chondrosarcoma (pp. 404–407)	Adulthood and old age	Maxilla favored slightly	Poorly defined, lucent to moderately opaque	Swelling, pain, or paresthesia may be present; prognosis fair to poor, better if in mandible; often misdiagnosed as benign cartilage lesions; rare
Ewing's sarcoma (pp. 407–409)	Children and young adults	Mandible favored	Diffuse lucency; poorly defined; periosteal "onionskin" reaction may be present; may be multilocular	Swelling, pain, or paresthesia may be present; prognosis is poor; malignant cell is of unknown origin; rare
Burkitt's lymphoma (Figs. 3 and 4) (pp. 409–411)	Children	Mandible or maxilla	Diffuse lucency	Malignancy of B lymphocytes linked to Epstein-Barr virus; pain or paresthesia may be presenting symptom; prognosis is fair; rare in the USA

Malignant Nonodontogenic Neoplasms of the Jaws

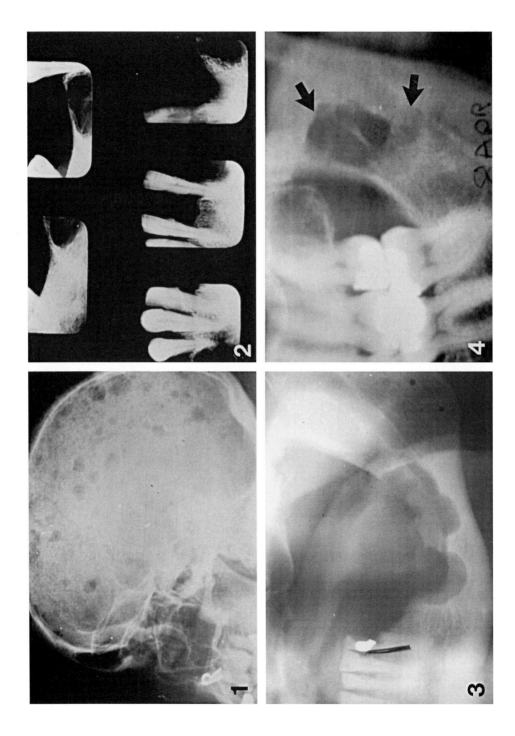

Malignant Nonodontogenic Neoplasms of the Jaws *Continued*

DISEASE	PATIENT AGE	LOCATION	RADIOGRAPHIC APPEARANCE	OTHER FEATURES
Plasma cell myeloma (Figs. 1 and 2) (pp. 411–413)	Adults	Mandible favored	Well-defined lucencies described as punched-out lesions; some lesions diffuse	Swelling, pain, or numbness may be presenting complaint; Bence Jones protein in urine of a majority of patients; rare to have only jaw lesions; prognosis is poor; solitary lesions eventually become disseminated
Metastatic carcinoma (Figs. 3 and 4) (p. 413)	Adults	Mandible favored; occasionally gingiva	Ill-defined, destructive lucency; may be multilocular; some tumors may have opaque foci (e.g., prostate, breast, lung)	Pain or paresthesia common; origin is most likely from a malignancy of breast, kidney, lung, colon, prostate, or thyroid; uncommon

15

Metabolic and Genetic Jaw Diseases

METABOLIC
Paget's Disease
Hyperparathyroidism
Infantile Cortical Hyperostosis
Phantom Bone Disease
Acromegaly
GENETIC
Cherubism
Osteopetrosis
Others (see text)
Osteogenesis Imperfecta
Cleidocranial Dysplasia
Crouzon's Syndrome
Treacher Collins Syndrome
Pierre Robin Syndrome
Marfan's Syndrome
Ehlers-Danlos Syndrome
Down Syndrome
Hemifacial Atrophy
Hemifacial Hypertrophy
Clefts of the Lip and Palate
Fragile X Syndrome

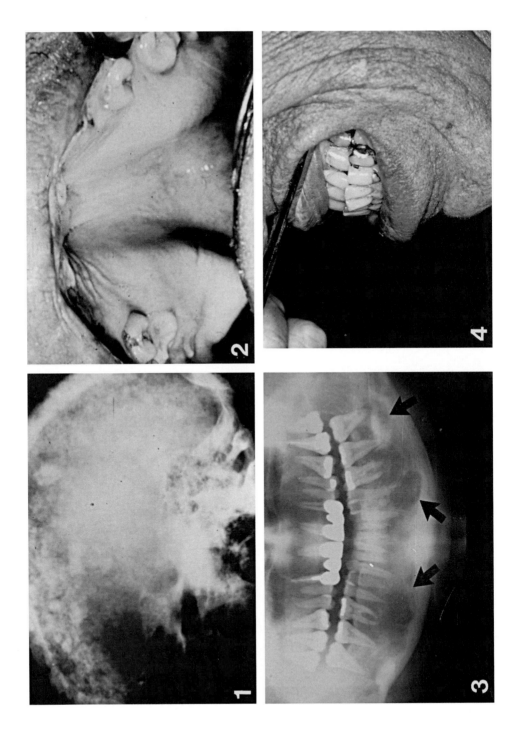

Metabolic and Genetic Jaw Diseases

DISEASE	PATIENT AGE	LOCATION	RADIOGRAPHIC APPEARANCE	OTHER FEATURES
Paget's disease (Figs. 1 and 2) (pp. 417–420)	Over 40 years of age	Maxilla favored, bilateral and symmetric	Diffuse lucent to opaque bone changes; opaque lesions described as cotton wool; hypercementosis, loss of lamina dura, obliteration of periodontal ligament space, and root resorption may be seen	Patients develop pain, deafness, blindness, and headache because of bone changes; initial complaint may be that denture is too tight; diastemas may develop; complications of hemorrhage early, infection and fracture late; alkaline phosphate elevated; cause unknown but affects bone metabolism
Hyperparathyroidism (Fig. 3) (pp. 420–423)	Any age	Mandible favored	Usually well-defined lucency(ies); may be multilocular; a minority of patients show loss of lamina dura	Usually asymptomatic; microscopically identical to central giant cell granuloma; serum calcium elevated; most caused by parathyroid adenoma; rare
Infantile cortical hyperostosis (pp. 424–425)	Infants	Mandible and other bones of the skeleton	Cortical thickening/sclerosis	Cause unknown; self-limited; treatment is supportive
Phantom bone disease (p. 425)	Young adults	Mandible more than maxilla	Gradual lucency of entire bone	Cause unknown; no treatment
Acromegaly (Fig. 4) (pp. 425–427)	Adults (after closure of epiphyses)	Mandible; uniform, bilateral	Large jaw	Excess production of growth hormone after closure of epiphyses (condylar growth becomes active); prognathism, diastemas may appear; rare

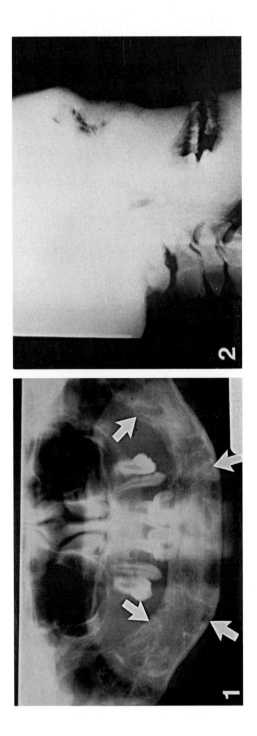

Metabolic and Genetic Jaw Diseases *Continued*

DISEASE	PATIENT AGE	LOCATION	RADIOGRAPHIC APPEARANCE	OTHER FEATURES
Cherubism (Fig. 1) (pp. 427–429)	Children	Mandible favored; uniform, bilateral	Bilateral multilocular lucencies	Autosomal dominant inheritance pattern; facies is cherub-like; microscopy similar to that for central giant cell granuloma; process stabilizes after puberty; rare
Osteopetrosis (Fig. 2) (pp. 429–432)	Children and adults	Both jaws (and skull)	Diffuse, homogeneous, and symmetric opacification; may cause arrested root development and delayed eruption	Infantile, recessive (severe) and adult, dominant forms; intermediate form also recessive but has mild presentation; results in inhibition of bone resorption; patients develop anemia, blindness, and deafness; dental complication of infection and fracture; rare

The authors make grateful acknowledgment to the following physicians for photographs used in the overview section: S.K. Young (p. O-4, Fig. 4, and p. O-14, Fig. 2), M.L. Bernstein (p. O-10, Fig. 4), R. Millard (p. O-12, Fig. 1), T. Osborn (p. O-20, Fig. 1), A. Plotzke (p. O-38, Fig. 1), R. Courtney (p. O-38, Fig. 3, and p. O-58, Fig. 2), C. Taylor (p. O-44, Fig. 2), M.M. Ash and H.D. Millard (p. O-64, Fig. 1), and K. Volz (p. O-96, Fig. 2).

1

Vesiculo-Bullous Diseases

VIRAL DISEASES

Oral mucous membranes may be infected by one of several different viruses, each producing a relatively distinct clinical-pathologic picture (Table 1–1).

The herpesviruses are a large family of viruses characterized by a DNA core surrounded by a capsid and an envelope. Seven types of herpesviruses are known to be pathogenic for humans, and 6 of 7 have been linked to diseases in the head and neck area. The Epstein-Barr virus has been linked to infectious mononucleosis, Burkitt's lymphoma, nasopharyngeal carcinoma, and oral "hairy" leukoplakia. Cytomegalovirus has been associated with salivary gland disease and systemic disease of immunocompromised patients. Varicella-zoster virus (VZV) has been shown to cause chickenpox and herpes zoster. Herpes simplex virus type I (HSV-I) has been shown to be responsible for oral, perioral, and occasionally genital infections. Herpes simplex virus type II (HSV-II) has been associated with genital infections and occasionally with oral and perioral lesions. HHV8 has been linked to Kaposi's sarcoma.

Herpes Simplex Virus Infections

HSV infections are common vesicular eruptions of the skin and mucosa. They occur in two forms: systemic or primary disease and localized or secondary disease. Both forms are self-limited, but exacerbations of the primary form are common, because the virus can sequester itself in ganglionic tissue. Control rather than cure is the usual treatment scenario.

Pathogenesis (Fig. 1–1). Physical contact with an infected individual is the typical route of HSV inoculation for someone (seronegative) who has not been previously exposed to the virus or possibly for someone with a low titer of protective antibody to HSV. Documentation of spread of infection through airborne droplets, through contaminated water, or through contact with inanimate objects is generally lacking. During the primary infection, only a small percentage of individuals show clinical signs and symptoms of infectious systemic disease while a vast majority experience only subclinical disease. This latter group, now seropositive, has been identified through the laboratory detection of circulating antibodies to HSV.

The incubation period after exposure ranges from several days to 2 weeks. In overt primary disease, a vesiculo-ulcerative eruption typically occurs in the oral and perioral tissues (primary gingivostomatitis). The focus of eruption is expected at the original site of contact.

After resolution of primary herpetic gingivostomatitis, the virus is believed to migrate, through some unknown mechanism, along the periaxon sheath of the trigeminal nerve to the trigeminal ganglion, where it is capable of remaining in a latent or sequestered state. Reactivation of virus may follow exposure to sunlight ("fever blisters"), exposure to cold ("cold sores"), trauma, stress, and immunosuppression causing a secondary or recurrent infection.

An immunocompromised host may develop severe secondary disease. HSV-seropositive patients being prepared for bone marrow transplants with chemotherapeutic drugs such as cyclophosphamide (with or without total body radiation) are at risk for a form of secondary herpes that is particularly severe. Posttransplant chemotherapy also predisposes seropositive patients to recurrent oral infections. HSV seropositive patients infected with human immunodeficiency virus (HIV) may also

Table 1–1. Viruses and Associated Conditions of Significance to Clinical Dentistry

VIRUS FAMILY	VIRUS	DISEASE
Herpesvirus	Herpes simplex virus type I	Primary herpes gingivostomatitis
		Secondary herpes (oral and herpes simplex labialis)
		Herpetic whitlow
		Occasionally, genital herpes
	Herpes simplex virus type II	Genital herpes
		Occasionally, oral herpes
	Varicella-zoster virus	Varicella, herpes zoster
	Epstein-Barr virus	Mononucleosis
		Burkitt's lymphoma
		Nasopharyngeal carcinoma
		Hairy leukoplakia
	Cytomegalovirus	Salivary gland disease
	Human herpesvirus-6	Roseola infantum
	Human herpesvirus-8	Kaposi's sarcoma
Papovavirus	Papilloma virus	Oral warts
		Oral papillomas
		Condyloma acuminatum
		Heck's disease
		? Carcinoma
Paramyxovirus	Measles virus	Measles
	Mumps virus	Mumps parotitis
	Parainfluenza virus	Respiratory infections
Orthomyxovirus	Influenza virus	Influenza
Picornavirus	Coxsackie virus	Hand-foot-and-mouth disease
		Herpangina
	Rhinovirus	Common cold

exhibit severe secondary disease. Uncommonly, HIV-positive patients may have lesions that are coinfected by both HSV and cytomegalovirus. The pathogenesis of dually infected ulcers is unclear. Seronegative patients may rarely be affected with herpetic disease during immunosuppressive transplant states.

The reactivated virus travels by way of the trigeminal nerve to the originally infected epithelial surface, where replication occurs, resulting in a focal vesiculo-ulcerative eruption. Presumably because the humoral and cell-mediated arms of the immune system have been sensitized to HSV antigens, the lesion is limited in extent and systemic symptoms usually do not occur. As the secondary lesion resolves, the virus returns to the trigeminal ganglion and evidence of viral particles can no longer be found within the epithelium. From one third to one half of the United States population experience recurrent herpetic lesions. It is believed that nearly all secondary lesions develop from reactivated latent virus, although reinfection by different strains of the same subtype is considered to be a remote possibility.

Most oral-facial herpetic lesions are due to HSV-I, although a small percentage may be caused

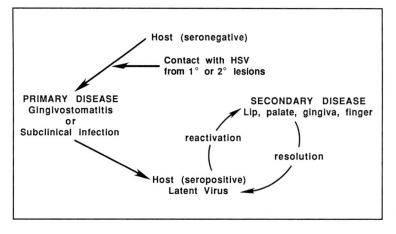

Figure 1–1. Pathogenesis of HSV-I infections.

by HSV-II secondary to oral-genital contact. Lesions caused by either virus are clinically indistinguishable. HSV-II has a predilection for genital mucosa, with infections having a pathogenesis similar to HSV-I infections of the head and neck. Latent virus, however, is sequestered in the lumbosacral ganglion. Occasional HSV-I infections of the genitalia have also been noted. Previous HSV-I infections may provide some protection against HSV-II infection because of antibody cross-reactivity.

One of the more disconcerting pieces of information to be uncovered about HSV infections is the asymptomatic shedding of intact virus particles in saliva of a small percentage of previously infected individuals (approximately 5%). Acquisition of genital herpes from an asymptomatic infected sexual partner has been documented, the infection believed to be due to transmission of virus through shedding in vaginal secretions. The level of risk of infection from such persons has not been measured, although it is probably very low and is certainly much less than the risk of infection from individuals with symptomatic disease.

Another problem with herpes infections is their possible carcinogenic potential. Considerable accumulated evidence has linked HSV-II to carcinoma of the cervix. Whether or not HSV-I (or HSV-II) has carcinogenic potential in the head and neck area has yet to be convincingly shown. Most evidence relates to HSV antibody titers in oral patients with cancer.

Clinical Features
Primary Herpetic Gingivostomatitis. Primary disease is usually seen in children, although adults who have not been previously exposed to HSV or who fail to mount an appropriate response to a previous infection may be affected. The vesicular eruption may appear on the skin, vermilion, or oral mucous membranes (Fig. 1–2). Intraorally, lesions may appear on any mucosal surface. This is in contradistinction to the recurrent form of the disease, in which lesions are confined to the hard palate and gingiva. The primary lesions are accompanied by fever, arthralgia, malaise, headache, and cervical lymphadenopathy.

After the systemic primary infection runs its course of about 1 week to 10 days, the lesions heal without scar. Also, by this time the virus may have migrated to the trigeminal ganglion to reside in a latent form. The number of individuals with primary clinical or subclinical infections in which virus assumes dormancy in nerve tissue is unknown.

Secondary or Recurrent HSV Infections. Secondary herpes represents the reactivation of latent virus. It is believed that only rarely does reinfection from an exogenous source occur in seropositive individuals. A large majority of the population (up to 90%) have antibodies to HSV, and up to 40% of this group may develop secondary herpes. The pathophysiology of recurrence has been related to either a breakdown in focal immunosurveillance or an alteration in local inflammatory mediators that allows the virus to replicate.

Patients usually have prodromal symptoms of tingling, burning, or pain in the site in which lesions will appear. Within a matter of hours, multiple fragile and short-lived vesicles appear. These become ulcerated and coalesce to form map-like superficial ulcers. The lesions heal with-

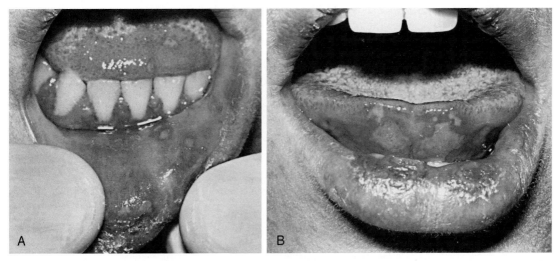

Figure 1–2. *A*, Primary herpes gingivostomatitis in a 14-year-old girl. Note the lip ulcers and inflamed gingiva. *B*, Same patient with confluent tongue ulcers.

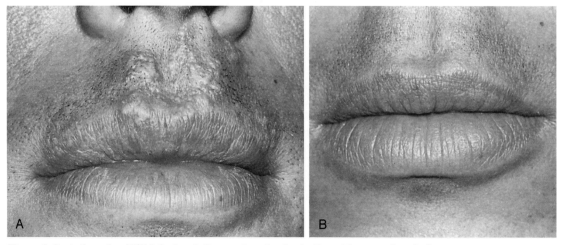

Figure 1–3. *A*, Secondary HSV infection. *B*, Same patient showing healing without scar 2 weeks later.

out scarring in 1 to 2 weeks and rarely become secondarily infected (Fig. 1–3). The number of recurrences is variable and ranges from one per year to as many as one per month. Recurrence rate appears to decline with age with each individual. The secondary lesions typically occur at or near the same site with each recurrence. Regionally, most secondary lesions occur on the vermilion and surrounding skin. This type of disease is usually referred to as *herpes simplex labialis* (HSL) (Fig. 1–4). When recurrences appear intraorally, they are almost always on the hard palate or gingiva (Fig. 1–5).

IMMUNODEFICIENCY. Secondary herpes in the context of immunosuppression results in significant pain and discomfort as well as a predisposition to secondary bacterial and fungal infections. Lesions may be atypical in that they may be chronic and destructive. They also are not site restricted orally.

Herpetic Whitlow. Herpetic whitlow refers to either a primary or a secondary HSV infection involving the finger(s) (Fig. 1–6). Before the universal use of examination gloves, this type of infection typically occurred in dental practitioners who had been in physical contact with infected individuals. In the case of a seronegative clinician, contact may result in a vesiculo-ulcerative eruption on the digit (rather than in the oral region) along with the signs and symptoms of primary systemic disease. Recurrent lesions, if they occur, would be expected on the finger(s). Herpetic whitlow in a seropositive clinician (e.g., one with a history of HSV infection) is believed to be possible although less likely because of previous immune stimulation by herpes simplex antigens. The

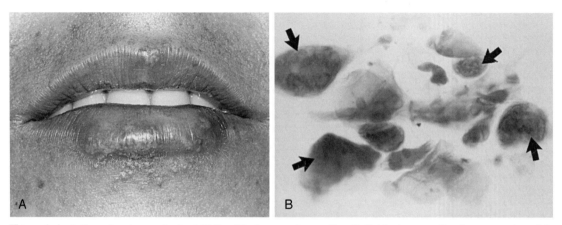

Figure 1–4. *A*, Secondary herpes simplex labialis of the lower and upper lips. *B*, Cytologic preparation from a scraping of the base of the vesicles. Note the numerous virus-infected multinucleated epithelial cells *(arrows)*. Normal keratinocytes are seen at bottom center.

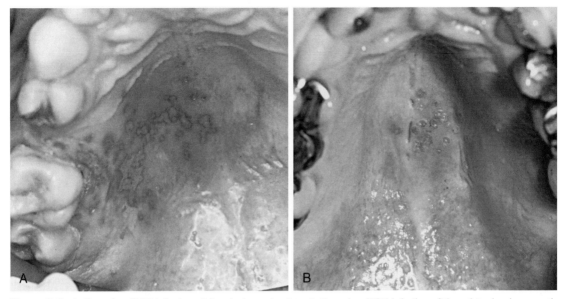

Figure 1–5. *A*, Secondary HSV infection of the gingiva and palate. *B*, Secondary HSV infection of the palate showing recently ruptured vesicles.

potential occupational hazard of contact with sero-positive patients who shed virus in saliva has not been adequately studied. If there is a risk, it is probably very slight.

Pain, redness, and swelling are prominent with herpetic whitlow and can be very pronounced. Vesicles or pustules eventually break and become ulcers. Lymphadenopathy may also be present. Duration of herpetic whitlow is protracted, as long as 4 to 6 weeks. Recurrences with this form of herpes infection would be expected in the same site.

HISTOPATHOLOGY. Microscopically, intra-epithelial vesicles containing exudate, inflammatory cells, and some virus-infected epithelial cells are seen (Figs. 1–7 and 1–8). Lining the vesicles are highly characteristic epithelial cells that show the effects of HSV infection. Some of these cells contain a single nucleus, and some are multinucleated. The nucleus is homogeneous and glassy in appearance, with nuclear material forced to the perimeter of the nuclear membrane. These features can also be readily found on cytologic preparations and are indicative of a herpes-type infection. On morphologic grounds, however, HSV-I cannot be differentiated from HSV-II or from the herpes-

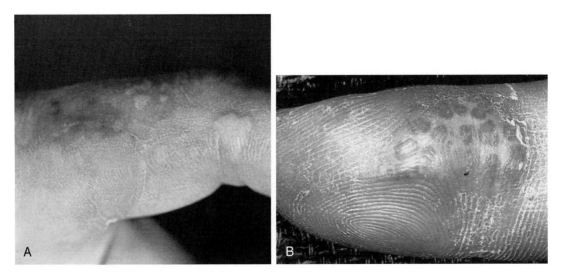

Figure 1–6. *A* and *B*, Herpes whitlow showing early vesicular eruption. (Courtesy of Dr. S. K. Young.)

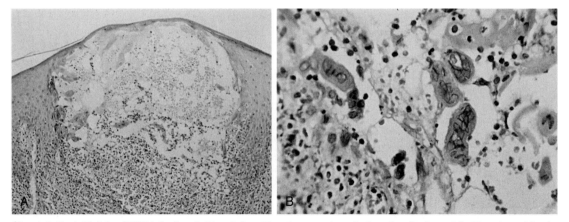

Figure 1–7. *A*, Vesicle of HSV infection. *B*, Virus-infected keratinocytes along the lateral wall of a vesicle. Note the multinucleated keratinocytes.

viruses responsible for herpes zoster. After several days, herpes-infected epithelial cells cannot be demonstrated in either cytologic or biopsy preparations. In HIV-positive patients with coinfected ulcers, lesions exhibit typical HSV-associated changes as well as cytomegaly of endothelial cells in the lesion base.

Differential Diagnosis. The diagnosis of primary herpetic gingivostomatitis is usually apparent from clinical features. It can be confirmed by a virus culture (which requires 2 to 4 days for positive identification). Immunologic methods using monoclonal antibodies or DNA *in situ* hybrid-

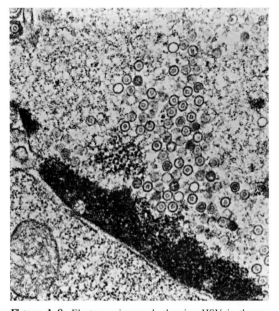

Figure 1–8. Electron micrograph showing HSV in the nucleus of a keratinocyte. Nucleic acid cores are surrounded by electron-dense protein capsid rings. (Courtesy of Dr. S. K. Young.)

ization techniques have also become useful for specific virus identification in tissue sections.

The systemic signs and symptoms coupled with the oral ulcers may require differentiation from streptococcal pharyngitis, erythema multiforme, and Vincent's infection. Clinically, streptococcal pharyngitis does not involve the lips or perioral tissues, and vesicles do not precede the ulcers. Oral ulcers of erythema multiforme are larger, usually without a vesicular stage, and are less likely to affect the gingiva. In Vincent's infection (acute necrotizing ulcerative gingivitis), oral lesions are limited to the gingiva, are not preceded by vesicles, and demonstrate tissue necrosis.

Intraorally, secondary herpes is often confused with aphthous stomatitis but can usually be distinguished from it on the basis of clinical features (Table 1–2). Multiple lesions, vesicles preceding ulcers, and palatal and gingival location are indicative of herpesvirus infection. Other oral conditions that may show clinical features similar to secondary herpes include trauma, chemical burns, and contact allergy. Lip lesions of secondary herpes may need to be distinguished from the pustules of impetigo.

Treatment. One of the most important factors in the treatment of HSV infections is timing. For any drug to be effective, it must be initiated as soon as possible. No later than 48 hours from the onset of symptoms is generally regarded as the ideal time for the start of therapeutic measures. Carriers or vehicles of topical medications are also apparently very important in the chemotherapy of HSV infections. Those agents that facilitate drug absorption are more likely to be successful than those that do not.

A number of virus-specific drugs have been developed, but at present no single therapeutic regimen has proved to be uniformly effective in

Table 1–2. Comparison of Secondary Oral Herpes Simplex Virus Infections and Minor Oral Aphthous Ulcers

PARAMETER	HERPES	MINOR APHTHAE
Cause	HSV-I	Focal immunodysregulation
Precipitating factors	Stress, trauma, ultraviolet light, change in immune status	Stress, trauma, hormonal changes, diet, immunologic alterations
Prodromal symptoms	Usually	Occasionally
Cytology	Virus-infected epithelial cells	Nonspecific
Vesicular stage	Yes	No
Number of ulcers	Multiple, confluent	Usually one, oval
Pain	Yes	Yes
Location	Vermilion, hard palate, gingiva (any site with immunosuppression)	All other mucosal sites (any site with immunosuppression)
Duration	1–2 weeks (prolonged with immunosuppression)	1–2 weeks (prolonged with immunosuppression)
Scar after healing	No	Major form only
Recurrent	Yes	Yes
Treatment	Antiviral drugs	Steroids

the treatment of oral and perioral HSV infections. Many remedies and nonspecific forms of treatment have been used. All have produced limited or inconsistent results. Development of virus-specific compounds has been slow because of the extreme difficulty in finding a selective virucidal agent that spares the cell.

Limited success has been obtained with some herpesvirus-specific drugs. Currently, acyclovir has shown the greatest efficacy in the treatment of mucocutaneous infections. A 5% acyclovir ointment applied five times per day when symptoms first appear reduces slightly the duration of HSL and may abort some lesions. It does not prevent recurrence, however, and may be ineffective in some patients. Oral acyclovir tablets (400 mg five times per day) are effective in the treatment of primary genital herpes and to a lesser degree in the treatment of recurrent genital disease. Oral acyclovir for the treatment of HSL is more effective than the ointment form.

Systemic acyclovir does not prevent recurrences, but it may shorten the course of the disease. Without prophylactic acyclovir in seropositive bone marrow transplant recipients, most develop secondary herpes. With prophylactic therapy, herpes infrequently affects this population.

The rationale for the use of acyclovir is its ability to interrupt viral replication through inhibition of DNA polymerization. In herpes-infected cells, acyclovir is converted by a virus-induced enzyme, thymidine kinase, and other cellular enzymes to a form that inhibits primarily viral DNA polymerase rather than host cell DNA polymerase. The end result is interruption of viral DNA synthesis and relative sparing of cellular DNA synthesis.

Until new, more effective drugs are developed and tested for mucocutaneous herpetic infections, therapy will necessarily be frustrating and unpre-

dictable. The typically occurring primary herpetic gingivostomatitis is currently best managed with supportive therapy: fluids, rest, oral lavage, and antipyretics. For more severe systemic infections, oral acyclovir may be required. Topical acyclovir, although it is only somewhat effective, is a rational approach to the treatment of secondary herpes. Control of problematic cases may require prophylactic acyclovir. In patients with minor recurrent herpetic lesions, the treatment, at this time, is empirical. In HIV-positive patients with severe disease, aggressive therapy that may include intravenous acyclovir or ganciclovir may be necessary.

Varicella-Zoster Infections

Etiology and Pathogenesis. VZV is one of the herpesviruses that is pathogenic for humans. The primary infection for the disease in seronegative individuals is known as *varicella* (chickenpox). The secondary disease or reactivation of latent VZV is known as *herpes zoster* (shingles). Structurally, VZV is very similar to HSV in that it has a DNA core, a protein capsid, and a lipid envelope. Thus, both have similar light and electron microscopic appearances. Some antigenic determinants are also shared by both viruses. Relative to pathogenesis, striking similarities can also be noted. The ability of the virus to remain quiescent in sensory ganglia for indefinite periods after a primary infection is common to both. A cutaneous or mucosal vesiculo-ulcerative eruption following reactivation of latent virus is also typical of VZV and HSV. A number of clinical signs and symptoms, however, appear to be unique to each infection and are discussed next. Immunosuppression predisposes patients to VZV infections.

Varicella. Transmission of varicella is believed

to be predominantly through the inspiration of contaminated droplets. Much less commonly, direct contact is an alternative way of acquiring the disease. During the 2-week incubation period, virus proliferates within macrophages, with subsequent viremia and dissemination to skin and other organs. Host defense mechanisms of nonspecific interferon production and specific humoral and cell-mediated immune responses are also triggered. Overt clinical disease then appears in most individuals. As the viremia overwhelms body defenses, systemic signs and symptoms develop. Eventually, in a normal host, the immune response is able to limit and halt the replication of virus, allowing recovery in 2 to 3 weeks. During the disease process, the VZV may progress along sensory nerves to the sensory ganglia, where it can reside in a latent, undetectable form.

Herpes Zoster. Reactivation of latent VZV is uncommon but characteristically follows such occurrences as immunosuppressive states due to malignancy (especially hematopoietic and lymphoid types) or drug administration, irradiation or surgery of the spinal cord, or local trauma. A depressed cellular immune state, especially in association with HIV infection, appears to be a major factor in the development of herpes zoster. Prodromal symptoms of pain or paresthesia develop and persist for several days as the virus infects the sensory nerve of a dermatome (usually of the trunk or head and neck). A vesicular skin eruption that becomes pustular and eventually ulcerated follows. The disease lasts several weeks and may be followed by a troublesome postherpetic neuralgia (in approximately 10% of patients) that takes several months to resolve. Local cutaneous hyperpigmentation may also be noted on occasion.

Clinical Features

Varicella. A majority of the population experiences a primary infection during childhood. Nearly all adults older than 60 years have had VZV infection. Fever, chills, malaise, and headache may accompany a rash that involves primarily the trunk and head and neck. The rash quickly develops into a vesicular eruption that becomes pustular and eventually ulcerates. Successive crops of new lesions appear, owing to repeated waves of viremia. This causes the presence, at any one time, of lesions in all stages of development (Fig. 1–9). The infection is self-limited and lasts several weeks. Oral mucous membranes may be involved in primary disease and usually demonstrate multiple shallow ulcers that are preceded by evanescent vesicles (Fig. 1–10). Because of the intense pruritic nature of the skin lesions, secondary bacterial infection is not uncommon and may result in healing with scar formation. Complications, including pneumonitis, encephalitis, and inflammation of other organs, may occur in a very small percentage of cases. If varicella is acquired during pregnancy, fetal abnormalities may occur. When older adults and immunocompromised patients are affected, varicella may be much more severe, protracted, and more likely to produce complications.

Herpes Zoster. Zoster is basically a condition of the older adult population and of individuals who have compromised immune responses. Risk is especially high in those who have lymphoid or hematopoietic malignancies (e.g., Hodgkin's disease, lymphocytic leukemia) and those who are also being treated with cytotoxic or immunosuppressive drugs. Other high-risk groups include patients receiving high-dose radiation or steroids or organ transplants and AIDS patients.

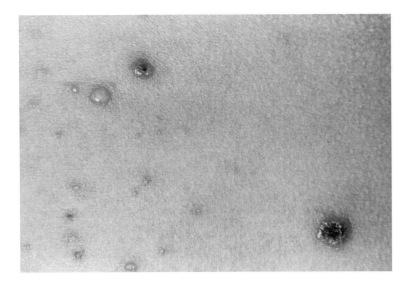

Figure 1–9. Varicella lesions of the trunk in all stages of development.

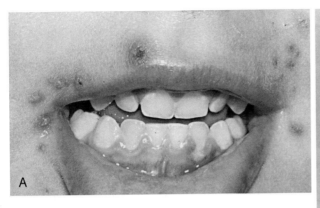

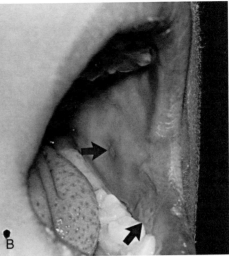

Figure 1-10. *A,* Perioral and gingival lesions in a 5-year-old child with varicella. *B,* Same patient with oral ulcers *(arrows).*

The sensory nerves of the trunk and head and neck are commonly affected. Involvement of the various branches of the trigeminal nerve may result in unilateral oral, facial, or ocular lesions (Fig. 1–11). Involvement of facial and auditory nerves produces the *Ramsay Hunt syndrome,* in which facial paralysis is accompanied by vesicles of the ipsilateral external ear, tinnitus, deafness, and vertigo.

After several days of prodromal symptoms of pain or paresthesia in the area of the involved dermatome, a well-delineated unilateral maculopapular rash appears. This may occasionally be accompanied by systemic symptoms as well. The rash quickly becomes vesicular, pustular, and then ulcerative. Remission usually occurs in several weeks. Complications include secondary infection of ulcers, postherpetic neuralgia (which may be refractory to analgesics), motor paralysis, and ocular inflammation when the ophthalmic division of the trigeminal nerve is involved.

Histopathology. The morphology of the VZV and the inflammatory response to its presence in both varicella and herpes zoster are essentially the same as those with HSV. Examination under a light microscope reveals virus-infected epithelial cells showing homogeneous nuclei, representing viral products, with margination of chromatin. Multinucleation of infected cells is also typical. Both cytologic smears and histologic specimens demonstrate these characteristic cellular changes. As infected cells swell, adhesive qualities are lost, resulting in acantholytic vesicles. Inflammatory cells and exudate add to the vesicle contents, with

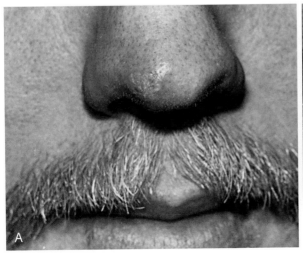

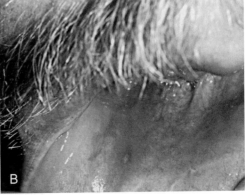

Figure 1-11. Herpes zoster in a 24-year-old man. The patient had conjunctivitis, a nose eruption *(A),* and lip ulcers *(B).*

eventual breakdown and ulceration. In uncomplicated cases, epithelium regenerates from the ulcer
margins with little or no scar.

Differential Diagnosis. Varicella is usually
clinically diagnosed when a history of exposure
and the type and distribution of lesions are carefully noted. Other primary viral infections that
may show some similarities include primary HSV
infection and hand-foot-and-mouth (HFM) disease.

Herpes zoster is most commonly confused with
recurrent HSV infections and may on clinical
grounds be indistinguishable from them. The
longer duration, the greater intensity of prodromal
symptoms, the unilateral distribution with abrupt
ending at the midline, and postherpetic neuralgia
all favor a clinical diagnosis of herpes zoster.
Diagnosis of equivocal cases can be definitively
made through virus antigen typing using laboratory immunologic tests (e.g., immunohistochemistry or DNA *in situ* hybridization).

Treatment. For varicella, supportive therapy is
generally indicated in normal individuals. However, in immunocompromised patients, more substantial measures are warranted. Virus-specific
drugs that are effective in treating HSV infections
have also shown efficacy in the treatment of VZV
infections. These include systemically administered acyclovir, vidarabine, and human leukocyte
interferon. Corticosteroids are generally contraindicated.

Patients with herpes zoster and intact immune
responses have generally been treated empirically.
However, it has been shown that oral acyclovir
used at high doses (800 mg five times per day for
7 to 10 days) can shorten the disease course and
reduce postherpetic pain. Analgesics provide only
limited relief from pain. Topically applied virus-
specific drugs may have some benefit if used early.
Topically applied substance P inhibitor (capsaicin)
may provide some relief from postherpetic pain.
The use of topical or systemic corticosteroids
cannot yet be recommended. In patients with compromised immune responses, systemically administered acyclovir, vidarabine, or interferon is indicated, although success is variable.

Hand, Foot, and Mouth Disease

Etiology and Pathogenesis. One of the subdivisions of another family of viruses known as
picornavirus (literally, small [pico] RNA [rna] virus) is a group known as Coxsackie virus (also
known as Coxsackievirus), named after the New
York town where the virus was first identified.

Certain subtypes of the Coxsackie group of picornaviruses are known to cause oral vesicular eruptions, two of which are HFM and herpangina.

HFM is a highly contagious viral infection that
is usually caused by Coxsackie type A16, although
serologic types A5, A9, A10, B2, and B5 and
enterovirus 71 (another group of picornaviruses)
have been isolated on occasion. The mode of
transfer of virus from one individual to another is
through either airborne spread or fecal-oral contamination. With subsequent viremia, the virus
exhibits a predilection for mucous membranes of
the mouth and cutaneous regions of the hands
and feet.

Clinical Features. This viral infection typically occurs in epidemic or endemic proportions
and affects predominantly children younger than
5 years. After a short incubation period, the condition resolves spontaneously in 1 to 2 weeks.

Signs and symptoms are usually mild to moderate in intensity and include low-grade fever, malaise, lymphadenopathy, and sore mouth. Pain from
oral lesions is often a patient's chief complaint.
The oral lesions begin as vesicles that quickly
rupture to become ulcers that are covered by a
yellow fibrinous membrane surrounded by an erythematous halo (Fig. 1–12). The lesions, which
are multiple, can occur anywhere in the mouth,
although the palate, tongue, and buccal mucosa
are favored sites. Multiple maculopapular lesions,
typically on the feet, toes, hands, and fingers,
appear concomitantly with or shortly after the oral
lesions (Fig. 1–13). These lesions progress to a
vesicular state and eventually become ulcerated
and encrusted.

Histopathology. The vesicles of this condition
are found within the epithelium because of obli-
gate viral replication in keratinocytes. Eosinophilic inclusions may be seen within some of the
infected epithelial cells. As the keratinocytes are
destroyed by virus, the vesicular cavity becomes
filled with proteinaceous debris and inflammatory
cells.

Differential Diagnosis. Because this disease
may express itself primarily within the oral cavity,
a differential diagnosis should include primary
herpes gingivostomatitis and possibly varicella.
The relatively mild symptoms, cutaneous distribution, and epidemic spread should help separate
this condition from the others. Virus culture or
detection of circulating antibodies may be done to
confirm clinical impression.

Treatment. Because of the relatively short duration, the self-limiting nature, and the general
lack of virus-specific therapy, treatment for HFM
is usually symptomatic. Nonspecific mouthwashes
may be used to help alleviate oral discomfort.

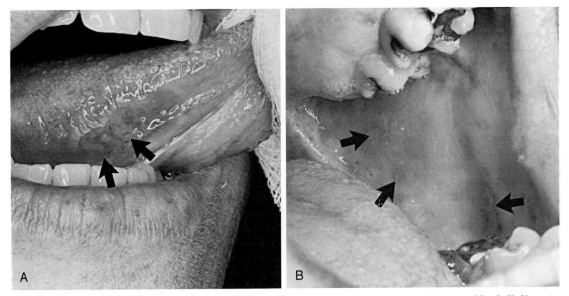

Figure 1–12. *A* and *B*, Hand-foot-and-mouth disease—oral ulcers *(arrows)* in a young woman. (Courtesy of Dr. S. K. Young.)

Herpangina

Etiology and Pathogenesis. This acute viral infection is caused by another Coxsackie type A virus (types A1–6, A8, A10, A22, B3, and possibly others). It is transmitted by contaminated saliva and occasionally through contaminated feces.

Clinical Features. Herpangina is usually endemic, with outbreaks occurring typically in summer or early fall. It occurs more often in children than in adults. They generally complain of malaise, fever, dysphagia, and sore throat after a short incubation period. Intraorally, a vesicular eruption appears on the soft palate, faucial pillars, and tonsils (Fig. 1–14). A diffuse erythematous pharyngitis is also present.

The signs and symptoms are usually mild to moderate and generally last less than a week. On occasion, the Coxsackie virus responsible for typical herpangina may be responsible for subclinical infections or for mild symptoms without evidence of pharyngeal lesions.

Differential Diagnosis. Diagnosis is usually based on historical and clinical information. The characteristic distribution and short duration of herpangina separate it from other primary viral infections such as herpetic gingivostomatitis, HFM, and varicella. The vesicular eruption, mild

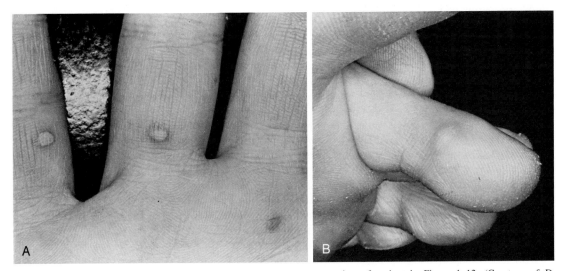

Figure 1–13. *A* and *B*, Hand-foot-and-mouth disease—cutaneous expression of patient in Figure 1–12. (Courtesy of Dr. S. K. Young.)

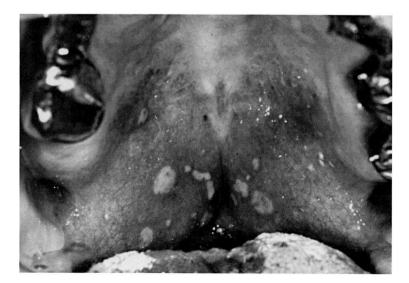

Figure 1–14. Herpangina. Multiple oral ulcers with erythematous bases are apparent in the soft palate.

symptoms, summer presentation, and diffuse pharyngitis also distinguish the condition from streptococcal pharyngitis, and the systemic symptoms distinguish it from aphthous stomatitis. Laboratory confirmation can be made by virus isolation or detection of serum antibodies.

Treatment. Because herpangina is self-limited, is mild and of short duration, and causes few complications, treatment usually is not required.

Measles (Rubeola)

Etiology and Pathogenesis. Measles is a highly contagious viral infection caused by a member of the paramyxovirus family of viruses. The virus, known simply as *measles virus*, is a DNA virus and is related structurally and biologically to viruses of the orthomyxovirus family, which cause mumps and influenza. The virus is spread by airborne droplets through the respiratory tract.

German measles, or rubella, is a contagious disease that is caused by an unrelated virus of the togavirus family. It shares some clinical features with measles, such as fever, respiratory symptoms, and rash. These features are, however, very mild and short lived in German measles. Also, Koplik's spots, which are characteristic of measles, do not appear in German measles. The significance of the German measles virus lies in its ability to cause congenital defects in a developing fetus. The abnormalities produced are varied and may be severe, especially if the intrauterine infection occurs during the first trimester of pregnancy.

Clinical Features. Measles is predominantly a disease of children, often appearing seasonally in winter and spring. After an incubation period of 7 to 10 days, prodromal symptoms of fever, malaise, coryza, conjunctivitis, photophobia, and cough develop. In 1 to 2 days, pathognomonic small erythematous macules with white necrotic centers appear in the buccal mucosa (Fig. 1–15). These herald spots, known as *Koplik's spots* after the pediatrician who first described them, usher in the characteristic maculopapular skin rash of measles. Koplik's spots generally precede the skin rash by 1 to 2 days. The rash initially affects the head and neck, followed by the trunk and then the extremities. Complications associated with the measles virus include encephalitis and thrombocytopenic purpura. Secondary infection may develop as otitis media or pneumonia.

Histopathology. Infected epithelial cells, which eventually become necrotic, overlie an inflamed dermis that contains dilated vascular channels and a focal inflammatory response. Lymphocytes are found in a perivascular distribution. In lymphoid tissues, large characteristic multinucleated macrophages, known as *Warthin-Finkeldey giant cells*, are seen (Fig. 1–16).

Differential Diagnosis. Diagnosis of measles is usually made on the basis of clinical signs and symptoms. Prodromal symptoms, Koplik's spots, and rash should provide sufficient evidence of measles. If necessary, laboratory confirmation can be made through virus culture or serologic tests for antibodies to measles virus.

Treatment. There is no specific treatment for measles. Supportive therapy of bed rest, fluids, adequate diet, and analgesics generally suffices.

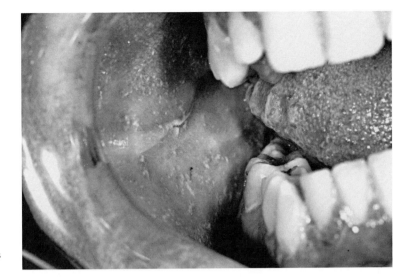

Figure 1–15. White Koplik's spots in the buccal mucosa.

CONDITIONS ASSOCIATED WITH IMMUNOLOGIC DEFECTS

Pemphigus Vulgaris

Pemphigus is a mucocutaneous disease characterized by intraepithelial blister formation. This results from a breakdown or loss of intercellular adhesion, thus producing epithelial cell separation known as *acantholysis*. Widespread ulceration following rupture of the blisters leads to painful debilitation, fluid loss, and electrolyte imbalance. Before the use of corticosteroids, death was a not uncommon outcome for patients with pemphigus vulgaris. Subsets of pemphigus include pemphigus

vegetans (a variant of pemphigus vulgaris), pemphigus foliaceus, and pemphigus erythematosus.

Etiology and Pathogenesis. All forms of the disease retain distinctive presentations both clinically and microscopically but share a common autoimmune etiology. Evident are circulating autoantibodies of the IgG type that are reactive against components of epithelial desmosome-tonofilament complexes. The specific molecular site has been identified as desmoglein 3, one of several proteins in the desmosomal cadherin family. The circulating autoantibodies are responsible for the earliest morphologic event: the dissolution or disruption of intercellular junctions and loss of cell-to-cell adhesion. The ease and extent of epithelial cell separation are, generally, directly proportional to the titer of circulating pemphigus antibody. It is

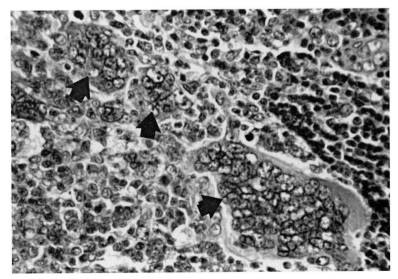

Figure 1–16. Warthin-Finkeldey giant cells *(arrows)* in tonsillar tissue.

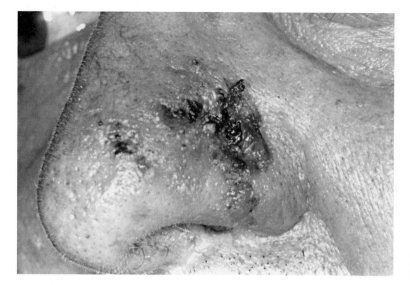

Figure 1–17. Skin ulcers of pemphigus vulgaris.

believed that the pemphigus antibody, once bound to the target antigen, activates an epithelial intracellular proteolytic enzyme or group of enzymes that act at the desmosome-tonofilament complex.

Clinical Features. Skin lesions present as ulcers preceded by bullae (Fig. 1–17). However, patients with pemphigus vulgaris present with the first signs of the disease in the oral mucosa in approximately 60% of cases. Such lesions may precede the onset of cutaneous lesions by periods of up to 1 year. Presentation of the lesions may initially be as fluid-filled bullae (or vesicles) or as shallow ulcers (Fig. 1–18). Bullae rapidly rupture, leaving a collapsed roof. This grayish membrane is easily removed with a gauze sponge, leaving a red, painful, ulcerated base. Ulcers range in appearance from small aphthous-like lesions (Fig. 1–19) to large map-like lesions (Fig. 1–20). Gentle traction on clinically unaffected mucosa may produce stripping of epithelium, a positive Nikolsky's sign. A great deal of discomfort often occurs with confluence and ulceration of smaller vesicles of the soft palate, buccal mucosa, and floor of the mouth.

The incidence of pemphigus vulgaris is equal in both sexes. Genetic and ethnic factors appear to predispose to the development of the disease. Pemphigus vulgaris, although generally rare, may be relatively common in some racial and ethnic groups. An increased incidence has been noted in Ashkenazic Jews and in individuals with certain histocompatibility antigen phenotypes (HLA-DR, HLA-A10, HLA-B, HLA-DQB, HLA-DRB1).

Other autoimmune diseases may occur in association with pemphigus vulgaris, such as myasthenia gravis, lupus erythematosus, rheumatoid

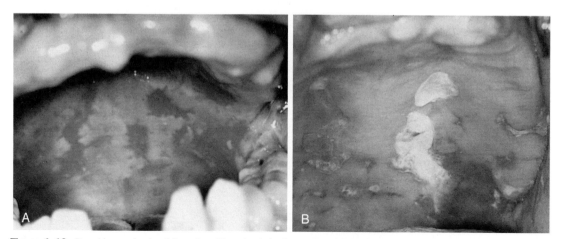

Figure 1–18. Pemphigus vulgaris of the palate. Note the dark ulcers *(A)* and light fibrin-covered ulcers *(B)*.

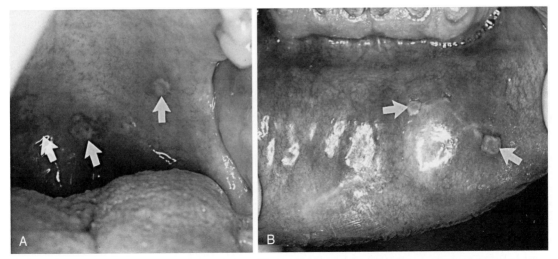

Figure 1–19. *A* and *B*, Pemphigus vulgaris in a 45-year-old man. Multiple aphthous-type ulcers are apparent *(arrows)*.

arthritis, Hashimoto's thyroiditis, thymoma, and Sjögren's syndrome. A wide range has been noted from childhood to the elderly age groups, although most cases are noted within the fourth and fifth decades of life.

Histopathology and Immunopathology. Pemphigus vulgaris represents the prototypical suprabasal or intraepithelial clefting morphology that generally characterizes all forms of pemphigus. Pathognomonic of pemphigus vulgaris is the acantholytic lesion that features squamous epithelial cells lying free within the bulla or vesicle cavity (Fig. 1–21). Loss of desmosomal attachments and retraction of tonofilaments result in assumption of a more spherical form by the acantholytic epithelial cells (Fig. 1–22). These cells,

also known as *Tzanck cells*, are further characterized by nuclear enlargement and hyperchromasia. Subsequent to formation of the suprabasal cleft, the intact basal layer remains attached to the lamina propria, producing a pattern that has been likened to a row of tombstones. In addition to fluid and Tzanck cells, the bulla or vesicle contains variable numbers of neutrophils and occasional eosinophils. When an intact lesion is evident clinically, a cytologic smear, prepared by unroofing the vesicle and gently scraping the base of the lesion, will enable rapid microscopic identification of the acantholytic cells. Initial diagnosis made from a cytologic smear must be confirmed by more definitive procedures.

In addition to a standard biopsy, confirmation

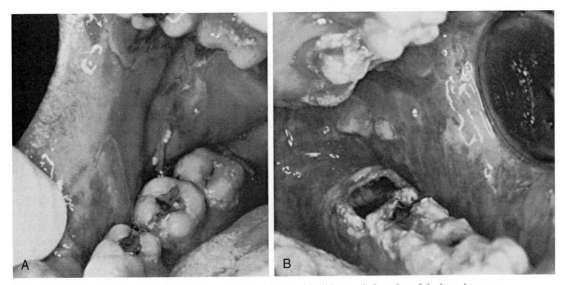

Figure 1–20. *A* and *B*, Pemphigus vulgaris in a 47-year-old man with widespread ulceration of the buccal mucosa.

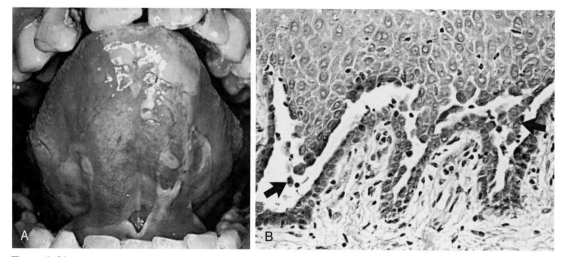

Figure 1–21. *A*, Pemphigus vulgaris of the ventral surface of the tongue. *B*, Biopsy specimen showing intraepithelial separation with free-floating epithelial (Tzanck) cells *(arrows)*.

of the diagnosis of pemphigus vulgaris can be made with the use of either direct or indirect immunofluorescence testing (Fig. 1–23). Direct immunofluorescence uses a biopsy specimen in an attempt to demonstrate autoantibody already attached to the tissue. In pemphigus vulgaris, direct immunofluorescence testing of perilesional tissue almost always demonstrates intercellular antibodies of the IgG type (Fig. 1–24). The greatest intensity of fluorescence is usually within the parabasal region, with a gradual diminution of fluorescence as the surface is approached. In addition to IgG antibodies, C3 and, less commonly, IgA can be detected in the same intercellular fluorescent pattern.

The indirect immunofluorescence technique uses the patient's serum reacted with normal control tissue in an effort to demonstrate the presence (and the concentration) of circulating antibody. Such circulating antibodies may be noted in approximately 80% of patients with pemphigus vulgaris. This indirect technique also permits assessment of disease severity, which has been related to titer (or concentration) of circulating antibody. Indirect immunofluorescence titers can then be practically used to adjust medication schedules and dosages.

Differential Diagnosis. Clinically the lesions of pemphigus vulgaris must be distinguished from other vesiculo-bullous disease processes such as bullous and cicatricial pemphigoid, erythema multiforme, bullous lichen planus, and dermatitis her-

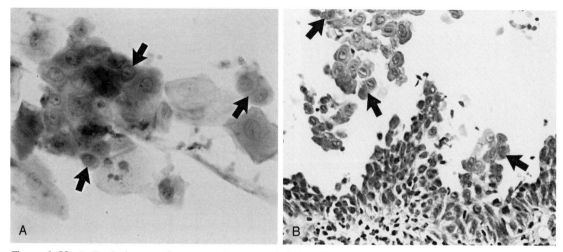

Figure 1–22. *A*, Cytologic smear from a pemphigus vulgaris lesion. Note the rounded epithelial cells characteristic of this condition *(arrows)*. *B*, Tissue biopsy specimen showing an intact basal layer and acantholytic keratinocytes (Tzanck cells) *(arrows)*.

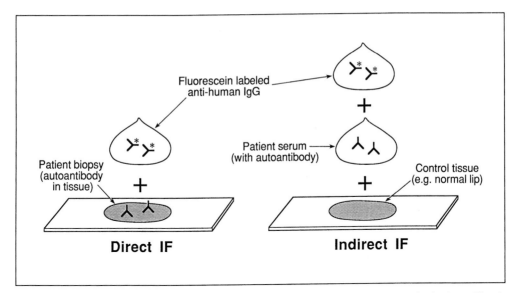

Figure 1–23. Immunofluorescence techniques for demonstrating autoantibodies in either the patient's tissue (direct) or the patient's serum (indirect).

petiformis. When lesions are small, aphthous stomatitis may be a consideration. Also, a syndrome known as *paraneoplastic pemphigus* may simulate pemphigus vulgaris. Patients with this syndrome have a lymphoma or other malignancy and a mucocutaneous pemphigus-like blistering disorder in which intraepithelial separation (acautholysis) is seen. Unlike pemphigus, the autoantibodies are directed at several antigenic targets, in both the attachment zones of the epithelium and basement membrane. The underlying malignancy is believed to be responsible for the induction of the autoimmune response.

A diagnosis of *pemphigus vegetans*, a variant or closely related form of pemphigus vulgaris, may also be entertained in some situations. Although originally regarded as an infectious disease, subsequent reclassification based on the presence of acantholysis placed it within the pemphigus group of disorders. It is predominantly a skin disease, but the vermilion and intraoral mucosa are frequently involved, often initially (Fig. 1–25). This rare variant of pemphigus is distinguished through its microscopic appearance. Early acantholytic bullae are followed by epithelial hyperplasia and intraepithelial abscess formation. These pustular "vegetations" contain abundant eosinophils. In general, this form of pemphigus tends to resemble a verrucous or hypertrophic excrescence rather than the blistering of acute pemphigus vulgaris. The course of this disease may parallel the course of pemphigus vulgaris. Pemphigus vegetans–type lesions may also be seen during a lull in the general course of pemphigus vulgaris. Spontaneous remissions may occur in pemphigus vegetans, with complete re-

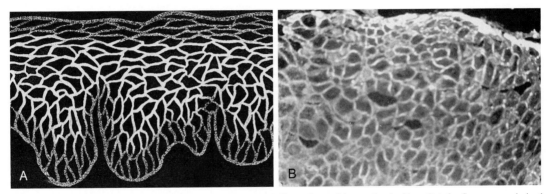

Figure 1–24. *A*, Immunofluorescence pattern seen in the epithelium of pemphigus vulgaris. Note that the fluorescence is in the intercellular desmosomal areas, predominantly in the prickle cell zone. *B*, Photomicrograph of actual fluorescence stain.

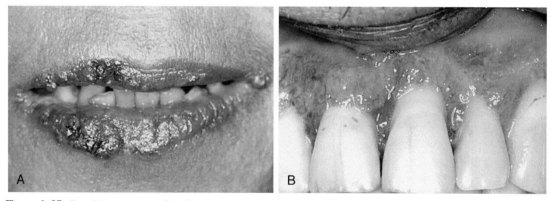

Figure 1–25. Pemphigus vegetans of the lips *(A)* and gingiva *(B)*.

covery noted—a phenomenon not characteristic of pemphigus vulgaris.

Treatment and Prognosis. The high morbidity and mortality rates previously associated with pemphigus vulgaris have been radically reduced since the introduction of systemic corticosteroids. The reduction in mortality, however, does carry a degree of iatrogenic morbidity associated with chronic corticosteroid use. Indeed, the 8 to 10% mortality per 5 years is generally secondary to long-term steroid therapy.

Disease control may be achieved with intermediate dose of steroid (prednisone). For more severely affected patients, high-dose corticosteroid use is followed by a combined drug approach that includes alternate-day prednisone plus a steroid-sparing immunosuppressant agent such as azathioprine, methotrexate, or cyclophosphamide. The latter regimen helps reduce both the suppressive effects of steroid on the pituitary-adrenal axis and other complications of high-dose steroid therapy such as immunosuppression, osteoporosis, hyperglycemia, and hypertension.

Overall, the prognosis for patients with pemphigus vulgaris is guarded because of the potential profound side effects of the drugs used for treatment. The major clinical problem, once the disease has been brought under control, is the proba-

ble lifelong treatment commitment, albeit at relatively low dosage, to these powerful drugs.

Cicatricial Pemphigoid (Mucous Membrane Pemphigoid)

Cicatricial pemphigoid represents a chronic blistering or vesiculo-bullous disease known by a host of synonymous terms, including *benign mucous membrane pemphigus, ocular pemphigus, childhood pemphigoid*, and *mucosal pemphigoid*. When the disorder affects the gingiva exclusively, the terms *gingivosis* and *desquamative gingivitis* have been used, although such terms are generally unacceptable because of lack of specificity.

Etiology and Pathogenesis. Cicatricial pemphigoid is idiopathic and is also considered an autoimmune process with an unknown stimulus (Table 1–3). Deposits of immunoglobulins and complement components along the basement zone (on direct immunofluorescence testing) are characteristic. The molecular targets are believed to be laminin 5 (kalinin) and a protein of 180 kd that is also known as *bullous pemphigoid antigen 180*. Circulating antibodies against the basement membrane zone antigens in cicatricial pemphigoid are

Table 1–3. General Features of Pemphigus and Pemphigoid

FEATURE	PEMPHIGUS	PEMPHIGOID
Detectable circulating antibody	Yes, IgG	No
Tissue-bound autoantibody	Yes, IgG (also complement)	Yes, IgG (also IgA, complement)
Target tissue	Desmosomes (desmoglein 3)	Basement membrane (laminin 5 and BP 180)
Vesicles	Intraepithelial	Subepithelial
Sites affected	Oral mucosa, skin	Oral mucosa (esp. gingiva), eye, genitals
Nikolsky's sign	Yes	Yes
Treatment	Systemic steroids and other immunosuppressive agents	Systemic or topical steroids
Prognosis	Fair to good	Good to excellent

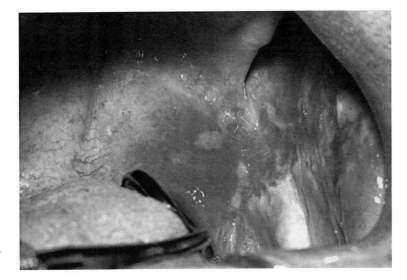

Figure 1–26. Cicatricial pemphigoid showing ulcers and erythema of the soft palate and buccal mucosa.

usually difficult to detect, presumably because of relatively low serum levels.

The cellular events in lesion production are more presumed than definitive, since the closely related condition, bullous pemphigoid, has served as a pathogenetic model (see the later section on the pathogenesis of bullous pemphigoid).

Clinical Features. This is a disease of adults and the elderly and tends to affect women more than men. Rarely, cicatricial pemphigoid has been reported in children. The oral mucosal presentation ranges from erosion or desquamation of attached gingival tissues to large areas of vesiculobullous eruptions involving gingiva, alveolar mucosa, palate, buccal mucosa, tongue, and floor of the mouth (Fig. 1–26). Bullae are rarely seen because the blisters are fragile and short lived.

Lesions are chronic and may heal with scarring (cicatrix), particularly skin and eye lesions. Extraoral sites in the order of frequency following oral mucosa are conjuctiva, larynx, genitalia, esophagus, and skin. Cutaneous lesions are uncommon and usually appear in the head and neck and extremities. The development of skin lesions typically follows the appearance of mucosal lesions.

Gingival lesions often present as patchy red zones with mild to moderate discomfort. Concomitant ulcers may be seen on marginal and attached gingiva (Fig. 1–27).

With chronicity, pain typically diminishes in intensity. Intact epithelium, especially adjacent to ulcers, can often be stripped away with ease, leaving a raw, denuded, bleeding substratum. This is

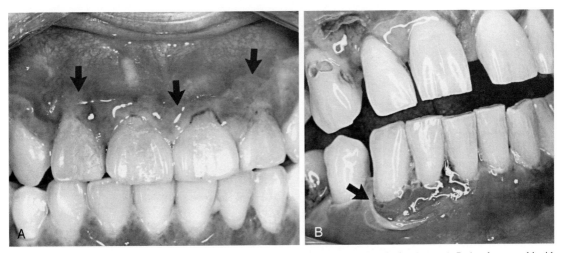

Figure 1–27. *A*, Cicatricial pemphigoid of the gingiva with ulceration of the attached gingiva *(arrows)*. *B*, Another pemphigoid-affected patient with maxillary gingival ulcers and traumatic denudation of the mandibular gingiva *(arrow)*.

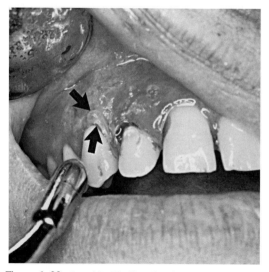

Figure 1–28. Pemphigoid-affected patient with induced bulla (Nikolsky's sign) *(arrows)*.

one of several mucocutaneous diseases in which a positive Nikolsky's sign may be seen. This involves the application of gentle massage or a shearing force on uninvolved tissue, producing a blister (Fig. 1–28). Symptoms often preclude performance of routine oral hygiene, resulting in considerable plaque accumulation, which in turn further aggravates the gingival tissues.

Histopathology and Immunopathology. Cicatricial pemphigoid is a subepithelial or sub-basal clefting disorder (Fig. 1–29). There is no evidence of acantholysis. The lamina propria is variably infiltrated by few lymphocytes. With time, the infiltrate becomes more intense and mixed.

Direct immunofluorescence studies of intact oral mucosa demonstrate a linear pattern of homogeneous IgG fluorescence (Fig. 1–30). C3 is commonly found in the same distribution. Although the fluorescent pattern is not distinguishable from that of bullous pemphigoid, the submicroscopic location of the antigenic target (lower part of the lamina lucida) is distinctive (Fig. 1–31). Results of indirect immunofluorescence studies are usually negative, but IgG and, less commonly, IgA have occasionally been demonstrated in the serum of patients with cicatricial pemphigoid.

Differential Diagnosis. The clinical differential diagnosis for this form of vesiculo-bullous disease must include pemphigus vulgaris. When the attached gingiva is the exclusive site of involvement, atrophic lichen planus, discoid lupus erythematosus, and contact allergy should also be included. Final diagnosis may require direct immunofluorescence examination.

Treatment and Prognosis. Topical or systemic corticosteroids are typically used to treat cicatricial pemphigoid. Prednisone, used for moderate to severe disease, often provides disappointing results, however. Very high doses may be required to achieve significant results. Because side effects of prednisone therapy may outweigh benefits, especially when lesions are only intraoral, high-potency topical steroids are often used (e.g., clobetasol, betamethasone dipropionate, fluocinonide, desoximetasone). An occlusive dressing of topical corticosteroids often enhances the local response. For gingival disease, a custom-made, flexible mouth guard may be used to keep the topical medication in place. Scrupulous oral hygiene further enhances the effectiveness of topical corticosteroids when gingival involvement is significant.

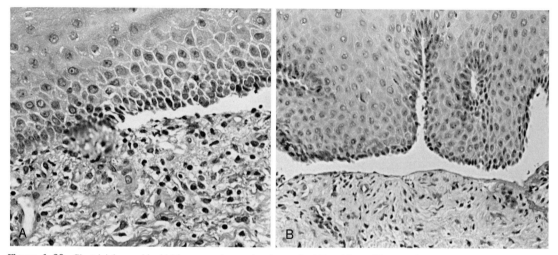

Figure 1–29. Cicatricial pemphigoid biopsy specimens showing early *(A)* and later *(B)* separation at the level of the basement membrane.

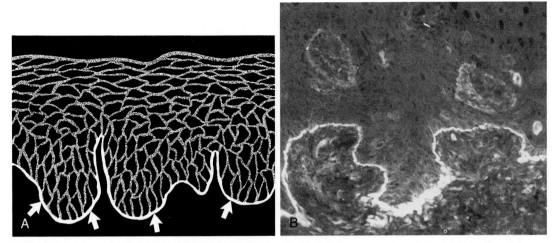

Figure 1–30. *A*, Immunofluorescence pattern of cicatricial pemphigoid. Staining appears along the basement membrane *(arrows)*. *B*, Photomicrograph of actual fluorescence stain.

Rinsing with chlorhexidine is often a useful adjunct.

In cases in which standard therapy has failed, other systemic agents have been used with varying success rates. These have included the use of sulfapyridine, sulfones, antibiotics, and nutritional supplementation. In severe cases, immunosuppressive agents (azathioprine, cyclophosphamide, cyclosporine) may occasionally be added to the prednisone regimen to reduce steroid dose and thus help avoid steroid-associated complications.

Although cicatricial pemphigoid has a relatively

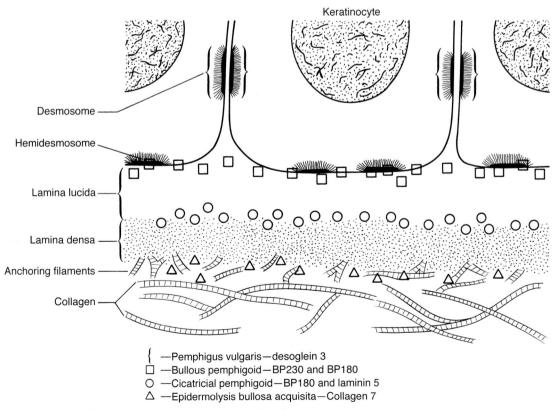

Figure 1–31. Location of antigenic targets in vesiculo-bullous diseases.

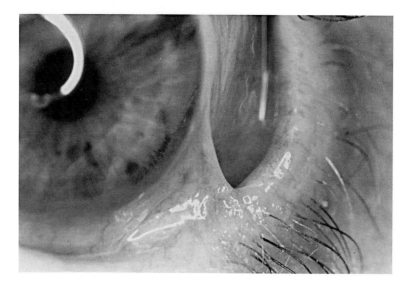

Figure 1–32. Symblepharon, a complication of cicatricial pemphigoid characterized by adhesion between contiguous conjunctival surfaces.

benign course, significant debilitation and morbidity can occur. Long-term prognosis is unpredictable. In some cases, a slow but spontaneous improvement may be noted, with complete resolution occurring over a few years. In other cases, however, the course may be protracted, with some patients exhibiting alternating periods of improvement and exacerbation. The prognosis for children is good in most cases, because the disease is usually self-limiting.

Of importance for patients with oral cicatricial pemphigoid is the possible appearance of ocular complications. When or if the eyes become affected, definitive early treatment is critical because corneal damage, conjunctival scarring, and eyelid changes can lead to blindness. Therefore, ophthalmologic examination should be part of the treatment plan for patients with oral cicatricial pemphigoid (Fig. 1–32).

Bullous Pemphigoid

Etiology and Pathogenesis. Bullous pemphigoid and its closely related mucosal counterpart, cicatricial pemphigoid (mucous membrane pemphigoid), appear to share similar etiologic and pathogenetic factors (Table 1–4). Unlike cicatricial pemphigoid, titers of circulating autoantibodies to basement membrane zone antigens are usually detectable in bullous pemphigoid. Such autoantibody titers do not, however, correlate well with the level of disease activity.

Autoantibodies have been demonstrated against

Table 1–4. Comparison and Contrast of Cicatricial and Bullous Pemphoigoid

PARAMETER	CICATRICIAL PEMPHIGOID	BULLOUS PEMPHIGOID
Cause	Autoimmune	Autoimmune
Age at onset	50–80 years	50–80 years
Gender	Females affected more than males	Females and males equally affected
Oral lesions	Oral cavity most common site	Oral mucosa infrequently affected
	Gingiva most common intraorally	Oral lesions do not appear before skin lesions
	Eye lesions may lead to blindness	Ulcers preceded by bullae
	Ulcers preceded by bullae	Lesions usually heal without scar
	Ulcers may heal with scar	
Skin lesions	Uncommon; head, neck, extremities	Trunk and extremities most common sites
	Ulcers preceded by bullae	Ulcers preceded by bullae; rash
Light microscopy	Subepithelial bullae	Subepithelial bullae
Ultrastructure	Separation below basal cells	Separation below basal cells
Immunology	Linear deposits of IgG and C3	Linear deposits of IgG and C3
	No circulating antibody detectable	Circulating antibody detectable
Treatment	Corticosteroids, immunosuppressives, dapsone	Corticosteroids, immunosuppressives, dapsone
Course	Chronic, remissions uncommon	Chronic, remissions not uncommon

basement membrane zone laminin, a glycoprotein and so-called bullous pemphigoid antigen, which is found in hemidesmosomes and in the lamina lucida of basement membrane. Subsequent to binding of circulating autoantibodies to tissue antigens, a series of events occur, one of which is complement activation. This attracts neutrophils and eosinophils to the basement membrane zone. These cells then release lysosomal proteases, which in turn participate in degradation of the basement membrane attachment complex. The final event is tissue separation at the epithelium-connective tissue interface. Detailed immunoelectron microscopic studies have demonstrated that the lamina lucida of the basal lamina complex is the actual cleavage plane.

Clinical Features. This bullous disease is seen primarily in the elderly, with the peak incidence in the seventh and eighth decades. The gender distribution is equal, and ethnic predilections are not seen in this condition. Lesions characteristically appear in skin, although concomitant vesiculo-bullous lesions of skin and oral mucosa (and other mucosal sites) occur in approximately one third of patients.

Skin lesions are characterized anatomically by a trunk and limb distribution (Fig. 1–33). Although tense vesicles and bullae are typically noted, they are often preceded by or associated with an erythematous papular eruption. Pruritus may be associated with the skin lesions. Oral mucosal lesions of bullous pemphigoid cannot be distinguished from those of cicatricial pemphigoid. Bullae and erosions may be noted, especially on the attached gingiva, a commonly affected site. Other areas of involvement may include the soft palate, buccal mucosa, and floor of the mouth.

Histopathology and Immunopathology. Bullae are subepithelial in bullous pemphigoid and appear similar to those in cicatricial pemphigoid under the light microscope. Ultrastructurally, the basement membrane is cleaved at the level of the lamina lucida.

Circulating autoantibody titers neither correlate with nor fluctuate with the level of clinical disease, as is the case with pemphigus vulgaris. Direct immunofluorescence shows a linear deposition of IgG and C3 along the basement membrane zone.

Studies indicate that the bullous pemphigoid antigen is located within the basal keratinocytes as a transmembrane molecule that extends into the basement membrane zone. A major bullous pemphigoid antigen is 230 kd, and a minor antigen is 180 kd in size. Both antigens are synthesized by basal keratinocytes.

Treatment. Periods of clinical remission have been noted with bullous pemphigoid. Systemic corticosteroids are generally used to control this disease. Nonsteroidal immunosuppressive agents may also effect control of the disease process as well as reduce steroid side effects. Antibiotics (tetracycline and erythromycin) and niacinamide have provided some clinical success.

Dermatitis Herpetiformis

This is a skin eruption that rarely affects the oral mucosa. The cause is unknown, but most patients have an associated gluten-sensitive enteropathy. There is no etiologic relationship to HSV or other member of the herpesvirus family.

Etiology and Pathogenesis. Although no demonstrable circulating autoantibodies are noted in

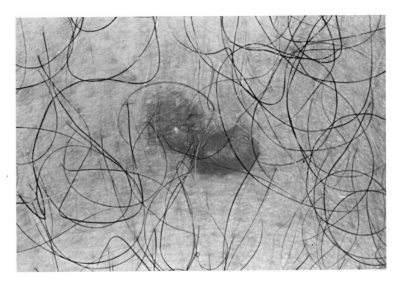

Figure 1–33. Bullous pemphigoid of the skin.

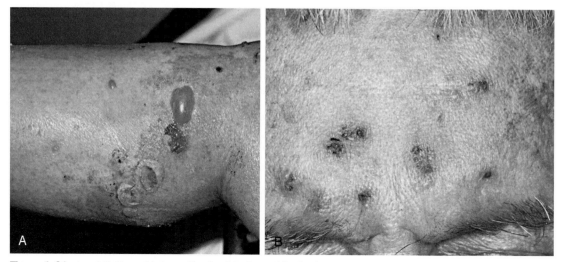

Figure 1–34. *A* and *B*, Dermatitis herpetiformis of the leg and forehead.

the sera of patients, deposits of IgA are evident in tissue sections. Cell-mediated immunity may also have a role in the pathogenesis of this disease. In most patients, an association is noted between skin disease and sensitivity to gluten that is related to malabsorption of fat. Improvement of the skin and fat absorption often occurs with a gluten-free diet. Substantiating this relationship is the relapse noted on reintroduction of gluten-containing foods. The etiologic relationship between cutaneous and intestinal diseases remains obscure, although certain common B lymphocyte–associated antigens are noted in most patients. Additionally, immunogenetic studies have demonstrated an increased incidence of HLA-B8, HLA-DR3, and HLA-DQ histocompatibility antigens in patients with dermatitis herpetiformis and ordinary gluten-sensitive enteropathy.

Clinical Features. Dermatitis herpetiformis is a chronic disease typically seen in young and middle-aged adults, with a slight male predilection. Periods of exacerbation and remission further characterize this disease. Cutaneous lesions are papular, erythematous, vesicular, and often intensely pruritic (Figs. 1–34 and 1–35). Lesions are usually symmetric in their distribution over the extensor surfaces, especially the elbows, shoulders, sacrum, and buttocks. Of diagnostic significance is the frequent involvement of the scalp and face. Lesions are usually aggregated (herpetiform) but often are individually disposed. In some patients, exacerbations may be associated with ingestion of foods or drugs containing iodide compounds. In others, a seasonal (summer months) peak may be seen.

In the oral cavity, vesicles and bullae are

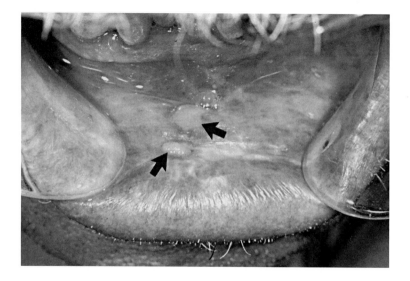

Figure 1–35. Dermatitis herpetiformis of the labial mucosa with postvesicular ulceration *(arrows)*.

evanescent. Subsequent to rupture, superficial nonspecific ulcers have a fibrinous base with erythematous margins. Lesions may involve both keratinized and nonkeratinized mucosa.

Histopathology and Immunopathology. Collections of neutrophils, eosinophils, and fibrin are seen at the papillary tips of the dermis. Subsequent exudation at this location contributes to epidermal separation. A lymphophagocytic infiltrate is seen in perivascular spaces.

The immunologic finding of IgA deposits at the tips of the connective tissue papillae is specific for dermatitis herpetiformis. The pattern of IgA deposition at the papillary tips is usually granular to speckled, although linear IgA patterns may be noted. In addition, it is possible to localize the third component of complement (C3) in lesional and perilesional tissue in a distribution similar to that of IgA.

Diagnosis. Characteristic histopathology and demonstration of specific IgA immunofluorescence enable clear separation of this disease from other vesiculo-bullous diseases.

Treatment and Prognosis. Dermatitis herpetiformis is generally treated with dapsone, sulfoxone, and sulfapyridine. Response is usually prompt in the presence of adequate doses. Because patients often have an associated enteropathy, a gluten-free diet may also be part of the therapeutic regimen. Elimination of gluten from the diet reduces small bowel pathology within months.

In most instances, dermatitis herpetiformis is a lifelong condition, often exhibiting long periods of remission. Many patients, however, may be relegated to long-term dietary restrictions or drug treatment or both.

Linear IgA Disease

Linear IgA is a chronic autoimmune disease of skin that frequently affects mucous membranes, including gingiva. Unlike dermatitis herpetiformis, it is not associated with gluten-sensitive enteropathy (and may not be responsive to dapsone therapy). Skin lesions may be urticarial, annular, targetoid, or bullous. Oral lesions, present in a majority of cases, are ulcerative (preceded by bullae) in nature (Fig. 1–36). Ocular lesions, also seen in a majority of cases, are in the form of ulcers. Patients respond to sulfones or corticosteroids.

Microscopically, separation at the basement membrane is seen (Fig. 1–37). With direct immunofluorescence, linear deposits of IgA are found at the epithelium-connective tissue interface. The molecular target is a 120-kd protein (Fig. 1–38).

Although clinicopathologically, linear IgA disease shares features with dermatitis herpetiformis, cicatricial pemphigoid, and bullous pemphigoid, it cannot be confidently subclassified under any one of these well-established entities. Until more is learned of linear IgA disease, it should probably be considered as a separate condition.

HEREDITARY DISEASES

Epidermolysis Bullosa

Etiology and Pathogenesis. Epidermolysis bullosa is a general term that encompasses one acquired and several genetic varieties (dystrophic, junctional, simplex) of disease that are basically

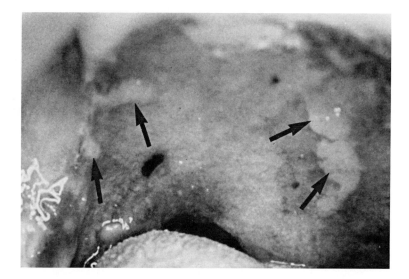

Figure 1–36. Palatal oral ulcers in an edentulous patient with linear IgA disease. (Courtesy of Dr. L. Chan.)

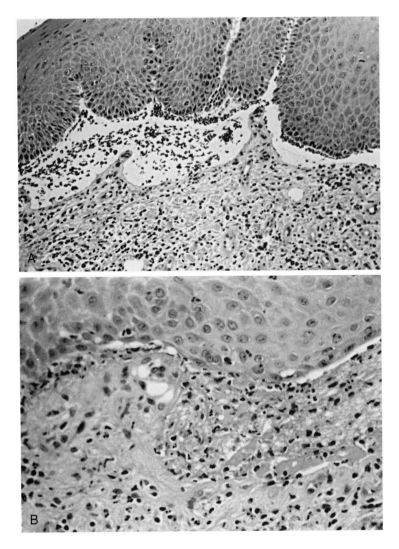

Figure 1–37. Photomicrographs of linear IgA disease. *A*, Separation at the basement membrane. *B*, Early separation with infiltration by eosinophils.

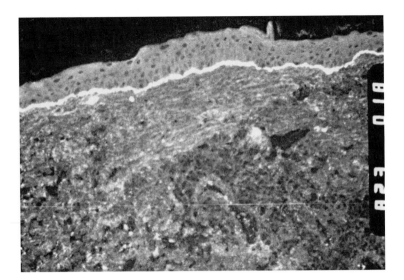

Figure 1–38. Immunofluorescent deposits (linear) at the epithelium-connective tissue junction. (Courtesy of Dr. L. Chan.)

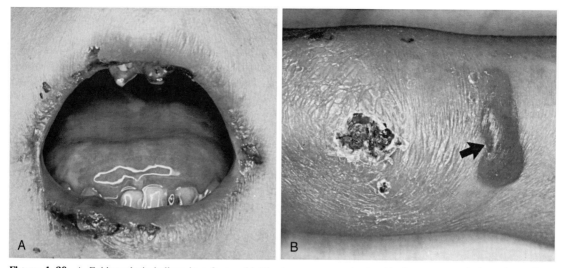

Figure 1–39. *A,* Epidermolysis bullosa in a 9-year-old. The tongue mucosa is atrophic from recurrent lesions, the teeth are hypoplastic, and the oral orifice is restricted because of recurrent lesions. *B,* Knee of the same patient showing flaccid bulla *(arrow)* and other residua of previous lesions.

characterized by the formation of blisters at sites of minor trauma. The several genetic types range from autosomal dominant to autosomal recessive in origin and are further distinguished by various clinical features, histopathology, and ultrastructure. The acquired nonhereditary form, known as *epidermolysis acquisita,* is unrelated to the other types, relative to etiologic and pathogenetic aspects. In this acquired type, IgG deposits are frequently found in sub–basement membrane tissue. These antibodies are thought to be a manifestation of the autoimmune nature of this form of the disease. Autoantibodies bind to type VII collagen located below the lamina densa component of the basement membrane complex.

In the hereditary forms of epidermolysis bullosa, circulating antibodies are not part of the mechanism of disease progression. Pathogenesis appears to be related rather to genetic defects in basal cells, hemidesmosomes, or anchoring connective tissue filaments, depending upon which form of the condition is present.

Clinical Features. The feature common to all subtypes of epidermolysis bullosa is bulla formation from minor provocation, usually over areas of stress such as the elbows and knees (Fig. 1–39). Onset of disease is during infancy or early childhood for the hereditary forms and during adulthood for the acquired type. Severity is generally greater with the inherited recessive forms. Blisters may be widespread and severe and may result in scarring and atrophy. Nails may be dystrophic in some forms of this disease.

Oral lesions are particularly common and severe in the recessive forms of this group of diseases

and uncommon in the acquired form. Oral manifestations include bullae that heal with scar, constricted oral orifice due to scar contracture, and hypoplastic teeth (Fig. 1–39). These changes are most pronounced in the type known as *recessive dystrophic epidermolysis bullosa.*

Treatment and Prognosis. Prognosis is dependent on the subtype of epidermolysis bullosa. The range of behavior varies from life-threatening in one of the recessive forms, known as *junctional epidermolysis bullosa,* to debilitating in most other forms. Therapy includes avoidance of trauma, supportive measures, and chemotherapeutic agents (none of which is consistently effective). Corticosteroids, vitamin E, phenytoin, retinoids, dapsone, and immunosuppressives all have been suggested as possibly being of some benefit to patients.

Bibliography

Viral Diseases

Axell T, Liedholm R. Occurrence of recurrent herpes labialis in an adult Swedish population. Acta Odontol Scand 48:119–123, 1990.

Bernstein J, Korman N, Bickers D, et al. Topical capsaicin treatment of chronic postherpetic neuralgia. J Am Acad Dermatol 21:265–270, 1989.

Corey L, Spear P. Infections with herpes simplex viruses. N Engl J Med 314:686–691; 749–757, 1986.

Dolin R. Antiviral chemotherapy and chemoprophylaxis. Science 227:1296–1303, 1985.

Douglas J, Critchlow C, Benedetti J, et al. A double-blind study of oral acyclovir for suppression of recurrences of genital herpes simplex virus infection. N Engl J Med 310:1551–1556, 1984.

Eversole R. Viral infections of the head and neck among

HIV-seropositive patients. Oral Surg Oral Med Oral Pathol 73:155–163, 1992.

Ficarra G, Shillitoe E. HIV-related infections of the oral cavity. Crit Rev Oral Biol Med 3:207–231, 1992.

Fiddian A, Ivanyi L. Topical acyclovir in the management of recurrent herpes labialis. Br J Dermatol 109:321–326, 1983.

Fiddian A, Yeo J, Stubbings R, Dean D. Successful treatment of herpes labialis with topical acyclovir. BMJ 286:1699–1701, 1983.

Flaitz CM, Nichols CM, Hicks MJ. Herpesviridae-associated persistent mucocutaneous ulcers in acquired immunodeficiency syndrome. Oral Surg Oral Med Oral Pathol 81:433–441, 1996.

Guinan M. Oral acyclovir for treatment and suppression of genital herpes simplex virus infection. JAMA 255:1747–1749, 1986.

Heimdahl A, Mattsson T, Dahllof G, et al. The oral cavity as a port of entry for early infections in patients treated with bone marrow transplantation. Oral Surg Oral Med Oral Pathol 68:711–716, 1989.

Herbert A, Berg J. Oral mucous membrane diseases of childhood. Semin Dermatol 11:80–87, 1992.

Huff J, Bean B, Balfor H, et al. Therapy of herpes zoster with oral acyclovir. Am J Med 85:84–89, 1988.

Ishimaru Y, Nakano S, Yamaoka K, Takami S. Outbreaks of hand, foot, and mouth disease by enterovirus 71. Arch Dis Child 55:583–588, 1980.

Jayasuriya A, Nash A. Pathogenesis and immunobiology of herpes simplex virus in mouse and man. Cancer Invest 3:199–207, 1985.

Morton P, Thompson A. Oral acyclovir in the treatment of herpes zoster in general practice. N Z Med J 102:93–95, 1989.

Nakayama T, Urano T, Osano M, et al. Outbreak of herpangina associated with coxsackie virus B3 infection. Pediatr Infect Dis J 8:495–498, 1989.

Pruksananonda P, Hall C, Insel R, et al. Primary human herpesvirus 6 infection in young children. N Engl J Med 326:1145–1150, 1992.

Raborn GW, Martel AY, Grace MGA, McGaw WT. Oral acyclovir in prevention of herpes labialis. Oral Surg Oral Med Oral Pathol 85:55–59, 1998.

Regezi JA, Eversole LR, Barker BF, et al. Herpes simplex and cytomegalovirus coinfected oral ulcers in HIV-positive patients. Oral Surg Oral Med Oral Pathol 81:55–62, 1996.

Reichman R, Badger G, Mertz G, et al. Treatment of recurrent genital herpes simplex infections with oral acyclovir. JAMA 251:2103–2107, 1984.

Rooney J, Bryson Y, Mannia M, et al. Prevention of ultraviolet light-induced herpes labialis by sunscreen. Lancet 338: 1419–1422, 1991.

Rooney J, Felser J, Ostrove J, Straus S. Acquisition of genital herpes from an asymptomatic sexual partner. N Engl J Med 314:1561–1564, 1986.

Schubert M, Peterson D, Flurnoy N, et al. Oral and pharyngeal herpes simplex virus infection after allogenic bone marrow transplantation: analysis of factors associated with infection. Oral Surg Oral Med Oral Pathol 70:286–293, 1990.

Scott DA, Coulter WA, Biagioni PA, et al. Detection of herpes simplex virus type 1 shedding in the oral cavity by polymerase chain reaction and enzyme-linked immunosorbent assay at the prodromal stage of recrudescent herpes labialis. J Oral Pathol Med 26:305–309, 1997.

Scully C. Orofacial herpes simplex virus infections: current concepts in the epidemiology, pathogenesis, and treatment, and disorders in which the virus may be implicated. Oral Surg Oral Med Oral Pathol 68:701–710, 1989.

Spruance S, Schnipper L, Overall J Jr, et al. Treatment of herpes simplex labialis with topical acyclovir in polyethylene glycol. J Infect Dis 146:85–90, 1982.

Spruance S, Stewart J, Freeman D. Early application of topical 15% idoxuridine in dimethyl sulfoxide shortens the course of herpes simplex labialis: a multicenter placebo-controlled trial. J Infect Dis 161:191–197, 1990.

Spruance S, Stewart J, Rowe N, et al. Treatment of recurrent herpes simplex labialis with oral acyclovir. J Infect Dis 161:185–190, 1990.

Immunologic and Hereditary Diseases

Anhalt G. Pemphigoid: bullous and cicatricial. Dermatol Clin 8:701–716, 1990.

Buxton RS, Cowin P, Franke WW, et al. Nomenclature of the desmosomal cadherins. J Cell Biol 121:481–483, 1993.

Chan L, Regezi J, Cooper K: Oral manifestations of linear IgA disease. J Acad Dermatol 22:362–365, 1990.

Economopoulou P, Laskaris G. Dermatitis herpetiformis: oral lesions as an early manifestation. Oral Surg Oral Med Oral Pathol 62:77–80, 1986.

Edelson R. Photopheresis: a new therapeutic concept. Yale J Biol Med 62:565–577, 1989.

Elder MJ, Lightman S, Dart JKG. Role of cyclophosphamide and high dose steroid in ocular cicatricial pemphigoid. Br J Ophthalmol 79:264–266, 1995.

Fine J. The skin basement membrane zone. Adv Dermatol 2:283–304, 1987.

Fine JD, Bauer EA, Briggaman RA, et al. Revised clinical and laboratory criteria for subtypes of inherited epidermolysis bullosa. J Am Acad Dermatol 24:119–135, 1991.

Fullerton S, Woodley D, Smoller B, Anhalt G. Paraneoplastic pemphigus with autoantibody deposition after autologous bone marrow transplantation. JAMA 267:1500–1502, 1992.

Helm TN, Camisa C, Valenzuela R, Allen C. Paraneoplastic pemphigus. Oral Surg Oral Med Oral Pathol 75:209–213, 1993.

Hietanen I, Reunala T. IgA deposits in the oral mucosa of patients with dermatitis herpetiformis and linear IgA disease. Scand J Dent Res 92:230–234, 1984.

Jonsson R, Mountz J, Koopman W. Elucidating the pathogenesis of autoimmune disease: recent advances at the molecular level and relevance to oral mucosal disease. J Oral Pathol Med 19:341–350, 1990.

Kawana S, Geoghegan WD, Jordan RE, Nishiyama S. Deposition of the membrane attack complex of complement in pemphigus vulgaris and pemphigus foliaceus skin. J Invest Dermatol 92:588–592, 1989.

Koch PJ, Mahoney MG, Ishikawa H, et al. Targeted disruption of the pemphigus vulgaris antigen (desmoglein 3) gene in mice causes loss of keratinocyte cell adhesion with a phenotype similar to pemphigus vulgaris. J Cell Biol 137:1091–1102, 1997.

Laskaris G, Triantafyllou A, Economopoulou P. Gingival manifestations of childhood cicatricial pemphigoid. Oral Surg Oral Med Oral Pathol 66:349–352, 1988.

Lawley T, Strober W, Yaoita H, Katz S. Small intestinal biopsies and HLA types in dermatitis herpetiformis patients with granular and linear IgA skin deposits. J Invest Dermatol 74:9–12, 1980.

Marinkovich MP. The molecular genetics of basement membrane diseases. Arch Dermatol 129:1557–1565, 1993.

Niimi Y, Zhu X-J, Bystryn JC. Identification of cicatricial pemphigoid antigens. Arch Dermatol 128:54–57, 1992.

Nisengard R, Chorzelski T, Maciejowska E, et al. Dermatitis herpetiformis: IgA deposits in gingiva, buccal mucosa, and skin. Oral Surg Oral Med Oral Pathol 54:22–25, 1982.

Oranje A, van Joost T. Pemphigoid in children. Pediatr Dermatol 6:267–274, 1989.

Otley C, Hall R. Dermatitis herpetiformis. Dermatol Clin 8:759–769, 1990.

Patel H, Anhalt G, Diaz L. Bullous pemphigoid and pemphigus vulgaris. Ann Allergy 50:144–150, 1983.

Porter S, Scully C, Midda M, Eveson J: Adult linear immunoglobulin A disease manifesting as desquamative gingivitis. Oral Surg Oral Med Oral Pathol 70:450–453, 1990.

Prost C, DeLeca A, Combemale P, et al. Diagnosis of adult linear IgA dermatosis by immunoelectronmicroscopy in 16 patients with linear IgA deposits. J Invest Dermatol 92:39–45, 1989.

Rantala I, Hietanen J, Soidinmaki H, Ruenala T. Immunoelectron microscopic findings in oral mucosa of patients with dermatitis herpetiformis and linear IgA disease. Scand J Dental Res 93:243–248, 1985.

Reginer M, Vaigot P, Michel S, et al. Localization of bullous pemphigoid antigen (BPA) in isolated human keratinocytes. J Invest Dermatol 85:187–190, 1985.

Rogers R, Seehafer J, Perry H. Treatment of cicatricial (benign mucous membrane) pemphigoid with dapsone. J Am Acad Dermatol 6:215–223, 1982.

Scharf J, Friedmann A, Steinman L, et al. Specific HLA-DQB and HLA-DRB1 alleles confer susceptibility to pemphigus vulgaris. Proc Natl Acad Sci U S A 86:6215–6219, 1989.

Singer K, Hashimoto K, Jensen P, et al. Pathogenesis of autoimmunity in pemphigus. Annu Rev Immunol 3:87–108, 1985.

Vincent SD, Lilly GE, Baker KA. Clinical, historic, and therapeutic features of cicatricial pemphigoid. Oral Surg Oral Med Oral Pathol 76:453–459, 1993.

Wiesenfeld D, Martin A, Scully C, Thomas J. Oral manifestations of linear IgA disease. Br Dent J 153:398–399, 1982.

Woodley D. Epidermolysis bullosa acquisita. Prog Dermatol 22:1–13, 1988.

Woodley D. Clearing of epidermolysis bullosa acquisita with cyclosporine. J Am Acad Dermatol 22:535–536, 1990.

Wojnarowska F, Marsden R, Bhogal B, Black M. Chronic bullous disease of childhood, childhood cicatricial pemphigoid and linear IgA disease of adults. J Am Acad Dermatol 19:792–805, 1988.

Wright J, Fine J, Johnson L. Oral soft tissues in hereditary epidermolysis bullosa. Oral Surg Oral Med Oral Pathol 71:440–446, 1991.

Yamani Y, Kitajima Y, Yaoita H. Characterization of a bullous pemphigoid antigen synthesized by cultured human squamous cell carcinoma cells. J Invest Dermatol 93:220–223, 1989.

Zhu X, Niimi Y, Bystryn J. Identification of a 160 kD molecule as a component of the basement membrane zone as a minor bullous pemphigoid antigen. J Invest Dermatol 94:817–821, 1990.

2

Ulcerative Conditions

An ulcer is defined simply as loss of epithelium. The term *erosion* generally implies a superficial defect producing some loss of epithelium. For all practical purposes, however, *erosion* and *ulcer* are used interchangeably. Ulcers that are preceded by blisters (vesicles or bullae) represent a distinct set of oral conditions, which are discussed in Chapter 1.

Ulcerative lesions are commonly encountered in dental patients. Although many oral ulcers have similar clinical appearances, their etiologies can range from reactive to neoplastic to oral manifestations of dermatologic disease. Diagnosis is important not only for the patient but also for the clinician. Infectious ulcers are potentially transmissible to dental personnel and should be approached with caution.

REACTIVE LESIONS

Etiology. Ulcers are the most common oral soft tissue lesion. Most are caused by simple mechanical trauma, and a cause-and-effect relationship is usually obvious. Most ulcers are a result of accidental trauma and generally appear in regions that are readily trapped between the teeth, such as the lower lip, tongue, and buccal mucosa (Fig. 2–1). A traumatic ulcer in the anterior portion of the tongue of infants with natal teeth is known as *Riga-Fede disease* (Fig. 2–2). Prostheses, most commonly dentures, are frequently associated with traumatic ulcers, which may be acute or chronic (Fig. 2–3).

In unusual circumstances, lesions may be self-induced because of an abnormal habit that is often associated with some psychologic problem (Fig. 2–4). These so-called *factitial injuries* are often as difficult to decipher as they are to treat. These lesions may prove to be frustrating clinical problems, especially if one has no suspicion of a self-induced cause. Psychologic counseling may ultimately be required to help resolve the problem.

Traumatic oral ulcers may also be iatrogenic. Respect for the fragility of oral soft tissues is, of course, of paramount importance in the treatment of dental patients. Overzealous tissue manipulation or concentration on treating primarily hard tissues may be related to accidental soft tissue injury that can be avoided. Ulcers induced by removal of adherent cotton rolls (Fig. 2–5), by the negative pressure of a saliva ejector, and by accidental striking of mucosa with rotary instruments are uncommon but preventable lesions.

Chemicals may be the cause of oral ulcers because of their acidic or basic nature or because of their ability to act as irritants or allergens. Lesions may be patient induced or iatrogenic (Fig. 2–6). Aspirin burns are still seen, although they are much less common than before. When acetylsalicylic acid is placed inappropriately against mucosa in an attempt by the patient to relieve toothache, a mucosal burn or coagulative necrosis occurs, the

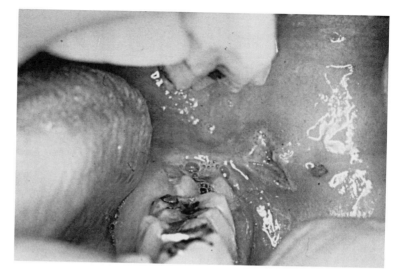

Figure 2–1. Acute traumatic ulcer.

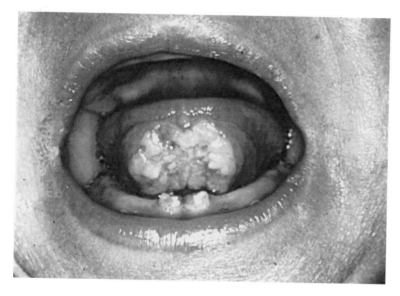

Figure 2–2. Riga-Fede ulceration in an infant.

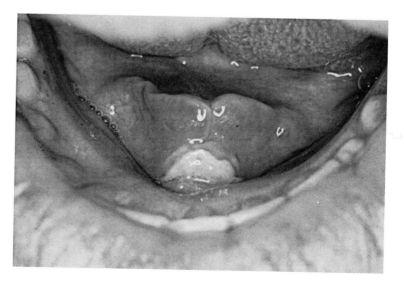

Figure 2–3. Fibrin-covered ulcer in the floor of the mouth, associated with denture flange trauma.

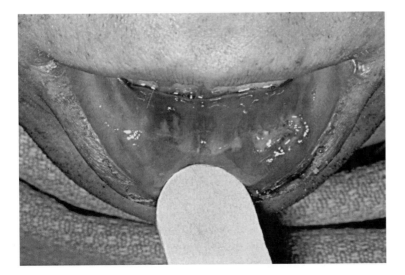

Figure 2–4. Acute self-induced ulcers associated with a lip-biting habit.

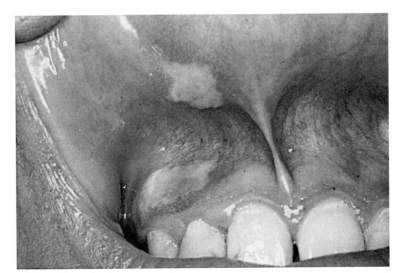

Figure 2–5. Acute iatrogenic cotton roll ulcers.

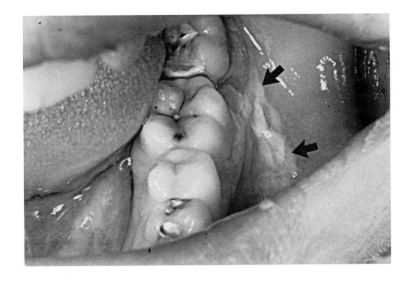

Figure 2–6. Iatrogenic phenol burn *(arrows)* associated with cavity medication of a second molar.

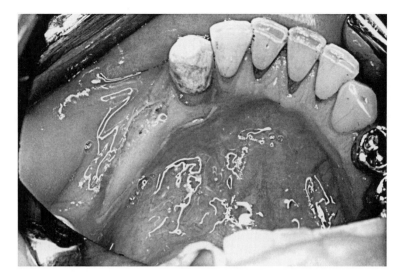

Figure 2–7. Hydrocolloid burn resulting in bone exposure of the mandibular ridge.

extent being dependent on the duration and number of aspirin applications. Many over-the-counter medications for toothache, aphthous ulcers, and denture-related injuries have the ability to damage oral mucosa if used injudiciously. Dental cavity medications, especially those containing phenol, may cause iatrogenic oral ulcers. Tooth-etching agents have been associated with mucosal burns of a chemical nature. Endodontic and vital bleaching procedures in which strong oxidizing agents are used (30% hydrogen peroxide) have also produced burns.

Ulcers following heat burns are relatively uncommon intraorally. Pizza burns, caused by hot cheese, have been noted in the palate. Iatrogenic heat burns may also be seen after injudicious use of tooth impression material, such as wax, hydrocolloid (Fig. 2–7), and dental compound.

Oral ulcerations are typically seen during the course of therapeutic radiation for head and neck cancers (Fig. 2–8). In those malignancies—namely, squamous cell carcinoma—that require large doses of radiation, in the range of 60 to 70 Gy, oral ulcers are invariably seen in tissues within the path of the beam. For malignancies such as lymphoma, in which lower doses of 40 to 50 Gy are tumoricidal, ulcers are likely but are less severe and of shorter duration. Radiation-induced ulcers persist through the course of therapy and for several weeks afterward, at which time spontaneous healing occurs without scar.

Clinical Features. Acute reactive ulcers of oral mucous membranes exhibit the clinical signs and symptoms of acute inflammation. The lesions are covered by a yellow-white fibrinous exudate and are surrounded by an erythematous halo. Varying

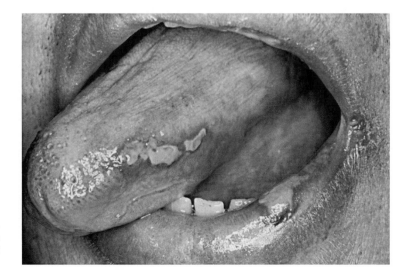

Figure 2–8. Acute radiation-induced ulcers of the lip and tongue associated with therapeutic radiation for lymphoma.

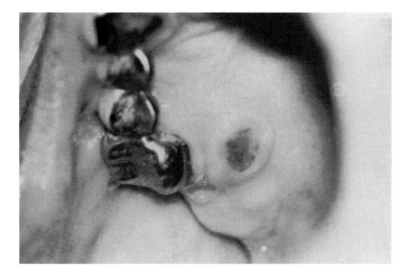

Figure 2–9. Chronic ulcer overlying exostosis of the hard palate.

degrees of pain and tenderness are associated with acute lesions.

Chronic reactive ulcers may cause little or no pain. They are covered by a yellow membrane and are surrounded by elevated margins that may show hyperkeratosis (Fig. 2–9). Induration often associated with these lesions is due to scar formation and chronic inflammatory cell infiltration.

A particularly ominous-appearing but benign chronic ulcer known as *traumatic granuloma,* occasionally may be seen in association with deep mucosal injury. This crateriform ulcer may measure 1 to 2 cm in diameter, and healing may take several weeks. It is usually found in the tongue. Another ominous-appearing chronic ulcer, characteristically seen in the hard palate, is known as *necrotizing sialometaplasia.* It is associated with ischemic necrosis of a minor salivary gland and heals spontaneously in several weeks (see Chapter 8).

Histopathology. Acute ulcers show a loss of surface epithelium that is replaced by a fibrin network containing predominately neutrophils. The ulcer base contains dilated capillaries and, with time, granulation tissue. Regeneration of the epithelium begins at the ulcer margins, with proliferating cells moving over the granulation tissue base and under the fibrin clot.

Chronic ulcers have a granulation tissue base, with scar found deeper in the tissue (Fig. 2–10). A mixed inflammatory cell infiltrate is seen throughout. Epithelial regeneration occasionally may not occur because of continued trauma or because of unfavorable local tissue factors. It has been speculated that these factors are related to inappropriate adhesion molecule expression (integrins) and/or inadequate extracellular matrix receptors for the keratinocyte integrins. In traumatic granulomas, tissue injury and inflammation extend into subjacent skeletal muscle. A characteristic

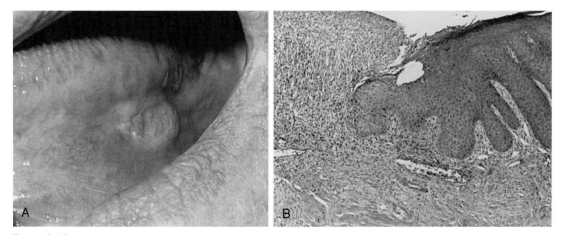

Figure 2–10. *A,* Chronic tongue ulcer. *B,* Ulcer margin showing abrupt transition from epithelium to fibrinous membrane.

lush eosinophil and macrophage infiltrate dominates the histologic picture.

Diagnosis. With acute reactive ulcers, the cause-and-effect relationship is usually apparent from the clinical examination and history. When there is a factitial overlay, diagnosis becomes a challenge.

The cause of chronic reactive ulcers may not be as readily apparent. In this circumstance, it is important that a differential diagnosis be developed. Conditions to consider are infection (syphilis, tuberculosis [TB], deep fungal infection) and malignancy. If the lesion is strongly suspected to be of traumatic origin, a 2-week observation period is warranted. If no change is seen or if the lesion increases in size, biopsy should be performed.

Treatment. Most reactive ulcers of oral mucous membranes are simply observed. If pain is considerable, symptomatic treatment may be of benefit. This could be in the form of a topical corticosteroid.

BACTERIAL CONDITIONS

Syphilis

Syphilis is a sexually transmitted disease that has been traced as far back as the time of Christopher Columbus. Whether Columbus's sailors who returned from the Indies were, in fact, responsible for the introduction of syphilis into the Old World is debatable, according to historians. Nonetheless, it was about this time that the virulent pandemic of the "great pox" began. Until Dr. Paul Ehrlich developed his "magic bullet," arsphenamine, around the turn of the century, there was no definitive treatment for syphilis. A stunning change in the control of syphilis followed the introduction of penicillin in the early forties. By 1940, approximately 600,000 new cases were reported annually in the United States; during the next 15 years, the rate declined to 6000 cases per year. More recently, there has been a slow increase; 35,000 cases were reported in 1987 and more than 50,000

in 1990. Increased numbers of cases are also found in the human immunodeficiency virus (HIV)–positive population. Further, a sharp increase in congenital syphilis has been recently documented. This has been associated, in large part, with maternal drug abuse, especially cocaine. Lack of prenatal care has also been important in the increased incidence of syphilis.

Etiology and Pathogenesis. Syphilis is caused by the spirochete *Treponema pallidum.* It is acquired by sexual contact with a partner with active lesions, by transfusion of infected blood, or by transplacental inoculation of the fetus by an infected mother.

When the disease is spread through contact, the infectious lesion of primary syphilis, known as a *chancre,* forms at the site of spirochete entry, with the subsequent development of painless, nonsuppurative regional lymphadenopathy (Fig. 2–11). The chancre heals spontaneously after several weeks without treatment, leaving the patient with no apparent signs of disease. After a latent period of several weeks, secondary syphilis develops (patients infected via transfusion bypass the primary stage and begin with secondary syphilis). This stage is marked by a spirochetemia with wide dissemination. Fever, flu-like symptoms, mucocutaneous lesions, and lymphadenopathy are typical. This stage also resolves spontaneously, and the patient enters another latency period. Relapses to secondary syphilis may occur in some patients. In about one third of those who have entered the latency phase and have not been treated, tertiary or late-stage syphilis develops. These patients may have central nervous system (CNS) involvement, cardiovascular lesions, or focal necrotic inflammatory lesions, known as *gummas,* of any organ.

Congenital syphilis occurs during the latter half of pregnancy, when the *T. pallidum* organism crosses the placenta from the infected mother. The spirochetemia that develops in the fetus may cause numerous inflammatory and destructive lesions in various fetal organs, or it may cause abortion.

Clinical Features. Primary syphilis results in a painless indurated ulcer(s) with rolled margins at the site of inoculation (Fig. 2–12). The lesion does

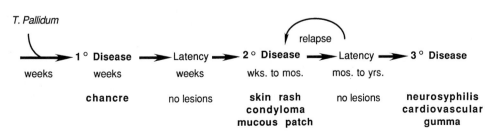

Figure 2–11. Pathogenesis of syphilis.

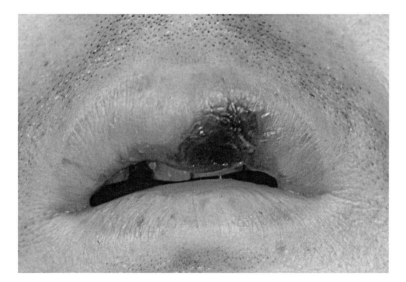

Figure 2–12. Chronic encrusted ulcer (chancre) of primary syphilis. (From Kerr DA, Ash MM Jr, Millard HD. Oral Diagnosis, 3rd ed. St. Louis, CV Mosby, 1983.)

not produce an exudate. The location is usually on the genitalia. Lip, oral, and finger lesions do occur occasionally and exhibit similar clinical characteristics. Regional lymphadenopathy, typified by firm, painless swelling, is often part of the clinical picture. The lesion heals without therapy in 3 to 12 weeks, with little or no scarring.

In untreated syphilis, secondary disease begins after about 2 to 10 weeks. The spirochetes are now disseminated widely and are the cause of a reddish-brown maculopapular cutaneous rash (Fig. 2–13) and ulcers covered by a mucoid exudate (mucous patches) on mucosal surfaces. Elevated broad-based verrucal plaques, known as *condylomata lata,* may also be seen on the skin and mucosal surfaces. Inflammatory lesions may potentially occur in any organ during secondary syphilis.

Manifestations of tertiary syphilis take many years to appear and can be profound, since there is a predilection for the cardiovascular system and the CNS. Fortunately, this stage of syphilis has become a rarity because of effective antibiotic treatment.

Manifestations of neural syphilis include general paresis (paralysis) and tabes dorsalis (locomotor ataxia). Inflammatory involvement of the cardiovascular system, especially the aorta, may result in aneurysms. Focal granulomatous lesions (gummas) may involve any organ. Intraorally, the palate is typically affected (Fig. 2–14). Development of generalized glossitis with mucosal atrophy has also been well documented in the tertiary stage of this disease. This so-called syphilitic glossitis has a predisposition for the development of squamous cell carcinoma.

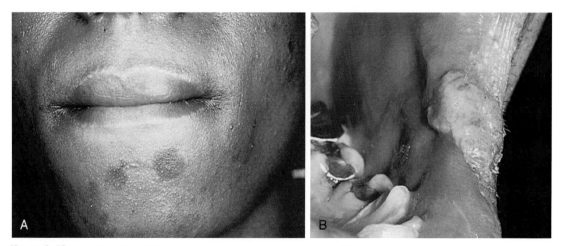

Figure 2–13. Macular lesions *(A)* and condyloma latum *(B)* of secondary syphilis.

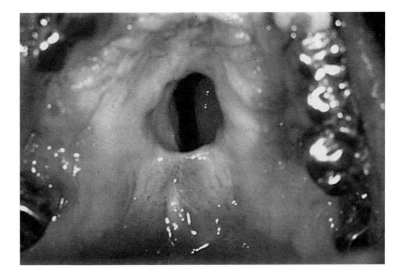

Figure 2–14. Palatal perforation as a result of gummatous inflammation of tertiary syphilis.

The generalized spirochetemia of congenital syphilis may result in numerous clinical manifestations that may affect any organ system in a developing fetus. A mucocutaneous rash may be seen early. When the infectious process involves the vomer, a nasal deformity known as *saddle nose* develops; or when periostitis of the tibia occurs, excessive anterior bone growth results in a deformity known as *saber shin.* Other late stigmata of congenital syphilis include three conditions known collectively as *Hutchinson's triad*: (1) an inflammatory reaction in the cornea (interstitial keratitis); (2) eighth nerve deafness; and (3) dental abnormalities consisting of notched or screwdriver-shaped incisors and mulberry molars (Fig. 2–15), presumably occurring because of spirochete infection of the enamel organ of teeth during amelogenesis.

Histopathology. The basic tissue response to *T. pallidum* infections consists of a proliferative endarteritis and infiltration of plasma cells. Endothelial cells proliferate within small arteries and arterioles, producing a concentric layering of cells that results in a narrowed lumen. Plasma cells, along with lymphocytes and macrophages, are typically found in a perivascular distribution. Spirochetes (silver stain) can be seen within the various lesions of syphilis, although they may be scant in tertiary lesions. Gummas may additionally show necrosis and greater numbers of macrophages, resulting in a granulomatous lesion that is similar to other conditions, such as TB.

Differential Diagnosis. Clinically as well as microscopically, syphilis is said to be the great imitator or mimicker because of its resemblance to many other unrelated conditions. When presenting

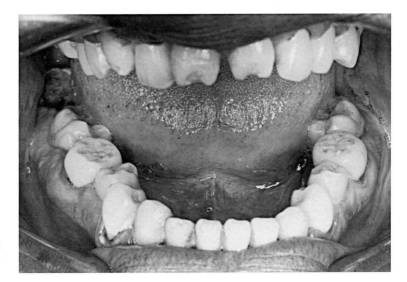

Figure 2–15. Notched incisors and mulberry molars, part of Hutchinson's triad.

orally, the chancre may be confused with and must be differentiated from squamous cell carcinoma, chronic traumatic lesions, and other infectious diseases, such as TB and histoplasmosis. The differential diagnosis of secondary syphilis would include many infectious and noninfectious conditions marked by a mucocutaneous eruption. Oral gummas, though rarely seen, may have a clinical appearance similar to the destructive lesions of midline granuloma.

Definitive diagnosis of syphilis is based on laboratory test confirmation of clinical impression. Among the several tests available are (1) darkfield examination of scrapings or exudate from active lesions, (2) special silver stain or immunologic preparation of biopsy tissue, and (3) serologic tests for antibodies to *T. pallidum.*

Treatment. The drug of choice for treating all stages of syphilis is penicillin. Through the years, *T. pallidum* has remained sensitive to penicillin as well as to other antibiotics, such as erythromycin and tetracycline.

Gonorrhea

Etiology. Gonorrhea is one of the most prevalent bacterial diseases in humans. It is caused by the gram-negative diplococcus *Neisseria gonorrhoeae.* Infection is transmitted by direct sexual contact with an infected partner. Containment of the number of infected individuals by tracing sexual contacts is enhanced by the short incubation period of less than 7 days but hampered by the absence of symptoms in many individuals, especially females. More than 690,000 civilian cases were reported in the United States in 1990, with the highest incidence in the 20- to 24-year-old age range.

Genital infections may be transmitted to the oral or pharyngeal mucous membranes through orogenital contact. Because oral mucosa is more resistant to physical trauma than pharyngeal mucosa, the latter site is much more commonly affected than the former. Risk of developing this form of disease is apparently much more likely with fellatio than with cunnilingus. Individuals may have concomitant genital and oral or pharyngeal infections that result from direct exposure to these areas rather than from spread through blood or lymphatics.

Transmission of gonorrhea from an infected patient to dental personnel is regarded as highly unlikely because the organism is very sensitive to drying and requires a break in the skin or mucosa to establish an infection. Gloves, protective eye-wear, and a mask should provide adequate protection from accidental infection.

Clinical Features. No specific clinical signs have been consistently associated with rarely occurring oral gonorrhea. However, multiple ulcerations and generalized erythema have been described. Symptoms range from none to generalized stomatitis.

In the more common pharyngeal gonococcal infection, presenting signs are usually general erythema with associated ulcers and cervical lymphadenopathy. The chief complaint may be sore throat, although many patients are asymptomatic.

Differential Diagnosis. Because of the lack of consistent and distinctive oral lesions, other conditions that cause multiple ulcers or generalized erythema should be included in a differential diagnosis. Aphthous ulcers, herpetic ulcers, erythema multiforme, pemphigus, pemphigoid, drug eruptions, and streptococcal infections should be considered. Diagnosis of gonorrhea is traditionally based on demonstration of the organism with Gram stains or culture on Thayer-Martin medium. Rapid identification of *N. gonorrhoeae* with immunofluorescent antibody techniques and other laboratory tests may also be used to support clinical impressions.

Treatment. The treatment of choice for gonorrhea is penicillin. Spectinomycin and third-generation cephalosporins (ceftriaxone and cefotaxime) are being used increasingly for treatment owing to strains that are resistant to penicillin. This may be supplemented by oral tetracycline. Ampicillin is apparently ineffective in the treatment of pharyngeal gonorrhea.

Tuberculosis

Etiology and Pathogenesis. TB is caused by the aerobic bacillus *Mycobacterium tuberculosis.* It does not react to Gram stain but appears red with Ziehl-Neelsen and Fite stains. With this latter stain, these organisms are not decolorized with acid-alcohol and are therefore also known as *acid-fast bacilli.*

Although TB has worldwide distribution, it has become much less prevalent than it was before the advent of antibiotics. However, significant numbers of patients (25,700 cases in the United States in 1990) continue to develop the active form of this disease, and a marked recent surge of new cases is noted. The case rate varies from one region to another and is dependent on factors that favor spread of communicable diseases, such as poor living conditions, low socioeconomic status, low native resistance, and compromised immunity from debilitating or immunosuppressed conditions. In the United States, a majority of cases can be found in densely populated urban areas, among immigrants from countries with high TB rates (e.g., Southeast Asia and Haiti), and among older individuals with compromised health. Of particular concern is the sharp rise of this disease within the acquired immunodeficiency syndrome (AIDS)–affected population and the implications for future control. Also, the emergence of multiple-drug-resistant forms of TB has raised concerns among health officials in many cities.

Spread of infection is through small airborne droplets, which carry the organism to pulmonary air spaces. Phagocytosis by alveolar macrophages follows, and the battle between bacterial virulence and host resistance begins. As the immune system is sensitized by the TB antigens, a positive tuberculin reactivity develops. The Mantoux test and the tine test are skin tests using a tubercle bacillus antigen, called *purified protein derivative,* to determine if the individual is hypersensitive to antigen challenge. A positive inflammatory skin reaction indicates that the individual's cell-mediated immune system has been sensitized, and it signifies previous exposure and subclinical infection but does not necessarily imply active disease.

A granulomatous inflammatory response to *M. tuberculosis* follows sensitization. In most cases, the cell-mediated immune response is able to control the infection, allowing subsequent arrest of the disease (Fig. 2–16). Inflammatory foci may eventually undergo dystrophic calcification. Latent organisms in these foci may become reactivated at a later date. In a small number of cases, the disease may progress through airborne, hematogenous, or lymphatic spread, so-called miliary spread.

Oral mucous membranes may become infected through implantation of organisms found in sputum or, less likely, through hematogenous deposition. Similar seeding of the oral cavity may also follow secondary or reactivated TB.

Clinical Features. Unless the primary infection becomes progressive, an infected patient will probably exhibit no symptoms. Skin testing and chest radiographs may provide the only indicators of infection. In reactivated disease, low-grade signs and symptoms of fever, night sweats, malaise, and weight loss may appear. With progression, cough, hemoptysis, and chest pain (pleural involvement) develop. As other organs become involved through spread of organisms, a highly varied clinical picture appears and is dependent on the organs involved.

Oral manifestations that usually follow implantation of *M. tuberculosis* from infected sputum may appear on any mucosal surface. The tongue and the palate are favored locations, however (Fig. 2–17). The typical lesion is an indurated, chronic, nonhealing ulcer that is usually painful. The causative organism is present in the base of these ulcers, making this a potential infectious hazard to dental personnel if barrier techniques are not used. Bony involvement of the maxilla and mandible may produce tuberculous osteomyelitis. This most likely follows hematogenous spread of the organism. Pharyngeal involvement results in painful ulcers, and laryngeal lesions may cause dysphagia and voice changes.

Histopathology. The basic microscopic lesion of TB is granulomatous inflammation, in which granulomas show central caseous necrosis. *M. tuberculosis* in tissue incites a characteristic macrophage response, due, at least in part, to bacterial wall lipids. Focal zones of macrophages become surrounded by lymphocytes and fibroblasts. The macrophages develop abundant eosinophilic cytoplasm, giving them a superficial resemblance to epithelial cells, in which case they are frequently called *epithelioid cells.* Fusion of macrophages results in the appearance of Langhans' giant cells, in which nuclei are distributed around the periphery of the cytoplasm. As the granulomas age, central necrosis occurs, usually referred to as case-

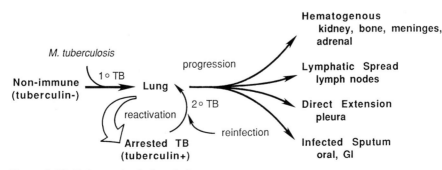

Figure 2–16. Pathogenesis of tuberculosis.

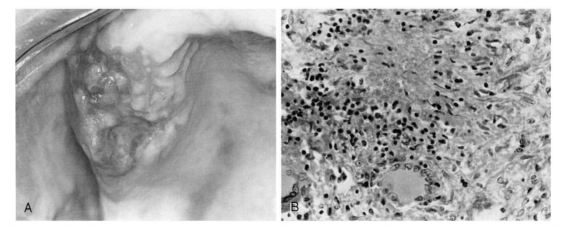

Figure 2–17. *A,* Tuberculous ulcer of the maxillary ridge. *B,* Typical granuloma showing central necrosis (top) and Langhans' giant cells (bottom).

ous necrosis because of the gross cheesy texture of these zones.

A Ziehl-Neelsen or Fite stain must be used to confirm the presence of the organism in the granulomas because several infectious and noninfectious conditions may also produce a similar granulomatous reaction. In the absence of acid-fast bacilli, other microscopic considerations would include syphilis, cat-scratch disease, tularemia, histoplasmosis, blastomycosis, coccidioidomycosis, sarcoidosis, and some foreign body reactions.

Differential Diagnosis. Based on clinical signs and symptoms alone, oral TB cannot be differentiated from several other conditions. A chronic indurated ulcer should prompt the clinician to consider primary syphilis and oral manifestations of deep fungal diseases. Noninfectious processes that should be considered clinically are squamous cell carcinoma and chronic traumatic ulcer. Major aphthae might also be included, although a history of recurrent disease should help separate this condition from the others.

Treatment. Before the advent of effective antibiotics, patients with TB were treated with bed rest and surgery. Chemotherapeutic regimens have now effectively replaced the earlier treatment approaches. Drugs likely to be employed for treatment of TB include isoniazid, rifampin, streptomycin, and ethambutol. Drug combinations are often used, and treatment may be extended as long as 2 years. Oral lesions would be expected to resolve with treatment of the patient's systemic disease. Unfortunately, infection with multidrug-resistant organisms appears to be increasing. Serious public health consequences could result.

Patients who convert from a negative to a positive skin test response may benefit from prophy-

lactic chemotherapy. This is dependent both on risk factors involved, such as age and immune status, and on the opinion of the attending internist.

Leprosy

Etiology and Pathogenesis. Leprosy, also known as *Hansen's disease,* is a rare granulomatous infection in the United States but relatively common in other parts of the world, such as Southeast Asia, South America, and India. It is caused by an acid-fast bacillus, *Mycobacterium leprae,* that is difficult to grow in culture. Growth has been possible in footpads of mice and in armadillos, both of which exhibit a relatively lower environmental temperature—apparently a requirement for growth of this organism. Leprosy is only moderately contagious, because transmission of the disease requires frequent direct contact with an infected individual for a long period. Inoculation through the respiratory tract is also believed to be a potential mode of transmission.

Clinical Features. There is a clinical spectrum of disease that ranges from a limited form (tuberculoid leprosy) to a generalized form (lepromatous leprosy); the latter has a more seriously damaging course. Generally, skin and peripheral nerves are affected. Lesions appear as erythematous plaques or nodules that represent a granulomatous response to the organism. Similar lesions may occur intraorally or intranasally. Damage to peripheral nerves results in anesthesia. In time, severe maxillofacial deformities can appear. Because of nerve dysfunction and anesthesia, the patient's extremities may suffer from trauma, ulceration, and bone resorption.

Histopathology. Microscopically, a granulomatous inflammatory response, in which macrophages and multinucleated giant cells predominate, is usually seen. Infiltration of nerves by mononuclear inflammatory cells is also expected. Acid-fast bacilli can be found within macrophages and are best demonstrated with the Fite stain. Organisms are most numerous in the lepromatous form of leprosy.

Diagnosis. Important for establishing a diagnosis is a history either of contact with a known infected patient or of living in a known endemic area. Signs and symptoms associated with skin and nerves should provide additional clues to the nature of the disease. The appearance of oral lesions without skin lesions seems highly improbable. Biopsy must be performed to confirm diagnosis because there is no laboratory test for leprosy.

Treatment. Current treatment centers on a chemotherapeutic approach in which several drugs are used for a period of years. The antileprosy drugs most commonly used include dapsone, rifampin, clofazimine, and thalidomide.

Actinomycosis

Etiology and Pathogenesis. Actinomycosis is a chronic bacterial disease that, as the name suggests, exhibits some clinical and microscopic features that are fungus-like. It is caused by *Actinomyces israelii,* an anaerobic or microaerophilic, gram-positive bacterium. On rare occasions, other *Actinomyces* species may be involved, or a related aerobic bacterium, *Nocardia asteroides,* may be responsible for a similar clinical picture. *A. israelii*

is a normal inhabitant of the oral cavity in a majority of healthy individuals. It is usually found in tonsillar crypts, gingival crevices, carious lesions, and nonvital dental root canals. Actinomycosis is not regarded as a contagious disease, because infection cannot be transmitted from one individual to another. Infections usually appear after trauma, surgery, or previous infection. Tooth extraction, gingival surgery, and oral infections predispose to the development of this condition. Evidence of other important predisposing factors has been slight, although actinomycotic infections have been recorded in osteoradionecrosis of the jaws and in patients with serious systemic illness.

Clinical Features. Most infections by *A. israelii* are seen in the thorax, abdomen, and head and neck and are usually preceded by trauma or direct extension of a contiguous infection. When occurring in the head and neck, the condition is usually designated *cervicofacial actinomycosis.* It typically presents as a swelling of the mandible that may simulate a pyogenic infection (Fig. 2–18). The lesion may become indurated and eventually form one or more draining sinuses, leading from the medullary spaces of the mandible to the skin of the neck. Less commonly the maxilla may be involved, resulting in an osteomyelitis that may drain through the gingiva. The pus draining from the chronic lesion may contain small yellow granules, known as *sulfur granules,* that represent aggregates of *A. israelii* organisms. Radiographically, this infection presents as a radiolucency with irregular and ill-defined margins.

Histopathology. A granulomatous inflammatory response with central abscess formation is expected in actinomycosis. In the center of the

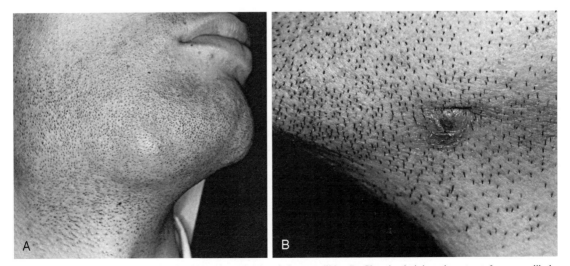

Figure 2–18. *A,* Swelling associated with actinomycosis of the mandible. *B,* Chronic draining sinus tract from mandibular actinomycosis.

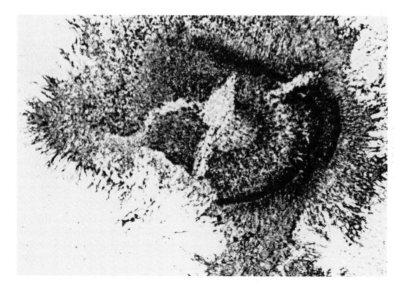

Figure 2–19. *Actinomyces* colony (sulfur granule). (Courtesy of Dr. W. G. Sprague.)

abscesses, distinctive colonies of organisms (sulfur granules) may be seen (Fig. 2–19). Radiating from the center of the colonies are numerous filaments with clubbed ends.

Differential Diagnosis. Clinically, actinomycosis may have to be differentiated from osteomyelitis caused by other bacterial or fungal organisms. Infections of the soft tissue of the neck, such as scrofula and *Staphylococcus* infections, may also be considered.

Definitive diagnosis is dependent on identification of the actinomycotic organism. This may be done through direct examination of exudate, microscopic evaluation of tissue sections, or microbiologic culture of pathologic material.

Treatment. Long-term, high-dose penicillin is the required antibiotic regimen for this disease. Intravenous penicillin (10 to 20 million units per day for 4 to 6 weeks) followed by oral penicillin (4 to 6 g per day for a period of weeks or months) is a standard regimen for actinomycosis. Tetracycline and erythromycin have also been used to effect cures. Additionally, drainage of abscesses and surgical excision of scar and sinus tracts is recommended to aerate tissue and to enhance penetration of antibiotics.

Noma

Noma, also known as *cancrum oris* and *gangrenous stomatitis,* is a rare disease of childhood that is characterized by a destructive process of orofacial tissues.

Etiology and Pathogenesis. Necrosis of tissue occurs as a consequence of invasion by anaerobic bacteria (fusiform bacilli and Vincent's spirochetes) in a host whose systemic health is significantly compromised. Malnutrition is the most frequently cited predisposing factor, although debilitation due to systemic disease, such as pneumonia or sepsis, has been described. The mechanism by which predisposing factors allow the microorganisms to become virulent pathogens is not understood.

Noma shares many features with the more limited and more benign acute necrotizing ulcerative gingivitis (Vincent's infection). Both are caused by the same organisms, both require compromised hosts, and both result in tissue necrosis.

Noma is rarely seen in the United States. It is typically found in relatively underdeveloped countries, especially those in which malnutrition or protein-deficient states are prevalent.

Clinical Features. The initial lesion of noma is a painful ulceration, usually of the gingiva or buccal mucosa, that spreads rapidly and eventually necrotizes (Fig. 2–20). Denudation of the involved bone may follow, eventually leading to necrosis and sequestration. Teeth in the affected area may become loose and may exfoliate. Penetration of organisms into the cheek, lip, or palate may also occur, resulting in fetid necrotic lesions. Before antibiotics were developed, fatalities from this disease were common.

Treatment. Therapy involves treating the underlying predisposing condition as well as the infection itself. Therefore, fluids, electrolytes, and general nutrition are restored, along with the introduction of antibiotics (usually penicillin). Débridement of necrotic tissue may also be beneficial if destruction is extensive.

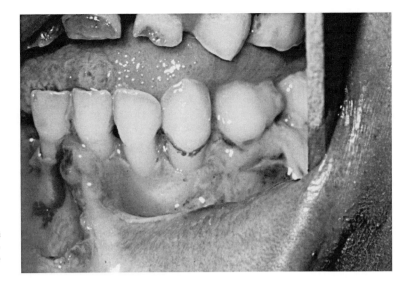

Figure 2–20. Noma involving the mandibular gingiva. Tissue is necrotic, resulting in exposure of mandibular bone.

FUNGAL DISEASES

Deep Fungal Diseases

Etiology and Pathogenesis. This group of fungal diseases is characterized by primary involvement of the lungs. Infections may potentially disseminate from this primary focus to involve other organ systems. Clinically, infections often mimic TB, relative to primary and secondary or reactivated disease.

The deep fungal infections having a significant incidence of oral expression include histoplasmosis, coccidioidomycosis, blastomycosis, and cryp-

tococcosis (Table 2–1). Oral infections typically follow implantation of oral mucous membranes by infected sputum. Oral infections may also follow hematogenous spread of fungus from a lung focus.

Histoplasmosis is endemic in the midwestern United States, although worldwide in distribution. Inhalation of yeasts from dust of dried pigeon droppings is regarded as a frequent source of infection. Coccidioidomycosis, on the other hand, is endemic in the West, especially in the San Joaquin Valley of California, where it has become known as *valley fever.* Blastomycosis is usually encountered in North America, especially in the Ohio-Mississippi river basin area. *Cryptococcus*

Table 2–1. Features of Deep Fungal Infections

	ORGANISM	PATHOGENESIS	SYMPTOMS	PRIMARY SITE	ORAL LESIONS	MICROSCOPY	TREATMENT
Histoplasmosis	*Histoplasma capsulatum*	Inhalation of spores in dust of bird excrement, endemic in midwestern USA	Cough, fever, night sweats, weight loss	Lung, may be asymptomatic	Chronic nonhealing ulcer(s), secondary to lung disease	Granulomatous reaction, 2–4 μm yeasts	Amphotericin B, ketoconazole
Coccidioido- mycosis	*Coccidioides immitis*	Inhalation of spores, endemic in western USA	Cough, fever, weight loss, chest pain, erythema multiforme	Lung, may be asymptomatic	Chronic nonhealing ulcer(s), secondary to lung disease	Granulomatous reaction, 20–60 μm spherules with endospores	Amphotericin B, ketoconazole
Blastomycosis	*Blastomyces dermatitidis*	Inhalation of spores, N. American distribution	Fever, weight loss, night sweats	Lung, some asymptomatic	Chronic nonhealing ulcers, draining sinus, secondary to lung disease	Granulomatous reaction, 5–20 μm budding yeasts	Amphotericin B, ketoconazole
Cryptococcosis	*Cryptococcus neoformans*	Inhalation of spores, pigeons are carriers	Cough, hemoptysis, headache	Lung, some asymptomatic	Chronic nonhealing ulcer(s), secondary to lung disease	Granulomatous reaction, 5–20 μm yeasts	Amphotericin B, flucytosine

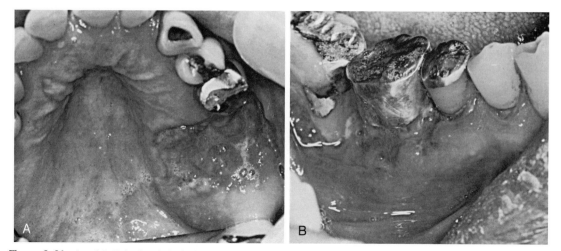

Figure 2–21. *A* and *B*, Palatal and gingival ulcers of oral histoplasmosis.

infections may be transmitted through inhalation of avian excrement. *Cryptococcus* also may occur in immunocompromised patients.

Clinical Features. The initial signs and symptoms of deep fungal infections are usually related to lung involvement and include cough, fever, night sweats, weight loss, chest pain, and hemoptysis. A skin eruption of erythema multiforme occasionally appears concomitantly with coccidioidomycosis.

Oral lesions are usually preceded by pulmonary infection. Primary involvement of oral mucous membranes is generally regarded as a highly unlikely route of infection. Swallowed infected sputum may potentially cause oral or gastrointestinal lesions. Also, erosion into pulmonary blood vessels by the inflammatory process may result in hematogenous spread to almost any organ. The usual oral lesion is ulcerative in nature (Fig. 2–21). Whether single or multiple, lesions are nonhealing, indurated, and frequently painful. Purulence may be an additional feature of blastomycotic lesions.

Histopathology. The basic inflammatory response to deep fungi is granulomatous in nature. In the presence of these microorganisms, macrophages and multinucleated giant cells dominate the histologic picture (Figs. 2–22 and 2–23). Purulence may be a feature of blastomycosis and, less likely, coccidioidomycosis and cryptococcosis. Peculiar to blastomycosis is pseudoepitheliomatous hyperplasia, associated with superficial infections in which ulceration has not yet occurred.

Differential Diagnosis. Clinically, the chronic, nonhealing oral ulcers caused by deep fungal infections may be similar to those of oral squamous

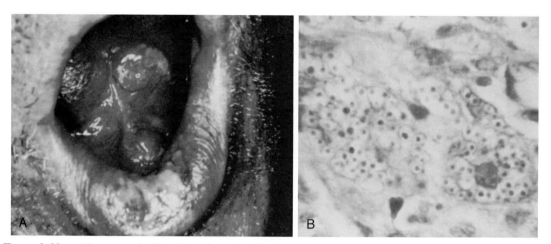

Figure 2–22. *A*, Histoplasmosis of the lip and tongue. (Courtesy of Dr. R. Millard.) *B*, Granulomatous inflammation. Tiny *Histoplasma capsulatum* organisms are seen within phagocytic cells. (Courtesy of Dr. W. G. Sprague.)

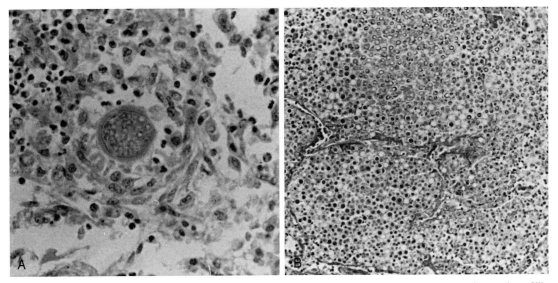

Figure 2–23. *A,* Spherule with endospores of coccidioidomycosis in a granulomatous focus. *B,* Blastomycotic organisms filling lung alveoli.

cell carcinoma, chronic trauma, oral TB, and primary syphilis. Blastomycosis may also produce a clinical picture that simulates cervicofacial actinomycosis. Culture of organisms from lesions or microscopic identification of organisms in biopsy tissue is required to establish definitive diagnosis. Skin tests and serologic tests are generally of little value in the diagnosis of deep fungal infections.

Treatment. Treatment of deep mycotic infections is generally chemotherapeutic. Surgical resection or incision and drainage may occasionally be used to enhance drug effects in treating some necrotic lung infections. Amphotericin B is the drug of choice, although this may be supported with or replaced by ketoconazole or fluconazole.

Subcutaneous Fungal Diseases—Sporotrichosis

Etiology and Pathogenesis. Some fungal infections affect primarily subcutaneous tissues. One of these, sporotrichosis, is of significance because it may have oral manifestations. It is caused by *Sporothrix schenckii* and results from inoculation of the skin or mucosa by contaminated soil or thorny plants. After an incubation period of several weeks, subcutaneous nodules that frequently become ulcerated develop. Systemic involvement is rare but may occur in individuals with defective or suppressed immune responses.

Clinical Features. Lesions appear at the site of inoculation and spread along lymphatic channels. On the skin, red nodules appear, with sub-

sequent breakdown, exudate production, and ulceration. Orally, lesions typically present as nonspecific chronic ulcers. Lymphadenopathy may also develop.

Histopathology. The inflammatory response to *S. schenckii* is basically granulomatous in nature. Central abscesses may be found in some of the granulomas, and overlying epithelium may exhibit pseudoepitheliomatous hyperplasia. The relatively small, round to oval fungus may be seen in tissue sections.

Diagnosis. Definitive diagnosis is based on culture of infected tissue on Sabouraud's agar. Special silver stains may also be used to identify the organism in tissue biopsy specimens.

Treatment. Sporotrichosis is usually treated with a solution of potassium iodide. In cases of toxicity or allergy to iodides, ketoconazole has been used with limited success. Generally, patients respond well to treatment, with little morbidity developing.

Opportunistic Fungal Infections—Phycomycosis

Etiology and Pathogenesis. *Phycomycosis,* also known as *mucormycosis,* is a generic term that includes fungal infections caused by the genera *Mucor* and *Rhizopus* and occasionally others. Organisms of this family of fungi, which normally are found in bread mold or decaying fruit and vegetables, are opportunistic, infecting humans when systemic health is compromised. Infections

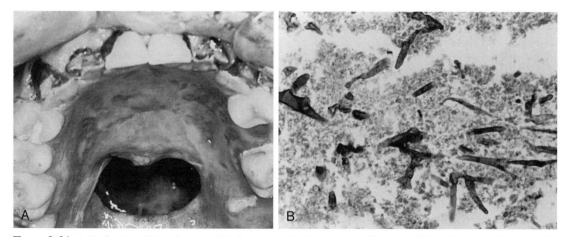

Figure 2–24. *A,* Perforation of the palate in a diabetic patient with phycomycosis. (Courtesy of Dr. J. Knapp.) *B,* Fungal hyphae in a necrotic focus.

typically occur in poorly controlled ketoacidotic diabetics, immunosuppressed transplant recipients, patients with advanced malignancies, patients being treated with steroids or radiation, or patients who are immunodepressed for any other reason, including AIDS.

Route of infection is through either the gastrointestinal tract or the respiratory tract. Infections may potentially occur anywhere along these routes.

Clinical Features. In the head and neck, lesions are most likely to occur in the nasal cavity, paranasal sinuses, and possibly the oropharynx. Pain and swelling precede ulceration. Tissue necrosis may result in perforation of the palate (Fig. 2–24). Extension into the orbit or brain is a common complication. The fungus has a propensity for arterial walls, where invasion may lead to hematogenous spread, thrombosis, or infarction.

Histopathology. Microscopically, an acute and chronic inflammatory infiltrate is seen in response to the fungus. The organism is usually readily identified in hematoxylin and eosin–stained sections in areas of tissue necrosis. Fungus in necrotic vessel walls in which thrombi may be evident is characteristic. Microscopically, the fungus appears as large, pale-staining, nonseptate hyphae that tend to branch at right angles.

Differential Diagnosis. It is important for clinicians to recognize that phycomycosis represents one of several opportunistic infections that may affect an immunocompromised host. Necrotic lesions of the nasal and paranasal sinuses should raise the suspicion of this type of infection. Confirmation must be made by identification of the fungus in biopsy tissue, exudates, or cultures. Because of the severity of underlying disease and the often rapid course that this infection may take,

diagnosis of phycomycosis may not be made until after death.

Perforating palatal lesions are rather rare but may be seen in association with other diseases. Inflammatory lesions would include gummatous necrosis of tertiary syphilis, midline granuloma, and Wegener's granulomatosis. Rarely, malignancies of nasal and sinus origin (squamous cell carcinoma and salivary gland adenocarcinoma) may present through the palate. Biopsy is required to differentiate these lesions.

Treatment. Amphotericin B is the drug of choice for treatment of phycomycosis. Surgical débridement of the upper respiratory tract lesions is also often required. Prognosis is generally dependent on the severity of underlying disease and the institution of appropriate therapy. Death is a relatively frequent consequence of this infection. Generally, lung infections are more likely than upper respiratory tract infections to be lethal.

CONDITIONS ASSOCIATED WITH IMMUNOLOGIC DYSFUNCTION

Aphthous Ulcers

Of all types of nontraumatic ulceration that affect mucous membranes, aphthous ulcers (canker sores) are probably the most common. Incidence ranges from 20 to 60%, depending on the population studied. Prevalence tends to be higher in professional persons and those in upper socioeconomic groups.

Etiology and Pathogenesis. Although the cause of aphthous ulcerations is unknown, several etiologic factors have been identified.

Immunologic Factors. Although somewhat conflicting, evidence that implicates a defect in the humoral immune system has been presented. Autoantibodies to oral mucous membranes have been demonstrated in patients with aphthous ulcers. These antibodies, however, react with prickle cells rather than with basal cells as would be expected from microscopic features, and they also cross-react with other epithelia in which aphthous ulcers do not occur.

Because some investigators believe that circulating immune complexes may be responsible for observed early extravasation of erythrocytes and infiltration of neutrophils in aphthous lesions, an immune-complex vasculitis has been postulated as a cause of this disease. In this theory, neutrophils responding to antigen-antibody complexes and complement in vessel walls release cytoplasmic enzymes, leading to destruction of overlying epithelium. This concept, which is analogous to leukocytoclastic vasculitis, is based on the presence of neutrophils early in this disease, a finding that has not been universally observed.

The most important immunologic findings have indicated that patients with this disease may have a defect in their cell-mediated immune response. CD4 lymphocytes are seen focally in the very early stages of the disease and, as such, are implicated as mediators. Basal cells in the area also express HLA-DR antigens early, suggesting a role for these cells as well. Because HLA-DR antigens are required for antigen presentation to immunocompetent cells, it could be speculated that these cells are presenting autoantigens to the infiltrating CD4 cells, leading to basal cell destruction.

In vitro tests that measure T cell sensitization to antigen have been performed on affected patients. Lymphocyte blast transformation studies have shown that when lymphocytes from affected patients are incubated with mucosal homogenates, blast transformation occurs. Another *in vitro* test, leukocyte migration inhibition, also produces positive results in patients with aphthous ulcers. T lymphocytes from affected patients have also been shown to be cytotoxic to cultured gingival epithelial cells but not to other epithelial cells. Further, patient T lymphocytes show increased antibody-dependent cellular cytotoxicity. Further support for an immunologic basis has been linked to alterations in T cell subset numbers in peripheral blood. As compared with controls, patients with aphthous ulcers have shown alterations in the ratio of CD4 to CD8 cells.

It is currently believed that aphthous ulcers are related to focal immune dysfunction in which T lymphocytes have a significant role. The nature of the initiating stimulus remains a mystery. The causative agent could be endogenous (autoimmune) antigen or exogenous (hyperimmune) antigen, or it could be a nonspecific factor, such as trauma in which chemical mediators may be involved.

Microbiologic Factors. Investigation into other possible causative factors has generally been unproductive. Because of the clinical similarity of oral aphthous ulcers to secondary herpes simplex virus (HSV) infections, a viral cause has been extensively investigated. The only supportive evidence has come from occasional isolation of adenovirus and HSV-I from some lesions and from the detection of part of the herpesvirus genome in peripheral mononuclear cells in some affected patients. Hypersensitivity to bacterial antigens on *Streptococcus sanguis* has generally been discarded.

Nutritional Factors. Deficiencies of vitamin B_{12}, folic acid, and iron as measured in serum have been found in a small percentage of patients with aphthous ulcers. Correction of these deficiencies has produced improvement or cures in this small group. The etiologic significance in all aphthous patients of this finding has been questioned because of the absence of uniform serum abnormalities, the absence of malabsorption symptoms, and the general absence of clinical improvement when these items are added to the diet of patients with aphthous ulcers. However, patients with malabsorption conditions such as *celiac disease* (*gluten-sensitive enteropathy* or *nontropical sprue*) and *Crohn's disease* have been reported as having occasional oral expression of aphthous-type ulcers. In such cases, deficiencies of folic acid and other factors may be part of the cause.

Other Factors. Other causes of aphthous ulcers that have been investigated include hormonal alterations, stress, trauma, and food allergies to substances in nuts, chocolate, and gluten. None of these is seriously regarded as being important in the primary causation of aphthous ulcers, although any of them may have a modifying or triggering role. Although HIV-positive patients may have more severe and protracted aphthous-like ulcers, the role of HIV and other agents is unknown.

Clinical Features. Three forms of aphthous ulcers have been recognized: minor, major, and herpetiform aphthous ulcers (Table 2–2). All are believed to be part of the same disease spectrum, and all are believed to have a common etiology. Differences are essentially clinical and correspond to degree of severity. All forms present as painful recurrent ulcers. Patients occasionally have prodromal symptoms of tingling or burning before the appearance of the lesions. The ulcers are not preceded by vesicles and characteristically appear

Table 2–2. Features of the Various Forms of Aphthous Ulcers

FEATURE	MINOR	MAJOR	HERPETIFORM	BEHÇET'S
Etiology	Immunologic defect	Immunologic defect	Immunologic defect	Immunologic defect, ?vasculitis
Area affected	All areas except gingiva, hard palate, and vermilion (any site in HIV+ patients)	All areas except gingiva, hard palate, and vermilion (any site in HIV+ patients)	Any intraoral area (any site in HIV+ patients)	All areas except gingiva, hard palate, and vermilion
Number of ulcers	Usually one	Several	Multiple (crops)	Few
Clinical appearance	Oval ulcer less than 0.5 cm	Oval, ragged ulcers, 0.5–2 cm, crateriform, several weeks' duration	Small ulcers in crops	Oval ulcers less than 1 cm
Vesicles preceding ulcers?	No	No	No	No
Extraoral sites	No	No	No	Yes—genitals, eyes
Treatment	None; symptomatic, topical steroids	Topical intralesional or systemic steroids	Topical or systemic steroids	Systemic steroids, immunosuppressives

on vestibular and buccal mucosa, tongue, soft palate, fauces, and floor of the mouth. Only rarely do these lesions occur on attached gingiva and hard palate, thus providing an important clinical sign for the separation of aphthous ulcers from secondary herpetic ulcers. In patients with AIDS, however, aphthous-like ulcers may occur in any mucosal site.

Minor Aphthous Ulcers. This is the most commonly encountered form of aphthous ulcers. It usually appears as a single painful, oval ulcer, less than 0.5 cm in diameter, that is covered by a yellow fibrinous membrane and surrounded by an erythematous halo (Fig. 2–25). Multiple oral aphthae may occasionally be seen. When the lateral or ventral surfaces of the tongue are affected, pain tends to be out of proportion to the size of

the lesion. Minor aphthous ulcers generally last 7 to 10 days and heal without scar formation. Recurrences vary from one individual to another. Periods of freedom from disease may range from a matter of weeks to as long as years.

Patients with underlying *Crohn's disease* may have, in addition to oral aphthae, mucosal fissures and nodules. This is most common in the buccal mucosa, vestibules, and lips, where it produces a cobblestone effect (Fig. 2–26). Biopsy of these mucosal nodules shows small noncaseating granulomas (Fig. 2–27). HIV-positive patients may develop minor aphthous ulcers, although proportionately more have major or herpetiform lesions.

Major Aphthous Ulcers. This form was previously thought to be a separate entity and was referred to as *periadenitis mucosa necrotica re-*

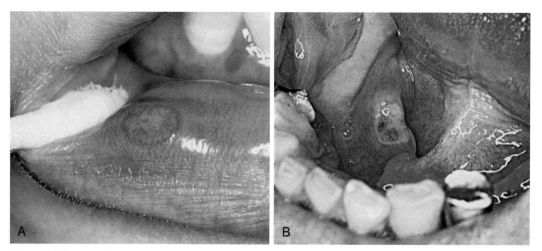

Figure 2–25. *A* and *B,* Minor aphthous ulcers.

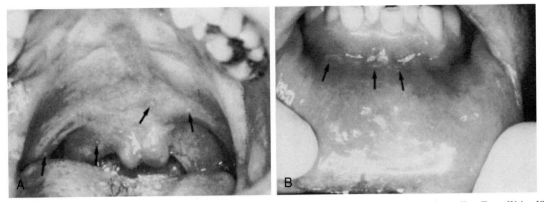

Figure 2–26. *A* and *B,* Crohn's disease. Note the multiple oral ulcers *(arrows)* and nodules of the lower lip. (From Weiss JS, Gupta AK, Regezi J, Rasmussen JE. Oral ulcers and cobblestone plaques. Oral Crohn's disease. Arch Dermatol 127:889, 892, 1991. Copyright 1991, American Medical Association.)

currens, or Sutton's disease. It is now regarded as the most severe expression of aphthous stomatitis. Lesions are larger (>0.5 cm) and more painful and persist longer than minor aphthae. Because of the depth of inflammation, major aphthous ulcers appear crateriform clinically and heal with scar formation (Fig. 2–28). Lesions may take as long as 6 weeks to heal, and as soon as one ulcer disappears, another one starts. In patients who experience an unremitting course with significant pain and discomfort, systemic health may be compromised because of difficulty in eating and psychologic stress. The predilection for movable oral mucosa is as typical for major aphthous ulcers as it is for minor aphthae (Fig. 2–29). HIV-positive patients may have aphthous lesions in any intraoral site.

Herpetiform Aphthous Ulcers. This form of

the disease presents clinically as recurrent crops of small ulcers (Fig. 2–30). Although movable mucosa is predominantly affected, palatal and gingival mucosa may also be involved. Pain may be considerable, and healing generally occurs in 1 to 2 weeks. Unlike herpetic infections, herpetiform aphthous ulcers are not preceded by vesicles and exhibit no virus-infected cells. Other than the clinical feature of crops of oral ulcers, there has been no finding that can link this disease to a viral infection.

Histopathology. It is generally accepted that important clues to the etiology and pathogenesis may be found during the early stages in the development of oral aphthous ulcers. Because these ulcers are usually clinically diagnosed, biopsies are unnecessary and rarely performed, resulting in the relatively limited availability of histopatho-

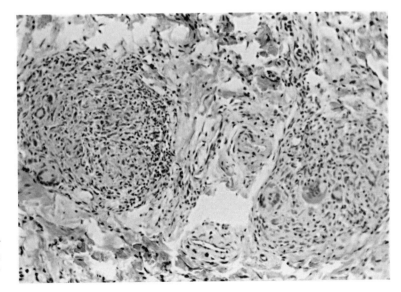

Figure 2–27. Biopsy specimen of the lip shown in Figure 2–26. Note the two small granulomas in the submucosa.

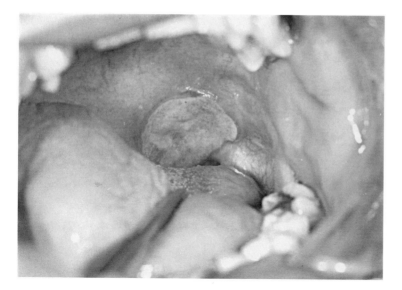

Figure 2–28. Major aphthous ulcers of the soft palate.

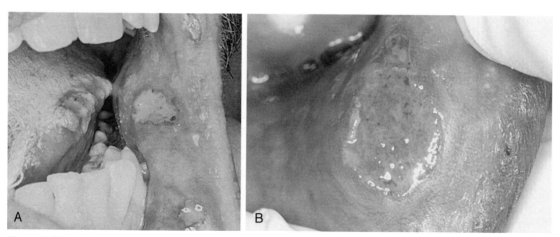

Figure 2–29. *A* and *B*, Major aphthous stomatitis.

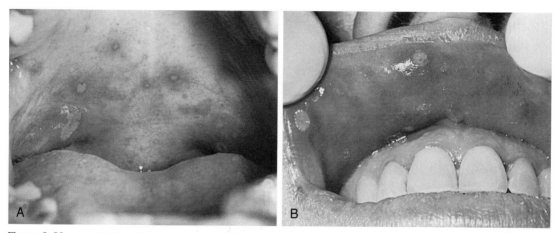

Figure 2–30. *A* and *B*, Herpetiform aphthous stomatitis.

logic material. Prospective studies have shown, however, that mononuclear cells are found in submucosa and perivascular tissues in the preulcerative stage. These cells are predominantly CD4 lymphocytes, which are soon outnumbered by CD8 lymphocytes as the ulcerative stage develops. Macrophages and mast cells are common inhabitants of the ulcer base. Extravasated erythrocytes and neutrophils have been described by some investigators in the early stages of these lesions, lending support for an immune-complex vasculitis etiology.

There are no microscopic diagnostic features of aphthous ulcers. At no time are virus-infected cells evident. Essentially, the same microscopic changes are found in all forms of aphthous ulcers, and all features support an immunologically mediated disease.

Differential Diagnosis. Diagnosis of aphthous ulcers is generally based on history and clinical appearance. Secondary (recurrent) oral herpes is often confused with aphthous ulcers but can usually be distinguished from it. History of vesicles preceding ulcers, location on hard gingiva and hard palate, and crops of lesions indicate herpes rather than aphthous ulcers. Other painful oral ulcerative conditions that may simulate the various forms of aphthous ulcers include trauma, pemphigus vulgaris, cicatricial pemphigoid, and oral expression of a systemic problem, such as Crohn's disease, neutropenia, and celiac disease.

Other aphthous-like ulcers may be associated with *cytomegalovirus* (CMV) (Fig. 2–31) or other opportunistic microorganisms. These ulcers are diagnosed through biopsy and possibly culture. Whether CMV is a primary or secondary agent in these ulcers is yet to be determined.

Treatment. In patients with occasional or few minor aphthous ulcers, usually no treatment is needed or sought because of the relatively minor discomfort. Also, a simple, inexpensive, and uniformly effective treatment is not available. However, when patients are more severely affected, some forms of treatment can provide significant control (but not necessarily a cure) of this disease. Reduction of healing time and pain has been reported with topically applied 5% amlexanox oral paste (Aphthasol). The number of remedies and over-the-counter agents used to treat aphthous ulcers rivals the number used for the treatment of secondary herpetic infections. Although some of these are occasionally effective, the rationale for their use is often obscure.

Because aphthous ulcers are most likely related to an immunologic defect, rational treatment would include drugs that can manipulate or regulate immune responses. In this category, corticosteroids currently offer the best chance for disease containment. In severely affected patients, systemic steroids may be used, but in patients with mild to moderate disease, only topical therapy appears justified. Intralesional injection of triamcinolone may be used for individual problematic lesions.

Systemic Steroids. Systemic steroids are appropriate for severe disease but should not be used unless the clinician has experience in this treatment area or is working with a knowledgeable consultant. The systemic effects and complications of glucocorticoids are numerous and can often be profound (Table 2–3).

For immediate control of severe aphthous stomatitis, a low to moderate dose of prednisone for a short period is recommended. A typical regimen might be 20 to 40 mg daily for 1 week, followed by another week at half the initial dose. Because the adrenals normally secrete most of their daily equivalent of 5 to 7 mg in the morning, all the

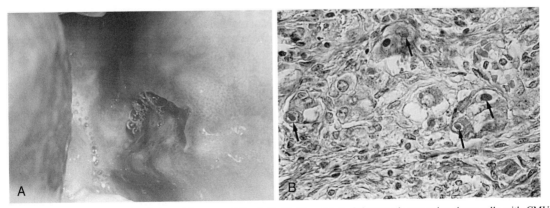

Figure 2–31. *A,* CMV-associated ulcer. (Courtesy of Dr. J. C. B. Stewart.) *B,* Submucosal connective tissue cells with CMV inclusion bodies *(arrows).*

Table 2–3. Systemic Effects and Side Effects of Glucocorticoid Therapy

EFFECT	SIDE EFFECT
Anti-inflammatory by stabilization of biologic membranes and capillaries	Therapeutic
Immunosuppression via lymphocytopenia and monocytopenia	Therapeutic, aggravation of TB and other infections, delayed wound healing
Gluconeogenesis from protein and fat breakdown	Aggravation of diabetes, muscle weakness, osteoporosis
Altered fat metabolism with redistribution in response to protein loss	Buffalo hump, hyperlipidemia
Fluid retention from Na resorption and K excretion	Moon face, weight gain
Potentiation of vasopressors	Blood pressure elevation, aggravation of congestion, heart failure
?Increased gastric secretions	Aggravation of peptic ulcer
Suppression of pituitary-adrenal axis	Adrenal atrophy
CNS effects	Psychologic changes
Ocular effects	Cataracts, glaucoma

CNS, central nervous system; TB, tuberculosis.

prednisone should be taken in one bolus early in the morning to simulate the physiologic process and thus minimize interference with the pituitary-adrenal axis and to minimize side effects. It is generally agreed that a slow steroid taper is not necessary if treatment lasts for less than 4 weeks, because adrenal suppression is likely to be minimal.

In patients requiring higher-dose, prolonged, or maintenance steroid therapy, an alternate-day regimen may be used after initial therapy. A short-acting steroid (24 to 36 hours), such as prednisone, is desired because it allows recovery or near-normal functioning of the pituitary-adrenal axis on the "off" (no prednisone) days. Additionally, the prednisone tissue effects outlast the adrenocorticotropic hormone suppression.

Topical Steroids. Topical steroids, if used judiciously, can be relatively efficacious and safe in the treatment of mild to moderate disease. Although nearly all topical compounds have been developed for use on the skin, it has been standard practice to prescribe these agents for use on mucous membranes. The science of topical steroid use in dentistry is relatively primitive when compared with use in dermatology. It has not been established for mucosal diseases whether more potent topical compounds are significantly more effective than less potent topical compounds, or whether more frequent application is more effective than less frequent application. Optimal vehi-

cles for intraoral use of steroids have also not been determined. Currently, empirical judgment is used to decide what type and strength of topical steroid to prescribe.

A number of factors determine the efficacy of a topical steroid. Intrinsic drug potency is significantly enhanced by halogenation of the parent compound, cortisol. Esterification makes it more lipophilic, providing greater penetrability. Increasing drug concentration can improve clinical efficacy, but there are limits beyond which no further gain is noted. For dermatologic use, ointments are probably the most effective because of their occlusive properties. Intraorally, ointments are not very useful because of their inability to adhere to mucous membranes. Creams and gels have received greater acceptance because they are more easily applied. Gels may, however, cause burning on application in some patients because of the alcohols used in their formulation. It should be noted that one vehicle, Orabase (Colgate-Hoyt), has been developed for oral use. It has, however, received only modest acceptance by clinicians and patients. Mixed with an equal amount of potent topical steroid, it may show clinical efficacy.

Commercially available topical steroids have been ranked in order of potency based on vasoconstriction assay and clinical trials by Cornell and Stoughton (1984). Table 2–4 is a reduced and modified version that should provide a rational basis for choosing an intraoral agent.

Numerous side effects of topical steroids have been recorded after prolonged or intense dermatologic use (Table 2–5). Most important are suppression of the pituitary-adrenal axis (as indicated by decreasing plasma cortisol) and Cushing's syndrome due to systemic steroid absorption. Other local skin effects include striae, atrophy, hypopigmentation, telangiectasia, induced acne, and folliculitis. Generally, the focal changes are difficult to assess and discern intraorally and are relatively insignificant. Systemic absorption, however, may be a concern if high-potency topical steroids are used liberally for extended periods.

Because only a relatively small amount of topical steroid is needed to cover most oral lesions, it is unlikely that significant systemic effects will occur with judicious intraoral use for short periods. Used over a 2- to 4-week period, 15 g of topical steroid should provide sufficient therapeutic effect for most oral ulcers (especially aphthous ulcers) with minimal risk of complication.

Because topical steroids can facilitate the overgrowth of *Candida albicans* orally, the concomitant use of an antifungal with high-potency corticosteroids is recommended. Use of a cream containing both steroid and antifungal, such as

Table 2-4. Potency Ranking of Topical Steroids*

	BRAND NAME	GENERIC NAME
1.	Temovate cream 0.05%	Clobetasol propionate
2.	Halog cream 0.1%	Halcinonide
	Lidex cream 0.05%	Fluocinonide
	Topicort cream 0.25%	Desoximetasone
	Lidex gel 0.05%	Fluocinonide
3.	Aristocort cream-HP 0.5%	Triamcinolone acetonide
	Diprosone cream 0.05%	Betamethasone dipropionate
	Florone cream 0.05%	Diflorasone diacetate
	Maxiflor cream 0.05%	Diflorasone diacetate
4.	Synalar cream-HP 0.2%	Fluocinolone acetonide
	Topicort-LP cream 0.05%	Desoximetasone
5.	Benisone cream 0.025%	Betamethasone benzoate
	Cordran cream 0.025%	Flurandrenolide
	Kenalog cream 0.1%	Triamcinolone acetonide
	Locoid cream 0.1%	Hydrocortisone butyrate
	Synalar cream 0.025%	Fluocinolone acetonide
	Valisone cream 0.1%	Betamethasone valerate
	Westcort cream 0.2%	
6.	Tridesilon cream 0.05%	Desonide
	Locorten cream 0.03%	Flumethasone pivalate
7.	[Several]	Hydrocortisone 1%

Modified from Cornell R, Stoughton R. The use of topical steroids in psoriasis. Dermatol Clin 2:397–409, 1984.
*Potency decreases from 1 to 7. Within each group, steroids are of approximately equal potency.

betamethasone and clotrimazole, makes treatment less costly and compliance more likely.

Antibiotics. Antibiotics have been used in the treatment of aphthous ulcers, with fair to good results. The effects may be systemic or topical and are most likely related to the elimination of secondary bacterial infection of the ulcers. An oral rinse containing chlorhexidine gluconate 0.12% (Peridex [Procter & Gamble]) has been used with mild success. The mechanism allowing for clinical improvement is perhaps related to diminishing the oral bacterial flora load and possibly to the binding to free nerve endings and epithelial cells.

Other Drugs. Immunosuppressive drugs, such as azathioprine and cyclophosphamide, because of their rather profound side effects, are generally justified only for the treatment of severely affected patients (to allow reduced prednisone dosages).

Table 2-5. Side Effects of Topical Corticosteroids

Systemic
    Suppression of pituitary-adrenal axis
    Iatrogenic Cushing's syndrome
Local (skin)
    Striae
    Atrophy
    Hypopigmentation
    Telangiectasia
    Induced acne
    Folliculitis
    Candidiasis

Preliminary results suggest that thalidomide may provide relief to severely affected patients, especially AIDS patients.

Behçet's Syndrome

Behçet's syndrome is a multisystem disease (gastrointestinal, cardiovascular, ocular, CNS, articular, pulmonary, dermal) in which recurrent oral aphthae are a consistent feature. Although the oral manifestations are relatively minor, involvement of other sites, especially the eyes and CNS, can be quite serious.

Etiology. The cause of this condition is basically unknown, although the underlying disease mechanism may likely be an immunodysfunction in which vasculitis has a part. Behçet's syndrome may have a genetic predisposition as well, particularly in reference to the frequent presence of HLA-B51 within this group. Also, some indirect evidence that has been presented suggests a viral etiology.

Clinical Features. The lesions of this syndrome typically affect the oral cavity, the eye, and the genitalia (Fig. 2-32). Other regions or systems are less commonly involved. Recurrent arthritis of the wrists, ankles, and knees may be associated. Cardiovascular manifestations are believed to result from vasculitis and thrombosis. CNS manifestations are frequently in the form of headaches, although infarcts have been reported. Pustular ery-

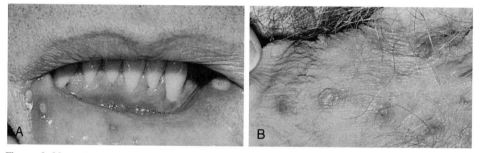

Figure 2–32. *A,* Oral ulcers of Behçet's syndrome. *B,* Penile ulcers in the same patient.

thema nodosum–like skin lesions have also been described. Relapsing polychondritis (e.g., auricular cartilage, nasal cartilage) in association with Behçet's stigmata has been designated as the *MAGIC syndrome* (*m*outh *a*nd *g*enital ulcers with *i*nflamed *c*artilage).

Oral manifestations of this syndrome appear identical to the ulcers of aphthous stomatitis. The ulcers are usually of the minor aphthous type and are found in the typical aphthous distribution.

Ocular changes are found in most patients with Behçet's. Uveitis, conjunctivitis, and retinitis are among the more common inflammatory processes.

Genital lesions are ulcerative in nature and may be the cause of significant pain and discomfort. Painful ulcerative lesions may also occur around the anus. Inflammatory bowel disease and neurologic problems have been described in some patients.

Histopathology. T lymphocytes are prominent in the ulcerative lesions of Behçet's syndrome. However, neutrophilic infiltrates in which the cells appear within vessel walls have also been described. Some believe that these changes are representative of a leukocytoclastic vasculitis. Immunopathologic support of a vascular target in this condition comes from the demonstration of immunoglobulins and complement in the vessel walls.

Diagnosis. The diagnosis of Behçet's syndrome is based on clinical signs and symptoms associated with the various regions described earlier. Biopsy and laboratory tests all produce nonspecific results.

Treatment. There is no standard therapy for Behçet's syndrome. Systemic steroids are often prescribed and immunosuppressive drugs, such as chlorambucil and azathioprine, may be used instead of or in addition to steroids. Dapsone, cyclosporine, thalidomide, and interferon may have a role in the treatment of these patients.

Reiter's Syndrome

Etiology. The underlying cause of this syndrome is unknown, although there appears to be

some genetic influence in some cases. An infectious process has been suspected but not substantiated. An abnormal immune response to microbial antigen(s) is now regarded as a likely mechanism for the multiple manifestations of this syndrome.

Clinical Features. The major components of Reiter's syndrome are arthritis, nongonococcal urethritis, and conjunctivitis or uveitis. The urethritis generally precedes the appearance of the other lesions. Mucocutaneous lesions may be seen in as many as half of the patients with Reiter's syndrome. Maculopapular lesions may occur on the genitalia as well as at other sites.

Oral lesions have been described as relatively painless aphthous-type ulcers occurring almost anywhere in the mouth. Tongue lesions have been likened to those of geographic tongue.

Highly characteristic of this syndrome is its occurrence predominantly in white men in their third decade. The duration of the disease varies from weeks to months, and recurrences are not uncommon.

Diagnosis. Diagnosis is dependent on recognition of the various signs and symptoms associated with this syndrome. There are no specific laboratory tests for Reiter's syndrome.

Treatment. Nonsteroidal anti-inflammatory agents are generally used in the treatment of this disease. Antibiotics have also been added to the treatment regimen, with varied success.

Erythema Multiforme

Erythema multiforme (EM) is a self-limiting eruption characterized by targetoid skin lesions and/or ulcerative oral lesions. It has been divided into two subtypes: a minor form, usually associated with an HSV trigger, and a major severe form, more often triggered by systemic drugs.

Etiology and Pathogenesis. The basic cause of EM is unknown, although a hypersensitivity reaction is suspected. Some evidence suggests that the disease mechanism may be related to antigen-antibody complexes that are targeted for small vessels in the skin or mucosa. In about half the cases, precipitating or triggering factors can be identified. These generally fall into the two large categories of infections and drugs. Other factors, such as malignancy, vaccination, autoimmune disease, and radiotherapy, are occasionally cited as possible triggers. Infections frequently reported include HSV (due to HSV-I and -II), TB, and histoplasmosis. Various types of drugs have precipitated EM, with barbiturates and sulfonamides among the more frequent offenders.

Clinical Features. EM is usually an acute self-limited process that affects the skin or mucous membranes or both. Between 25 and 50% of the patients with cutaneous EM have oral manifestations of this disease. It may on occasion be chronic, or it may be a recurring, acute problem. In recurrent disease, prodromal symptoms may be experienced before any eruption. Young adults are most commonly affected. Individuals often develop EM in the spring or fall and may have recrudescences seasonally. The term *erythema multiforme* was coined to include the multiple and varied clinical appearances that are associated with the cutaneous manifestations of this disease. The classic skin lesion of EM is the target or iris lesion (Fig. 2–33). It consists of concentric erythematous rings separated by rings of near-normal color. Typically, the extremities are involved, usually in a symmetric distribution. Other types of skin manifestations of EM include macules, papules, vesicles, bullae, and urticarial plaques.

Orally, EM characteristically presents as an ulcerative disease, varying from a few aphthous-type lesions to multiple superficial, widespread ulcers in EM major (Figs. 2–34 and 2–35). Short-lived vesicles or bullae are infrequently seen at the initial presentation. Any area of the mouth may be involved, with lips, buccal mucosa, palate, and tongue being most frequently affected. Recur-rent oral lesions may appear as multiple painful ulcers similar to the initial episode or as less symptomatic erythematous patches with limited ulceration.

Symptoms range from mild discomfort to severe pain. Considerable apprehension may also be associated with this condition initially because of the occasional explosive onset occurring in some patients. Systemic signs and symptoms of headache, slightly elevated temperature, and lymphadenopathy may accompany more intense disease.

At the severe end of the EM spectrum, intense involvement of the mouth, eyes, skin, genitalia, and occasionally the esophagus and respiratory tract may be seen concurrently. This severe variant of EM major is sometimes called *Stevens-Johnson syndrome.* Systemic signs and symptoms in this syndrome are more pronounced, and cutaneous and mucosal lesions may be more extensive. The lips may become encrusted, and oral lesions may cause exquisite pain. Superficial ulceration, often preceded by bullae, is common to all the sites affected. Ocular inflammation (conjunctivitis and uveitis) may lead to scarring and blindness in some patients.

Histopathology. The microscopic pattern for EM consists of epithelial hyperplasia and spongiosis. Basal and parabasal apoptotic keratinocytes are also usually seen (Fig. 2–36). Vesicles occur at the epithelium–connective tissue interface, although intraepithelial vesiculation may be seen. Connective tissue changes usually appear as infiltrates of lymphocytes and macrophages in perivascular spaces and in connective tissue papillae.

Immunopathologic studies are nonspecific for EM. The epithelium shows negative staining for immunoglobulins. Vessels have, however, been shown to have IgM, complement, and fibrin in their walls. This latter finding has been used to support an immune-complex vasculitis cause for EM. Autoantibodies to desmoplakins I and II have

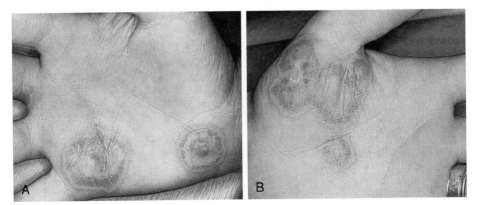

Figure 2–33. *A* and *B*, Target or iris lesions of erythema multiforme.

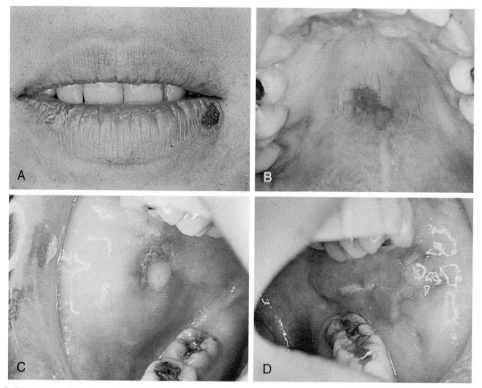

Figure 2–34. *A,* Resolving herpetic lip lesion that triggered oral *(B–D)* and cutaneous (Fig. 2–33) erythema multiforme in a 26-year-old woman.

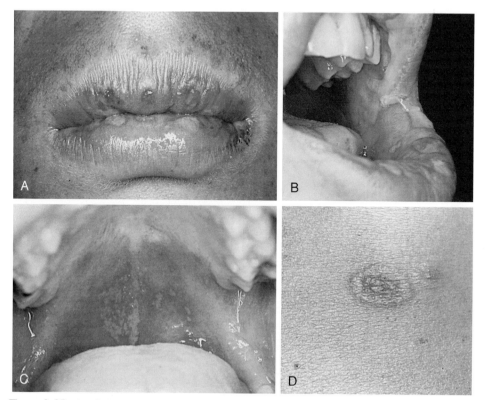

Figure 2–35. *A* to *D,* Recurrent oral and cutaneous (back) erythema multiforme in a young man.

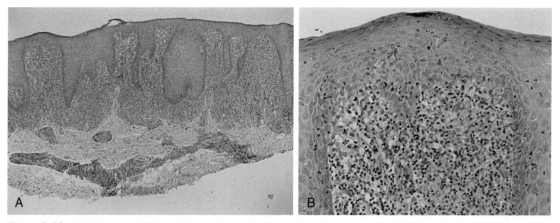

Figure 2–36. *A,* Erythema multiforme. The interface and a deep perivascular mononuclear infiltrate are seen. *B,* High magnification showing macrophages and lymphocytes in the connective tissue papillae.

been identified in a subset of EM major–affected patients, suggesting that both cell-mediated and humoral immune systems may contribute to the pathogenesis of EM.

Differential Diagnosis. When target, or iris, skin lesions are present, clinical diagnosis is usually straightforward. However, in the absence of these or any skin lesions, several possibilities should be considered for the oral expression of this disease. Included would be primary HSV infections (Table 2–6), aphthous ulcers, pemphigus vulgaris, cicatricial pemphigoid, and erosive lichen planus. The general lack of systemic symptoms; the favored oral location of lips, buccal mucosa, tongue, and palate (rarely gingiva); the larger ulcers (usually not preceded by blisters); the presence of target skin lesions; and a history of recent drug ingestion or infection should favor a diagnosis of EM. Cytologic smears of scrapings of the base of one or two ulcers early in the course of the disease could be diagnostic for a herpetic infection. Sudden onset and limited duration would help separate EM from pemphigus vulgaris, cicatricial pemphigoid, and lichen planus. Hema-

toxylin and eosin–stained sections from early lesions should help separate EM from pemphigus, pemphigoid, and lichen planus. Aphthous ulcers could be ruled out on historical and clinical grounds.

Treatment. In EM minor, symptomatic treatment may be all that is necessary. In EM major, topical corticosteroids with antifungals may help control disease. The use of systemic corticosteroids is controversial and is believed by some to be contraindicated. Acyclovir at 400 to 600 mg daily may be effective in preventing recurrences in patients who have an HSV-triggered disease. Supportive measures, such as oral irrigation, adequate fluid intake, and use of antipyretics, may provide patients with substantial benefit.

Lupus Erythematosus

Lupus erythematosus (LE) may be seen in one of two well-recognized forms—systemic (acute) LE, and discoid (chronic) LE—both of which may have oral manifestations. A third form known as

Table 2–6. Differentiating Features of Erythema Multiforme and Primary Herpes

FEATURE	ERYTHEMA MULTIFORME	PRIMARY HERPES
Systemic symptoms	None to slight	Pronounced
Typical clinical appearance	Oral—ulcers	Oral—multiple small lesions
	Skin—target lesions	Skin—multiple small ulcers
Areas typically affected	Buccal mucosa, tongue, palate, lips, extremities	Gingiva, lips, perioral skin
Cytology	Nonspecific	Virus-infected cells
Age	Young adults	Children
Precipitating factors	Recent drug use or infection (especially herpes simplex labialis)	Exposure to infected patient

subacute lupus has also been described. In the spectrum of LE, systemic lupus erythematosus (SLE) is of particular importance because of the profound impact it has on many organ systems. Discoid lupus erythematosus (DLE) is the less aggressive form, affecting predominantly the skin and rarely progressing to the systemic form. It may, however, be of great cosmetic significance because of its predilection for the face. Subacute cutaneous lupus erythematosus, described as lying intermediate between SLE and DLE, results in skin lesions of mild to moderate severity. It is marked by mild systemic involvement and the appearance of some abnormal autoantibodies.

Etiology and Pathogenesis. LE is thought to result from an autoimmune process that may be influenced by genetic or viral factors. Both the humoral and the cell-mediated arms of the immune system are involved in the etiology and pathogenesis of this condition.

A large number of autoantibodies directed against various cellular antigens in both the nucleus and the cytoplasm have been identified. These antibodies may be found in the serum or in tissue bound to antigens. Circulating antibodies are responsible for the positive reactions noted in the antinuclear antibody (ANA) and LE cell tests that are performed to help confirm the diagnosis of lupus. Also circulating in serum are antigen-antibody complexes that mediate disease in many organ systems.

Indications that the cell-mediated system has an important role in the pathogenesis of LE are found in the histology of lupus lesions, in which T lymphocytes may appear in prominent numbers, and in the results of abnormal T cell function test results in affected patients. The prevalence of laboratory immunologic abnormalities in LE varies. Only rarely are serologic alterations demonstrable in DLE.

Clinical Features

Discoid Lupus Erythematosus. DLE is a disease characteristically seen in middle age, especially in women. Lesions frequently appear solely on the skin, most commonly on the face and scalp. Oral and vermilion lesions are also frequently seen but usually in the company of cutaneous lesions. On the skin, lesions appear as disk-shaped erythematous plaques with hyperpigmented margins (Fig. 2–37). As the lesions expand peripherally, the center heals, with the formation of scar and loss of pigment. Involvement of hair follicles results in permanent hair loss (alopecia).

Mucous membrane lesions appear in about 25% of patients with cutaneous DLE. The buccal mucosa, gingiva, and vermilion are most frequently affected (Figs. 2–38 and 2–39). Lesions may appear as erythematous plaques or erosions. Usually present are delicate white, keratotic striae radiating from the periphery of the lesions, similar to those of oral lichen planus. Keratotic papules may also be seen throughout the lesions. The diagnosis of oral lesions may not be evident on the basis of clinical appearance, but it is often suspected in the presence of skin lesions. Progression of DLE to SLE is very unlikely, although the potential does exist.

Systemic Lupus Erythematosus. In this form of LE, skin and mucosal lesions are relatively mild, and patients' complaints are dominated by multiple system involvement. Numerous autoantibodies directed against nuclear and cytoplasmic antigens are found in SLE-affected patients. These antibodies, when complexed to their corresponding antigens either in serum or in the target organ, can cause lesions in nearly any tissue, resulting in a wide variety of clinical signs and symptoms.

Involvement of the skin results in an erythematous rash, classically seen over the malar processes and bridge of the nose. This results in the characteristic butterfly distribution usually associated with SLE. Other areas of the face, trunk, and hands may also be involved. The lesions are non-scarring and may flare as systemic involvement progresses. Occasionally, disk-shaped skin lesions, similar to those seen in DLE, appear in SLE.

Oral lesions of SLE are generally similar to those seen in DLE. Ulceration, erythema, and keratosis may be seen (Fig. 2–40). In addition to the vermilion, the buccal mucosa, gingiva, and palate are frequently involved.

Systemic expression of SLE may initially be in the form of fever, weight loss, and malaise. Typically, with disease progression many organ systems become involved. Joints, kidneys, heart, and lungs are most frequently affected, although many other organs may express manifestations of this disease. The inflammatory lesions of the variously involved tissues result in a wide array of signs and symptoms. Kidney lesions (glomerulopathy) are, however, the most important, because they are most commonly responsible for the death of SLE-affected patients (Table 2–7).

Serologic tests for autoantibodies yield positive results in patients with SLE. The ANA test is regarded as a reliable and relatively specific test for SLE. Among the antibodies that may cause a positive ANA test result are anti–single-stranded DNA, anti–double-stranded DNA, and antinuclear ribonuclear protein. Specific tests for these and other autoantibodies of SLE are also available. Another serologic test for SLE is the LE cell test,

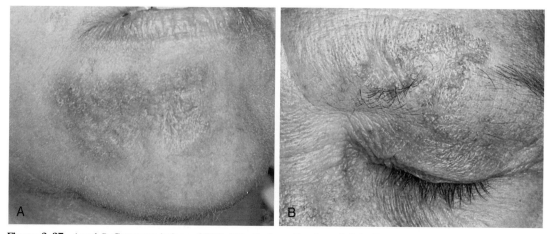

Figure 2–37. *A* and *B,* Cutaneous lesions of DLE. Note the loss of eyebrow hair in *B.*

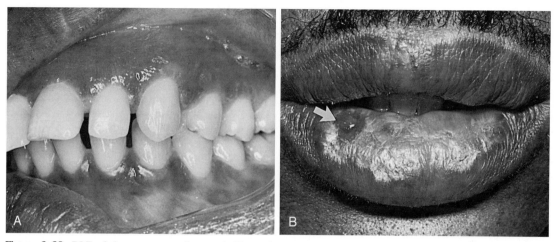

Figure 2–38. DLE of the mucous membranes. *A,* The entire maxillary gingiva is erythematous, with faint keratotic striae. Mandibular gingiva is unaffected. *B,* The lower lip is keratotic, with one area of ulceration *(arrow).*

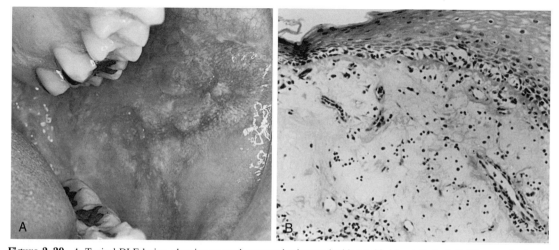

Figure 2–39. *A,* Typical DLE lesion, showing an erythematous background with speckled keratotic foci. *B,* Microscopic changes include edema, interface change, and epithelial atrophy.

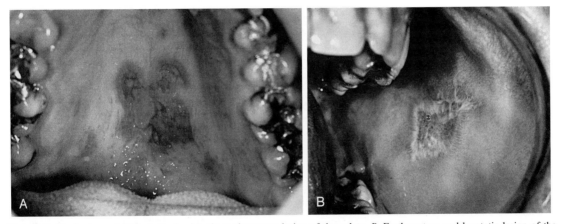

Figure 2–40. Lesions of SLE. *A,* Predominantly erythematous lesion of the palate. *B,* Erythematous and keratotic lesion of the buccal mucosa.

although it is less sensitive and less specific than the ANA test.

Antibodies to Ro (SS-A) and La (SS-B) cytoplasmic antigens may also be present in SLE.

Histopathology. In DLE, several microscopic changes are seen with relative consistency. Basal cell destruction, hyperkeratosis, epithelial atrophy, lymphocytic infiltration (often in a perivascular distribution), and vascular dilatation with edema of the upper dermis or submucosa are characteristic features. The most important microscopic feature diagnostically is the interface change, because it appears that the basal cell layer is the primary target in skin and mucous membrane disease. Because this is also the case for lichen planus, the two diseases may be difficult to separate microscopically (Table 2–8).

In SLE, oral lesions are microscopically similar to lesions of DLE, although inflammatory cell infiltrates are less evident and more diffuse.

Changes in skin lesions vary from slight to marked, depending on whether lesions are erythematous or "discoid." Interface change, lymphocytic infiltrates, and fibrinoid vascular changes are usually seen.

Other organs, when involved in SLE, show some individual histologic variations. Generally, however, basic underlying histologic changes are common to all locations. These consist of vasculitis, mononuclear infiltrates, and fibrinoid change.

Direct immunofluorescent testing of skin and mucosal lesions shows granular-linear deposits of immunoglobulins (IgG, IgM, IgA), complement (C3), and fibrinogen along the basement membrane zone in a majority of patients. Because C3 and fibrinogen deposits may appear in several other conditions, immunostaining for these components is believed to be of little value in the diagnosis of LE. Demonstration of immunoglobulin deposits in a granular-linear subepidermal pat-

Table 2–7. Comparison of Discoid and Systemic Lupus Erythematosus

PARAMETER	DISCOID LUPUS ERYTHEMATOSUS	SYSTEMIC LUPUS ERYTHEMATOSUS
Organs involved		
Skin	Almost always	Usually
Oral	Frequently	Occasionally
Joints	No	Usually
Kidneys	No	Usually
Heart	No	Usually
Other	No	Often
Symptoms	No	Fever, weight loss, malaise
Serology		
ANA test	Negative	Positive
LE cell test	Negative	Positive
Immunopathology		
Direct immunofluorescence	Positive, granular-linear basement membrane deposits of Ig	Positive, granular-linear basement membrane deposits of Ig

Table 2–8. Comparison of Lupus Erythematosus and Lichen Planus

PARAMETER	LUPUS ERYTHEMATOSUS	LICHEN PLANUS
Histopathology		
Basal cell destruction	Yes	Yes
Lymphocytic infiltrate	Yes	Yes
Subepithelial band	No	Yes
Perivascular	Yes	No
Hyperkeratosis	Yes	Yes
Epithelial atrophy	Yes	Occasionally
Submucosal edema	Yes	No
Vasodilatation	Yes	No
Immunopathology (basement membrane)		
Immunoglobulins	Yes	No
Complement	Fine granular deposits	Coarse granular deposits
Fibrinogen	Usually	Usually
Serology		
ANA test	SLE positive DLE negative	Negative
LE cell test	SLE positive DLE negative	Negative

tern is, however, thought to be relatively specific. This is also the basis of the lupus band test, which uses biopsy specimens of involved and uninvolved skin and immunofluorescent staining for immuno-globulins. Positive lupus band staining is seen in lesional skin of most patients with DLE and SLE. Uninvolved skin usually reacts positively in SLE and negatively in DLE.

Differential Diagnosis. Clinically, lesions of oral LE most often resemble erosive lichen planus (Fig. 2–41). Oral lupus lesions tend to be less symmetrically distributed than lichen planus. Also, the keratotic striae of LE are much more delicate and subtle than Wickham's striae of lichen planus. When significant ulceration is present, pemphigus vulgaris, cicatricial pemphigoid, erythema multiforme, and drug reaction might also be considerations. Also, lupus might be confused with erythroplakia, in which there are foci of keratosis (speckled erythroplakia). The presence of characteristic skin lesions or systemic signs and symptoms may help in the diagnosis of LE. Biopsy and direct immunofluorescent testing should confirm the clinical impression. Negative serologic tests for autoantibodies (e.g., ANA test) would rule out systemic involvement.

Treatment. DLE is usually treated with topical steroids. High-potency creams can be used intraor-

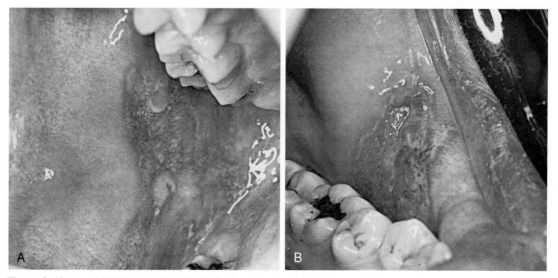

Figure 2–41. *A* and *B*, DLE in a lichenoid distribution. Note the dark background with associated delicate white striae.

ally but should be used with caution on facial skin because of secondary cutaneous changes. In refractory cases, antimalarials or sulfones may be used.

Systemic steroids may be used in the treatment of SLE. The prednisone dose is generally dependent on the severity of the disease, and prednisone may be combined with immunosuppressive agents for their therapeutic and steroid-sparing effects. Antimalarials and nonsteroidal anti-inflammatories may also be used in the control of this disease.

Drug Reactions

Etiology and Pathogenesis. Although the skin is more commonly involved in adverse reactions to drugs, the oral mucosa may occasionally be the target. Oral mucous membranes may be the sole site of involvement, or they may be part of a skin reaction to the offending drug. Virtually any drug has the potential to cause an untoward reaction, but some have a greater ability to do so than others. Also, some patients have a greater tendency than others to react to drugs. Some of the drugs that are more commonly cited as being involved in adverse reactions are listed in Table 2–9.

Pathogenesis of drug reactions may be related to either immunologic or nonimmunologic mechanisms. With the immunologic route, a patient's immune response is triggered by an antigenic component on the drug molecule, resulting in a hyperimmune response or drug allergy. In this type of reaction, the humoral arm of the immune system is predominantly involved. The potential for drug allergy is directly dependent on the immunogenicity of the drug, the frequency of exposure, the route of administration (topical more likely than oral), and the innate reactivity of the patient's immune system.

One of several mechanisms may be involved in drug allergy. IgE-mediated reactions occur when the drug (allergen) reacts with IgE antibody bound to mast cells. Subsequently, release of chemical mediators from the mast cells produces the clinical disease, which may range from a localized rash to anaphylaxis.

Another pathway for drug reactions involves a cytotoxic reaction in which an antibody binds to a drug (antigen) that is already attached to a cell surface. The target cells may be specific or nonspecific and may cause pathologic changes in any organ. If, for example, red blood cells are the cells involved, the result of this type of reaction would be anemia.

A third pathogenetic mechanism in drug allergy involves circulation of the antigen for extended periods, allowing sensitization of the patient's immune system and production of new antibody. Subsequent binding of antigen and antibody results in circulating complexes that may be deposited in various sites, producing allergic organopathies, such as nephritis, arthritis, and dermatitis. Disease caused by this mechanism is also known as *serum sickness.*

Drug reactions that are nonimmunologic in nature do not stimulate an immune response in the patient and are not antibody dependent. In this type of response, drugs may directly affect mast cells, causing the release of chemical mediators. The reactions may also be a result of overdose, toxicity, or side effects of the drugs.

Clinical Features. Cutaneous manifestations of drug reactions are widely varied and are dependent on many factors, some of which include the type of drug, drug dose, and individual patient differences. Changes may appear rapidly, as in anaphylaxis, angioedema, and urticaria, or, more likely, appear several days after drug use.

Acquired angioedema is an IgE-mediated allergic reaction that is precipitated by drugs or foods such as nuts and shellfish. These substances may act as sensitizing agents (antigens) that elicit IgE production. On antigenic rechallenge, mast cells bound with IgE in the skin or mucosa release their contents to cause the clinical picture of angioedema. *Hereditary angioedema* produces similar clinical changes but through a different mechanism. Individuals who inherit this rare autosomal dominant trait or spontaneous mutation have a qualitative or quantitative deficiency of the inhibitor of the first component of complement, C1 esterase. Absent or dysfunctional C1 inhibitor leads ultimately to release of vasoactive peptides and the often serious clinical manifestations that characterize this condition.

Angioedema, by either an acquired or a hereditary pathway, appears as a soft, diffuse, painless swelling, usually of the lips, neck, or face (Fig. 2–42). There is typically no color change. The

Table 2–9. Representative Drugs Known to Cause Adverse Reactions

Antimalarials	Local anesthetics
Aspirin	Meprobamate
Barbiturates	Methyldopa
Chlorpromazine	Oxprenolol hydrochloride
Cimetidine	Penicillin
Codeine	Phenytoin
Erythromycin	Retinoids
Gold compounds	Streptomycin
Indomethacin	Sulfonamides
Ketoconazole	Tetracycline

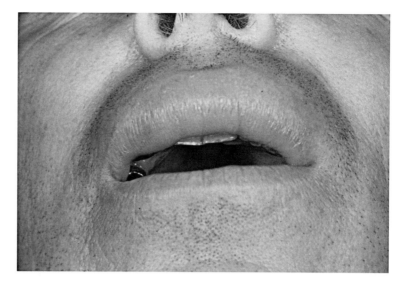

Figure 2–42. Angioedema of the upper lip.

condition generally subsides after 1 to 2 days and may recur at a later date. Emergency treatment may be required if the process has led to respiratory distress because of glottic or laryngeal involvement. Antihistamines and, in problematic cases, corticosteroids are used to treat this form of allergy.

Other cutaneous manifestations of drug reactions include urticaria, maculopapular rash, erythema, vesicles, ulcers, and target lesions (EM) (Fig. 2–43). An unusual form of drug reaction is known as *fixed drug reaction.* In patients with this condition, an erythematous lesion appears in the same cutaneous location with each antigenic challenge (Fig. 2–44).

Oral manifestations of drug reactions may be erythematous, vesicular, or ulcerative in nature (Fig. 2–45). They may also mimic erosive lichen planus, in which case they are known as *lichenoid drug reactions* (Fig. 2–46 and Table 2–10). The widespread ulcers typical of EM are often representative of a drug reaction.

Histopathology. The microscopy of drug reactions includes such nonspecific features as spongiosis, apoptotic keratinocytes, lymphoid infiltrates, eosinophils, and ulceration. An interface pattern of mucositis (i.e., a lymphoid infiltrate focused at the epithelial-connective tissue interface) is often seen in mucosal allergic reactions. Although biopsy may not be diagnostic, it may be helpful in ruling out other diagnostic considerations. Nonetheless, many of these microscopic changes may be seen in the various types of drug reactions: mononuclear or polymorphonuclear infiltration in a subepithelial or perivascular distribution, basal cell destruction, edema, and keratinocyte necrosis.

Diagnosis. Because the clinical and histologic features of drug reactions are highly variable and nonspecific, the diagnosis of drug reaction re-

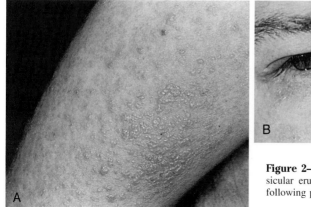

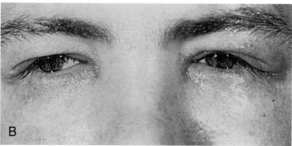

Figure 2–43. Extraoral manifestations of drug reactions. *A,* Vesicular eruption on arm due to phenobarbital. *B,* Conjunctivitis following penicillin ingestion.

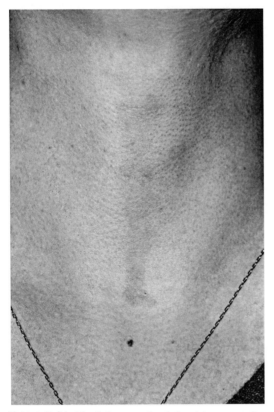

Figure 2–44. Fixed drug reaction induced by tetracycline. (Courtesy of Dr. J. C. B. Stewart.)

Table 2–10. Drugs with Potential to Cause Oral Lichenoid Changes

Allopurinol
Angiotensin-converting enzyme inhibitors
Enalapril
Furosemide
Gold salts
Hydroxychloroquine
Mercury
Methyldopa
Nonsteroidal anti-inflammatory agents
Palladium
Para-aminosalicylic acid
Penicillamine
Phenothiazine
Propranolol
Quinidine
Streptomycin
Tetracyclines
Thiazides
Tolbutamide
Triprolidine

quires a high index of suspicion and careful history taking. Recent use of a drug is important, because reaction after several days tends to rule against drug reaction. An exception is the delayed reaction (up to 2 weeks) noted after the use of ampicillin. Withdrawal of the suspected drug should result in improvement, and reinstitution of the drug (a procedure that is usually ill advised for the patient's safety) should exacerbate the patient's condition. If rechallenge is performed, minute amounts of the offending drug or a structurally related drug should cause a reaction. Another consideration that would support a drug reaction is the clinical expression of lesions that are generally regarded as being typically allergic in nature.

Treatment. The most important measure in the management of drug reactions is identification and withdrawal of the causative agent. If this is impossible or undesirable, alternative drugs may have to be substituted or the eruption may have to be dealt with on an empirical basis. Antihistamines and occasionally corticosteroids may be useful in the management of oral and cutaneous eruptions due to drug reactions.

Contact Allergy

Etiology and Pathogenesis. Contact allergic reactions can be caused by antigenic stimulation

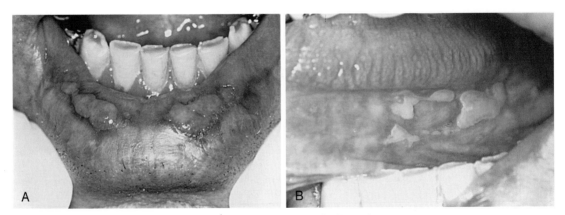

Figure 2–45. *A* and *B*, Mucosal ulcers due to a drug reaction to captopril (Capoten).

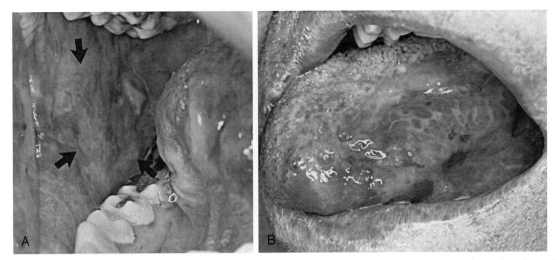

Figure 2–46. Lichenoid drug reaction. *A,* Most of the buccal mucosa is ulcerated *(arrows). B,* The tongue shows ulceration and keratotic striae.

by a vast array of foreign substances. The immune response is predominantly cell mediated in nature. In the sensitization phase, the Langerhans cells appear to have a major role in the recognition of foreign antigen. The Langerhans cells differ from their relatives the macrophages in that they are widely distributed throughout epidermis and mucosa. They are dendritic cells found usually midway in the epithelium among keratinocytes; they are responsible for processing antigens that enter the epithelium from the external environment. The Langerhans cells subsequently present the appropriate antigenic determinants to T lymphocytes. After antigenic rechallenge, local lymphocytes secrete chemical mediators of inflammation (lym-

phokines) that produce the clinical and histologic changes characteristic of this process.

Clinical Features. Lesions of contact allergy occur directly adjacent to the causative agent (Fig. 2–47), unless the material is volatile, in which case distant tissue may be affected. Presenting lesions range from erythematous to vesicular to ulcerative.

Although contact allergy is frequently seen on the skin, it is relatively uncommon intraorally. Some of the many materials containing agents known to cause oral contact allergic reactions are toothpaste, mouthwash, candy, chewing gum, topical antimicrobials, topical steroids, iodine, essential oils, and denture base material (Fig. 2–48).

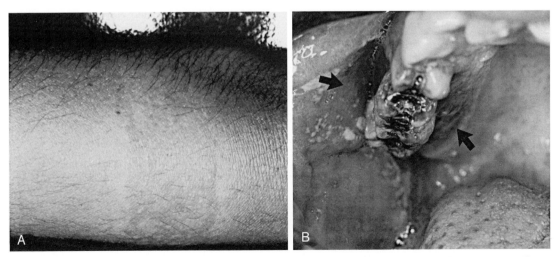

Figure 2–47. *A,* Contact allergic lesion on the wrist associated with a watch band. (Courtesy of Dr. S. K. Young.) *B,* Contact allergic reaction of the gingiva and buccal mucosa *(arrows)* caused by a periodontal pack.

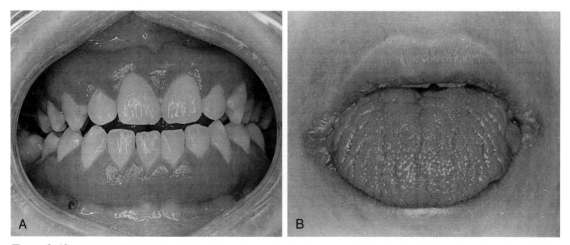

Figure 2–48. *A* and *B,* Oral lesions attributed to an allergen in chewing gum. *A,* The gingiva is intensely erythematous. *B,* The tongue epithelium is atrophic, and commissures are fissured.

Cinnamon has been specifically identified as an etiologic agent in oral contact stomatitis. Lesions associated with this offender are usually white or even lichenoid, although ulcerative and red lesions may be seen.

Although denture acrylic is frequently held accountable for allergic contact reactions in the palate, this is probably a misconception. These red lesions are more likely related to chronic candidiasis. If a component of the denture material, especially unpolymerized monomer, were responsible for allergic change, tissue reaction would be seen not only in the palate but also on the alveolar ridge and on the buccal mucosa where contact is made.

Histopathology. Microscopically, the epithelium and connective tissue show inflammatory changes. Spongiosis and vesiculation may be seen within the epithelium. A perivascular lymphophagocytic infiltrate is found in the immediate supporting connective tissue. Blood vessels may be dilated, and occasional eosinophils may be seen.

Diagnosis. Careful history taking is essential. Establishing a cause and effect relationship between offending agent and tissue change may not always be possible. Biopsy may be helpful. Patch testing may be helpful but should be performed by an expert in the area because of the possibility of producing false-positive results when done on skin and false-negative results when attempted on mucosa.

Treatment. Primary treatment should be directed at elimination of the offending material if it can be identified. In uncomplicated cases, lesions should heal in 1 to 2 weeks. Topical steroids may hasten the healing process.

Wegener's Granulomatosis

Etiology. Wegener's granulomatosis is an inflammatory condition of unknown etiology. Efforts to identify a cause have generally focused on infection and immunologic dysfunction but have been unproductive.

Clinical Features. Typically, the triad of upper respiratory tract, lung, and kidney involvement is seen in this condition. Occasionally, only two of the three sites are affected. Lesions may also present in the oral cavity and skin and, potentially, in any other organ system. The basic pathologic process that is common to all foci is necrotizing vasculitis and granulomatous inflammation.

This is a rare disease of middle age. Initial presentation often occurs with head and neck symptoms. Symptoms typical of sinusitis, rhinorrhea, nasal stuffiness, and epistaxis may be seen with or without nonspecific complaints of fever, arthralgia, and weight loss. In a majority of cases, nasal or sinus (usually maxillary) involvement is seen and is often present early in the course of the disease. Destructive lesions are typically ulcerated; necrosis and perforation of the nasal septum are occasionally seen. Perforation of the hard palate is uncommonly seen in Wegener's granulomatosis. Intraorally, red granular gingival lesions have been reported (Fig. 2–49). The process is generalized and results in relatively uniform enlargement. Most patients have kidney involvement that consists of a focal necrotizing glomerulitis. Renal failure is the final outcome of kidney disease. Inflammatory lung lesions, varying in intensity from slight to severe, may eventually lead to respiratory failure.

Histopathology. The basic pathologic process

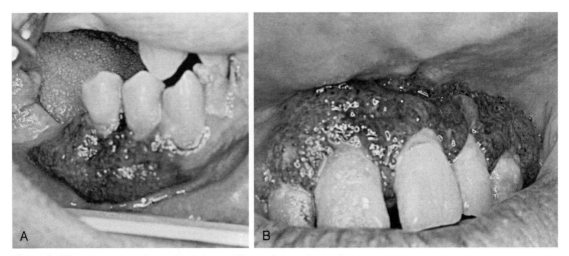

Figure 2–49. *A* and *B,* Granular erosive lesions of Wegener's granulomatosis.

is granulomatous, with necrotizing vasculitis usually present. Variable numbers of acute and chronic inflammatory cells are seen in the granulomatous zones. Necrosis and multinucleated giant cells may be seen in the granulomatous areas. The affected small vessels show a mononuclear infiltrate within their walls in the presence of fibrinoid necrosis. Definitive diagnosis in the absence of vascular changes is difficult, because the microscopy findings would be nonspecific. Diagnosis may be made by exclusion of other diseases.

Diagnosis. Diagnosis is generally dependent on the finding of granulomatous vasculitis in biopsy tissue of upper respiratory tract lesions, evidence of involvement of lung, or kidney lesions. Development of labeled antineutrophil cytoplasmic antibodies has provided serologic correlation with biopsy-proven vasculitis. On both a clinical and a microscopic level, chronic infectious processes, such as TB, syphilis, histoplasmosis, and blastomycosis, and neoplastic processes, such as lymphoma and undifferentiated squamous cell carcinoma, might be serious considerations in a differential diagnosis of this disease. Culture and tissue identification of microorganisms, when negative, would help rule out infectious processes.

Immunohistochemical staining could be used to help rule out neoplasia.

Treatment. Before the development of chemotherapeutic agents, renal failure and death were frequent outcomes of this disease process. The use of the cytotoxic agent cyclophosphamide and corticosteroids has provided patients having this disease with a relatively favorable prognosis. Remissions occur in approximately 75% of cases.

Midline Granuloma

Midline granuloma is a diagnosis made by exclusion of other granulomatous and necrotizing midfacial lesions. Some investigators believe that this condition represents an atypical or unrecognized lymphoma.

Etiology. Because midline granuloma has many features that overlap with Wegener's granulomatosis, these two conditions were at one time classified together (Table 2–11). Midline granuloma, like Wegener's granulomatosis, is of unknown cause, although a hyperimmune response to a yet unidentified antigen is suspected. Lym-

Table 2–11. Comparison of Wegener's Granulomatosis and Midline Granuloma

FEATURE	WEGENER'S GRANULOMATOSIS	MIDLINE GRANULOMA
Etiology	Unknown	Unknown
Location	Upper respiratory tract, lung, kidney	Upper respiratory tract, oral (may have palate perforation)
Histology	Granulomatous	Nonspecific
	Necrotizing vasculitis	Inflammation
Treatment	Cyclophosphamide/prednisone	Radiation

phoid neoplasia from chronic immune stimulation has also been suggested.

Clinical Features. Midline granuloma is a unifocal destructive process, generally in the midline of the oronasal region, that does not affect other organ systems. Lesions appear clinically as aggressive necrotic ulcers that are progressive and nonhealing (Fig. 2–50). Extension through soft tissue, cartilage, and bone is typical. Perforation of the nasal septum and hard palate is characteristic as well. Without treatment, the inflammatory process eventually consumes the patient, and because of continuous erosion into vital structures, especially blood vessels, death has been a typical outcome.

Histopathology. Microscopically, the process is nonspecific and typically appears as acute and chronic inflammation in partially necrotic tissue. Because of the almost trivial inflammatory appearance of this condition, several biopsies may be required before one may be confident or comfortable with the diagnosis of midline granuloma.

Differential Diagnosis. Clinically, destructive processes of the midline of the nose or palate would include Wegener's granulomatosis, infectious disease, and neoplasia. Bacterial infection, such as TB and syphilis (gumma), may present as a chronic ulcerative process. This is also possible for deep fungal diseases such as histoplasmosis, blastomycosis, and phycomycosis. Neoplasia (poorly differentiated squamous cell carcinoma, sarcomas, and lymphomas) could also present as a destructive midline process.

Treatment. The treatment of choice is high-dose local radiation. It is relatively effective and has produced a reasonably optimistic prognosis.

Corticosteroids also have been used with partial success.

Chronic Granulomatous Disease

Etiology and Pathogenesis. This rare systemic disease is inherited in an X-linked manner and occasionally in an autosomal recessive mode. The resulting clinical defect is altered neutrophil and macrophage function. These cells have the capacity to phagocytose microorganisms but lack the ability to kill certain bacteria and fungi owing to insufficient intracellular enzymatic function.

Clinical Features. Manifestations of chronic granulomatous disease appear during childhood and, because of the more frequent X-linked inheritance pattern, occur predominantly in males. The process may affect many organs, including lymph nodes, lung, liver, spleen, bone, and skin, as recurrent or persistent infections. Oral lesions are frequently seen in the form of multiple ulcers that are also recurrent or persistent.

Histopathology. Microscopically, the lesions of chronic granulomatous disease are granular or nodular. Granulomas may exhibit central necrosis.

Diagnosis. The clinical features of recurrent or persistent infections in young patients and the presence in tissue samples of granulomatous inflammation suggest a diagnosis of chronic granulomatous disease. Neutrophil function tests would help confirm the diagnosis. In the differential diagnosis, other granulomatous diseases, such as Crohn's disease, TB, histoplasmosis, blastomycosis, and tularemia, could be included.

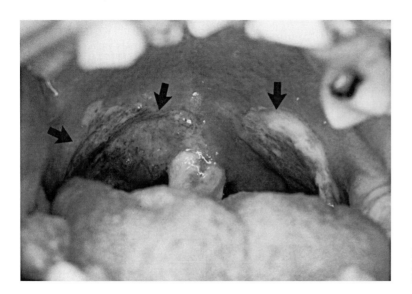

Figure 2–50. Soft palate and uvular ulcers *(arrows)* of midline granuloma.

Treatment. Treatment is based on the use of specific antimicrobial agents that are directed against the appropriate organism. Those agents that are capable of penetrating mononuclear cell membranes to reach the cytoplasm, where the organisms reside, are especially useful.

Cyclic Neutropenia

This rare blood dyscrasia of unknown cause is manifested as severe cyclic depletions of neutrophils from the blood and marrow, with a mean cycle or periodicity of about 21 days. Fever, malaise, oral ulcers, cervical lymphadenopathy, and infections may appear during neutropenic episodes. Patients are also prone to exaggeration of periodontal disease. There is no definitive treatment. Early recognition of infections is important in management, as is judicious use of antibiotics.

NEOPLASMS

Squamous Cell Carcinoma

Relative to incidence of all cancers, oral and oropharyngeal squamous cell carcinomas represent about 3% of the total in men and 2% in women. When stated as numbers, however, the statistics seem more impressive. Annually, nearly 30,000 new cases of oral and oropharyngeal cancer are expected to occur in men and women in the United States. The ratio of men to women is now about 2 to 1. This shift from 3 to 1 has been related to an increase in smoking by women and to their longer life expectancy.

Deaths due to oral and oropharyngeal cancer represent approximately 2% of the total in men and 1% in women. The total number of annual deaths are as great as 9500.

The trend in survival of patients with this malignancy has been rather disappointing during the past several decades, improving only slightly from 45% to about 50%. The survival rates for blacks were estimated to be significantly and consistently lower. Geographic variations in oral and oropharyngeal carcinoma survival rates exist in the United States and around the world and are most likely connected to habits related to the etiology of this condition.

The survival rate of oral and oropharyngeal cancer has remained disappointingly low and relatively constant, despite advances in detection and treatment of many other malignancies. Currently, improvement of survival rate lies in early detection, an area in which dental practitioners must

have a primary role. The oral cavity is readily accessible for examination and biopsy, making early diagnosis a realistic and achievable goal in oral cancer control.

Etiology. Of all factors believed to contribute to the etiology of oral cancer, tobacco is regarded as the most important. All forms of tobacco smoking as well as the use of smokeless tobacco have been strongly linked to the cause of oral cancer. Cigar and pipe smoking is linked to greater risk for the development of oral cancer than cigarette smoking, unless "reverse smoking" is done, as may be the habit in India and some South American countries. In this form of smoking, the lighted end of the cigarette is held inside the mouth. The risk then becomes exceedingly high because of the intensity of tobacco combustion adjacent to palatal and lingual tissues. In any event, the time-dose relationship of carcinogens found in tobacco smoke as well as in the tobacco itself is of paramount importance in the cause of oral cancer. The greater the length of time tobacco is used and the greater the amount used, the greater the risk. In addition to an overall increased risk of development of cancer in all regions of the mouth, pipe smokers appear to have a special predilection for squamous cell carcinoma of the lower lip.

With the use of smokeless tobacco, whether in the form of snuff (ground and finely cut tobacco) or chewing tobacco (loose-leaf tobacco), the risk of developing oral cancer is increased, especially relative to buccal mucosa and gingiva. Increased sales and use of smokeless tobacco are believed to be due largely to marketing campaigns and peer pressure. Advocated by few to be a relatively safe substitute for cigarettes, the use of smokeless tobacco cannot be condoned and must be regarded as a health hazard. An additional new concern is that young smokeless tobacco users will eventually switch to cigarettes. The use of smokeless tobacco has not only a relationship to oral cancer but also a direct relationship to elevation of blood pressure, physiologic dependence, and periodontal disease.

In India and some other Asian countries, oral cancer is the most common type of malignancy and may account for more than 50% of all cancer cases. This is generally linked to the use of smokeless tobacco mixed with other materials and to the prevalence of its use. The tobacco, typically used with betel nut, slaked lime, and spices, is known as the quid, or pan, and is held in the buccal vestibule for long periods. This combination of ingredients, which may vary from one locale to another, is more carcinogenic than tobacco used alone.

Alcohol consumption also appears to add to the

risk of oral cancer development. Identification of alcohol alone as a carcinogenic factor has been somewhat difficult because of mixed smoking and drinking habits by most patients with oral cancer. Nonetheless, most authorities regard alcohol as at least a modifier if not an initiator of oral cancer. Its effects are simplistically thought to occur through its ability to irritate mucosa and its ability to act as a solvent for carcinogens, especially those in tobacco. Carcinogenic contaminants in alcoholic drinks are also thought to have a role in cancer development.

Some microorganisms have been implicated in oral cancer. The fungus *C. albicans* has been suggested as a possible causative agent; this theory is based on its potential to produce a carcinogen, *N*-nitrosobenzylmethylamine. The link between some viruses and some types of oral cancer has been shown to be relatively strong. Epstein-Barr virus has been linked to Burkitt's lymphoma and nasopharyngeal carcinoma. Its effects seem to be related, in part, to the suppression of apoptosis in tumor cells. Human herpesvirus type 8 (HHV8) has been linked to Kaposi's sarcoma. Studies have demonstrated the presence of human papillomavirus (HPV) subtypes 16 and 18 in oral squamous cell carcinomas, suggesting a role for this virus in oral cancers. Verrucous carcinoma has also been identified as a lesion possibly related to HPV infection. The mechanism by which HPV contributes to carcinogenesis is through viral proteins, E6 and E7, which can complex to p53 protein and retinoblastoma proteins, respectively. In oral cancer, inhibition of native or wild-type p53 would lead to acceleration of cell cycle and a compromised DNA repair mechanism.

The only convincing nutritional problem that has been associated with oral cancer is iron deficiency associated with *Plummer-Vinson syndrome,* which typically affects middle-aged women. The syndrome components include a painful red tongue, mucosal atrophy, dysphagia, and a predisposition to the development of oral squamous cell carcinoma.

Ultraviolet light is a known carcinogenic agent that is a significant factor in basal cell carcinomas of the skin and squamous cell carcinomas of the skin and lip. The cumulative dose of sunlight and the amount of protection by natural pigmentation are of great significance in the development of these cancers. In the ultraviolet light spectrum, radiation with a wavelength of 2900 to 3200 nm (UVB) is more carcinogenic than light of 3200 to 3400 nm (UVA).

A compromised immune system puts patients at risk for oral cancer (as well as lymphoproliferative diseases). This increased risk has been docu-

mented for bone marrow transplant recipients. The total body radiation and high-dose chemotherapy that are used to condition patients for transplants puts patients at lifelong risk for solid and lymphoid malignancies.

Chronic irritation is generally regarded as a modifier rather than an initiator of oral cancer. Mechanical trauma from ill-fitting dentures, broken fillings, and other frictional rubs is unlikely to cause oral cancer. If, however, a cancer is started from another cause, these factors will probably hasten the process. Poor oral hygiene is also regarded as having a comparable modifying effect.

Molecular Basis of Oral Cancer. The common denominator to all the etiologic factors of oral cancer is their ability to alter the mucosal keratinocyte genome permanently. These factors, through mutation, amplification, or deactivation of oncogenes and tumor suppressor genes, can lead to the phenomenon known as cancer. The protein products of these genes are crucial to the control of cell cycle (proliferation, suppression, signaling), cell survival (apoptosis, antiapoptosis), and cell mobility. In general, it is believed that malignancy is the accumulation of many sustained unrepaired genetic events in a cell line. The products of these mutated or modified genes give the malignant cells a proliferation and motility advantage over normally regulated cells.

It is becoming apparent that in different cell types of different organ systems, malignancy arises from a different combination of mutated/dysregulated genes. Among the genetic events that give rise to cancer is a mutation that is common to almost all cancers: mutation (and occasionally dysregulation) of the *p53* gene. This is a key genetic alteration because the protein product of *p53* normally arrests cell proliferation to allow repair of damaged DNA so that mutations are not perpetuated. Other oncoproteins that seem to have some role in oral carcinomas through mutation or dysregulation include those associated with genes known as *c-Myc, Ras, Bcl-2, MDM-2,* and *p16.* Undoubtedly, additional genes (and gene products) will be found to contribute to oral carcinogenesis. Determining how frequent and how important these changes are in the malignant transformation process is an important objective of current cancer research. Modern cancer therapy may eventually be based on control of the altered genes or their protein products.

Clinical Features
Carcinoma of the Lips. From a biologic viewpoint, carcinomas of the lower lip should be separated from carcinomas of the upper lip. Carcinomas of the lower lip are far more common than

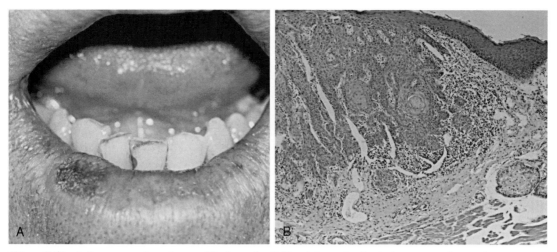

Figure 2–51. *A,* Squamous cell carcinoma of the lower lip. *B,* Elevated margins due to the presence of a neoplasm.

upper lip lesions. Ultraviolet light and pipe smoking are much more important in the cause of lower lip cancer than upper lip cancer. The growth rate is slower for lower lip cancers than for upper lip cancers. The prognosis for lower lip lesions is generally very favorable, whereas the prognosis for upper lip lesions is only fair.

Lip carcinomas account for 25 to 30% of all oral cancers. They appear most commonly between 50 and 70 years of age and affect men much more often than women. Lesions arise on vermilion and may appear as chronic nonhealing ulcers (Fig. 2–51) or as exophytic lesions that are occasionally verrucous in nature (Fig. 2–52). Deep invasion generally appears later in the course of the disease. Metastasis to local submental or sub-

mandibular lymph nodes is uncommon but is more likely with larger, more poorly differentiated lesions.

Carcinoma of the Tongue. Squamous cell carcinoma of the tongue is the most common intraoral malignancy. Excluding lip lesions, it accounts for between 25 and 40% of oral carcinomas. It has a definite predilection for males in their sixth, seventh, and eighth decades. However, lesions may uncommonly be found in the very young. These lesions often exhibit a particularly aggressive behavior.

Lingual carcinoma is typically asymptomatic. In later stages, as deep invasion occurs, pain or dysphagia may be a prominent patient complaint. The characteristic clinical appearance is one of an

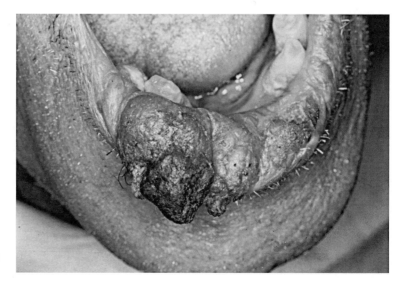

Figure 2–52. Exophytic squamous cell carcinoma of the lip.

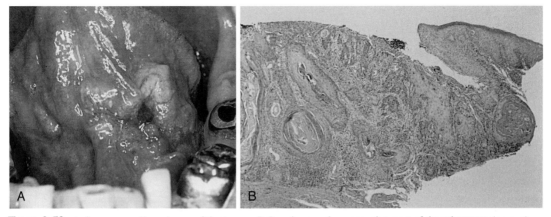

Figure 2–53. *A,* Squamous cell carcinoma of the tongue. *B,* Invasive neoplasm occupies most of the submucosa *(arrows).*

indurated, nonhealing ulcer with elevated margins (Figs. 2–53 and 2–54). The neoplasm may occasionally have a prominent exophytic as well as an endophytic growth pattern. A small percentage of leukoplakias of the tongue represent invasive squamous cell carcinoma or eventually become squamous cell carcinoma. Most erythroplakic patches that appear on the tongue are either *in situ* or invasive squamous cell carcinomas at the time of discovery.

The most common location of cancer of the tongue is the posterior lateral border, accounting for as many as 45% of tongue lesions. Lesions very uncommonly develop on the dorsum or in the tip of the tongue. Approximately 25% of tongue cancers occur in the posterior one third or base of the tongue. These lesions are more troublesome than the others because of their silent progression in an area that is difficult to visualize. Accordingly, these lesions are more often advanced or have metastasized regionally by the time they are discovered, reflecting a significantly poorer prognosis than for lesions of the anterior two thirds.

Metastases from tongue cancer are relatively common at the time of primary treatment. In general, metastatic deposits from squamous cell carcinoma of the tongue are found in the lymph nodes of the neck, usually on the ipsilateral side. The first nodes to become involved are the submandibular or jugulodigastric nodes at the angle of the mandible. Uncommonly, distant metastatic deposits may be seen in the lung or the liver.

Carcinoma of the Floor of the Mouth. The floor of the mouth is the second most common intraoral location of squamous cell carcinomas, accounting for 15 to 20% of cases. Again, carcinomas in this location occur predominantly in older men, especially those who are chronic alcoholics and smokers. The usual presenting appearance is that of a painless, nonhealing, indurated ulcer (Fig. 2–55). It may also appear as a white or red patch (Fig. 2–56). The lesion occasionally may widely infiltrate the soft tissues of the floor of the mouth, causing decreased mobility of the tongue. Metastasis to submandibular lymph nodes is not uncommon for lesions of the floor of the mouth.

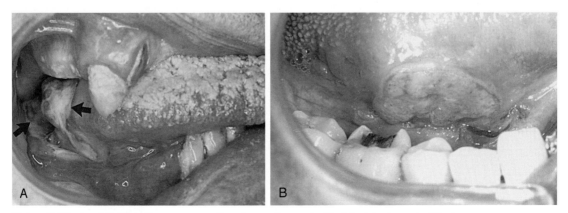

Figure 2–54. *A* and *B,* Ulcerative squamous cell carcinomas *(arrows* in *A)* of the lateral aspect of the tongue.

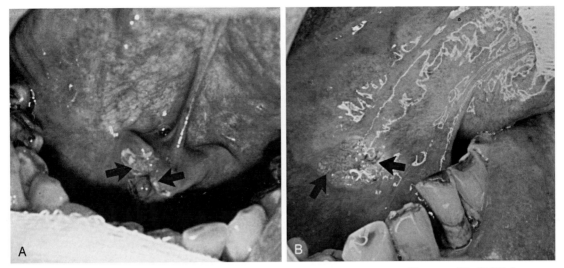

Figure 2–55. *A* and *B,* Early squamous cell carcinomas of the floor of the mouth *(arrows).* (Courtesy of Dr. E. Ellis.)

Carcinoma of the Buccal Mucosa and Gingiva. Lesions of the buccal mucosa and gingiva each account for approximately 10% of oral squamous cell carcinomas. Men in their seventh decade typify the group affected. Smokeless tobacco is an important etiologic factor in malignant change in these regions. The presenting clinical appearance varies from a white patch to a nonhealing ulcer to an exophytic lesion (Fig. 2–57). In the last-mentioned group is the clinical pathologic entity *verrucous carcinoma.* This subset of squamous cell carcinoma, most often associated with the use of smokeless tobacco, presents as a broad-based, wart-like mass (Fig. 2–58). It is slow growing and very well differentiated, rarely metastasizes, and has a very favorable prognosis.

Carcinoma of the Palate. There is some justi-fication for the separation of cancers of the hard palate from those of the soft palate. In the soft palate and contiguous faucial tissues, squamous cell carcinoma is a fairly common occurrence, accounting for 10 to 20% of intraoral lesions. In the hard palate, squamous cell carcinomas are relatively uncommon but adenocarcinomas are relatively common. However, palatal carcinomas are frequently encountered in countries such as India where reverse smoking is the custom.

Palatal squamous cell carcinomas generally present as asymptomatic red or white plaques or as ulcerated and keratotic masses (adenocarcinomas initially appear as nonulcerated masses) in older men (Figs. 2–59 and 2–60). Metastasis to cervical nodes or large lesions signifies an ominous course.

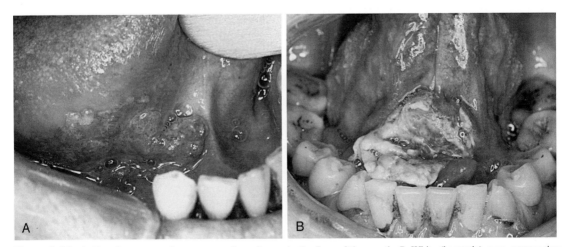

Figure 2–56. *A,* Granular pattern of squamous cell carcinoma in the floor of the mouth. *B,* White (keratotic) mass representing advanced carcinoma.

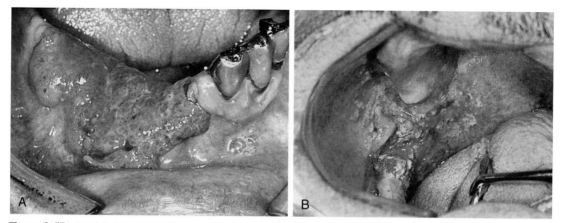

Figure 2–57. *A* and *B,* Squamous cell carcinoma of the alveolar ridge and retromolar pad.

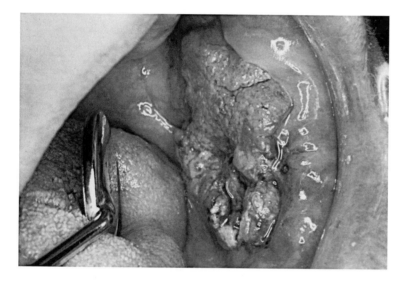

Figure 2–58. Verrucous carcinoma of the buccal mucosa. (Courtesy of Dr. J. R. Hayward.)

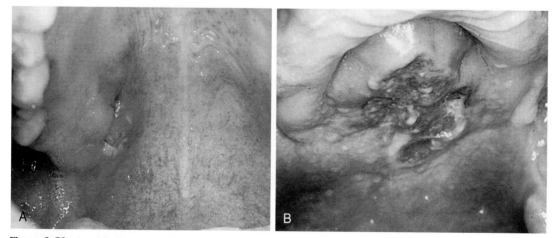

Figure 2–59. *A* and *B,* Squamous cell carcinoma of the palate.

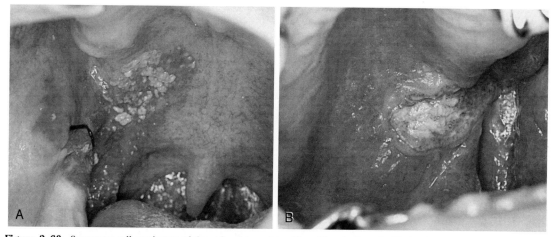

Figure 2–60. Squamous cell carcinoma of the soft palate and tonsillar pillar. *A,* Note the black silk suture at the biopsy site. *B,* Second primary oral cancer in a 58-year-old man.

Histopathology. Most oral squamous cell carcinomas are moderately or well-differentiated lesions. Keratin pearls and individual cell keratinization are usually evident. Invasion into subjacent structures in the form of small nests of hyperchromatic cells is also typical. *In situ* carcinoma extension into salivary excretory ducts can be regarded as a high-risk microscopic sign for potential recurrence. It probably equates with invasion. Considerable variation between tumors is seen relative to numbers of mitoses, nuclear pleomorphism, and amount of keratinization. In hematoxylin and eosin–stained sections of poorly differentiated lesions, keratin is absent or is seen in minute amounts. It can, however, be identified using immunohistochemical techniques for the demonstration of antigenic determinants on otherwise occult keratin intermediate filaments. A significant inflammatory host response is usually found surrounding the nests of invading tumor cells. Lymphocytes, plasma cells, and macrophages all may be seen in large numbers.

Rarely, an oral squamous cell carcinoma appears as a proliferation of spindle cells that may be mistaken for a sarcoma. This type of tumor, known as *spindle cell carcinoma,* arises from the surface epithelium usually of the lips and occasionally of the tongue. Immunohistochemical staining can be used to identify keratin antigens in this lesion when hematoxylin and eosin–stained sections show equivocal findings.

Verrucous carcinoma is characterized by very well-differentiated epithelial cells that appear more hyperplastic than neoplastic. A key feature is the invasive nature of the lesion in the form of broad pushing margins. The advancing front is usually surrounded by lymphocytes, plasma cells, and macrophages. Diagnosis based solely on mi-

croscopic features is often difficult; it is frequently necessary to consider the lesion in the context of clinical presentation.

Another microscopic variant that has a predilection for base of tongue and pharynx is biologically highly malignant and is known as *basaloid-squamous carcinoma.* In these tumors, a basaloid pattern of tumor cells is seen adjacent to tumor cells that exhibit squamous differentiation. This tumor may be confused microscopically with basaloid adenoidcystic carcinoma and adenosquamous carcinoma.

Differential Diagnosis. When oral squamous cell carcinomas present in their typical clinical form of chronic nonhealing ulcers, other ulcerative conditions should be considered. An undiagnosed chronic ulcer must always be considered potentially infectious until biopsy proves otherwise. It may be impossible on clinical grounds to separate TB, syphilis, and deep fungal infections expressing oral manifestations from oral cancer. Chronic trauma, including factitial injuries, may also mimic squamous cell carcinoma. Careful history taking is especially important, and biopsy confirms the diagnosis. In the palate and contiguous tissues, midline granuloma and necrotizing sialometaplasia would be serious diagnostic considerations.

Treatment. Generally, oral cancers are best treated with surgery or radiation or both. Smaller lesions are typically treated with surgery alone, with radiation used as a backup in the event of recurrence. Factors that determine which is to be used include lesion location, histologic type, institution facilities and philosophy, referral patterns, and therapist skills. All things being equal, cure rates are essentially similar, particularly in stage I and early stage II lesions. Larger lesions may

Table 2–12. Side Effects of Therapeutic Radiation

TEMPORARY SIDE EFFECTS	PERMANENT SIDE EFFECTS
Mucosal ulcers	Xerostomia
Pain	Cervical caries
Dysgeusia/hypogeusia	Osteonecrosis
Candidiasis	Telangiectasia
Dermatitis	Epithelial atrophy
Erythema	Alopecia (higher doses)
Alopecia (lower doses)	

be treated with either modality or with surgery followed by radiation. Elective or prophylactic neck dissection or radiation is advocated by many in order to eliminate subclinical or occult metastases. Oral squamous cell carcinomas are generally resistant to chemotherapeutic measures. Effects are generally measured in terms of tumor regression rather than elimination. Although anticancer drugs may reduce tumor bulk and delay spread, the profound morbidity associated with this type of treatment may not justify its use. When chemotherapy is used to treat oral squamous cell carcinoma, it is usually used as adjunctive therapy in advanced cases.

Therapeutic Radiation Regimens and Complications. In the head and neck, therapeutic radiation is most commonly used in the treatment of squamous cell carcinomas and lymphomas. It tends to be more effective on less well-differentiated lesions. Early reports indicated that verrucous lesions were radioresistant, but this concept has been challenged.

The radiation level needed to kill malignant cells ranges from 40 to 70 Gy. In order to make this tolerable to patients, radiation is fractionated into daily doses of approximately 2 Gy. This allows delivery over a 4- to 7-week period of a total tumor dose of 40 to 50 Gy for lymphomas and 60 to 70 Gy for squamous cell carcinomas.

Along with the therapeutic effects of radiation are side effects that are dose dependent (Table 2–12). Some of these are reversible, although others are not. Radiation-induced mucositis and ulcers and the accompanying pain, xerostomia, loss of taste, and dysgeusia are common side effects (Fig. 2–61). Radiation mucositis is a reversible condition that begins 1 to 2 weeks after the start of therapy and ends several weeks after the termination of therapy. Oral candidiasis often accompanies the mucositis. Use of antifungals, chlorhexidine rinses, or salt-soda rinses helps reduce morbidity.

Permanent damage to salivary gland tissue situated in the beam path may produce significant levels of xerostomia. Some recovery is often noted, especially at lower radiation levels. Xerostomia is frequently a patient's chief complaint during the postradiation period. The frequent use of water or artificial saliva is of minimal benefit to these patients. Pilocarpine, used during the course of radiation, may provide some protective measure of salivary function. With the dryness also comes the potential for the development of cervical or so-called radiation caries (Figs. 2–62 and 2–63). This problem can be minimized with regular follow-up dental care and scrupulous oral hygiene (Fig. 2–64).

Skin in the path of the radiation beam also suffers some damage. Alopecia is temporary at lower radiation levels but permanent at the higher levels required in the treatment of squamous cell

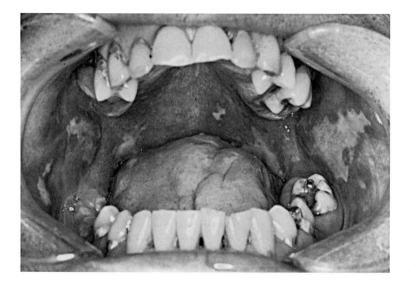

Figure 2–61. Acute radiation-induced ulcers (mucositis).

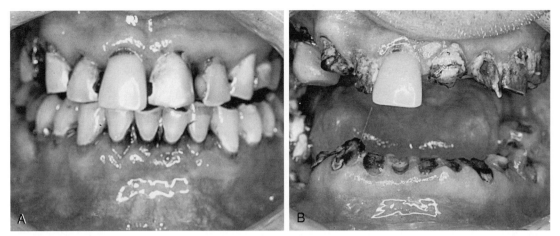

Figure 2–62. *A,* Cervical radiation caries resulting from xerostomia and poor oral hygiene. *B,* Same patient 3 years later.

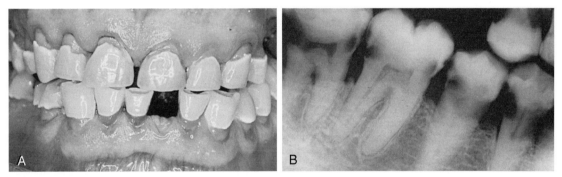

Figure 2–63. *A* and *B,* Radiation-associated cervical caries.

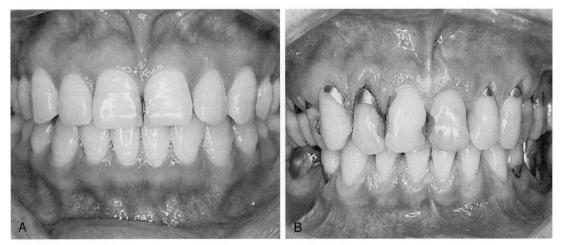

Figure 2–64. *A* and *B,* Postirrradiation-status patients with xerostomia but excellent oral hygiene and follow-up care.

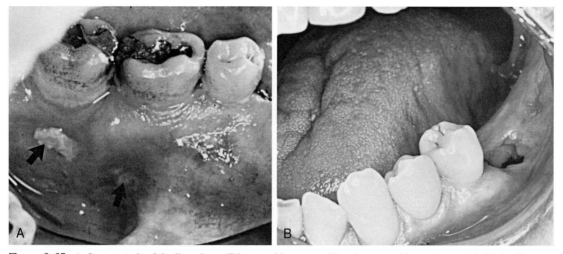

Figure 2–65. *A,* Osteonecrosis of the lingual mandible caused by trauma. Note the exposed bone *(arrows). B,* Nonhealing bone of 2 years' duration in site of postradiation extraction.

carcinoma. Skin erythema is temporary, but the telangiectasias and atrophy that follow are permanent.

A more insidious and hidden problem lies in the damage that radiation causes to bone, which may result in osteonecrosis. Radiation apparently has deleterious effects on osteocytes, osteoblasts, and endothelial cells, causing reduced capacity of bone to recover from injury. Injury may come in the form of trauma (such as extractions), advancing periodontal disease, and periapical inflammation associated with nonvital teeth (Fig. 2–65). Once osteonecrosis occurs, varying amounts of bone (usually in the mandible) are lost. This may be an area as small as a few millimeters in size to

as large as half the jaw or more (Fig. 2–66). The most important factor responsible for osteonecrosis is the amount of radiation directed through bone on the path to the tumor. Oral health is also of considerable significance. Poor nutrition and chronic alcoholism appear to be influential in the progression of this complication. Conservative surgical removal of necrotic bone may assist in the healing process. Also, if available, the use of a hyperbaric oxygen chamber may provide the patients with a healing advantage.

Because osteonecrosis is a danger that is always present after radiation, tooth extractions should be avoided after therapy. If absolutely necessary, tooth removal should be performed as atraumati-

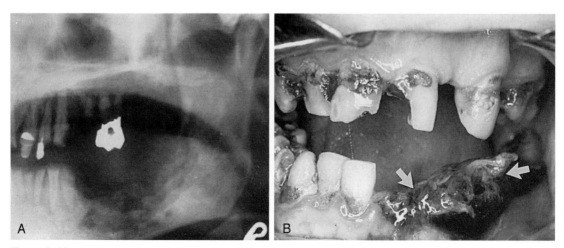

Figure 2–66. *A,* Advanced osteonecrosis of the mandible in the same patient as in Figure 2–60. *B,* Advanced cervical caries and necrosis of the mandibular bone *(arrows).*

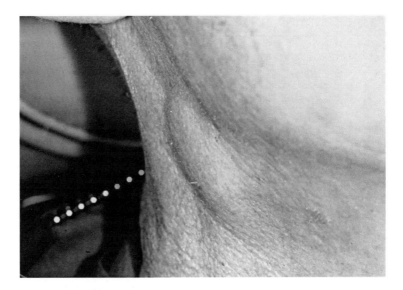

Figure 2–67. Lymph node metastasis from oral squamous cell carcinoma (stage III disease).

cally as possible, using antibiotic coverage. It is preferable to commit to a treatment plan that schedules tooth removal before radiation therapy begins. Initial soft tissue healing before beginning therapy reduces the risk of nonhealing of the extraction sites. Prosthetic devices such as dentures and partial dentures, if carefully constructed and monitored, can be worn without difficulty. Xerostomia does not seem to cause difficulty in wearing these prostheses. Continued careful surveillance of the patient's oral health, during and after radiation therapy, helps keep complications to an acceptable minimum.

Prognosis. The prognosis for patients with oral squamous cell carcinoma is dependent on both histologic subtype (grade) and clinical extent (stage) of the tumor. Of the two, clinical stage is more important. Other, more abstract factors that may influence clinical course include age, gender, general health, immune system status, and mental attitude.

The grading of a tumor is the microscopic determination of the differentiation of the tumor cells. Well-differentiated lesions generally have a less aggressive biologic course than poorly differentiated lesions. Of all squamous cell carcinoma histologic subtypes, the most well differentiated, verrucous carcinoma, has the most favorable prognosis. The less-differentiated lesions have a correspondingly poorer prognosis.

The most important indicator of prognosis is the clinical stage of the disease. Once metastasis to cervical nodes has occurred, the 5-year survival rate is reduced by approximately half. The overall 5-year survival rate for oral squamous cell carcinoma is around 45 to 50%. If the neoplasm is small and localized, the 5-year cure rate may be

as high as 60 to 70% (lower lip lesions may rate as high as 80 to 90%). However, if cervical metastases are present at the time of diagnosis, the survival figures drop precipitously to about 25% (Fig. 2–67).

A numeric system for the clinical staging of oral squamous cell carcinoma has been devised to provide clinical uniformity. It is known as the TNM system—T is a measure of the primary tumor size, N is an estimation of the regional lymph node metastasis, and M is a determination of distant metastases (Table 2–13). Use of this system allows more meaningful comparison of data from different institutions and helps guide therapeutic decisions. As the clinical stage advances from I to IV, prognosis worsens (Table 2–14).

Another factor that comes into play in the overall prognosis of oral cancer is the increased risk for the development of a second primary lesion.

Table 2–13. TNM Staging System for Oral Squamous Cell Carcinoma

T—Tumor
T_1—Tumor less than 2 cm in diameter
T_2—Tumor 2–4 cm in diameter
T_3—Tumor greater than 4 cm in diameter
T_4—Tumor invades adjacent structures

N—Node
N_0—No palpable nodes
N_1—Ipsilateral palpable nodes
N_2—Contralateral or bilateral nodes
N_3—Fixed palpable nodes

M—Metastasis
M_0—No distant metastasis
M_1—Clinical or radiographic evidence of metastasis

Table 2-14. TNM Staging System

Stage I	$T_1 N_0 M_0$
Stage II	$T_2 N_0 M_0$
Stage III	$T_3 N_0 M_0$
	$T_1 N_1 M_0$
	$T_2 N_1 M_0$
	$T_3 N_1 M_0$
Stage IV	$T_1 N_2 M_0$
	$T_2 N_2 M_0$
	$T_3 N_2 M_0$
	$T_1 N_3 M_0$
	$T_2 N_3 M_0$
	$T_3 N_3 M_0$
	$T_4 N_0 M_0$
	Any patients with M_1

These lesions represent not recurrence or persistence of the original tumor but new, geographically separate lesions of the upper alimentary tract or even of other organ systems. Approximately 10% of patients with oral cancer develop a second primary lesion, often in the first or second follow-up year. The single most important factor that accounts for this phenomenon probably is the conditioning by etiologic factors of large areas of mucosa (field effect).

Carcinoma of the Maxillary Sinus

Etiology. Malignancies of the paranasal sinuses occur most commonly in the maxillary sinus. The cause is unknown, although squamous metaplasia of sinus epithelium associated with chronic sinusitis and oral antral fistulas is believed by some investigators to be a predisposing factor.

Clinical Features. This is a disease of older age, affecting predominantly patients older than 40 years. Men are generally afflicted more than women. Past history in these patients frequently includes symptoms of sinusitis. As the neoplasm progresses, a dull ache in the area occurs, with eventual development of overt pain. Specific signs and symptoms referable to oral structures are common, especially when the neoplasm has its origin in the sinus floor. As the neoplasm extends toward the apices of the maxillary posterior teeth, referred pain may occur. Toothache, which actually represents neoplastic involvement of the superior alveolar nerve, is a not uncommon symptom in patients with maxillary sinus malignancies. In ruling out dental disease by history and clinical tests, it is imperative that the dental practitioner be aware that sinus neoplasms may present through the alveolus. Without this suspicion, unfortunate delays in definitive treatment may occur. Other clinical signs of invasion of the alveolar process include recently acquired malocclusion, displacement of teeth, and vertical mobility of teeth (teeth undermined by neoplasm). Failure of a socket to heal after an extraction may be indicative of tumor involvement. Paresthesia should always be viewed as an ominous sign and should cause the clinician to consider malignancy within bone. Occasional maxillary sinus cancers may present as a palatal ulcer and mass representing extension through the bone and soft tissue of the palate (Fig. 2–68).

Histopathology. Of the malignancies that originate in the maxillary sinus, squamous cell carcinoma is the most common histologic type. These lesions are generally less differentiated than those occurring in oral mucous membranes. Infrequently, adenocarcinomas arising presumably from mucous glands in the sinus lining may be seen.

Diagnosis. From a clinical standpoint, when oral signs and symptoms appear to be related to

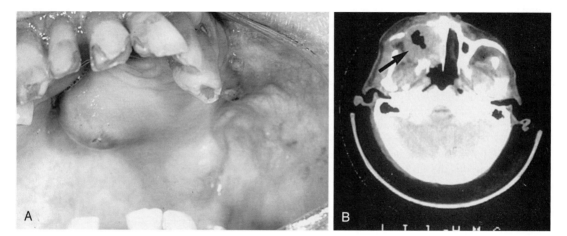

Figure 2–68. *A,* Carcinoma of the maxillary sinus presenting through the palate. *B,* Tomogram showing a maxillary sinus mass *(arrow).*

antral carcinoma, dental origin must be ruled out. This is best accomplished by the dental practitioner because of familiarity with normal tooth-jaw relationships and experience in interpretation of vitality tests. Other clinical considerations related to malignancies in the age group in which antral carcinomas occur are metastatic disease and plasma cell myeloma. Osteosarcoma and other less common sarcomas that are usually found in a younger age group might also be included. Palatal involvement should also cause the clinician to consider adenocarcinoma of minor salivary gland origin, lymphoma, and squamous cell carcinoma.

Treatment and Prognosis. Maxillary sinus carcinomas are generally treated with surgery or radiation or both. A combination of the two seems to be somewhat more effective than either modality alone. Radiation is often completed first, with surgical resection following. Chemotherapy used in conjunction with radiation has been somewhat successful.

In any event, the prognosis is only fair at best. Cure is directly dependent on the clinical stage of the disease at the time of initial treatment. Compared with oral lesions, sinus lesions are discovered in a more advanced stage because of delays in seeking treatment and delays in making a definitive diagnosis. The anatomy of the area also influences prognosis. The 5-year survival rate is about 25%. If the disease is discovered early, the likelihood of survival increases.

Bibliography

Infectious Diseases

Alfieri N, Fleury R, Opromolla D, et al. Oral lesions in borderline and reactional tuberculoid leprosy. Oral Surg Oral Med Oral Pathol 55:52–57, 1983.

Centers for Disease Control. Summaries of notifiable diseases in the United States. MMWR 39:10, 1991.

Frieden TR, Sterling T, Pablos-Mendez A, et al. The emergence of drug-resistant tuberculosis in New York City. N Engl J Med 328:521–532, 1993.

Giunta J, Fiumara N. Facts about gonorrhea and dentistry. Oral Surg Oral Med Oral Pathol 62:529–531, 1986.

Gobel M, Iseman MD, Madsen LA. Treatment of 171 patients with pulmonary tuberculosis resistant to isoniazid and rifampin. N Engl J Med 328:527–532, 1993.

Griffin J, Bach D, Nespeca J, et al. Noma. Oral Surg Oral Med Oral Pathol 56:605–607, 1983.

Happonen R, Viander M, Pelliriemi L. *Actinomyces israelii* in osteoradionecrosis of the jaws. Oral Surg 55:580–588, 1983.

Jamsky R, Christen A. Oral gonococcal infections. Oral Surg Oral Med Oral Pathol 53:358–362, 1982.

Mani N. Secondary syphilis initially diagnosed from oral lesions. Oral Surg Oral Med Oral Pathol 58:47–50, 1984.

Michaud M, Blanchette G, Tomich C. Chronic ulceration of the hard palate: first clinical sign of undiagnosed pulmonary tuberculosis. Oral Surg Oral Med Oral Pathol 57:63–67, 1984.

Morbidity and mortality report, Centers for Disease Control, Atlanta, GA. Congenital syphilis—New York City, 1986–1988. Arch Dermatol 126:288–289, 1990.

Immunologic Diseases

Alpsoy E, Yilmaz E, Basaran E. Interferon therapy for Behçet's disease. J Am Acad Dermatol 31:617–619, 1994.

Aslanzadeh J, Heim K, Espy M, et al. Detection of HSV-specific DNA in biopsy tissue of patients with erythema multiforme by polymerase chain reaction. Br J Dermatol 126:19–23, 1992.

Bangert J, Freeman R, Sontheimer R, et al. Subacute cutaneous lupus erythematosus and discoid lupus erythematosus. Arch Dermatol 120:332–337, 1984.

Batsakis J, Luna M. Midfacial necrotizing lesions. Semin Diagn Pathol 4:90–116, 1987.

Buchner A, Lozada F, Silverman S. Histopathologic spectrum of oral erythema multiforme. Oral Surg Oral Med Oral Pathol 49:221–228, 1980.

Coenen C, Borsch G, Muller K, Fabry H. Oral inflammatory changes as an initial manifestation of Crohn's disease antedating abdominal diagnosis. Dis Colon Rectum 31:548–552, 1988.

Cornell R, Stoughton R. The use of topical steroids in psoriasis. Dermatol Clin 2:397–409, 1984.

Devaney K, Travis W, Hoffman G, et al. Interpretation of head and neck biopsies in Wegener's granulomatosis. Am J Surg Pathol 14:555–564, 1990.

Ferguson M, Wray D, Carmichael H, et al. Coeliac disease associated with recurrent aphthae. Gut 21:223–226, 1980.

Firth N, Reade P. Angiotensin-converting enzyme inhibitors implicated in oral mucosal lichenoid reactions. Oral Surg Oral Med Oral Pathol 67:41–44, 1989.

Foedinger D, Sterniczky B, Elbe A, et al. Autoantibodies against desmoplakin I and II define a subset of patients with erythema multiforme major. J Invest Dermatol 106:1012–1016.

Fritz K, Weston W. Topical glucocorticosteroids. Ann Allergy 50:68–76, 1983.

Gallant C, Kenny P. Oral glucocorticoids and their complications. J Am Acad Dermatol 14:161–177, 1986.

Glenert U. Drug stomatitis due to gold therapy. Oral Surg Oral Med Oral Pathol 58:52–56, 1984.

Greenspan J, Gadol N, Olson J, et al. Lymphocyte function in recurrent aphthous ulceration. J Oral Pathol 14:592–602, 1985.

Hamuryudan V, Yurdakul S, Serdaroglu S, et al. Topical alpha interferon in the treatment of oral ulcers in Behçet's syndrome: a preliminary report. Clin Exp Rheumatol 8:51–54, 1990.

Hoffman G, Kerr G, Leavitt R, et al. Wegener's granulomatosis: an analysis of 158 patients. Ann Intern Med 116:488–498, 1992.

Jorizzo J. Behçet's disease. Arch Dermatol 122:556–558, 1986.

Kallenberg CG. Antineutrophil cytoplasmic antibodies (ANCA) and vasculitis. Clin Rheumatol 9(Suppl):132–135, 1990.

Kanas R, Jensen J, Abrams A, Wuerker R. Oral mucosal cytomegalovirus as a manifestation of the acquired immune deficiency syndrome. Oral Surg Oral Med Oral Pathol 64:183–189, 1987.

Kazmierowski J, Wuepper K. Erythema multiforme: immune-complex vasculitis of the superficial cutaneous micro-vasculature. J Invest Dermatol 71:366–369, 1978.

Khandwala A, VanInwegen RG, Alfano MC. 5% amlexanox oral paste, a new treatment for recurrent minor aphthous ulcers: I. Clinical demonstration of acceleration of wound healing and resolution of pain. Oral Surg Oral Med Oral Pathol 83:222–230, 1997.

Landesberg R, Fallon M, Insel R. Alterations of T helper/

inducer and T suppressor/inducer cells in patients with recurrent aphthous ulcers. Oral Surg Oral Med Oral Pathol 69:205–208, 1990.

Lindemann R, Riviere G, Sapp P. Oral mucosal antigen reactivity during exacerbation and remission phase of recurrent aphthous ulceration. Oral Surg Oral Med Oral Pathol 60:281–284, 1985.

Lo J, Berg R, Tomecki K. Treatment of discoid lupus erythematosus. Int J Dermatol 28:497–507, 1989.

Lozada-Nur F, Gorsky M, Silverman S. Oral erythema multiforme: clinical observations and treatment of 95 patients. Oral Surg Oral Med Oral Pathol 67:36–40, 1989.

Lozada-Nur F, Miranda C, Maliksi R. Double-blind clinical trial of 0.05% clobetasol proprionate ointment in orabase and 0.05% fluocinonide ointment in orabase in the treatment of patients with oral vesiculoerosive diseases. Oral Surg Oral Med Oral Pathol 77:598–604, 1994.

MacPhail LA, Greenspan D, Feigal DW, et al. Recurrent aphthous ulcers in association with HIV infection. Oral Surg Oral Med Oral Pathol 71:678–683, 1991.

MacPhail L, Greenspan D, Feigal D, et al. Recurrent aphthous ulcers in association with HIV infection. Oral Surg Oral Med Oral Pathol 71:678–683, 1991.

Miller R, Gould A, Bernstein M. Cinnamon-induced stomatitis venenata. Oral Surg Oral Med Oral Pathol 73:708–716, 1992.

O'Duffy J. Behçet's syndrome. N Engl J Med 323:326–327, 1990.

Olson J, Feinberg I, Silverman S Jr, et al. Serum vitamin B$_{12}$, folate, and iron levels in recurrent aphthous ulceration. Oral Surg Oral Med Oral Pathol 54:517–520, 1982.

Orme R, Nordlund J, Barich L, Brown T. The MAGIC syndrome (mouth and genital ulcers with inflamed cartilage). Arch Dermatol 126:940–944, 1990.

Pedersen A. Recurrent aphthous ulceration: virologic and immunologic aspects. APMIS suppl. 37:1–37, 1993.

Pederson A, Klausen B, Hougen H, Stenvang J. T-lymphocyte subsets in recurrent aphthous ulceration. J Oral Pathol 18:59–60, 1989.

Phelan J, Eisig S, Freedman P, et al. Major aphthous-like ulcers in patients with AIDS. Oral Surg Oral Med Oral Pathol 71:68–72, 1991.

Plemons J, Rees T, Zachariah N. Absorption of a topical steroid and evaluation of adrenal suppression in patients with erosive lichen planus. Oral Surg Oral Med Oral Pathol 69:688–693, 1990.

Porter S, Scully C, Flint S. Hematologic status in recurrent aphthous stomatitis compared with other oral disease. Oral Surg Oral Med Oral Pathol 66:41–44, 1988.

Savage N, Mohananda R, Seymour G, et al. The proportion of suppressor-inducer T-lymphocytes is reduced in recurrent aphthous stomatitis. J Oral Pathol 17:293–297, 1988.

Savage N, Seymour G, Kruger B. T-lymphocyte subset changes in recurrent aphthous stomatitis. Oral Surg Oral Med Oral Pathol 60:175–181, 1985.

Schiodt M. Oral discoid lupus erythematosus. II. Skin lesions and systemic lupus erythematosus in sixty-six patients with six-year follow-up. Oral Surg Oral Med Oral Pathol 57:177–180, 1984.

Schiodt M. Oral discoid lupus erythematosus. III. A histopathologic study of sixty-six patients. Oral Surg Oral Med Oral Pathol 57:281–293, 1984.

Schiodt M, Holmstrup P, Dabelsteen E, Ullman S. Deposits of immunoglobulins, complement, and fibrinogen in oral lupus erythematosus, lichen planus, and leukoplakia. Oral Surg Oral Med Oral Pathol 51:603–608, 1981.

Ship JA. Recurrent aphthous stomatitis. An update. Oral Surg Oral Med Oral Pathol 81:141–147, 1996.

Storrs F. Use and abuse of systemic corticosteroid therapy. J Am Acad Dermatol 1:95–105, 1979.

Wermuth D, Geoghegan W, Jordon R. Anti-Ro/SSA antibodies. Arch Dermatol 121:335–338, 1985.

Wray D, Vlagopoulos T, Siraganian R. Food allergens and basophil histamine release in recurrent aphthous stomatitis. Oral Surg Oral Med Oral Pathol 54:388–400, 1982.

Wysocki G, Brooke R. Oral manifestations of chronic granulomatous disease. Oral Surg Oral Med Oral Pathol 46:815–819, 1978.

Neoplasms

Beahrs O, Henson D, Hutter R, et al. Manual for Staging of Cancer, 3rd ed. Philadelphia, JB Lippincott, 1988, pp 27–30.

Connolly G, Winn D, Hecht S, et al. The reemergence of smokeless tobacco. N Engl J Med 314:1020–1027, 1986.

Curtis RE, Rowlings PA, Deeg HJ, et al. N Engl J Med 336:897–904, 1997.

Daley TD, Lovas JG, Peters E, et al. Salivary gland duct involvement in oral epithelial dysplasia and squamous cell carcinoma. Oral Surg Oral Med Oral Pathol 81:186–192, 1996.

Ferretti G, Raybould T, Brown A, et al. Chlorhexidine prophylaxis for chemotherapy and radiotherapy-induced stomatitis: a randomized double-blind trial. Oral Surg Oral Med Oral Pathol 69:331–338, 1990.

Flaitz CM, Nichols CM, Adler-Storthz K, Hicks MJ. Intraoral squamous cell carcinoma in human immunodeficiency virus infection. Oral Surg Oral Med Oral Pathol 80:55–62, 1995.

Gopalakrisnan R, Weghorst CM, Lehman TA, et al. Mutated and wild-type p53 expression and HPV integration in proliferative verrucous leukoplakia and oral squamous cell carcinoma. Oral Surg Oral Med Oral Pathol 83:471–477, 1997.

Jones J, Watt FM, Speight PM. Changes in the expression of alpha-V integrins in oral squamous cell carcinomas. J Oral Pathol 26:63–68, 1997.

Krogh P, Hald B, Holmstrup P. Possible mycological etiology of oral cancer: catalytic potential of infecting *Candida albicans* and other yeasts in production of *N*-nitrosobenzylmethylamine. Carcinogenesis 8:1543–1548, 1987.

Kropveld A, van Mansfield ADM, Nabben N, et al. Discordance of p53 status in matched primary tumors and metastases in head and neck squamous cell carcinoma patients. Eur J Cancer B Oral Oncol 6:388–393, 1996.

McDonald JS, Jones H, Pavelic LJ, et al. Immunohistochemical detection of the H-ras, K-ras, and N-ras oncogenes in squamous cell carcinoma of the head and neck. J Oral Pathol Med 23:342–346, 1994.

Riethdorf S, Friedrich RE, Ostwald C, et al. P53 gene mutations and HPV infection in primary head and neck squamous cell carcinomas do not correlate with overall survival: a long-term follow-up study. J Oral Pathol Med 26:315–321, 1997.

Sankaranarayanan R. Oral cancer in India: an epidemiologic and clinical review. Oral Surg Oral Med Oral Pathol 69:325–330, 1990.

Shibuya H, Amagasa T, Seta K. Leukoplakia-associated multiple carcinomas in patients with tongue carcinoma. Cancer 57:843–846, 1986.

Sugerman PB, Joseph BK, Savage NW. Review article: the role of oncogenes, tumor suppressor genes and growth factors in oral squamous cell carcinoma: a case of apoptosis versus proliferation. Oral Diseases 1:172–188, 1995.

Valdez IH, Wolff A, Atkinson JC, et al. Use of pilocarpine during head and neck radiation therapy to reduce xerostomia and salivary dysfunction. Cancer 71:1848–1851, 1993.

Watts S, Brewer Erin, Fry T. Human papillomavirus DNA types in squamous cell carcinomas of the head and neck. Oral Surg Oral Med Oral Pathol 71:701–707, 1991.

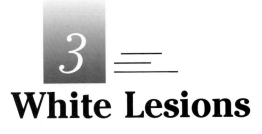

White Lesions

White-appearing lesions of the oral mucosa obtain their characteristic appearance from the scattering of light through an altered mucosal surface. Such alterations may be the result of a thickened layer of keratin, epithelial hyperplasia of the stratum malpighii, intracellular edema of epithelial cells, and reduced vascularity of subjacent connective tissue. White or yellow-white lesions may be due to a fibrin exudate covering an ulcer, submucosal deposits, surface debris, or fungal colonies.

HEREDITARY CONDITIONS

Several hereditary disorders of the oral mucosa are characterized by hyperkeratosis resulting in the common clinical finding of a mucosal white lesion. These conditions have also been termed *genokeratoses* or a more general term, *genodermatosis*.

Leukoedema

Leukoedema is a generalized buccal mucosa opacification that can be regarded as a variation of normal. It can be identified in the majority of the population.

Etiology and Pathogenesis. To date, the cause of leukoedema has not been established. Attempts to implicate factors such as smoking, alcohol ingestion, bacterial infection, salivary conditions, and electrochemical interactions have been unsuccessful. Some studies, however, indicate a possible relationship between poor oral hygiene and abnormal masticatory patterns.

Clinical Features. Leukoedema is usually discovered as an incidental finding. It is asymptomatic, is symmetric in distribution, and occurs on the buccal mucosa (Fig. 3–1). It appears as a gray-white, diffuse, filmy or milky surface. In more exaggerated cases, a whitish cast with surface textural changes, including wrinkling or corrugation, may be seen. With stretching of the buccal mucosa, the opaque changes dissipate, except in more advanced cases. It is seen more commonly in nonwhites, especially African-Americans.

Histopathology. In leukoedema, the epithelium is parakeratotic and acanthotic, with marked intracellular edema of spinous cells. The enlarged epithelial cells have small, pyknotic nuclei in optically clear cytoplasm. Alterations in the germinative layer are absent, as are inflammatory changes in the lamina propria.

Differential Diagnosis. Leukoplakia, white sponge nevus, hereditary benign intraepithelial dyskeratosis, and the response to chronic cheek biting may show clinical similarities to leukoedema. The overall thickness of these lesions, their persistence on stretching, and specific microscopic features help separate them from leukoedema.

Treatment and Prognosis. No treatment is necessary because the changes are innocuous. The lesion has no malignant potential and suggests no

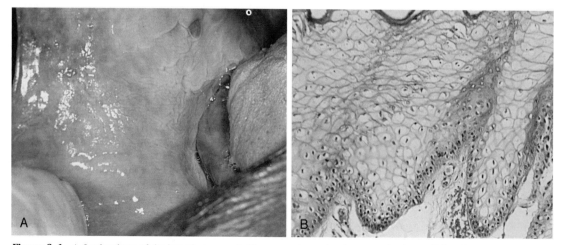

Figure 3–1. *A,* Leukoedema of the buccal mucosa. *B,* Biopsy specimen showing extensive intracellular edema.

predisposition to the development of leukoplakia. It is important to recognize this process and avoid unnecessary intervention.

White Sponge Nevus

White sponge nevus is an autosomal dominant condition that appears to be due to keratin 4 and/or 13 point mutations. It affects the buccal mucosa bilaterally, and no treatment is required.

Clinical Features. It presents as an asymptomatic, deeply folded, white or gray lesion that may affect several mucosal sites. Lesions tend to be somewhat thickened and have a spongy consistency. The presentation intraorally is almost always bilateral and symmetric and usually appears early in life, typically before puberty. The characteristic clinical manifestations of this particular form of keratosis are usually best observed on the buccal mucosa, although other areas such as the tongue, especially along the lateral margins, and vestibular mucosa may also be involved (Fig. 3–2). Although the conjunctival mucosa is usually spared, a variable degree of involvement of the esophageal, anal, vulval, and vaginal mucosa occurs.

Histopathology. Microscopically, the epithelium is greatly thickened, with marked spongiosis, acanthosis, and parakeratosis. Within the stratum spinosum, marked hydropic or clear cell change may be noted, often beginning in the parabasal region and extending very close to the surface. Perinuclear eosinophilic condensation of cytoplasm is characteristic of prickle cells in white sponge nevus. Occasional individual cells demonstrate premature keratinization within the spinous layer. It is often possible to see columns of para-

keratin extending from the spinous layer to the surface. The lamina propria and submucosa are unremarkable.

Differential Diagnosis. The differential diagnosis includes hereditary benign epithelial dyskeratosis, pachyonychia congenita, lichen planus, and cheek chewing. Once tissue diagnosis is confirmed, no additional biopsies are necessary.

Treatment. There is no specific treatment for this particular condition, because it is asymptomatic and benign and has no malignant potential.

Hereditary Benign Intraepithelial Dyskeratosis

Etiology. Hereditary benign intraepithelial dyskeratosis (HBID), also known as *Witkop's disease,* is a rare, heritable condition of an autosomal dominant, highly penetrant nature. This condition was noted within a triracial isolate of white, Indian, and African-American composition in Halifax County, North Carolina. The initial cohort of 75 patients was traced to a single common female ancestor who lived nearly 130 years earlier.

Clinical Features. HBID is a syndrome that includes the early onset (usually within the first year of life) of bulbar conjunctivitis and oral white lesions (Fig. 3–3). Precipitating the bulbar conjunctivitis are foamy gelatinous plaques that represent the ocular counterpart of the oral mucosal lesions.

Oral lesions consist of soft, asymptomatic, white folds and plaques of spongy mucosa. Areas characteristically involved include the buccal and labial mucosa and labial commissures as well as the floor of the mouth and lateral surfaces of the tongue, gingiva, and palate. The dorsum of the

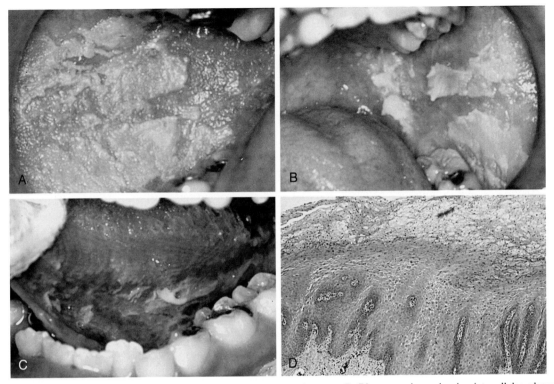

Figure 3–2. *A* to *C*, White sponge nevus of the buccal mucosa and tongue. *D*, Biopsy specimen showing intracellular edema and perinuclear condensation in the lower epithelial cells.

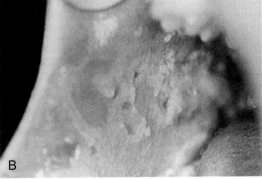

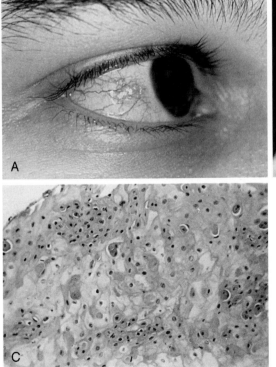

Figure 3–3. *A* and *B*, Hereditary benign intraepithelial dyskeratosis of the conjunctiva and buccal mucosa. (*A* and *B*, Courtesy of Dr. J. R. Jacoway.) *C*, Biopsy sample of a buccal mucosa lesion of HBID. Epithelium shows intracellular edema and dyskeratosis (dark cells).

tongue is usually spared. Oral lesions are generally detected within the first year of life, with a gradual increase in intensity until midadolescence. Involved areas along the occlusal line frequently are macerated, further enhancing their shaggy surface texture.

In some patients, ocular lesions may vary seasonally. Some patients may complain of photophobia, especially in early life. Blindness, secondary to corneal vascularization, has been reported. In others, spontaneous shedding of the conjunctival plaques occurs on a seasonal basis.

Histopathology. Similarities between oral and conjunctival lesions are noted microscopically. Epithelial hyperplasia and acanthosis are present, with significant hydropic change (Fig. 3–3). Enlarged, hyaline, and so-called waxy eosinophilic cells, which are the dyskeratotic elements, are present in the superficial half of the epithelium. Nondyskeratotic cells are enlarged and edematous. Normal cellular features are noted within the lower spinous and basal layers. Inflammatory cell infiltration within the lamina propria is minimal, and the epithelial-connective tissue junction is well defined.

Differential Diagnosis. The oral features of HBID are remarkably similar to those of white sponge nevus. Adequate history and biopsy are necessary to establish a diagnosis. *Pachyonychia congenita* and hypertrophic lichen planus might also be considered in a clinical differential. In pachyonychia congenita, however, distinctive fingernail and toenail changes—extreme thickening along the free nail edge—are present. Additionally, defects of teeth, angular cheilitis, follicular keratosis, and corneal dyskeratosis may be noted. In lichen planus, no inheritance pattern is evident and the microscopy findings are distinctive. Lichen planus nail changes are related to nail fold destruction. Eye changes are not seen in lichen planus.

Treatment. No treatment is necessary, because this condition is self-limiting. It appears to pose no risk of malignant transformation.

Follicular Keratosis

Etiology and Pathogenesis. Follicular keratosis (Darier's disease, Darier-White disease) is a genetically transmitted disorder with an autosomal dominant mode of inheritance. In a large series of 200 kindred, the chance of an affected offspring developing the disease was 50%, with an equal gender distribution. Many cases also appear sporadically or as new mutations. Although the etiology of follicular keratosis is well established, con-

cepts concerning pathogenesis are less well understood.

Clinical Features. Onset of this disease is usually noted in childhood or adolescence. Skin manifestations are characterized by small, skin-colored papular lesions symmetrically distributed over the face, trunk, and intertriginous areas. The papules eventually coalesce and feel greasy because of excessive keratin production. The coalesced areas subsequently form patches of vegetating to verrucous growths that have a tendency to become infected and malodorous. Lesions may also occur unilaterally or in a zosteriform pattern. Thickening of the palms and soles (hyperkeratosis palmaris et plantaris) by excessive keratotic tissue is not uncommon. On the dorsa of the hands, the lesions are similar to flat warts or verruca plana and acrokeratosis verruciformis (Hopf's keratosis). Fingernail changes may include fragility, splintering, and subungual keratosis. Nail changes are often helpful in establishing a diagnosis.

Oral involvement by this disease is well established (Fig. 3–4). The extent of the oral lesions may parallel the extent of skin involvement. Favored oral mucosal sites include keratinized regions, such as attached gingiva and hard palate, although nearly all oral sites have been reported to be involved. The lesions typically appear as small, whitish papules, producing an overall cobblestone appearance. Papules range from 2 to 3 mm in diameter and may become coalescent. Extension beyond the oral cavity into the oropharynx and pharynx may occur.

Histopathology. Oral lesions closely resemble the cutaneous lesions (Fig. 3–5). Features include (1) suprabasal lacunae (clefts) formation containing acantholytic epithelial cells, (2) basal layer proliferation immediately below and adjacent to the lacunae or clefts, (3) formation of vertical clefts that show a lining of parakeratotic and dyskeratotic cells, and (4) the presence of specific benign dyskeratotic cells—*corps ronds* and *grains*. Corps ronds are large, keratinized squamous cells with round, uniformly basophilic nuclei and intensely eosinophilic cytoplasm. Grains are smaller parakeratotic cells with pyknotic, hyperchromatic nuclei.

Differential Diagnosis. Follicular keratosis, when affecting the oral mucosa, may bear some clinical resemblance to the rarely occurring conditions dyskeratosis congenita and acanthosis nigricans. Other conditions to be excluded from follicular keratosis are condyloma acuminatum and nicotine stomatitis. Microscopically, Hailey-Hailey disease might be included in the differential diagnosis.

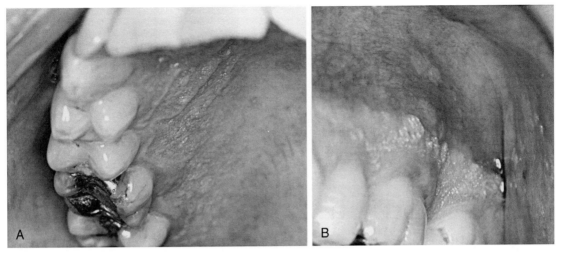

Figure 3–4. *A* and *B*, Follicular keratosis of the right hard palate and upper gingiva.

Treatment and Prognosis. Vitamin A analogues or retinoids, in the form of etretinate (aromatic retinoid) and isotretinoin (13-*cis*-retinoic acid), have been used effectively. Side effects, including cheilitis, elevation of serum liver enzyme and triglyceride levels, and severe dryness of the skin, have also placed some limitations on this treatment method. Discontinuation of treatment usually produces variable periods of remission, with an eventual return to the original level of involvement.

Although the disease is chronic and slowly progressive, remissions may be noted in some patients. Malignant change within oral mucosal lesions has not been reported.

REACTIVE LESIONS

Focal (Frictional) Hyperkeratosis

Etiology. Focal (frictional) hyperkeratosis is a white lesion that is often classified under the general clinical term *leukoplakia*. In this chapter, however, because there may be an obvious cause-and-effect relationship for this lesion, it is separated from the idiopathic (unknown etiology) leukoplakias.

Chronic rubbing or friction against an oral mucosal surface may result in a presumably protec-

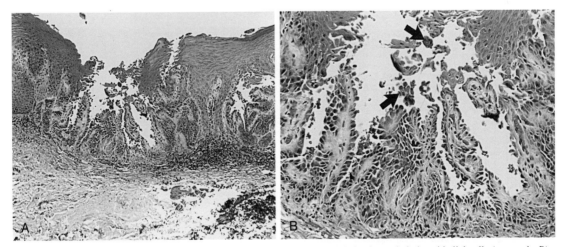

Figure 3–5. *A* and *B*, Micrograph of follicular keratosis showing vertical clefts and acantholytic epithelial cells *(arrows* in *B).*

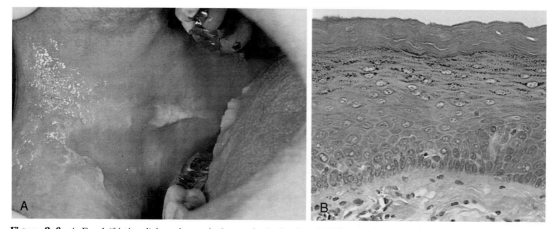

Figure 3–6. *A*, Focal (frictional) hyperkeratosis due to cheek chewing. *B*, Micrograph showing hyperkeratosis.

tive hyperkeratotic white lesion that is analogous to a callus on the skin.

Clinical Features. Friction-induced hyperkeratoses occur in areas that are commonly traumatized, such as lips, lateral margins of the tongue, buccal mucosa along the occlusal line, and edentulous ridges (Figs. 3–6 and 3–7). Chronic cheek or lip chewing may result in opacification (keratinization) of the area affected. Chewing on edentulous alveolar ridges produces the same effect.

Histopathology. As the name indicates, the primary microscopic change is hyperkeratosis. A few chronic inflammatory cells may be seen in the subjacent connective tissue. Dysplastic epithelial changes are not seen in simple frictional hyperkeratotic lesions.

Diagnosis. Careful history taking and examination should indicate the nature of this lesion. If the practitioner is clinically confident of a traumatic cause, no biopsy may be required. Patients should be advised to discontinue the causative habit, however. The lesion should resolve or at least reduce in intensity with time, confirming the clinical diagnosis. Resolution of the lesion would also allow unmasking of any underlying lesion that may not be related to trauma.

Treatment. Observation is generally all that is required for simple frictional hyperkeratotic lesions. Control of the habit causing the lesion should result in clinical improvement. Any lesion of questionable cause should undergo biopsy.

White Lesions Associated with Smokeless Tobacco

In the United States, geographic and gender differences in tobacco use have been noted. Numbers of frequent users, which typically have been high in the southern states, have significantly in-

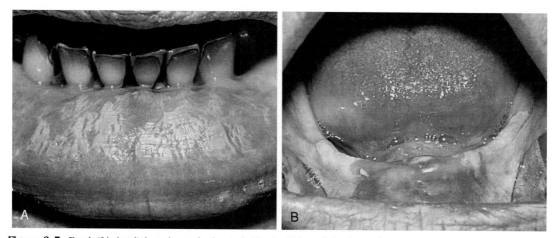

Figure 3–7. Focal (frictional) hyperkeratosis due to habitual rubbing of the lip against the teeth *(A)* and wearing ill-fitting dentures *(B)*.

creased in other areas, especially western states. Usage by men in New York and Rhode Island is less than 1% of the population, but in West Virginia it exceeds 20%. In a 1986 survey of 25 states and the District of Columbia, 6.5% of men and 0.3% of women were regular users of smokeless tobacco. Among teenagers, whites are the predominant users of smokeless tobacco, with males making up nearly all of this group.

In other parts of the world, different forms of smokeless tobacco are used. The tobacco preparations are generally of higher (alkaline) pH. In older populations, with a longer exposure to tobacco and other agents, keratinized ridges or spikes of tissue often develop, frequently producing a characteristic pumice-like pattern of keratinization. This pattern has been noted on areas of the oral mucosa that normally do not keratinize.

The general increase in smokeless tobacco consumption has been related to both peer pressure and increased media advertising, which often glamorizes the use of smokeless tobacco or snuff dipping. Additionally, individuals who have been intense smokers or those who wish to avoid smoking may gravitate to this alternative. The clinical results of long-term exposure to smokeless tobacco include the development of oral mucosal white patches, dependence, alterations of taste and smell, increased periodontal disease, and significant amounts of dental abrasion.

Etiology. A causal relationship has been documented between smokeless tobacco and tissue changes. Although all forms of smokeless tobacco may potentially cause alterations in the oral mucosa, snuff (finely divided tobacco) appears to be much more likely to cause oral lesions than chewing tobacco. Oral mucosa responds to the irritating effects of tobacco with inflammation and kerato-

sis. Dysplastic changes may follow, with an associated risk of malignant change. The use of any form of tobacco increases the risk of subsequent development of oral mucosal dysplasia. Although most investigators believe there is significant risk of malignant transformation, the level of risk has not been satisfactorily measured. This biologic alteration in tissues is thought to be a response to tobacco constituents and perhaps other agents that are added to tobacco for flavoring or moisture retention. Carcinogens, such as nitrosonornicotine, an organic component of chewing tobacco and snuff, have been identified in the tobacco. The pH of snuff, which ranges between 8.2 and 9.3, may be another factor that relates to the alteration of mucosa.

Duration of exposure to smokeless tobacco that is necessary to produce mucosal damage is measured in terms of years. It has been demonstrated that leukoplakia can be predicted with use of three tins of tobacco per week or duration of the habit for more than 2 years.

Clinical Features. The white lesions of the oral mucosa associated with smokeless tobacco use develop in the immediate area where the tobacco is habitually placed (Figs. 3–8 and 3–9). The most common area of involvement is the mucobuccal fold of the mandible, in either the incisor or the molar region. The altered epithelium generally has a granular to wrinkled appearance. In advanced cases, a heavy folded character may be seen. Less frequently, an erythroplakic or red component may be admixed with the white keratotic component. The lesions are generally painless and asymptomatic, and their discovery is often incidental to routine oral examination.

Histopathology. Slight to moderate parakeratosis is noted over the surface of the affected

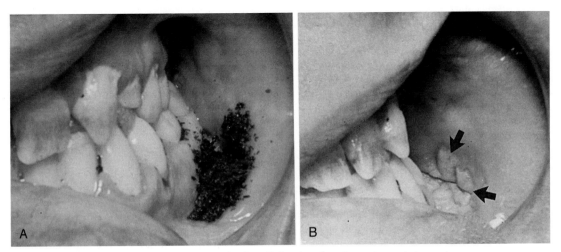

Figure 3–8. Smokeless tobacco user. *A*, Tobacco in place. *B*, Resultant hyperkeratotic pouch *(arrows)*.

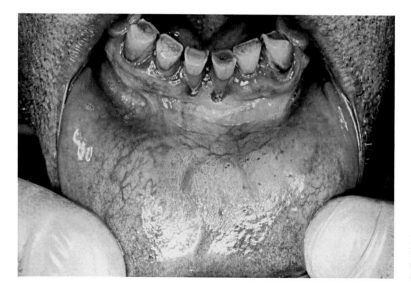

Figure 3–9. Hyperkeratosis caused by smokeless tobacco. Note the associated periodontal disease and tooth abrasion.

mucosa. Superficial levels of epithelium may demonstrate vacuolization or edema. Epithelial hyperplasia is typical, and atrophy and ulceration are unusual. A slight to moderate chronic inflammatory cell infiltrate is typically present. Epithelial dysplasia may occasionally develop in these lesions, especially in long-time users. Salivary gland alterations are primarily inflammatory and are seen in approximately 40% of biopsy specimens. Such changes include acinar atrophy, interstitial fibrosis, and dilated excretory ducts. On occasion, a diffuse zone of basophilic stromal alteration may be seen, usually adjacent to minor salivary glands.

Differential Diagnosis. Focal (frictional) hyperkeratosis and idiopathic leukoplakia might clinically resemble this condition. Historical information should help rule out these. In the early phases of development, snuff or smokeless tobacco–induced lesions may resemble the diffuse, filmy character of leukoedema, although in leukoedema the change is bilateral and symmetric. The surface alterations in white sponge nevus may approximate the character of lesions related to snuff dipping; however, the bilateral and more general distribution of lesions in white sponge nevus distinguishes the two processes.

Treatment and Prognosis. With discontinuation of tobacco use, some lesions may disappear after several weeks, indicative of an excellent prognosis. Persistent lesions should be removed and examined histologically. A long period of exposure to smokeless tobacco appears necessary for malignant transformation to develop. These lesions are generally of low-grade malignancy, ranging from verrucous carcinoma to ulcerated squamous cell carcinoma.

Nicotine Stomatitis

Etiology. This is a common tobacco-related form of keratosis. Nicotine stomatitis is most typically associated with pipe and cigar smoking, with a positive correlation between severity of the condition and intensity of smoking. The importance of the direct topical effect of smoke can be appreciated in instances in which the hard palate is covered by a removable prosthesis, resulting in sparing of the mucosa beneath the appliance and hyperkeratosis of exposed areas. The combination of tobacco carcinogens and heat is markedly intensified in *reverse smoking* (lit end positioned inside the mouth), adding a significant risk for malignant conversion.

Clinical Features. The palatal mucosa initially responds with an erythematous-type reaction and over time with increased keratinization. Subsequent to the opacification or keratinization of the surface, red dots surrounded by white keratotic rings appear (Fig. 3–10). The dots represent inflammation of the salivary gland excretory ducts.

Histopathology. Nicotine stomatitis is generally characterized by a thickened epithelium, with moderate levels of acanthosis and a significant increase in the thickness of the overlying orthokeratin. The minor salivary glands in the area demonstrate mild to severe inflammatory change. Excretory ducts may show squamous metaplasia, and glandular tissue contains chronic inflammatory cells, acinar atrophy, and scar.

Treatment and Prognosis. The overall significance of nicotine stomatitis in comparison with keratosis in other portions of the oral cavity is minimal. This condition rarely evolves into malig-

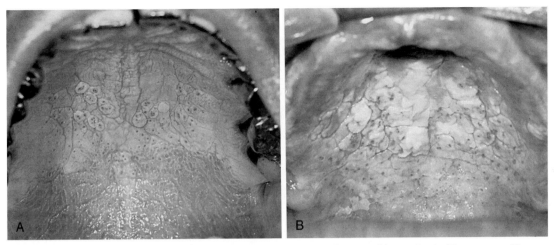

Figure 3–10. *A*, Nicotine stomatitis associated with pipe smoking. *B*, Nicotine stomatitis associated with reverse smoking.

nancy except in individuals who *reverse smoke*. This habit, which is common in other countries (e.g., India), intensifies the carcinogenic effect of heat, smoke, and possibly other tobacco constituents on the palate, resulting in considerable risk of cancer development.

Although the risk of carcinoma development in the palate is minimal, the risk of malignancy elsewhere in the oral cavity and upper respiratory tract is increased. Nicotine stomatitis might be viewed as a potential indicator of significant epithelial change at sites other than the hard palate.

Solar Cheilitis

Solar or actinic cheilitis represents accelerated tissue degeneration of the vermilion portion of the lips, especially the lower lip, secondary to regular and prolonged exposure to sunlight. This particular condition occurs almost exclusively in whites and is especially prevalent in those with fair skin. It is closely correlated with total cumulative exposure to sunlight and amount of skin pigmentation.

Etiology and Pathogenesis. The wavelengths of light most responsible for actinic cheilitis and, in general, other degenerative actinically related skin conditions are usually considered to be those between 2900 and 3200 nm (UVB). This radiant energy affects not only the epithelium but also the supporting connective tissue.

Clinical Features. The affected vermilion portion of the lips takes on an atrophic, pale to silvery gray, glossy appearance, often with fissuring and wrinkling at right angles to the cutaneous-vermilion junction (Fig. 3–11). In advanced cases, the junction is irregular or totally effaced, with a degree of epidermization of the vermilion evident.

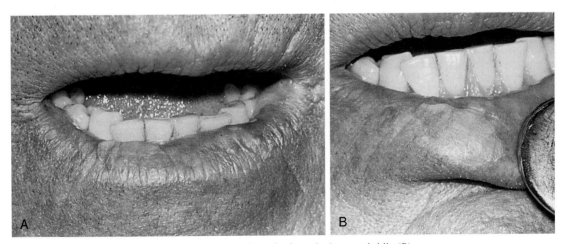

Figure 3–11. *A* and *B*, Solar cheilitis. Note the hyperkeratotic plaque in the extended lip *(B)*.

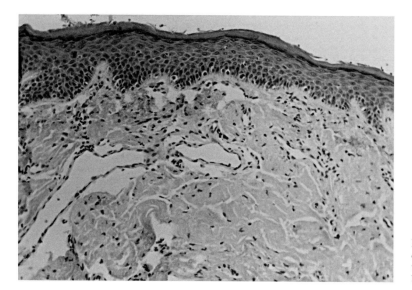

Figure 3–12. Micrograph of solar cheilitis showing hyperkeratosis, epithelial atrophy, telangiectasia, and basophilic change of the submucosa.

Mottled areas of hyperpigmentation and keratosis are often noted as well as superficial scaling, cracking, erosion, ulceration, and crusting.

Histopathology. The overlying epithelium may be atrophic or focally and irregularly hyperplastic with surface parakeratosis or orthokeratosis of variable thickness. Various dysplastic changes may be seen, from slight atypia to carcinoma *in situ*, often with a wide spectrum of change within the same specimen. Characteristic is a striking basophilia of the submucosa (elastin replacement of collagen) and the appearance of telangiectatic vessels (Fig. 3–12).

Treatment. Because of the positive relationship between exposure to ultraviolet light and carcinoma, lip protection may be indicated. The use of lip balm containing the sunscreen agent *para*-aminobenzoic acid (PABA) or its derivatives is indicated during periods of sun exposure in high-risk patients. Sun-blocking opaque agents also boost the effectiveness of the balm (Table 3–1).

Chronic sun damage mandates periodic examination and biopsy if ulceration persists or if induration becomes evident. If atypical changes are noted within the epithelium, a vermilionectomy may be performed in association with mucosal advancement to replace the damaged vermilion. Acceptable results are also obtainable with use of laser surgery or cryosurgery.

OTHER WHITE LESIONS

Idiopathic Leukoplakia

Leukoplakia is a clinical term indicating a white patch or plaque of oral mucosa that cannot be rubbed off and cannot be characterized clinically as any other disease. This definition excludes lesions that may be clinically diagnostic, such as lichen planus, candidiasis, leukoedema, and white sponge nevus. Leukoplakias may have similar clinical appearances but have a considerable degree of microscopic heterogeneity. The absence of any specific histologic connotation for leukoplakia is an important concept intended to eliminate some of the former confusion about this term. Because leukoplakias may range microscopically from benign hyperkeratosis to invasive squamous cell carcinomas, biopsy is mandatory to establish a definitive diagnosis. It is important to note that premalignant lesions are not always white and that persistent leukoplakias are usually not premalignant or malignant.

Etiology and Pathogenesis. Many cases of leukoplakia are etiologically related to the use of tobacco in smoked or smokeless forms and may regress after discontinuation of tobacco use. The point of irreversibility, however, cannot be defined in terms of duration of tobacco use, forms of tobacco used, or clinical presentation. Other fac-

Table 3–1. Agents Used to Protect Tissue from Damaging Effects of Ultraviolet Light

SUNSCREEN	SUNBLOCK
Absorbs light	Scatters light
Protects from <3200 nm light	Protects from >3200 nm light
Reduces burning (erythema)	Reduces tanning (melanogenesis)
e.g., *p*-aminobenzoate, *p*-aminobenzoic acid	e.g., zinc oxide, titanium dioxide

tors, such as alcohol abuse, trauma, and *Candida albicans* infection, may have a role in the etiology of leukoplakia. Nutritional factors have also been cited as important, especially relative to iron deficiency anemia and development of sideropenic dysphagia (Plummer-Vinson or Paterson-Kelly syndrome).

There is no doubt that some leukoplakias develop into oral squamous cell carcinoma. Rates of transformation vary considerably from study to study, in part because of cultural habits of tobacco use. Geographic differences in transformation rate as well as prevalence and location of oral leukoplakias are likely related to these differences in tobacco habits in various parts of the world. In studies of United States populations, the majority of oral leukoplakias are benign and probably never become malignant. Studies indicate that malignant transformation of leukoplakia occurs over a range from about 1% to as high as 17%, averaging 4 to 5%. There are wide ranges of risk of transformation from one anatomic site to another.

Clinical Features. Leukoplakia is a condition associated with a middle-aged and older population, with the vast majority of cases occurring after the age of 40 years. Trends in the use of smokeless tobacco by high-school students may ultimately result in a shift of this age toward a younger population. Over time there has also been a shift in gender predilection, with near parity in incidence of leukoplakia due apparently to the change in smoking habits of women.

Predominant sites of occurrence have changed through the years. At one time, the tongue was the most common site for leukoplakia, although this area has given way to the mandibular mucosa and the buccal mucosa, which account for almost half of the leukoplakias (Fig. 3–13). The palate, maxillary ridge, and lower lip are somewhat less frequently involved, and the floor of the mouth and retromolar sites are involved comparatively infrequently.

The relative risk of neoplastic transformation varies from one region to another. Although the floor of the mouth accounts for a relatively small percentage (10%) of leukoplakias, a large percentage are dysplastic, carcinoma *in situ*, or invasive lesions when examined microscopically (Table 3–2). Leukoplakia of the lips and tongue also exhibits a relatively high percentage of dysplastic or neoplastic change. In contrast to these sites, the retromolar area exhibits these changes in only about 10% of cases.

On visual examination, leukoplakia may vary from a barely evident, vague whiteness on a base of uninflamed, normal-appearing tissue to a definitive white, thickened, leathery, fissured, verrucous or wart-like lesion. Red zones may also be seen in some leukoplakias, prompting use of the term *speckled leukoplakia*. On palpation, some lesions may be soft, smooth, or finely granular in texture. Other lesions may be roughened, nodular, or indurated.

Proliferative verrucous leukoplakia has been segregated from other leukoplakias. This type of leukoplakia begins as simple keratosis and eventually becomes verrucous in nature. Some lesions can become clinically aggressive. It is persistent, becomes multifocal, and is recurrent. The cause is unknown, although some may be associated with human papillomavirus and some with tobacco use. The diagnosis is determined clinicopathologically and is usually made retrospectively. Malignant transformation to verrucous or squamous cell carcinoma is seen in as many as 15% of cases.

Histopathology. Histologic changes for idiopathic leukoplakia range from hyperkeratosis, acanthosis, dysplasia, and carcinoma *in situ* to invasive squamous cell carcinoma (Fig. 3–14). By definition, the term *dysplasia* refers to disordered growth whereas the term *atypia* refers to abnormal cellular features. Various degrees of dysplasia may be described in which the epithelial pattern shows mild, moderate, or severe change. This is a subjective determination, and it indicates that the changes do not appear abnormal enough to qualify as neoplastic (Fig. 3–15). Specific microscopic characteristics of dysplasia include (1) drop-shaped epithelial ridges, (2) basal layer hyperplasia, (3) irregular stratification, (4) increased and abnormal mitotic figures, (5) individual or cell-group keratinization (epithelial pearl formation) within the spinous layer, (6) cellular pleomorphism, (7) nuclear hyperchromatism, (8) altered nuclear-cytoplasmic ratio, (9) enlarged nucleoli, (10) loss of basal cell polarity and "streaming" of spinous layer cells, and (11) loss or diminished intercellular adherence.

Table 3–2. Leukoplakia

SITE	DYSPLASIA OR CARCINOMA (%)
Floor of mouth	43
Lateral and ventral tongue	24
Lower lip	24
Palate	19
Buccal mucosa	17
Maxillary/mandibular mucosa/sulcus	15
Retromolar	12

From Waldron CA, Shafer WG. Leukoplakia revisited. A clinicopathologic study of 3256 oral leukoplakias. Cancer 36:1386–1392, 1975.

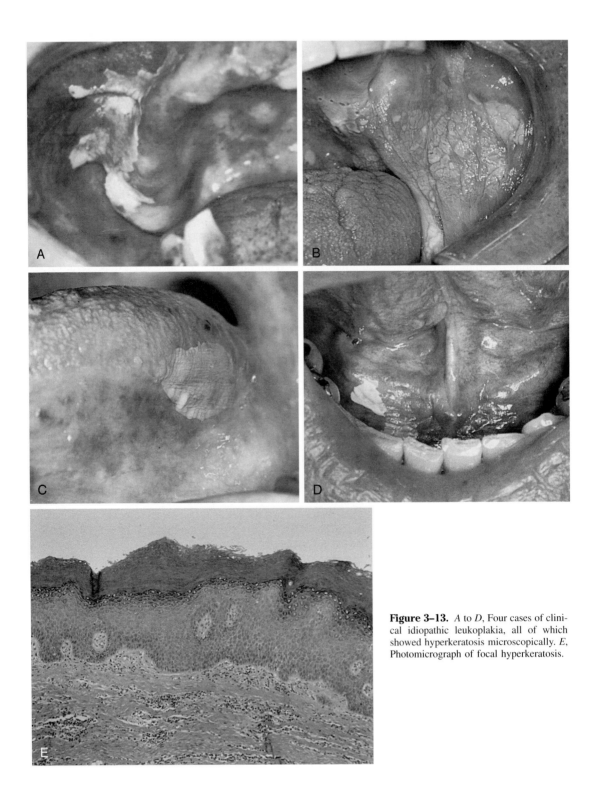

Figure 3–13. *A* to *D*, Four cases of clinical idiopathic leukoplakia, all of which showed hyperkeratosis microscopically. *E*, Photomicrograph of focal hyperkeratosis.

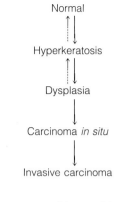

Normal

↑↓

Hyperkeratosis

↑↓

Dysplasia

↓

Carcinoma *in situ*

↓

Invasive carcinoma

↑ represents possible reversible process

Figure 3–14. Microscopic spectrum of idiopathic leukoplakia. Oral lesions may be found anywhere along this spectrum. Some may progress through the various stages over time, whereas others may apparently skip some or all stages to become invasive squamous cell carcinoma.

When the entire thickness of epithelium is involved with these changes in the so-called top-to-bottom effect, the term *carcinoma in situ* may be used (Fig. 3–16). Carcinoma *in situ* may also be identified when cellular atypia is particularly severe, even though the changes may not be evident from basement membrane to surface.

Progression of dysplasia to carcinoma has not been fully documented. It is generally accepted that the more severe the change, the more likely a lesion is to evolve to cancer. Also, some lesions can persist for indefinite periods without changing microscopically, and a few others apparently revert to normal. Carcinoma *in situ* is not regarded as a reversible lesion, although it may take many years for invasion to occur. It has been shown that a majority of squamous cell carcinomas of the upper aerodigestive tract, including the oral cavity, were preceded by severe dysplasia. Conceptually, invasive carcinoma begins when a microfocus of epithelial cell invades the lamina propria 1 to 2 mm beyond the basal lamina. At this early stage, the risk of regional metastasis is low.

About 5% of leukoplakias are invasive squamous cell carcinoma. There is, however, considerable variation in this figure because of variances in study design and population. The overall malignant transformation of benign leukoplakias accounts for approximately another 5% of the lesions.

Differential Diagnosis. The first step in developing a differential diagnosis for a white patch (leukoplakia) in the oral mucosa is determining whether the lesion can be eliminated with a gauze square or tongue blade. If the lesion can be removed, it represents a pseudomembrane, fungus colony, or debris. If there is evidence of bilateral buccal mucosa disease, hereditary conditions, cheek chewing, lichen planus, and lupus erythematosus (LE) should be included in the differential. Concomitant cutaneous lesions would give weight to the latter two. If either chronic trauma or tobacco use is elicited in the patient's history, frictional or tobacco-associated hyperkeratoses should be considered. Elimination of a suspected cause should result in some clinical improvement. Also included in a differential for tongue leukoplakia would be hairy leukoplakia and geographic tongue.

If the lesion in question is not removable and is not clinically diagnostic, it can then be generally classified as idiopathic, and biopsy becomes mandatory. In extensive lesions, multiple biopsies may be necessary to avoid sample error. The clinically

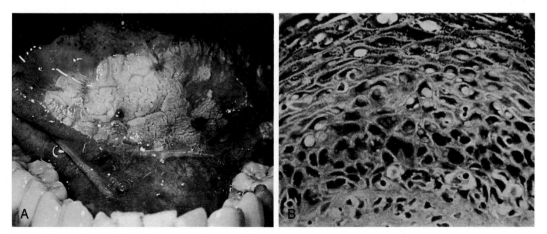

Figure 3–15. *A*, Clinical idiopathic leukoplakia of the left lateral surface of the tongue. *B*, Biopsy showing dysplastic changes of nuclear hyperchromatism and irregular epithelial maturation.

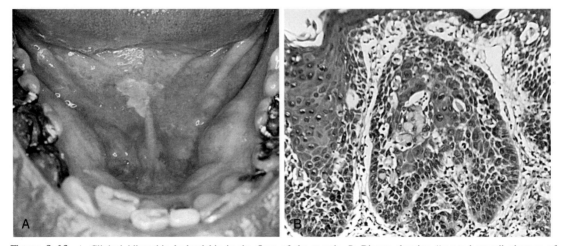

Figure 3–16. *A*, Clinical idiopathic leukoplakia in the floor of the mouth. *B*, Biopsy showing "top-to-bottom" changes of carcinoma *in situ*.

most suspicious areas (red, ulcerated, or indurated areas) should be included in the biopsy plan.

Treatment and Prognosis. In the absence of dysplastic or atypical epithelial changes, periodic examinations and rebiopsy of new suspicious areas would be appropriate. If the lesion is mildly dysplastic, some clinical judgment should be exercised in patient management. Potential etiologic factors should be considered. Removal of mildly dysplastic lesions would be in a patient's best interest if there is no apparent causative factor and the lesion is small. If considerable morbidity would result because of lesion size or location, follow-up surveillance would be desirable.

If leukoplakia is diagnosed as moderate to severe dysplasia, removal becomes obligatory. Various surgical methods such as scalpel excision, cryosurgery, electrosurgery, and laser surgery seem to be equally effective in ablating these lesions. In cases of extensive lesions, grafting procedures may be necessary after surgery. It is important to note that some idiopathic leukoplakias may recur after complete removal. It is impossible to predict which lesions will return and which will not.

Hairy Leukoplakia

Etiology and Pathogenesis. In 1981, an unusual white lesion was first described along the lateral margins of the tongue, predominantly in male homosexuals. Evidence indicates that this particular form of leukoplakia, known as *hairy leukoplakia*, represents an opportunistic infection related to the presence of Epstein-Barr virus (EBV) found almost exclusively in human immu-

nodeficiency virus (HIV)–infected individuals. Its prevalence in this population is approximately 20% and increases to as high as 80% in patients with acquired immunodeficiency syndrome (AIDS). Of importance is the fact that this lesion has been associated with subsequent or concomitant development of the clinical and laboratory features of AIDS in as many as 80% of cases. There is a positive correlation with depletion of peripheral CD4 cells. Several other oral conditions have also been described as having a greater than expected frequency in patients with AIDS (Table 3–3). In a small percentage of cases, confirmed diagnoses of hairy leukoplakia have been made in patients with other forms of immunosuppression, in particular, those associated with organ transplantation (medically induced immunosuppression). A few cases have been reported in patients who are apparently immunocompetent.

The presence of EBV in this lesion, as well as normal epithelium of patients with AIDS, has been confirmed. Viral particles have been localized within the nuclei and cytoplasm of the oral epithelial cells of hairy leukoplakia, with DNA hybrid-

Table 3–3. Oral Manifestations of AIDS

Hairy leukoplakia
Candidiasis
Aphthous ulcers
Kaposi's sarcoma
Lymphoma
Gingivitis/periodontal disease
Xerostomia
Viral infections (cytomegalovirus, herpesvirus, varicella-zoster)
?Squamous cell carcinoma

ization studies confirming the presence of the EBV genome. Studies further indicate that this particular virus replicates within the oral hairy leukoplakia lesion. It is not understood why the lateral surface of the tongue is the favored site.

Clinical Features. Hairy leukoplakia presents as a well-demarcated white lesion that varies in architecture from a flat, plaque-like lesion to one with papillary/filiform hair-like projections. It may be unilateral or bilateral (Fig. 3–17). The vast majority of reported cases have been located along the lateral margins of the tongue, with occasional extention onto the dorsal surface. Rarely hairy leukoplakia may be seen on the buccal mucosa, the floor of the mouth, or the palate. Lesions have not been seen in the vaginal or anal mucosa.

In general, there are no associated symptoms, although a suprainfection with *C. albicans* might call attention to the presence of this condition. In more severe cases, when the entire dorsum of the tongue is involved by the process, the patient may become visually aware of the lesion and may seek dental consultation.

Histopathology. The characteristic micro-scopic feature of hairy leukoplakia is found in the nuclei of upper level keratinocytes. Viral inclusions or peripheral displacement of chromatin with a resultant smudgy nucleus is evident. This is seen in the context of a markedly hyperparakeratotic surface, often with the formation of keratotic surface irregularities and ridges (Fig. 3–18). *C. albicans* hyphae are often seen extending into the superficial epithelial cell layers. Beneath the surface, within the spinous cell layer, cells show ballooning degeneration and perinuclear clearing. There is a general paucity of subepithelial inflammatory cells, and Langerhans cells are sparse.

Immunopathologic studies have demonstrated the presence of EBV within the cells showing nuclear inclusions and basophilic homogenization. Further confirmation has been accomplished by ultrastructural demonstration of intranuclear virions of EBV (Fig. 3–19).

Differential Diagnosis. The clinical differential diagnosis of hairy leukoplakia includes the more common idiopathic leukoplakia, frictional hyperkeratosis (tongue chewing), and leukoplakia associated with tobacco use. Other entities that

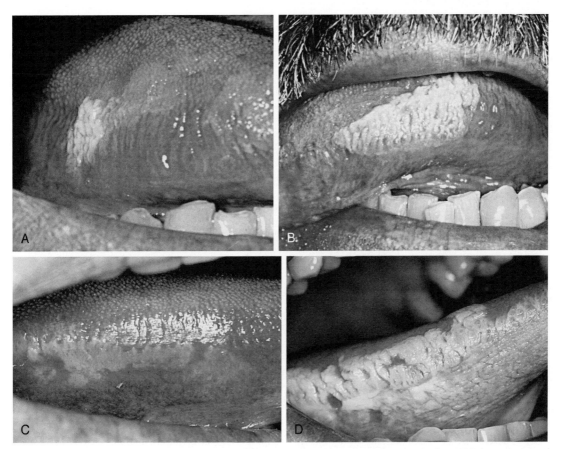

Figure 3–17. *A* and *B*, Bilateral hairy leukoplakia of the tongue. This patient was diagnosed as having AIDS 3 months later. (*A* and *B*, Courtesy of Dr. J. C. B. Stewart.) *C* and *D*, Other patterns of hairy leukoplakia.

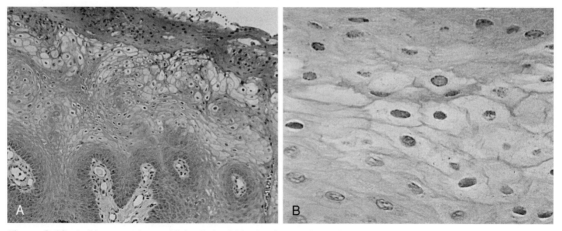

Figure 3–18. *A,* Biopsy specimen of hairy leukoplakia showing parakeratosis and balloon cell change. *B,* High magnification showing characteristic EBV-induced nuclear change.

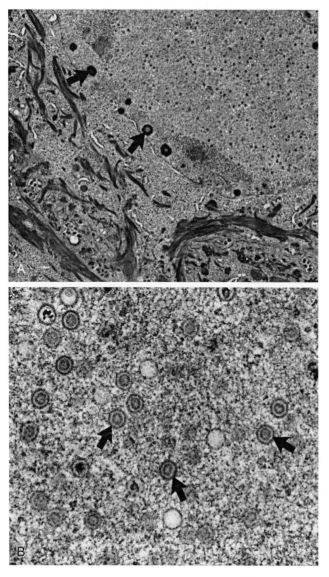

Figure 3–19. Electron micrographs of EBV in hairy leukoplakia. *A,* Keratinocyte containing bundles of dark tonofilaments. Chromatin fragments *(arrows)* are located along the nuclear membrane, and smaller dark viral particles occupy the nucleus (× 8000). *B,* Higher magnification of the nucleus showing detail of viral particles. The outer ring represents the viral capsid *(arrows)* surrounding a DNA core (× 60,000).

might also be considered are lichen planus, lupus erythematosus, chronic hyperplastic candidiasis, and possibly the keratotic reaction associated with electrochemical interactions.

Treatment and Prognosis. There is no specific treatment for hairy leukoplakia. It is critical, though, for this diagnosis to be confirmed subsequent to its clinical identification, because it may be a pre-AIDS sign. Responses to acyclovir ganciclovir, tretinoin, and podophyllin have been reported, with a return of lesions often noted on discontinuation of therapy.

Approximately 10% of individuals with diagnosed hairy leukoplakia have AIDS at the time of diagnosis, and an additional 18% develop this disease within 8 months. The probability of AIDS developing in individuals with hairy leukoplakia is nearly 50% at 16 months and as great as 80% by 30 months after the diagnosis of hairy leukoplakia is established.

Hairy Tongue

Etiology. The term *hairy tongue* is a nonspecific, clinically descriptive term referring to a condition occurring on the dorsal surface of the tongue. Although hairy tongue is generally idiopathic, there are numerous initiating or contributing factors. Broad-spectrum antibiotics, such as penicillin, and systemic corticosteroids are often identified in the clinical history of patients with this condition. Additionally, oxygenating mouth rinses containing hydrogen peroxide, sodium perborate, and carbamide peroxide have also been cited as possible contributing factors in this condition. Hairy tongue may also be seen in individuals who are intense smokers and in individuals who have undergone radiotherapy to the head and neck region for malignant disease. The basic problem

is believed to be related to an alteration in microbial flora, with an attendant overgrowth of fungi and chromogenic bacteria. However, numerous attempts at culture and identification of these organisms have not produced consistent results.

Clinical Features. The clinical alteration relates to hyperplasia of the filiform papillae, with concomitant retardation of the normal rate of desquamation. The result is a thick matted surface that serves to trap bacteria, fungi, cellular debris, and foreign material. Careful examination allows identification of individual elongated filiform papillae, some as long as several millimeters.

Symptoms are generally minimal, although when elongation of the papillae becomes exaggerated, a gagging or a tickling sensation may be felt. Depending on diet, oral hygiene, and the composition of the bacteria inhabiting the papillary surface, the color may range from white to tan to deep brown or black (Fig. 3–20).

Histopathology. Microscopic examination of a biopsy specimen confirms the presence of elongated filiform papillae, with surface contamination by clusters of microorganisms and fungi. Keratinization may extend into the midportions of the stratum spinosum. An orderly sequence of differentiation is noted from the basal region through the more superficial elements of the spinous layer. The underlying lamina propria is generally mildly inflamed.

Diagnosis. Because the clinical features of this lesion are usually quite characteristic, confirmation by biopsy is not necessary. Cytologic or culture studies are of little value.

Treatment and Prognosis. When taking a patient's history, identification of a possible etiologic factor, such as antibiotics or oxygenating mouth rinses, would be helpful. Discontinuing one of these agents should result in improvement within a few weeks. In cases in which individuals have

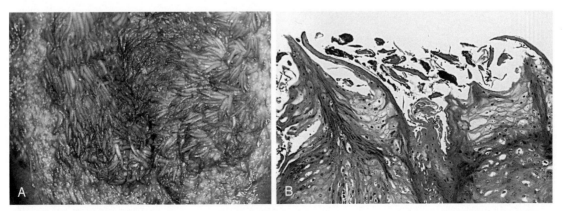

Figure 3–20. *A*, Hairy tongue stained dark by exogenous elements in a patient receiving radiation treatment for cancer. *B*, Biopsy specimen showing elongation of papillae and trapped bacterial colonies.

undergone radiotherapy, with resultant xerostomia and altered bacterial flora, management is more difficult. Brushing the tongue and maintaining fastidious oral hygiene should be of some benefit (application of a 1% solution of podophyllum resin has also been described as a useful treatment). It is important to emphasize to affected patients that this process is entirely benign and self-limiting and that the tongue should return to normal after institution of physical débridement and proper oral hygiene.

Geographic Tongue

Etiology. Geographic tongue, also known as *erythema migrans* and *benign migratory glossitis*, is a condition of unknown cause. Numerous theories have attempted to link this disease to emotional stress or infection by fungus or bacteria. Geographic tongue has been associated, probably coincidentally, with several different conditions, including psoriasis, seborrheic dermatitis, Reiter's syndrome, and atopy. In support of atopy, a significant difference has been noted between the prevalence of this condition in atopic patients having intrinsic asthma and rhinitis and its prevalence in patients with negative skin test reactions to various allergens. HLA-B15 antigens may be more commonly associated with an atopic patient and geographic tongue.

Clinical Features. Geographic tongue is seen in approximately 2% of the United States population, affecting women slightly more often than men. Children may occasionally be affected. This condition is characterized initially by the presence of small, round to irregular areas of dekeratinization and desquamation of filiform papillae (Fig. 3–21). The desquamated areas appear red and may be slightly tender. The elevated margins around the red zones are white to slightly yellowish white, often exhibiting a circinate pattern. Characteristically, the condition, when noted over a period of days or weeks, changes in pattern, appearing to

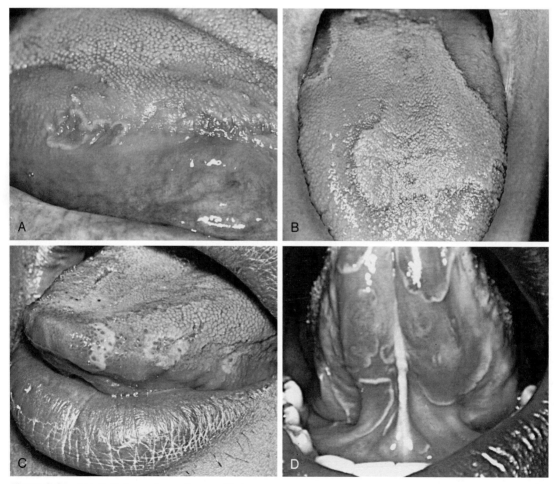

Figure 3–21. *A* to *D*, Various patterns of geographic tongue.

move across the dorsum of the tongue. As healing occurs in one area, the process extends to adjacent areas. A positive clinical correlation exists between geographic tongue and *plicated or fissured tongue.* The significance of this association is unknown, although symptoms may be more common when fissured tongue is present, presumably because of secondary fungal infection.

Rare cases of similar alterations of mucosa have been described in the floor of the mouth, the buccal mucosa, and the gingiva. The red atrophic lesions and white keratotic margins are similar to lingual counterparts.

Most patients with geographic tongue are asymptomatic. Occasionally, however, patients complain of irritation or tenderness, especially in relation to consumption of spicy foods and alcoholic beverages. Severity of symptoms varies with time and is often an indicator of the intensity of lesional activity. Lesions may periodically disappear and recur for no apparent reason.

Histopathology. Filiform papillae are reduced in number and prominence, and the margins of the lesion demonstrate hyperkeratosis and acanthosis. Closer to the central portion of the lesion, corresponding to the circinate erythematous areas, there is loss of superficial parakeratin, with significant migration of neutrophils and lymphocytes into the epithelium (Fig. 3–22). The leukocytes are often noted within a microabscess near the surface. An inflammatory cell infiltrate within the underlying lamina propria, consisting chiefly of neutrophils, lymphocytes, and plasma cells, can be seen. The histologic picture is reminiscent of psoriasis—indeed it has been described as a psoriasiform type of intraoral eruption. The clinical link, however, between geographic tongue and cutaneous psoriasis has not been substantiated.

Differential Diagnosis. Based on clinical appearance, geographic tongue is usually diagnostic. Only rarely might biopsy be required for a definitive diagnosis. In equivocal cases, clinical differential diagnosis might include candidiasis, leukoplakia, lichen planus, and lupus erythematosus.

Treatment and Prognosis. Because of the self-limiting and usually asymptomatic nature of this condition, treatment is not required. However, when symptoms occur, treatment is empirical. Topical steroids, especially ones containing an antifungal agent, may be helpful. Reassuring patients that this condition is totally benign and does not portend more serious disease helps relieve anxiety.

Lichen Planus

Lichen planus is a relatively common, chronic mucocutaneous disease of unknown cause. It was first described clinically by Wilson in 1869 and histologically by Dubreuilh in 1906. In oral mucosa, it typically presents as bilateral white lesions, occasionally with associated ulcers. The importance of this disease relates to its degree of frequency of occurrence, its occasional similarity to other mucosal diseases, its occasional painful nature, and its possible connection to malignancy.

Etiology and Pathogenesis. Although the cause of lichen planus is unknown, it is generally considered to be an immunologically mediated process that microscopically resembles a hypersensitivity reaction. It is characterized by an intense T cell infiltrate (CD4+ and especially CD8+ cells) located at the epithelial-connective tissue interface. Other immune-regulating cells (macrophages, XIIIa+ dendrocytes, Langerhans cells) are seen in increased numbers in lichen planus tissue. The

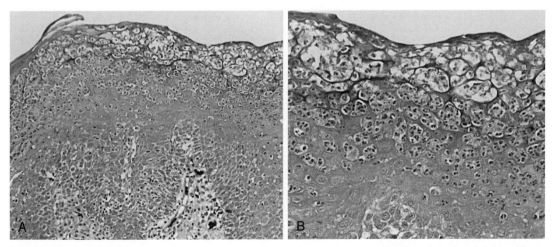

Figure 3–22. *A* and *B*, Biopsy specimen of an erythematous zone of geographic tongue showing relative keratin loss and intense neutrophilic infiltration.

disease mechanism appears to involve several steps that could be described as follows: an initiating factor/event, focal release of regulatory cytokines, up-regulation of vascular adhesion molecules, recruitment and retention of T lymphocytes, and cytotoxicity of basal keratinocytes mediated by the T lymphocytes.

The factor that initiates lichen planus is unknown. It is apparent, however, that recruitment and retention of lymphocytes is a requisite process. From what is known of leukocyte kinetics in tissue, attraction of lymphocytes to a particular site would require cytokine-mediated up-regulation of adhesion molecules on endothelial cells and concomitant expression of receptor molecules by circulating lymphocytes. In oral lichen planus, there is, in fact, increased expression of vascular adhesion molecules (known by acronyms ELAM-1, ICAM-1, VCAM-1), and infiltrating lymphocytes that express reciprocal receptors (known as L-selectin, LFA-1, and VLA4), supporting the hypothesis that there is activation of a lymphocyte homing mechanism in lichen planus. Some of the cytokines that are believed to be responsible for the up-regulated adhesion molecules are tumor necrosis factor (TNF-α), interleukin-1, and interferon-γ. The source of these cytokines is thought to be from resident macrophages, factor XIIIa dendrocytes, Langerhans cells, and the lymphocytes themselves.

The overlying keratinocytes in lichen planus have a significant role in disease pathogenesis. They may be another source of chemoattractive and proinflammatory cytokines mentioned earlier, and more importantly, they appear to be the immunologic target of the recruited lymphocytes. This latter role seems to be enhanced through keratinocyte expression of the adhesion molecule ICAM-1, which would be attractive to lymphocytes with corresponding receptor molecules (LFA-1). This could set up a favorable relationship between T cells and keratinocytes for cytotoxicity. The T cells appear to mediate basal cell death through the triggering of apoptosis.

Clinical Features. Lichen planus is a disease of middle age that affects men and women in nearly equal numbers. Children are rarely affected. The severity of the disease frequently parallels the patient's level of stress. An association between lichen planus and hepatitis C infection has been suggested. There appears to be no relationship between lichen planus and either hypertension or diabetes mellitus, as previously proposed.

Several types of lichen planus within the oral cavity have been described. The most common type is the *reticular form,* which is characterized by numerous interlacing white keratotic lines or striae (so-called Wickham's striae) that produce an annular or lacy pattern (Figs. 3–23 and 3–24). The buccal mucosa is the site most commonly involved. The striae, although occurring typically in a symmetric pattern on the buccal mucosae, may also be noted on the tongue and less frequently on the gingiva and the lips (Fig. 3–25). Almost any mucosal tissue may demonstrate manifestations of lichen planus. This form generally presents with minimal clinical symptoms and is often an incidental discovery.

The *plaque form* of lichen planus tends to resemble leukoplakia clinically but has a multifocal distribution. Such plaques generally range from slightly elevated to smooth and flat (Fig. 3–26).

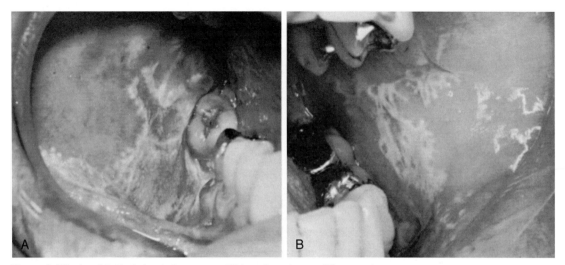

Figure 3–23. *A* and *B,* Typical reticular pattern of lichen planus in two different patients.

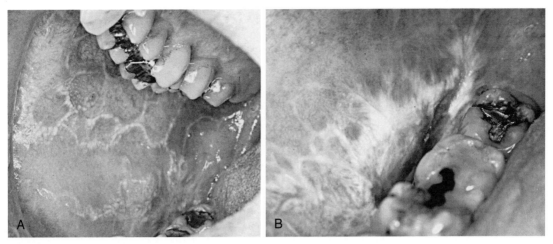

Figure 3–24. *A* and *B*, Lichen planus. Reticular pattern in two different patients.

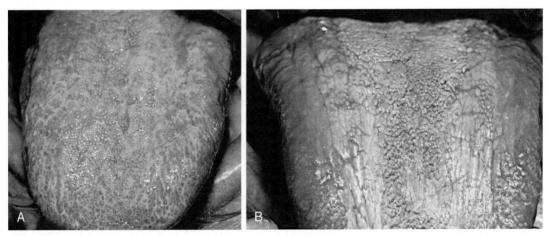

Figure 3–25. Lichen planus of the tongue. *A*, Reticular pattern. *B*, Plaque pattern with atrophy of the tongue papillae.

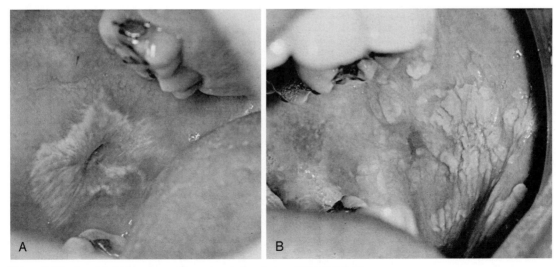

Figure 3–26. *A* and *B*, Lichen planus. Plaque-type lesions in two different patients.

The primary sites for this variant are the dorsum of the tongue and the buccal mucosa.

The *atrophic form* of lichen planus appears as red patches with very fine white striae. It may be seen in conjunction with reticular or erosive variants. The proportion of keratinized to atrophic areas varies from one area to another. The attached gingiva, frequently involved in this form of lichen planus, exhibits a patchy distribution, often in four quadrants (Fig. 3–27). Patients may complain of burning, sensitivity, and generalized discomfort.

In the *erosive form* of lichen planus, the central area of the lesion is ulcerated. A fibrinous plaque or pseudomembrane covers the ulcer. The process is a rather dynamic one, with changing patterns of involvement noted from week to week. Careful examination usually demonstrates keratotic striae, peripheral to the site of erosion, and erythema.

The rarely observed form of lichen planus is the *bullous variant*. The bullae or vesicles range from a few millimeters to centimeters in diameter. Such bullae are generally short lived and, on rupturing, leave an ulcerated, extremely uncomfortable surface. Lesions are usually seen on the buccal mucosa, especially in the posterior and inferior regions adjacent to the second and third molars. Lesions are less on the tongue, gingiva, and inner aspect of the lips. Reticular or striated keratotic areas should be seen with this variant of lichen planus.

On the skin, lichen planus is characterized by the presence of small, violaceous, polygonal, flat-topped papules on the flexor surfaces (Fig. 3–28). Other clinical varieties include hypertrophic, atrophic, bullous, follicular, and linear forms. Cutaneous lesions are noted in approximately 20 to 60% of patients presenting with oral lichen planus. Although the oral changes are more constant over time, it has been noted that the corresponding skin lesions wax and wane.

Histopathology. The microscopic criteria for lichen planus include hyperkeratosis, basal layer vacuolization with apoptotic keratinocytes, and a lymphophagocytic infiltrate at the epithelial-connective tissue interface (Fig. 3–29). With time, the epithelium undergoes gradual remodeling, resulting in reduced thickness and occasionally a sawtooth rete ridge pattern. Within the epithelium are increased numbers of Langerhans cells (as demonstrated with immunohistochemistry), presumably processing and presenting antigens to the subjacent T lymphocytes (Fig. 3–30). Discrete eosinophilic ovoid bodies representing the apoptotic keratinocytes are noted at the basal zone. These colloid or Civatte bodies are seen in other conditions such as drug reactions, lupus erythematosus, and some nonspecific inflammatory reactions.

Direct immunofluorescence demonstrates the presence of fibrinogen in the basement membrane zone in 90 to 100% of cases. Although immunoglobulins and complement factors may be found as well, they are far less common than fibrinogen deposition. The immunofluorescence pattern in this disease is not diagnostic, because such patterns may also be seen in lupus erythematosus and erythema multiforme.

Differential Diagnosis. Other diseases with a multifocal bilateral presentation that should be included in a clinical differential are lichenoid drug reaction, lupus erythematosus, cheek chewing, graft-versus-host disease, and candidiasis. Idiopathic leukoplakia and squamous cell carcinoma

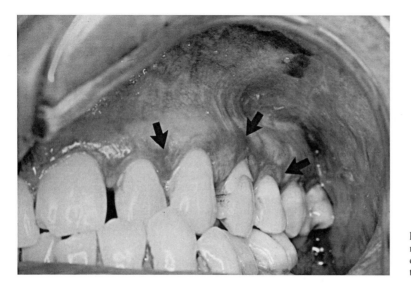

Figure 3–27. Atrophic lichen planus of the gingiva. Note atrophic dark areas *(arrows)* from which keratotic striae radiate.

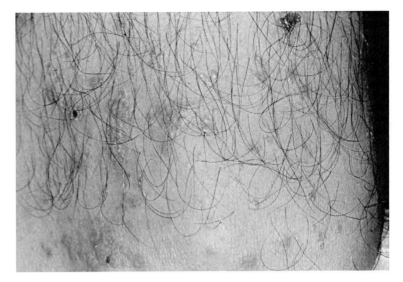

Figure 3–28. Lichen planus of the skin of the ankle presenting as an excoriated papular eruption.

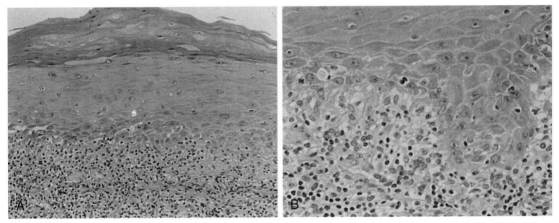

Figure 3–29. *A*, Micrograph of lichen planus showing hyperkeratosis and interface changes of lymphocyte infiltration and basal layer vacuolization. *B*, High magnification of the epithelial-connective tissue interface.

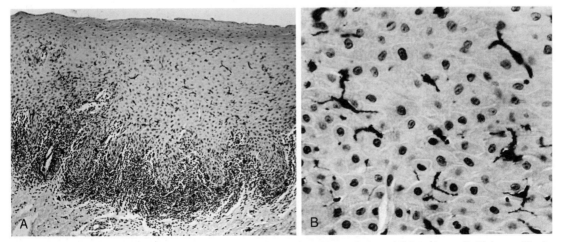

Figure 3–30. *A*, Immunohistochemical stain (S-100 protein) of Langerhans cells in oral lichen planus. *B*, High-magnification detail of dendritic Langerhans cells in the midepithelial zone.

might be considered when lesions are plaque-like. Erosive or atrophic lichen planus affecting the attached gingiva must be differentiated from cicatricial pemphigoid, chronic lupus erythematosus, contact hypersensitivity, and chronic candidiasis.

Treatment and Prognosis. Although lichen planus cannot generally be cured, some drugs can provide satisfactory control. Corticosteroids are the single most useful group of drugs in the management of patients with lichen planus. The rationale for their use is their ability to modulate inflammation and the immune response. Topical application and local injection of steroids have been successfully used in controlling but not curing this disease. In circumstances in which symptoms are severe, systemic steroids may be used for initial management. The addition of antifungal therapy to a corticosteroid regimen typically enhances clinical results. This is likely a result of elimination of secondary *C. albicans* growth in lichen planus–involved tissue. Antifungals also prevent the overgrowth of *C. albicans* that may be associated with corticosteroid use.

Because of their antikeratinizing and immunomodulating effects, systemic and topical vitamin A analogues (retinoids) have been used in the management of the keratinized reticular and plaque variants of lichen planus (Fig. 3–31). Reversal of white striae can be achieved with topical retinoids, although the effects may be only temporary. Systemic retinoids have been used in cases of severe lichen planus with various degrees of success. The benefits of systemic therapy must be carefully weighed against the rather significant side effects—cheilitis, elevation of serum liver enzyme and triglyceride levels, and teratogenicity. In cases with significant tissue involvement, more than one drug may be indicated. Various combinations of systemic steroids, topical steroids, and retinoids may be used with some success.

Although there is some debate about the malignant potential of oral lichen planus, it appears that the rate of oral squamous cell carcinoma is slightly higher in patients with lichen planus as compared with the general population. The actual frequency of malignant transformation appears to be rather low overall, and malignant transformation is more commonly noted in the erosive and the atrophic forms of the disease. Because lichen planus is a chronic condition, patients should be observed periodically and should be offered education about the clinical course, rationale of therapy, and risk of malignant transformation. This is particularly important for those with the erosive or the atrophic form of the disease and for those with a history of tobacco or alcohol abuse.

Dentifrice-Associated Slough

This is a relatively common phenomenon that has been associated with the use of several different brands of toothpaste. It is believed to be a superficial chemical burn or reaction to a component in the dentifrice, possibly the detergent or flavoring compounds. Clinically, it appears as a superficial whitish slough of the buccal mucosa (Fig. 3–32), typically detected by the patient as oral peeling. The condition is painless and is not known to progress to anything significant. The problem resolves with a switch to another, blander toothpaste.

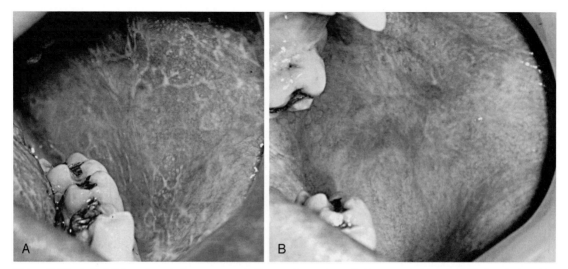

Figure 3–31. *A*, Oral lichen planus before treatment. *B*, Same patient at the end of treatment with topical 13-*cis*-retinoic acid.

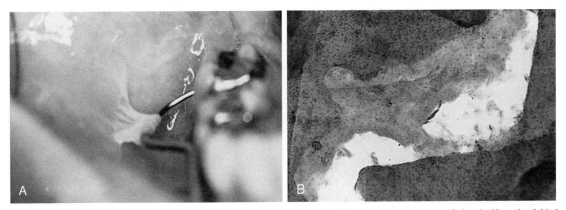

Figure 3–32. *A*, Dentifrice-associated slough captured with an explorer. *B*, Microscopic appearance of slough. Note the folded sheets of parakeratin.

NONEPITHELIAL WHITE-YELLOW LESIONS

Candidiasis

Candidiasis encompasses a group of mucosal and cutaneous conditions with a common etiologic agent from the *Candida* genus of fungi. It is the most common oral mycotic infection, although frequency rates are difficult to determine because of the prevalence of the causative organism in a large proportion of the population. The relationship between the commensal state and pathogenicity is a complex one, being based on local factors in some cases and local plus systemic factors in others. Oral manifestations may be acute or chronic, with various degrees of severity. Numerous systems of classification have been formulated, indicating the complexity of this condition, the many modes of clinical presentation, and the interrelationship with local and systemic factors. In addition, a relationship has been reported between a subset known as *candidal leukoplakia* and squamous cell carcinoma.

Etiology and Pathogenesis. Candidiasis is caused by *C. albicans* and the related but far less common species *C. parapsilosis*, *C. tropicalis*, *C. glabrata*, *C. krusei*, *C. pseudotropicalis*, and *C. guilliermondi*. *C. albicans* is a commensal organism residing in the oral cavity in a majority of healthy persons. Transformation or escape from a state of commensalism to that of a pathogen by this organism relates to local and systemic factors that are extremely difficult to create experimentally. The organism is a unicellular yeast of the Cryptococcaceae family and may exist in three distinct biologic and morphologic forms: the vegetative or yeast form of oval cells (blastospores), measuring 1.5 to 5 μm in diameter; the elongated cellular form (pseudohyphae); and the chlamydospore form, which consists of cell bodies measuring 7 to 17 μm in diameter, with a thick, refractile, enclosing wall. The persistence of this organism in its vegetative state is noted intraorally (and intravaginally) and is stated to be related in part to its symbiotic partnership with *Lactobacillus acidophilus*. As evidenced by its frequency in the general population, *C. albicans* is of weak pathogenicity, thereby reflecting the necessity for local or systemic predisposing factors (Table 3–4) to produce a disease state.

Infection with this organism is usually superficial, affecting the outer aspects of the involved oral mucosa or skin. In severely debilitated and immunocompromised patients, such as patients with AIDS, infection may extend into the alimentary tract (candidal esophagitis), bronchopulmonary tract, or other organ systems. The opportunistic nature of this organism is observed in the frequency of mild forms of the disease secondary to short-term use of systemic antibiotic therapy for minor bacterial infections.

Table 3–4. Predisposing Factors for *Candida* Infection

Immunologic immaturity of infancy
Endocrine disturbances
   Diabetes mellitus
   Hypoparathyroidism
   Pregnancy
   Systemic steroid therapy/hypoadrenalism
Topical corticosteroid therapy
Xerostomia
Poor oral hygiene
Advanced malignancy
Malabsorption and malnutrition
Systemic antibiotic therapy
Cancer chemotherapy and radiation therapy
Other forms of immunosuppression (e.g., AIDS)

Table 3–5. Oral Candidiasis Classification

Acute candidiasis
  Pseudomembranous
  Atrophic
Chronic candidiasis
  Atrophic
  Hypertrophic/hyperplastic
Mucocutaneous forms
  Localized (oral, face, scalp, nails)
  Familial
  Syndrome-associated

Clinical Features. Oral manifestations of this disease are variable, with numerous forms noted (Table 3–5). The most common form is the acute pseudomembranous form also known as *thrush* (Fig. 3–33). Young infants and the elderly are frequently affected. Estimates of disease frequency range up to 5% of neonates, 5% of cancer patients, and 10% of institutionalized, debilitated elderly patients. This infection is common in patients being treated with radiation or chemotherapy for leukemia and solid tumors, with up to half of those in the former group and 70% in the latter group affected. Candidiasis has also been recognized in patients who suffer from AIDS and those who have HIV infections.

Oral lesions of *acute candidiasis* are characteristically white, soft to gelatinous plaques or nodules that grow centrifugally and merge. Plaques are composed of fungal organisms, keratotic debris, inflammatory cells, desquamated epithelial cells, bacteria, and fibrin. Wiping away the plaques or pseudomembranes with a gauze sponge or cotton-tipped applicator leaves an erythematous, eroded, or ulcerated surface that is often tender. Although lesions of thrush may develop at any location, favored sites include the buccal mu-

cosa and mucobuccal folds, the oropharynx, and the lateral aspects of the dorsal tongue surface. In most instances in which the pseudomembrane has not been disturbed, the associated symptoms are minimal. In severe cases, patients may complain of tenderness, burning, and dysphagia.

Persistence of acute pseudomembranous candidiasis may eventually result in loss of the pseudomembrane, with presentation as a more generalized red lesion, known as acute *atrophic candidiasis* (Fig. 3–34). Along the dorsum of the tongue, patches of depapillation and dekeratinization may be noted. In the past, this particular form of candidiasis was known as *antibiotic stomatitis* or *antibiotic glossitis* because of its frequent relationship to antibiotic treatment of acute infections. Of interest is that broad-spectrum antibiotics or concurrent administration of multiple narrow-spectrum antibiotics may produce this secondary infection to a much greater degree than do single narrow-spectrum antibiotics. Withdrawal of the offending antibiotic and institution of appropriate oral hygiene leads to improvement. in contrast to the acute pseudomembranous form, oral symptoms of the acute atrophic form are quite marked because of numerous erosions and intense inflammation.

Chronic atrophic candidiasis is a commonly seen atrophic subset (Fig. 3–35). This particular form of candidiasis occurs in as many as 65% of geriatric individuals who wear complete maxillary dentures (denture sore mouth). Expression of this form of candidiasis depends on the conditioning of the oral mucosa by a covering prosthesis. There is a distinct predilection for the palatal mucosa as compared with the mandibular alveolar arch. Women show a greater propensity for developing this form of the disease than men. Chronic low-grade trauma secondary to poor prosthesis fit, less

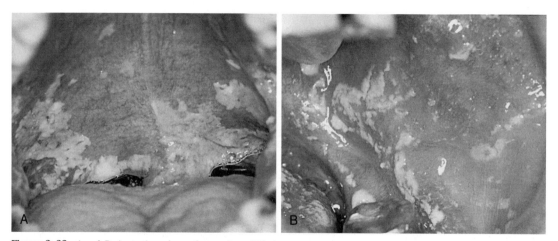

Figure 3–33. *A* and *B*, Acute (pseudomembranous) candidiasis.

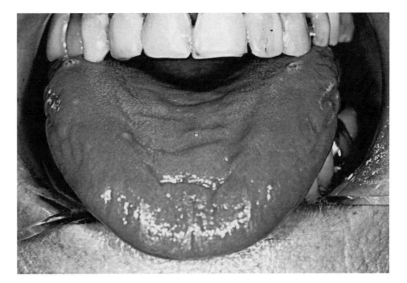

Figure 3–34. Acute atrophic candidiasis.

than ideal occlusal relationships, and failure to remove the appliance at night all contribute to the development of this condition. The clinical appearance is that of a bright red, somewhat velvety to pebbly surface, with relatively little keratinization.

Also seen in individuals with denture-related chronic atrophic candidiasis is *angular cheilitis* (Fig. 3–35). This condition is especially prevalent in individuals who demonstrate deep folds at the commissures secondary to overclosure. In such circumstances, small accumulations of saliva gather in the skin folds at the commissural angles and are subsequently colonized by yeast organisms (and frequently *Staphylococcus aureus*). Clinically, the lesions are moderately painful, fissured, eroded, and encrusted. Angular cheilitis may also occur in individuals who habitually lick their lips and deposit small amounts of saliva in the commissural angles.

A circumoral type of atrophic candidiasis may be noted in those with severe lip-licking habits with extension of the process onto the surrounding skin. The skin is fissured and demonstrates a degree of brown discoloration on a slightly erythematous base. This condition is to be separated from *perioral dermatitis,* which characteristically shows less crusting and a zone of uninvolved skin immediately adjacent to the cutaneous-vermilion junction.

Chronic candidal infections are also capable of producing a hyperplastic tissue response *(chronic hypertrophic candidiasis).* When occurring in the retrocommissural area, the lesion resembles speckled leukoplakia and, in some classifications, is known as *candidal leukoplakia.* It occurs in adults with no apparent predisposition to infection by *C.*

albicans, and it is believed by some clinicians to represent a premalignant lesion.

Hyperplastic candidiasis may involve the dorsum of the tongue in a pattern referred to as *median rhomboid glossitis* (Fig. 3–36). It is usually asymptomatic and is generally discovered on routine oral examination. The lesion is found anterior to the circumvallate papillae and has a rhomboid outline. It may have a smooth, nodular, or fissured surface. It may be slightly indurated and may range in color from white to a more characteristic red. In the past, this particular condition was believed to be a developmental anomaly, presumably secondary to persistence of the tuberculum impar of the developing tongue. Evidence indicates, however, that this is more likely a hypertrophic form of candidiasis.

Nodular papillary lesions of the hard palatal mucosa predominantly seen beneath maxillary complete dentures are thought to represent, at least in part, a response to chronic yeast infection (Fig. 3–36). The *papillary hyperplasia* is composed of individual nodules that are ovoid to spherical and form excrescences measuring 2 to 3 mm in diameter on an erythematous background.

Mucocutaneous candidiasis is a rather diverse group of conditions. The localized form of mucocutaneous candidiasis is characterized by longstanding and persistent candidiasis of the oral mucosa, nails, skin, and vaginal mucosa (Fig. 3–37). This form of candidiasis is often resistant to treatment, with only temporary remission following the use of standard antifungal therapy. This form begins early in life, usually within the first 2 decades. The disease begins as a pseudomembranous type of candidiasis and is soon followed by nail and cutaneous involvement. Nail changes

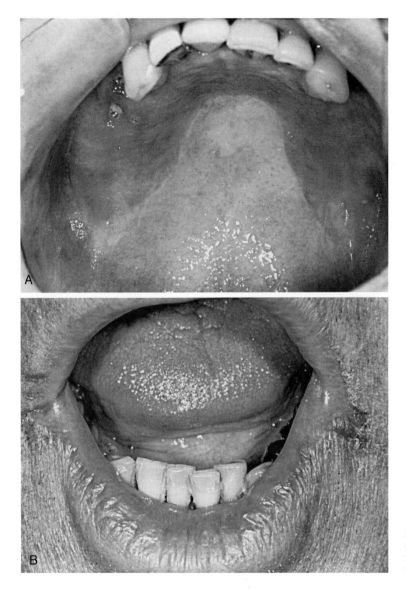

Figure 3–35. Chronic atrophic candidiasis. *A*, Denture "sore mouth" type. *B*, Angular cheilitis or perlèche type.

range from slight involvement of a single nail to severe disfigurement of all nails. Secondary granulomatous changes occur in the nail bed as well as in the associated skin lesions.

A familial form of mucocutaneous candidiasis, believed to be transmitted in an autosomal recessive fashion, demonstrates in nearly 50% of patients an associated endocrinopathy. This endocrinopathy usually consists of hypoparathyroidism, Addison's disease, and occasionally hypothyroidism or diabetes mellitus. Other forms of familial mucocutaneous candidiasis have associated defects in iron metabolism and cell-mediated immunity.

The triad of chronic mucocutaneous candidiasis, myositis, and thymoma was initially reported in 1968. Several cases have been reported since then.

Myositis usually is the initial manifestation, followed by mucocutaneous expression of the disease. Muscle biopsy specimens in this disorder demonstrate sharply demarcated, intense lymphocytic infiltration between bundles of striated muscle. The role of the thymus relates to a deficiency in T cell–mediated immunologic function, hence providing an opportunity for yeast proliferation. It is theorized that appropriately armed T lymphocytes may control *Candida* infections by manufacturing and releasing a lymphokine-like substance that is reported to be toxic for the organism.

A final form of candidiasis, both acute and chronic, is becoming increasingly evident within the immunosuppressed population of patients, in particular those infected with HIV. This form of candidiasis was originally described in 1981 and

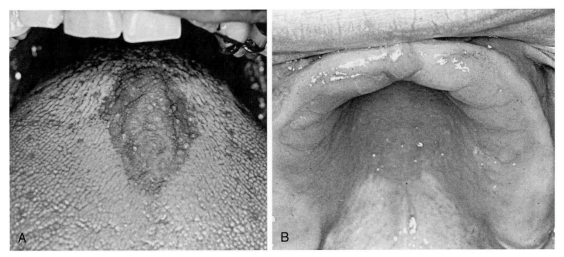

Figure 3–36. Chronic hypertrophic/hyperplastic candidiasis. *A*, Median rhomboid glossitis type. *B*, Palatal papillary type.

is now well recognized as being one of the more important opportunistic infections that afflict this group of patients. The significantly depleted cell-mediated arm of the immune mechanism is believed to be responsible for allowing the development of severe candidiasis in these patients.

Laboratory Findings. Clinical laboratory tests for this organism involve removal of a portion of the candidal plaque, which is then smeared on a microscope slide and macerated with 20% potassium hydroxide or stained with PAS. The slide is subsequently examined for typical hyphae. Culture identification and quantification of organisms may be performed with various media, including Sabouraud's broth, blood agar, and cornmeal agar. Immunofluorescent identification may be necessary in forms of the disease in which no colonies are clinically evident, especially in the chronic atrophic form of the disease. Traditional methods

of laboratory characterization of *C. albicans* and other species relate to viable carbohydrate fermentation and assimilation studies as well as microscopic characteristics.

Histopathology. In superficial infections, fungi are limited to the surface layers of the epithelium; in more severe examples, hyphae extend deeper into the epithelium (Fig. 3–38). Neutrophilic infiltration of the epithelium with superficial microabscess formation is typically seen. Yeast elements may be morphologically enhanced by staining with methenamine silver or periodic acid–Schiff (PAS) reagent. The predominant fungal forms growing in this particular form of the disease are pseudohyphae. These pseudohyphae penetrate the epithelium and may actually enter keratinocytes to become intracellular parasites. The chronic varieties of candidiasis have epithelial hyperplasia in common. Epithelial hyperplasia is a rather charac-

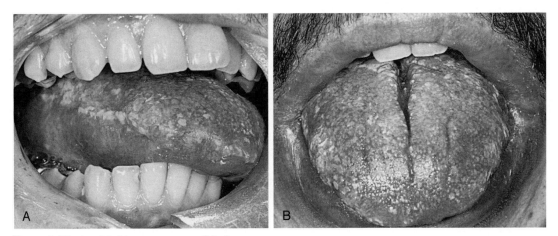

Figure 3–37. *A* and *B*, Mucocutaneous candidiasis.

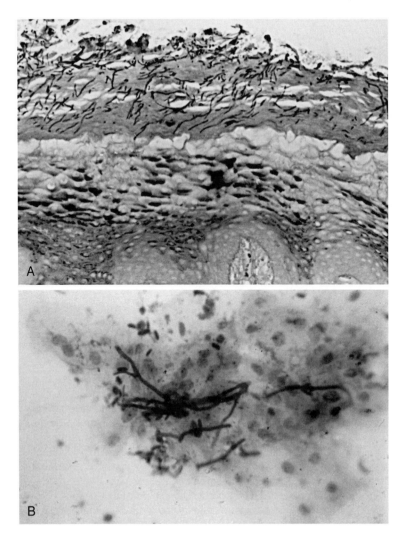

A

B

Figure 3–38. *A*, Microscopic section (PAS stain) of acute candidiasis. Numerous dark-stained hyphae and spore forms of *C. albicans* are present in the parakeratotic layer. *B*, Cytology smear showing hyphae over a background of parakeratotic cells. (*B*, Courtesy of Dr. W. G. Sprague.)

teristic feature of this form of the disease and has been shown to be induced by the presence of the yeast organism. Although chronic candidiasis may give rise to oral leukoplakia, there is no clear evidence that chronic candidiasis is in and of itself a precancerous state. It is possible, however, that epithelial invasion by this organism and subsequent proliferation may contribute to neoplastic change.

Differential Diagnosis. Candidal infections must be differentiated from several entities, including slough associated with chemical burns, traumatic ulcerations, mucous patches of syphilis, and white keratotic lesions. When isolated red lesions of the acute atrophic form of candidiasis are present, they must be differentiated from drug reactions and thermal burns. In addition, these red lesions may resemble erosive lichen planus, discoid lupus erythematosus, and early or mild cases of erythema multiforme.

Treatment and Prognosis. The majority of *C. albicans* infections may be simply treated with topical applications of nystatin suspension. In denture-related disease, nystatin cream may be used on the affected tissue and in the denture itself to provide prolonged contact and eliminate organisms in the denture material. Withdrawal of broad-spectrum antibiotics usually produces resolution of the oral yeast infection. If oxygenating agents, such as hydrogen peroxide, have been used continuously, withdrawal of these particular substances should allow for reestablishment of normal oral bacterial flora and relief of symptoms. Clotrimazole can be conveniently administered in lozenge or troche form. Topical applications of either nystatin or clotrimazole should be continued for at least 1 week beyond the disappearance of clinical manifestations of the disease. It is important to note that antifungals designed specifically for oral use contain considerable amounts of sugar, making them undesirable for the treatment of candidiasis in dentulous patients with xerostomia. Sugar-free antifungal vaginal tablets (dissolved in the mouth) are an excellent treatment alternative to avoid the complication of dental caries.

In cases of chronic mucocutaneous candidiasis or oral candidiasis associated with immunosuppression, topical agents may not be effective. In such instances, systemic administration of medications such as amphotericin B, ketoconazole, fluconazole, or itraconazole may be necessary. Caution must be exercised, however, because these drugs may be hepatotoxic.

The prognosis for acute and most other forms of chronic candidiasis is excellent. The underlying defect in most types of mucocutaneous candidiasis, however, militates against cure, although intermittent improvement may be noted after the use of systemic antifungal agents.

Mucosal Burns

Etiology. The most common form of superficial burn of the oral mucosa is associated with topical applications of chemicals, such as aspirin or caustic agents. Topical abuse of drugs, accidental placement of phosphoric acid–etching solutions or gel by a dentist, or overly fastidious use of alcohol-containing mouthwashes may produce similar effects.

Clinical Features. In cases of short-term exposure to agents capable of inducing tissue necrosis, a localized mild erythema may occur. As the concentration of the offending agent increases and as the contact time increases, surface coagulative necrosis is more likely to occur, resulting in a white slough or membrane (Fig. 3–39). Beneath the membrane is a friable, painful surface that bleeds easily on manipulation. With gentle traction, the surface slough peels from the denuded connective tissue, producing considerable tenderness and pain.

Thermal burns are commonly noted on the hard palatal mucosa and are generally associated with hot, sticky foods. Hot liquids are more likely to burn the tongue or the soft palate. Such lesions are generally erythematous rather than white (necrosis), as is seen with chemical burns.

Another form of burn that is potentially quite serious is the electrical burn. In particular, children who chew through electrical cords receive rather characteristic initial burns that are often symmetric. The result of these accidents is significant tissue damage, frequently followed by scarring and reduction in the size of the oral opening. The surface of these lesions tends to be characterized by a thickened slough that extends deep into the surrounding connective tissue.

Histopathology. In cases of chemical and thermal burns in which an obvious clinical slough has developed, the epithelial component shows coagulative necrosis through its entire thickness. A fibrinous exudate is also evident. The underlying connective tissue is intensely inflamed. Electrical burns are more destructive, showing deep extension of necrosis, often into muscle.

Differential Diagnosis. The fundamental element in establishing the diagnosis of a mucosal burn relates to obtaining an accurate history, with the identification of an agent that may produce tissue damage. Among the most frequent agents involved with localized mucosal sloughs traditionally has been aspirin, used as topical treatment for toothache.

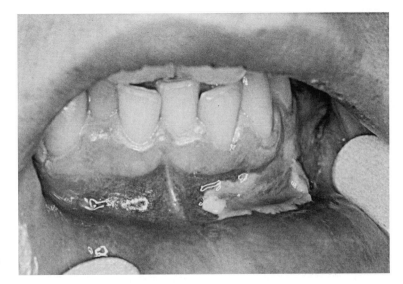

Figure 3–39. Chemical burn of the vestibular mucosa.

In the absence of a history of use of a chemical likely to produce a burn or a history of ingestion of excessively hot food, a fibrinous exudate over an ulcerated pyogenic granuloma or a pseudomembrane associated with acute necrotizing ulcerative gingivitis or noma-like lesion might be included in a differential diagnosis.

Treatment. Management of chemical, thermal, or electrical burns is quite variable. For patients with thermal or chemical burn, local symptomatic therapy with or without the use of systemic analgesics is appropriate. Topical therapy using hydrocortisone acetate with or without benzocaine may be helpful. Application of dilute solutions of topical anesthetic such as 1% dyclonine hydrochloride (Dyclone) also reduces symptoms. For patients with electrical burns, management may be much more difficult. The services of a pediatric dentist, the oral and maxillofacial surgeon, and, on occasion, a plastic surgeon may be necessary in more severe cases. Pressure stents may be required over the damaged areas to prevent early contracture of the wounds. After healing, further definitive surgical or reconstructive treatment may be necessary because of extensive scar formation or loss of significant amounts of tissue.

Submucous Fibrosis

Etiology. Several factors contributing to etiologic submucous fibrosis include general nutritional or vitamin deficiencies and hypersensitivity to various dietary constituents. The primary factor appears to be chronic and frequent chewing of the areca (betel) nut. From the dietary perspective, chronic exposure to chili peppers or chronic and prolonged deficiency of iron and B complex vitamins, especially folic acid, alters the oral mucosa. The alteration increases the risk or rate of hypersensitivity to many potential irritants, such as dietary spices and tobacco, with an attendant inflammatory reaction and fibrotic response.

Experimental models for the study of submucous fibrosis have been developed; *in vitro* studies have demonstrated that components of the betel nut *(Areca catecha)* increase collagen synthesis by 170% as compared with controls.

Clinical Features. This disease is rarely seen in North America. It is generally noted in individuals who have emigrated from Southeast Asia or India. Other ethnic clustering may be noted in Pakistanis and Burmese, with sporadic cases observed in South Vietnamese, Thais, Chinese, and Nepalese. Those affected are typically between the ages of 20 and 40, although the condition may be seen in younger and older individuals as well.

Oral submucous fibrosis presents as a whitish-yellow lesion that has a chronic insidious biologic course. It is typically seen within the oral cavity but on occasion may extend into the pharynx and the esophagus. Submucous fibrosis may occasionally be preceded by or be associated with vesicle formation. In time, the affected mucosa, especially the soft palate and the buccal mucosa, loses its resilience and elasticity, with resultant trismus and considerable difficulty in eating. The process progresses from the lamina propria initially to the underlying musculature.

Histopathology. Microscopically, the principal feature is atrophy of the epithelium, with variable degrees of dysplastic change. The superficial portions of the lamina propria are poorly vascularized and hyalinized (Fig. 3–40). Fibroblasts are few,

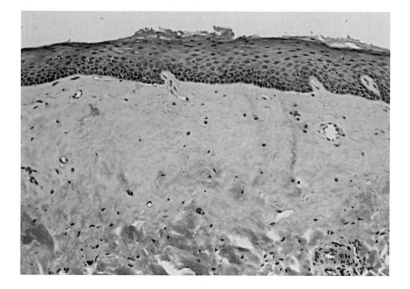

Figure 3–40. Biopsy of oral submucous fibrosis showing hyalinization of connective tissue and epithelial atrophy.

and there is a chronic inflammatory infiltrate ranging from minimal to moderate. Ultrastructural and immunofluorescence studies have shown that type I collagen predominates while type III collagen tends to localize at the epithelial-connective tissue interface, around blood vessels, salivary glands, and muscle. All forms of collagen, although excessive, are morphologically normal.

Differential Diagnosis. The clinical differential diagnosis of submucous fibrosis includes a relatively small number of entities. Radiation-related subepithelial fibrosis and mucosal scarring secondary to thermal or chemical burns may produce similar clinical features.

Treatment and Prognosis. Treatment has included stretching exercises and intralesional injections of corticosteroids. Surgical releasing procedures likewise have been used. Success has been reported with local injections of chymotrypsin, hyaluronidase, and dexamethasone, with surgical excision of fibrous bands and submucosal placement of placental grafts. All methods of treatment, however, have proved to be of only modest help in this essentially irreversible condition.

The primary importance of submucous fibrosis relates to its reported premalignant nature. The development of squamous cell carcinoma has been noted in as many as one third of patients with submucous fibrosis. It has been speculated that fibroblastic degeneration and epithelial atrophy form the physical basis for carcinogen penetration through the epithelium. The restriction or elimination of tobacco use should be attempted, and etiologic dietary agents should be withdrawn.

Fordyce's Granules

Etiology. Fordyce's granules represent ectopic sebaceous glands or sebaceous choristomas (normal tissue in an abnormal location). The origin of such granules is thought to be developmental.

Clinical Features. Fordyce's granules are multiple, often seen in aggregates or in confluent arrangements (Fig. 3–41). The sites of predilection include the buccal mucosa and the vermilion of the upper lip. The lesions generally are symmetrically distributed. Men show larger numbers of lesions per unit area than do women. The age of appearance generally is postpubertal, with numbers of lesions reaching a peak between 20 and 30 years of age. The lesions are asymptomatic and are often discovered incidentally by the patient or by the practitioner during a routine oral examination. A large proportion of the population is affected by this particular condition; it is seen in approximately 80% of individuals.

Histopathology. Superficially located lobules of sebaceous glands are aggregated around or adjacent to excretory ducts. The ducts themselves contain sebaceous and keratinous debris. The heterotopic glands are well formed and appear functional. Individual cells demonstrate a granular, rel-

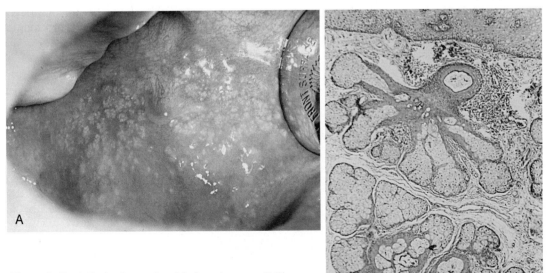

Figure 3–41. *A*, Fordyce's granules of the buccal mucosa. *B*, Biopsy specimen showing numerous lobules of sebaceous glands.

atively clear cytoplasm with nuclei that are slightly pyknotic in nature. Except for the relationship of sebaceous glands to hair in the skin, there is virtual identity of the oral glands with cutaneous glands.

Differential Diagnosis. The appearance and distribution of the glands may on occasion be mistaken for small clusters of *C. albicans* organisms. Simple wiping of the surface of the Fordyce's granules, however, would not result in their disappearance as would be the case with candidal colonies. Very few other conditions could be mistaken for this particular entity.

Treatment and Prognosis. No treatment is indicated for this particular condition, because the glands are normal in character and do not cause any untoward effects.

Ectopic Lymphoid Tissue

Ectopic lymphoid tissue may be found in numerous oral locations. It is normally found in the posterolateral aspect of the tongue, where it is known as the *lingual tonsil.* Aggregates of lymphoid tissue may commonly be seen in the soft palate, the floor of the mouth, and the tonsillar pillars, although they may occur in other sites as well.

Lymphoid tissue appears yellow or yellow-white clinically and typically produces small, dome-shaped elevations (Fig. 3–42). The tissue appears uninflamed, and the patient is unaware of its presence. Crypts in the lymphoid tissue may on occasion become obstructed, causing "cystic" dilatation of the area. These lesions may then be called *lymphoepithelial cysts.* In a strict sense, however, lymphoepithelial cysts are believed to be derived from cystic change of embryonically entrapped epithelium within lymphoid tissue.

Generally, lymphoid tissue can be diagnosed on clinical features alone. Because this is basically normal tissue, no biopsy is necessary.

Gingival Cysts

Gingival cysts of odontogenic origin occur in adults as well as infants. In infants, the relative frequency is highest in the neonatal phase, and by 3 months the cysts are rarely noted. Observations of such cysts in the neonatal period and later indicate that the vast majority involute spontaneously or rupture and exfoliate. Two eponyms have been commonly used as synonyms for gingival cysts (Epstein's pearls and Bohn's nodules), although these eponyms were originally intended to designate different neonatal cysts. The term *Epstein's pearls* was used to designate cysts noted along the palatal midline that had no relationship to the tooth-forming apparatus. The term *Bohn's nodules* referred to cysts noted along the alveolar ridges that were believed to be related to salivary gland remnants.

Etiology and Pathogenesis. Neonatal gingival cysts are thought to arise from the dental lamina remnants. Fetal tissues between 10 and 12 weeks of age show small amounts of keratin within elements of the dental lamina. Toward the end of the twelfth week of gestation, disruption of the dental lamina is evident, with many fragments demonstrating central cystification and keratin accumulation. Gingival cysts are generally numerous in the fetus and infant, increasing in number to the twenty-second week of gestation.

Midline palatal cysts, or Epstein's pearls, are

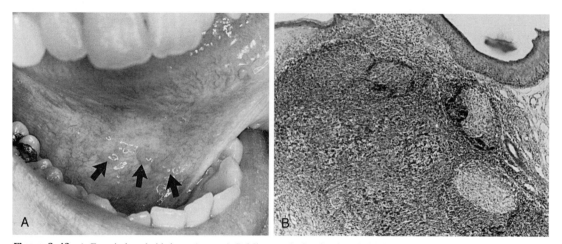

Figure 3–42. *A,* Ectopic lymphoid tissue *(arrows). B,* Micrograph showing lymphoid tissue covered by intact epithelium.

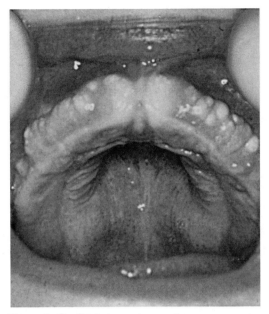

Figure 3–43. Gingival cysts in a newborn.

multilocular lesion. An alternative theory of pathogenesis relates to the traumatic implantation of surface epithelium into gingival connective tissue.

Clinical Features. Gingival cyst in a neonate presents as a white or off-white broad-based nodule approximately 2 mm in diameter. One to many cysts are evident along the alveolar crests (Fig. 3–43). Midline palatal cysts, on the other hand, present along the midpalatal raphe toward the junction of the hard and soft palate. The overall incidence has been estimated at 76%.

The gingival cyst of adults occurs chiefly during the fifth and sixth decades. It appears more frequently in the mandible than in the maxilla (Fig. 3–44). There is a great deal of similarity between the gingival cyst in the adult and the lateral periodontal cyst, including site of predilection, age of occurrence, clinical behavior, and overall morphology.

The gingival cyst of adults is painless, well circumscribed, and slow growing. The lesions generally occur in the attached gingiva, often within the interdental papilla. Only rarely are such lesions found along the lingual gingiva. Premolar and bicuspid regions of the mandible are favored locations. The overlying epithelium is intact and smooth. The lesion may appear white-yellow to blue. In cases of long duration and large size (approaching 1 cm in diameter), slight saucerization of the underlying alveolar crestal bone may occur, especially in the interdental region. In these cases, a subtle semilunar shadow or lucency, indicating erosion of the superior aspect of the alveolar crest, may be seen.

Histopathology. In the neonatal gingival cyst, subepithelial cystic structures demonstrate an epi-

thought to result from epithelial entrapment within the midline of palatal fusion. Small epithelial inclusions within the line of fusion produce microcysts that contain keratin and usually rupture early in life. Detailed developmental studies have shown that fewer than 20 midline palatal keratinizing cysts are noted in any fetus by the fourteenth week of gestation, with no increased tendency to exceed that number with time.

The origin of the gingival cyst of the adult is probably from remnants of the dental lamina (rests of Serres) within the gingival submucosa. Cystic change of these rests may occasionally result in a

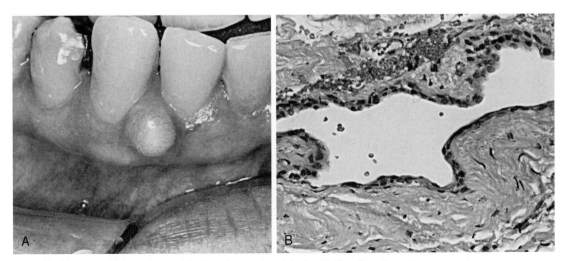

Figure 3–44. *A*, Gingival cyst in an adult. *B*, A thin, nonkeratinized epithelium lines the cyst.

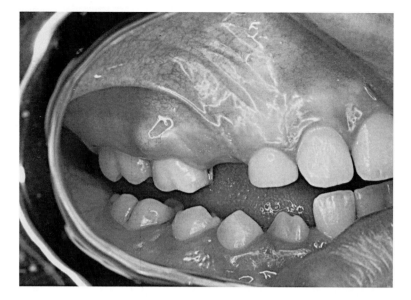

Figure 3–45. Parulis adjacent to an upper molar.

thelial lining that is often thin and attenuated. The basal layer is characteristically flattened, and the surface parakeratinized squames fill the lumen. Dystrophic mineralization is occasionally noted within the cystic contents as well as within the cyst wall.

A thin layer of cuboidal or flattened epithelial cells lines the gingival cyst of adults. Nuclei tend to be hyperchromatic but are uniform from one cell to another. The epithelial-connective tissue junction is flattened, with some cysts demonstrating plaques or focal epithelial thickenings, often with clear cell changes. Infrequently, the cyst lining keratinizes. Small, solid clusters of epithelium may also be seen within the connective tissue wall of the cyst, apart and separate from the epithelial lining.

Treatment. No treatment is indicated for gingival or palatal cysts of the newborn because they spontaneously rupture early in life or at the time of tooth eruption. Treatment of gingival cysts of the adult is surgical excision, with inclusion of the overlying epithelium recommended. Recurrence is unlikely.

Parulis

A parulis or "gum boil" represents a focus of pus in the gingival connective tissue. It is derived from an acute infection, either at the base of an occluded periodontal pocket or at the apex of a nonvital tooth. If the path of least resistance leads to gingival submucosa, a soft tissue abscess or

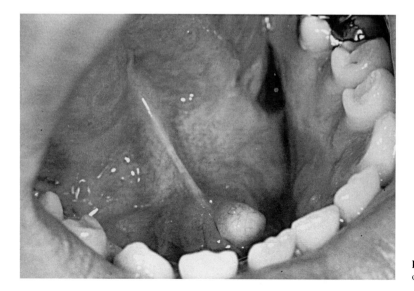

Figure 3–46. Lipoma on the floor of the mouth.

parulis results. The lesion presents as a yellow-white gingival tumescence with variable amounts of erythema (Fig. 3–45). Pain is typical, and once the pus escapes to the surface, symptoms are temporarily relieved. Treatment of the underlying condition (periodontal pocket or nonvital tooth) is required to achieve resolution of the gingival abscess.

Lipoma

Lipoma presents as a yellow or yellow-white uninflamed submucosal mass (Fig. 3–46) and is included in this section for completeness. Detailed discussion of this lesion is found in Chapter 7.

Bibliography

Hereditary Conditions

Burge SM, Fenton DA, Dawber RP, Leigh IM. Darier's disease: an immunohistochemical study using monoclonal antibodies to human cytokeratins. Br J Dermatol 118:629–640, 1988.

Burge SM, Millard PR, Wojnarowska F, Ryan TJ. Darier's disease: a focal abnormality of cell adhesion. J Cutan Pathol 17:160–169, 1990.

Burge SM, Wilkinson JD, Miller AJ, et al. The efficacy of an aromatic retinoid, Tigason (etretinate), in the treatment of Darier's disease. Br J Dermatol 104:675–679, 1981.

Dicken CH, Bauer EA, Hazen PG, et al. Isotretinoin treatment of Darier's disease. J Am Acad Dermatol 118:278–279, 1982.

Feinstein A, Friedman J, Schewach-Miller M. Pachyonychia congenita. J Am Acad Dermatol 19:705–711, 1988.

Lim J, Ng S. Oral tetracycline rinse improves symptoms of white sponge nevus. J Am Acad Dermatol 26:1003–1005, 1992.

Miller RL, Bernstein ML, Arm RN. Darier's disease of the oral mucosa: clinical case report with ultrastructural evaluation. J Oral Pathol 11:79–89, 1982.

Nichols GE, Cooper PH, Underwood PB, Greer KE. White sponge nevus. Obstet Gynecol 76:545–548, 1990.

Richard G, De Laurenzi V, Didona B, et al. Keratin 13 point mutation underlies the hereditary mucosal epithelial disorder white sponge nevus. Nat Genet 11:453–455, 1995.

Rugg E, McLean WH, Allison WE, et al. A mutation in the mucosal keratin K4 is associated with oral white sponge nevus. Nat Genet 11:450–452, 1995.

Reactive Lesions

Baric JM, Alman JE, Feldman RS, Chauncey HH. Influence of cigarette, pipe and cigar smoking on removable partial dentures, and age on oral leukoplakia. Oral Surg 54:424–429, 1982.

Centers for Disease Control. Smokeless tobacco use in the United States—behavioral risk factor surveillance system, 1986. MMWR 36:337–340, 1987.

Christen AG. The case against smokeless tobacco: five facts for the professional to consider. J Am Dent Assoc 101:464–469, 1980.

Connolly G, Winn D, Hecht S, et al. The reemergence of smokeless tobacco. N Engl J Med 314:1020–1027, 1986.

Creath CJ, Shelton WO, Wright JT, et al. The prevalence of smokeless tobacco use among adolescent male athletes. J Am Dent Assoc 116:43–48, 1988.

Daniels TE, Hansen LS, Greenspan JS, et al. Histopathology of smokeless tobacco lesions in professional baseball players. Oral Surg Oral Med Oral Pathol 73:720–725, 1992.

Grady P, Greene J, Daniels TE, et al. Oral mucosal lesions found in smokeless tobacco users. J Am Dent Assoc 121:117–123, 1990.

Kaugers GE, Mehailescu WL, Gunsolley JC. Smokeless tobacco use and oral epithelial dysplasia. Cancer 64:1527–1530, 1989.

Koop C. The campaign against smokeless tobacco. N Engl J Med 314:1042–1044, 1986.

Lindemann RA, Park N-H. Inhibition of human lymphokine-activated killer activity by smokeless tobacco (snuff) extract. Arch Oral Biol 33:317–321, 1988.

Mattson ME, Winn DM. Smokeless tobacco: association with increased cancer risk. NCI Monogr 1989(8):13–16.

Robertson PB, Walsh M, Greene J, et al. Periodontal effects associated with the use of smokeless tobacco. J Periodontol 61:438–443, 1990.

Rossie KM, Guggenheimer J. Thermally induced "nicotine" stomatitis. A case report. Oral Surg Oral Med Oral Pathol 70:597–599, 1990.

Sundstrom B, Mornstad H, Axell T. Oral carcinoma associated with snuff dipping. J Oral Pathol 11:245–251, 1982.

Winn DM. Smokeless tobacco and cancer: the epidemiologic evidence. CA 38:236–243, 1988.

Zakrzewska JM, Lopes V, Speight P, Hopper C. Proliferative verrucous leukoplakia. Oral Surg Oral Med Oral Pathol 82:396–401, 1996.

Zelickson BD, Roenigk RK. Actinic cheilitis. Treatment with the carbon dioxide laser. Cancer 65:1307–1311, 1990.

Other White Lesions

Barker J, Mitra R, Griffiths C, et al. Keratinocytes as initiators of inflammation. Lancet 337:211–214, 1991.

Barnard NA, Scully C, Eveson JW, et al. Oral cancer development in patients with oral lichen planus. J Oral Pathol Med 22:421–424, 1993.

Boehncke W, Kellner I, Konter U, Sterry W. Differential expression of adhesion molecules on infiltrating cells in inflammatory dermatoses. J Am Acad Dermatol 26:907–913, 1992.

Boisnic S, Francis C, Branchet M-C, et al. Immunohistochemical study of oral lesions of lichen planus: diagnostic and pathophysiologic aspects. Oral Surg Oral Med Oral Pathol 70:462–465, 1990.

Bolewska J, Holmstrup P, Moller-Madsen B, et al. Amalgam-associated mercury accumulations in normal oral mucosa, oral mucosal lesions of lichen planus and contact lesions associated with amalgam. J Oral Pathol Med 19:39–42, 1990.

Chou MJ, Daniels TE. Langerhans cells expressing HLA-DQ, HLA-DR and T6 antigens in normal oral mucosa and lichen planus. J Oral Pathol Med 18:573–576, 1989.

Corso B, Eversole LR, Hutt-Fletcher L. Hairy leukoplakia: Epstein-Barr virus receptors on oral keratinocyte plasma membranes. Oral Surg Oral Med Oral Pathol 67:416–421, 1989.

Crissman JD, Zarbo RJ. Dysplasia, in situ carcinoma, and progression to invasive squamous cell carcinoma of the upper aerodigestive tract. Am J Surg Pathol 13(Suppl 1):5–16, 1989.

Dekker NP, Lozada-Nur F, Lagenauer LA, et al. Apoptosis-associated markers in oral lichen planus. J Oral Pathol Med 26:170–175, 1997.

Ficarra G, Flaitz CM, Gaglioti D, et al. White lichenoid lesions of the buccal mucosa in patients with HIV infection. Oral Surg Oral Med Oral Pathol 76:460–466, 1993.

Gandolfo S, Carbone M, Carrozzo M, Gallo V. Oral lichen planus and hepatitis C virus (HCV) infection: is there a relationship? A report of 10 cases. J Oral Pathol Med 23:119–122, 1994.

Gilhar A, Pillar T, Winterstein G, Etzioni A. The pathogenesis of lichen planus. Br J Dermatol 120:541–544, 1989.

Giustina TA, Stewart JCB, Ellis CN, et al. Topical application of isotretinoin gel improves oral lichen planus. Arch Dermatol 122:534–536, 1986.

Green TL, Greenspan JL, Greenspan D, DeSouza YG. Oral lesions mimicking hairy leukoplakia: a diagnostic dilemma. Oral Surg Oral Med Oral Pathol 67:422–426, 1989.

Greenspan D, Greenspan J, Hearst N, et al. Relation of oral hairy leukoplakia to infection with the human immunodeficiency virus and the risk of developing AIDS. J Infect Dis 155:475–481, 1987.

Greenspan J, Greenspan D, Lennette ET, et al. Replication of Epstein-Barr virus within the epithelial cells of oral "hairy" leukoplakia, an AIDS-associated lesion. N Engl J Med 313:1564–1571, 1986.

Greenspan JS, Greenspan D, Palefsky JM. Oral hairy leukoplakia after a decade. Epstein-Barr Virus Report 2:123–128, 1995.

Gupta D, Sharma SC. Oral submucous fibrosis—a new treatment regimen. J Oral Maxillofac Surg 46:830–833, 1988.

Hansen L, Olson J, Silverman S. Proliferative verrucous leukoplakia. Oral Surg Oral Med Oral Pathol 60:285–298, 1985.

Holmstrup P, Scholtz AW, Westergaard J. Effect of dental plaque control on gingival lichen planus. Oral Surg Oral Med Oral Pathol 69:585–590, 1990.

Hong WK. Chemoprevention in oral premalignant lesions. Cancer Bull 38:145–148, 1986.

Hong WK, Endicott J, Itri LM, et al. 13-*cis*-Retinoic acid in the treatment of oral leukoplakia. N Engl J Med 315:1501–1505, 1986.

Hong WK, Lippman SM, Itri LM, et al. Prevention of second primary tumors with isotretinioin in squamous cell carcinoma of the head and neck. N Engl J Med 323:795–801, 1990.

Hunter J. The Langerhans cell: from gold to glitter. Clin Exp Dermatol 8:569–592, 1983.

Jarvinen J, Kullaa-Mikkonen A, Kotilainen R. Some local and systemic factors related to tongue inflammation. Proc Finn Dent Soc 85:197–209, 1990.

Krogh P, Holmstrup P, Thorn J. Yeast species and biotypes associated with oral leukoplakia and lichen planus. Oral Surg Oral Med Oral Pathol 63:48–54, 1987.

Lozada-Nur F, Robinson J, Regezi JA. Oral hairy leukoplakia in immunosuppressed patients. Oral Surg Oral Med Oral Pathol 78:599–602, 1994.

Nakamura S, Hiroki A, Shinohara M, et al. Oral involvement in chronic graft-versus host disease after allogenic bone marrow transplantation. Oral Surg Oral Med Oral Pathol 82:556–563, 1996.

Patton DF, Shirley P, Raab-Traub N, et al. Defective viral DNA in Epstein-Barr virus-associated oral hairy leukoplakia. J Virol 64:397–400, 1990.

Podzamczer D, Bolao F, Gudiol F. Oral hairy leukoplakia and zidovudine therapy. Arch Intern Med 150:689, 1990.

Porter SR, Kirby A, Olsen I, Barrett W. Immunologic aspects of dermal and oral lichen planus. Oral Surg Oral Med Oral Pathol 83:358–366, 1997.

Rajendran R, Vijayakumar T, Vasudevan DM. An alternative pathogenetic pathway for oral submucous fibrosis (OSMF). Med Hypotheses 30:35–37, 1989.

Ramirez-Amador V, Dekker NP, Lozada-Nur F, et al. Altered interface adhesion molecules in oral lichen planus. Oral Diseases 2:188–192, 1996.

Regezi JA, Daniels TE, Saeb F, Nickoloff BJ. Increased submucosal factor XIIIa-positive dendrocytes in oral lichen planus. J Oral Pathol Med 23:114–118, 1994.

Regezi JA, Dekker NP, MacPhail LA, et al: Vascular adhesion molecules in oral lichen planus. Oral Surg Oral Med Oral Pathol 81:682–690, 1996.

Salonen L, Axell T, Hellden L. Occurrence of oral mucosal lesions, the influence of tobacco habits and an estimate of treatment time in an adult Swedish population. J Oral Pathol Med 19:170–176, 1990.

Schubert MM, Sullivan KM, Morton TH, et al. Oral manifestations of chronic graft vs host disease. Arch Intern Med 144:1591–1595, 1984.

Sciubba JJ, Brandsma J, Schwartz M. Hairy leukoplakia: an AIDS-associated oportunistic infection. Oral Surg Oral Med Oral Pathol 67:404–410, 1989.

Shear M, Pindborg JJ. Verrucous hyperplasia of the oral mucosa. Cancer 46:1855–1862, 1980.

Shiohara T, Moriya N, Nagashima M. Induction and control of lichenoid tissue reactions. Springer Semin Immunopathol 13:369–385, 1992.

Silverman S Jr, Gorsky M, Lozada F. Oral leukoplakia and malignant transformation. Cancer 53:563–568, 1984.

Silverman S Jr, Gorsky M, Lozada-Nur F. A prospective follow-up study of 570 patients with oral lichen planus: persistence, remission, and malignant association. Oral Surg Oral Med Oral Pathol 60:30–34, 1985.

Silverman S, Migliorati C, Lozada-Nur F, et al. Oral findings in people with or at high risk for AIDS: a study of 375 homosexual males. J Am Dent Assoc 112:187–192, 1986.

Simon M, Hornstein OP. Prevalence rate of candida in the oral cavity of patients with oral lichen planus. Arch Dermatol Res 267:317–318, 1980.

Simon M, Reimer G, Schardt M, et al. Lymphocytotoxicity for oral mucosa in lichen planus. Dermatologica 167:11–15, 1983.

Sinor PN, Gupta PC, Murti PR, et al. A case-control study of oral submucous fibrosis with special reference to the etiologic role of areca nut. J Oral Pathol Med 19:94–98, 1990.

Slobert K, Jonsson R, Jontell M. Assessment of Langerhans' cells in oral lichen planus. J Oral Pathol 13:516–524, 1984.

Sniiders PJ, Schulten EA, Mullink H, et al. Detection of human papillomavirus and Epstein-Barr virus DNA sequences in oral mucosa of HIV-infected patients by the polymerase chain reaction. Am J Pathol 137:659–666, 1990.

Standish SM, Moorman WC. Treatment of hairy tongue with podophyllin resin. J Am Dent Assoc 68:535–540, 1964.

Sugerman PB, Savage NW, Seymour GJ, Walsh LJ. Is there a role for tumor necrosis factor-alpha in oral lichen planus? J Oral Pathol Med 25:21–24, 1996.

Syrjanen S, Laine P, Niemela M, Happonen RP. Oral hairy leukoplakia is not a specific sign of HIV-infection but related to immunosuppression in general. J Oral Pathol Med 18:28–31, 1989.

Van Wyk CW, Seedat HA, Phillips VM. Collagen in submucous fibrosis: an electron microscopic study. J Oral Pathol Med 19:182–187, 1990.

Vincent SD, Fotos PG, Baker KA, Williams TP. Oral lichen planus: the clinical, historical and therapeutic features of 100 cases. Oral Surg Oral Med Oral Pathol 70:165–171, 1990.

Waldron CA, Shafer WG. Leukoplakia revisited. Cancer 36:1386–1392, 1975.

Walton LJ, Thornhill MH, Macey MG, et al. Cutaneous lymphocyte-associated antigen (CLA) and $\alpha e\beta 7$ integrins are expressed by mononuclear cells in skin and oral lichen planus. J Oral Pathol Med 26:402–407, 1997.

Winzer M, Gilliar U, Ackerman AB. Hairy lesions of the oral cavity. Am J Dermatopathol 10:155–159, 1988.

Workshop on Oral Healthcare in HIV Disease (various authors). Oral Surg Oral Med Oral Pathol 73:137–247, 1992.

Zegarelli DJ. Ulcerative and erosive lichen planus: treated by modified topical steroid and injection steroid therapy. NY State Dent J 53(3):23–25, 1987.

Zunt SL, Tomich CE. Erythema migrans—a psoriasiform lesion of the oral mucosa. J Dermatol Surg Oncol 15:1067–1070, 1989.

Nonepithelial White-Yellow Lesions

Buchner A, Hansen L. The histomorphologic spectrum of the gingival cyst in the adult. Oral Surg Oral Med Oral Pathol 48:531–539, 1979.

Canniff JP, Harvey W. The aetiology of oral submucous fibrosis: the stimulation of collagen synthesis by extracts of areca nut. Int J Oral Surg 10:163–167, 1981.

Challacombe SJ. Immunologic aspects of oral candidiasis. Oral Surg Oral Med Oral Pathol 78:202–210, 1994.

Dreizen S. Oral candidiasis. Am J Med 77:28–33, 1984.

Greenspan D. Treatment of oral candidiasis in HIV infection. Oral Surg Oral Med Oral Pathol 78:211–215, 1994.

Klein R, Harris C, Small C, et al. Oral candidiasis in high-risk patients as the initial manifestation of the acquired immunodeficiency syndrome. N Engl J Med 311:354–358, 1984.

Pindborg JJ, Bhonsle RB, Murti PR, et al. Incidence and early forms of submucous fibrosis. Oral Surg Oral Med Oral Pathol 50:40–44, 1980.

Wysocki GP, Brannon RB, Gardner DG, et al. Histogenesis of the lateral periodontal cyst and the gingival cyst of the adult. Oral Surg Oral Med Oral Pathol 50:327–334, 1980.

4

Red-Blue Lesions

INTRAVASCULAR

Developmental Lesions

HEMANGIOMA

Etiology. The term *hemangioma* is used here in the generic sense to encompass various vascular neoplasms, hamartomas, and malformations that appear predominantly at or around birth. Because of the confusion surrounding the basic origin of many of these lesions, classification of clinical and microscopic varieties has been difficult. None of the numerous proposed classifications has had uniform acceptance, although there is merit in separating benign neoplasms from vascular malformations because of different clinical and behavioral characteristics. Using this approach, the term *congenital hemangioma* is used in a more restricted sense to identify benign congenital neoplasms of proliferating endothelial cells. Vascular

malformations include lesions resulting from abnormal vessel morphogenesis (Table 4–1). Separation of vascular lesions into one of these two groups can be of considerable significance relative to the treatment of patients. Unfortunately, in actual practice, some difficulty may be encountered in classifying lesions in this way because of overlapping clinical and histologic features.

In any event, congenital hemangiomas have traditionally been subdivided into two microscopic types—capillary and cavernous—that essentially reflect differences in vessel diameter. Vascular malformations may exhibit similar features but may also show vascular channels that represent arteries and veins.

Clinical Features. The congenital hemangioma, also known as *strawberry nevus,* usually presents around the time of birth but may not be apparent until childhood (Fig. 4–1). This lesion may exhibit a rapid growth phase followed several years later by an involution phase. In contrast, vascular malformations are generally persistent lesions that grow with the individual and do not involute (Figs. 4–2 and 4–3). Both types of lesions may range in color from red to blue, depending on the degree of congestion and their depth in tissue. When they are compressed, blanching occurs. This simple clinical test can be used to separate these lesions from hemorrhagic lesions in soft tissue (ecchymoses). Congenital hemangiomas and vascular malformations may be flat, nodular, or bosselated. Other clinical signs include the presence of a bruit or a thrill, features associated predominantly with vascular malformations. Lesions are most commonly found in lips, tongue, and buccal mucosa. Lesions that affect bone are probably vascular malformations rather than congenital hemangiomas.

Sturge-Weber syndrome, or *encephalotrigeminal angiomatosis,* is a condition that includes vascular malformations. In this syndrome, venous malformations involve the leptomeninges of the cerebral cortex, usually with similar vascular malformations of the face. The associated facial lesion, also known as *port-wine stain* or *nevus flammeus,* involves the skin innervated by one or more branches of the trigeminal nerve (Fig. 4–4). Port-wine stains may also occur as isolated lesions of

Table 4–1. Features of Hemangiomas

CONGENITAL HEMANGIOMA	VASCULAR MALFORMATION
Abnormality of endothelial cell proliferation	Abnormality of vessel morphogenesis
Results from increased number of capillaries	Results from dilatation of arteries, veins, or capillaries
Appears weeks after birth	Usually present at birth
Rapid growth	Progressive enlargement—grows with the patient
Spontaneous involution	Persistent
Rarely affects bone	Frequently affects bone
Resectable	Difficult to resect
Surgical bleeding controllable	Surgical hemorrhage a potential problem
Often circumscribed	Poorly circumscribed
Recurrence uncommon	Recurrence common
No bruit or thrill	May produce bruit or thrill

the skin without the other stigmata of Sturge-Weber syndrome. The vascular defect of Sturge-Weber syndrome may extend intraorally to involve the buccal mucosa and the gingiva. Ocular lesions may also appear.

Neurologic defects of Sturge-Weber syndrome may include mental retardation, hemiparesis, and seizure disorders. Patients may be taking phenytoin (Dilantin) for control of the latter problem, with possible secondary development of drug-induced generalized gingival hyperplasia. Calcification of the intracranial vascular lesion may provide radiologic evidence of the process in the leptomeninges.

Differential diagnosis would include *angioosteohypertrophy syndrome,* which is characterized by vascular malformations of the face (port-wine stains), varices, and hypertrophy of bone. The bony abnormality usually affects long bones but may also involve the mandible or maxilla, re-

sulting in asymmetry, malocclusion, and altered eruption pattern.

Rendu-Osler-Weber syndrome, or *hereditary hemorrhagic telangiectasia,* is a rare condition featuring abnormal vascular dilatations of terminal vessels in skin, mucous membranes, and occasionally viscera (Fig. 4–5). The telangiectatic vessels in this autosomal dominant condition appear clinically as red macules or papules, typically on the face, chest, and oral mucosa. Lesions appear early in life and persist throughout adulthood.

Intranasal lesions are responsible for epistaxis, the most common presenting sign of Rendu-Osler-Weber syndrome. Bleeding from oral lesions is also a frequent occurrence in affected patients. Control of bleeding may on occasion be a difficult problem. Chronic bleeding may also result in anemia.

Diagnosis of Rendu-Osler-Weber syndrome is based on clinical findings, hemorrhagic history,

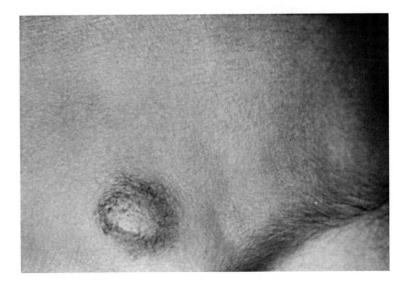

Figure 4–1. Congenital hemangioma on the forehead of an infant.

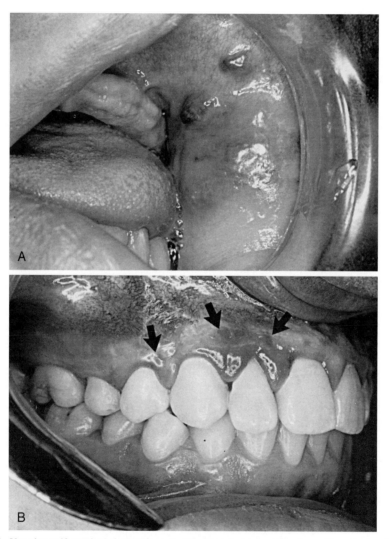

Figure 4–2. Vascular malformations (hemangiomas) of the buccal mucosa *(A)* and maxillary gingiva *(B)* *(arrows)*.

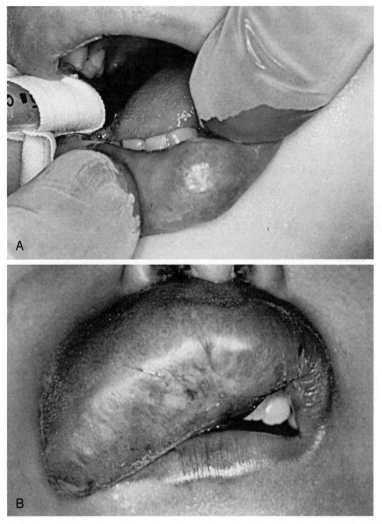

Figure 4–3. *A* and *B*, Vascular malformations (hemangiomas) of the lips. (Courtesy of Dr. W. Wade.)

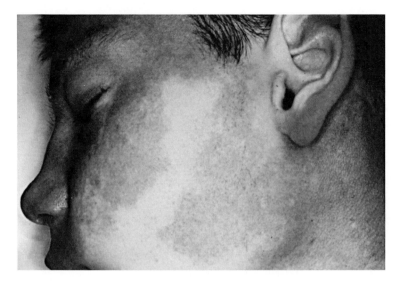

Figure 4–4. Vascular malformation (hemangioma) or port-wine stain of the type associated with Sturge-Weber syndrome.

and family history. Another condition that might be considered in a differential diagnosis is the *CREST syndrome.* This includes calcinosis cutis, Raynaud's phenomenon, esophageal dysfunction, sclerodactyly, and telangiectasia.

A *venous varix* or varicosity is an abnormal vascular dilatation. It is a relatively trivial vascular malformation when it appears in the oral mucosa (Fig. 4–6). Varices in the ventral aspect of the tongue are common developmental abnormalities. Varices are also common on the lower lip in older adults, especially those with chronic sun exposure. Varices are typically blue and blanch with compression. Thrombosis, insignificant in these lesions, occasionally occurs, giving them a firm texture. No treatment is required for venous varix,

unless it is frequently traumatized or is cosmetically objectionable.

Histopathology. Congenital hemangiomas have been classified microscopically as capillary or cavernous, depending on the size of the vascular spaces (Fig. 4–7). Spaces are lined by endothelium without muscular support. Clinically, no significant difference is noted between capillary and cavernous hemangiomas.

Vascular malformations may consist not only of capillaries but also of venous, arteriolar, and lymphatic channels. Lesions may be of purely one type of vessel, or they may be combinations of two or more.

Diagnosis. As a generic group, hemangiomas are usually self-evident on clinical examination.

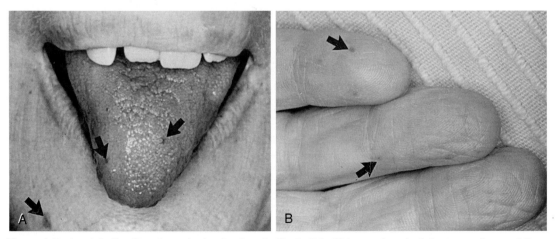

Figure 4–5. *A* and *B*, Hereditary hemorrhagic telangiectasis (Rendu-Osler-Weber syndrome) of the tongue, face, and fingers *(arrows).*

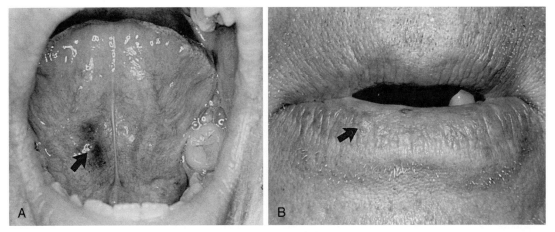

Figure 4–6. Venous varix of the ventral tongue surface *(A)* and the lip *(B) (arrows).*

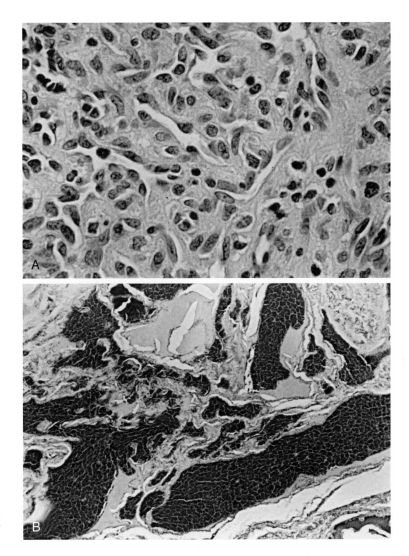

Figure 4–7. Micrographs of capillary *(A)* and cavernous *(B)* hemangiomas.

When they affect the mandible or the maxilla, a radiolucent lesion with a honeycomb pattern is expected. Differentiation between congenital hemangiomas and vascular malformations can be difficult and occasionally impossible. A complete history, a clinical examination, and angiography should be definitive.

Treatment. Spontaneous involution during early childhood is likely for congenital hemangiomas. If these lesions persist into the later years of childhood, involution is improbable and definitive treatment may be required. Vascular malformations generally do not involute and require intervention if eradication is the goal. Because the margins of these lesions are frequently ill defined, total elimination may not be practical or possible.

Treatment of vascular lesions continues to center around a careful surgical approach. Adjuncts include selective arteriole embolization and sclerosant therapy. Laser therapy is now a valid form of primary treatment of selected vascular lesions.

Reactive Lesions

PYOGENIC GRANULOMA

Etiology. This lesion represents an overexuberant connective tissue reaction to a known stimulus or injury. It appears as a red mass because it is composed predominantly of hyperplastic granulation tissue in which capillaries are very prominent. The term *pyogenic granuloma* is somewhat of a misnomer in that it is not pus producing, as *pyogenic* implies. It is, however, a tumor of granulation tissue, as *granuloma* implies.

Clinical Features. Pyogenic granulomas are commonly seen on the gingiva, where they are

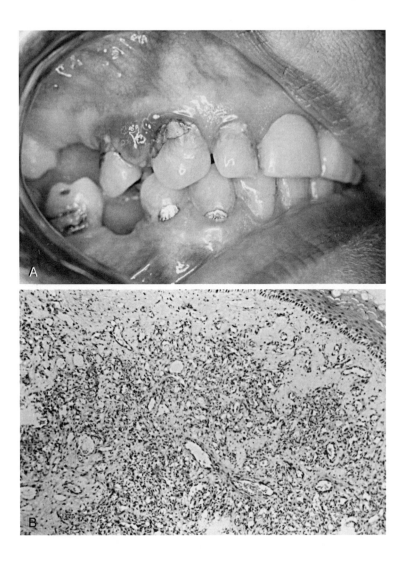

Figure 4–8. *A*, Pyogenic granuloma of the gingiva. *B*, Micrograph showing numerous capillaries responsible clinically for the dark color.

presumably caused by calculus or foreign material within the gingival crevice (Figs. 4–8 and 4–9). Hormonal changes of puberty and pregnancy may modify the gingival reparative response to injury. Under these circumstances, multiple gingival lesions or generalized gingival hyperplasia may be seen. Pyogenic granulomas are uncommonly seen elsewhere in the mouth but may appear in areas of frequent trauma, such as the lower lip, the buccal mucosa, and the tongue.

Pyogenic granulomas are typically red. Occasionally, they may become ulcerated because of secondary trauma. The ulcerated lesion may then become covered by a yellow, fibrinous membrane. They may be pedunculated or broad based and may range in size from a few millimeters to several centimeters. These lesions may be seen at any age and tend to occur in females more frequently than in males.

Histopathology. Microscopically, these lesions are composed of lobular masses of hyperplastic granulation tissue. Some scarring may be noted in some of these lesions, suggesting that there occasionally may be maturation of the connective tissue repair process. Variable numbers of chronic inflammatory cells may be seen. Neutrophils are present in the superficial zone of ulcerated pyogenic granulomas.

Differential Diagnosis. Clinically, this lesion must be differentiated from the peripheral giant cell granuloma, which also occurs as a red gingival mass. A peripheral fibroma may be another consideration, although these tend to be much lighter in color. Rarely, metastatic cancer may present as a red gingival mass. Biopsy is definitive.

Treatment. Pyogenic granulomas should be surgically excised to include the connective tissue

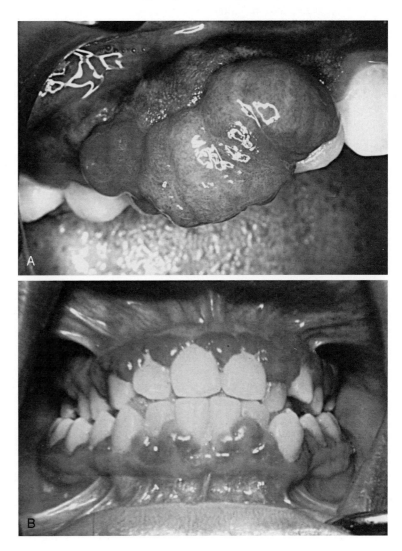

Figure 4–9. *A*, Large pyogenic granuloma of the gingiva. *B*, Generalized gingival hyperplasia (multiple pyogenic granulomas) associated with pregnancy.

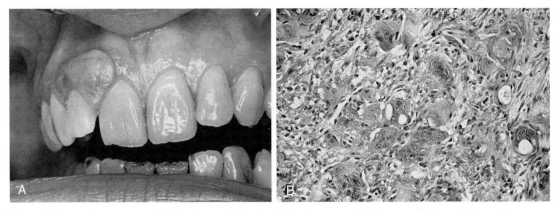

Figure 4–10. *A*, Peripheral giant cell granuloma. *B*, Micrograph showing young fibroblasts, capillaries, and giant cells.

from which the lesion arises as well as removal of any local etiologic factors, such as calculus. Recurrence is occasional and is believed to result from incomplete excision, failure to remove etiologic factors, or reinjury of the area.

PERIPHERAL GIANT CELL GRANULOMA

Etiology. The peripheral giant cell granuloma represents a relatively uncommon and unusual hyperplastic connective tissue response to injury of gingival tissues. It is one of the "reactive hyperplasias" commonly seen in oral mucous membranes, representing an exuberant reparative response. The feature that sets this lesion apart from the others is the appearance of multinucleated giant cells. The reason for their presence remains a mystery.

Clinical Features. Peripheral giant cell granu-lomas are seen exclusively in gingiva, usually in the area between the first permanent molars and the incisors (Fig. 4–10). They presumably arise from periodontal ligament or periosteum and cause, on occasion, resorption of alveolar bone. When this process occurs on the edentulous ridge, a superficial, cup-shaped radiolucency may be seen (Fig. 4–11). Peripheral giant cell granulomas typically present as red to blue broad-based masses. Secondary ulceration due to trauma may give the lesions a focal yellow zone caused by the formation of a fibrin clot over the ulcer. These lesions, most of which are about 1 cm in diameter, may occur at any age and tend to be seen more frequently in females than in males.

Histopathology. Hyperplastic granulation tissue is a basic element of the peripheral giant cell granuloma. Scattered throughout the lobulated granulation tissue mass are abundant multinucleated giant cells, the origin of which is unknown. Ultrastructural and immunologic studies have

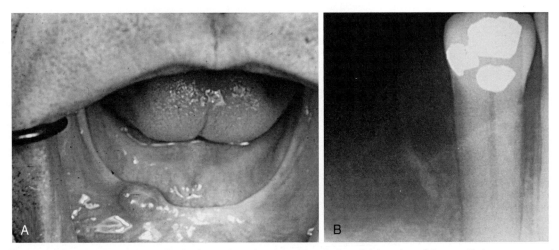

Figure 4–11. *A*, Peripheral giant cell granuloma of an edentulous ridge. *B*, Superficial erosion of the mandibular cortex caused by peripheral giant cell granuloma.

shown that the giant cells are derived from either macrophages, osteoclasts, or their precursors. The giant cells appear to be nonfunctional in the usual sense of phagocytosis and bone resorption.

Islands of metaplastic bone occasionally may be seen in these lesions. This finding has no clinical significance. Variable numbers of chronic inflammatory cells are present, and neutrophils are found in ulcer bases.

Differential Diagnosis. Generally, this lesion is clinically indistinguishable from a pyogenic granuloma. Although a peripheral giant cell granuloma is more likely to cause bone resorption than is a pyogenic granuloma, the differences are otherwise slight. Biopsy provides definitive results. Microscopically, a peripheral giant cell granuloma is identical to its central or intraosseous counterpart, a central giant cell granuloma, which is derived from the medullary tissue of the mandible and the maxilla. Clinical features adequately distinguish these two microscopically identical lesions.

Treatment. Surgical excision is the preferred treatment for peripheral giant cell granulomas. Removal of local factors or irritants is also required. Recurrence is uncommon.

MEDIAN RHOMBOID GLOSSITIS

Etiology. This entity was once thought to be a congenital abnormality related to the persistence of an embryonic midline tongue structure known as the *tuberculum impar.* This lesion is now believed to be related to a chronic infection by *Candida albicans.* The exact role of this fungus in the pathogenesis of the lesion is yet to be established.

Clinical Features. This lesion usually presents as a red elevated rhomboid or oval lesion in the dorsal midline of the tongue, just anterior to the circumvallate papillae (Fig. 4–12). The lesion may occasionally be mildly painful, although most are asymptomatic.

Histopathology. Microscopically, epithelial hyperplasia is evident in the form of bulbous rete ridges (Fig. 4–13). *C. albicans* hyphae can usually be found in the upper levels of the epithelium. A thick band of hyalinized connective tissue separates the epithelium from deeper structures.

Diagnosis. The diagnosis of median rhomboid glossitis is generally evident from clinical appearance. Because oral cancer rarely occurs at this location, squamous cell carcinoma is usually not a serious clinical consideration.

Treatment. No treatment generally is necessary for median rhomboid glossitis. If the lesion is painful, symptomatic treatment or use of clotrimazole troches may be necessary. If malignancy is part of a clinical differential diagnosis, biopsy should be performed. Median rhomboid glossitis itself is generally regarded as having no malignant potential.

Neoplasms

ERYTHROPLAKIA

Etiology. *Erythroplakia* is a clinical term that refers to a red patch on oral mucous membranes. It does not indicate a particular microscopic diagnosis, although after biopsy most are found to be severe dysplasia or carcinoma. The cause of this lesion is unknown. It is generally assumed, however, that the etiologic factors for erythroplakia are similar to those responsible for oral cancer.

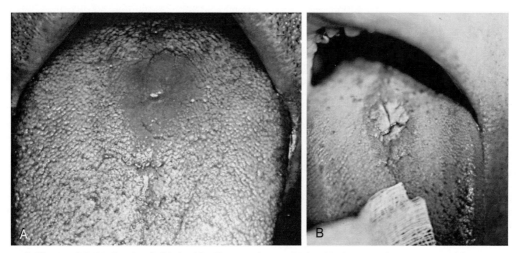

Figure 4–12. *A* and *B*, Median rhomboid glossitis. The central area of *B* is white because of secondary candidiasis.

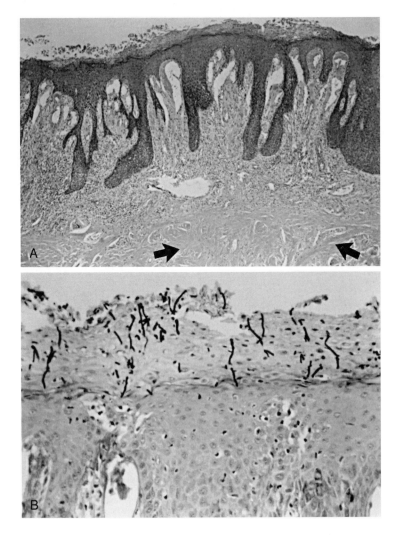

Figure 4–13. *A,* Micrograph of median rhomboid glossitis showing epithelial hyperplasia, prominent capillaries, and a band of hyalinized connective tissue at the base *(arrows). B,* PAS stain showing hyphae of *C. albicans* in the parakeratotic layer.

Therefore, tobacco probably has a significant role in the induction of many of these lesions. Alcohol, nutritional defects, chronic irritation, and other factors may also have contributing or modifying roles.

Clinical Features. Erythroplakia is seen much less frequently than its leukoplakia counterpart. It should, however, be viewed as a more serious lesion because of the significantly higher percentage of malignancies associated with it. The lesion appears as a red patch with fairly well defined margins (Fig. 4–14). High-risks sites are the floor of the mouth, the tongue, and the retromolar mucosa. Individuals between 50 and 70 years of age are usually affected, and there appears to be no gender predilection. Focal white areas representing keratosis may also be seen in some lesions. Erythroplakia is usually supple to the touch, although some induration may be noted in invasive lesions.

Histopathology. On biopsy, approximately 90% of erythroplakias show at least severe dysplastic change—about half are invasive squamous cell carcinomas, and 40% are severe dysplasias or *in situ* carcinomas (Fig. 4–15). The remainder are mild to moderate dysplasias. A relative reduction in keratin production and a relative increase in vascularity accounts for the clinical color of these lesions. Products of keratinocyte terminal differentiation, such as keratin, involucrin, and filaggrin, are found in reduced or negligible amounts in these lesions when stained immunohistochemically.

A rare histologic subtype of carcinoma *in situ,* known as *Bowen's disease,* may be seen as a red (or white) patch in the oral mucosa. When this process occurs on the glans penis, it is known as *erythroplasia of Queyrat.* Microscopic features that separate this lesion from the usual carcinoma *in situ* include marked disordered growth, multi-

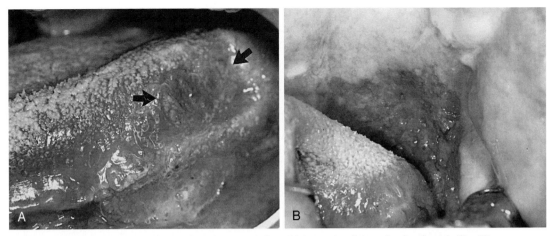

Figure 4–14. Erythroplakia of the posterolateral tongue surface *(A) (arrows)* and the soft palate/faucial pillar *(B).*

nucleated keratinocytes, large hyperchromatic keratinocyte nuclei, and atypical individual cell keratinization.

Differential Diagnosis. The clinical features of erythroplakia may occasionally be shared by several other red lesions. Atrophic candidiasis results in a red mucosal lesion, but symptoms are usually present. An expanded differential diagnosis would include Kaposi's sarcoma, ecchymosis, contact allergic reaction, vascular malformation, and psoriasis. A careful clinical history and examination should distinguish most of these lesions. Biopsy provides a definitive answer.

Treatment. The treatment of choice for erythroplakia is surgical excision. It is generally more important to excise widely than deeply in dysplastic and *in situ* lesions, because of their superficial nature. However, because the epithelial changes may extend down the salivary gland excretory ducts in the area, the deep surgical margin should not be too shallow. Several histologic sections

may be necessary to assess adequately the involvement of ducts.

It is generally accepted that severely dysplastic and *in situ* lesions eventually become invasive. The time required for this event can range from months to years. Follow-up examinations are critical for patients with these lesions, because of the potential field effect caused by etiologic agents.

KAPOSI'S SARCOMA

Etiology. Kaposi's sarcoma is a proliferation of endothelial cell origin, although dermal/submucosal dendrocytes, macrophages, lymphocytes, and probably mast cells may have a role in the genesis of these lesions. The various etiologic factors cited as possibly having significance include genetic predisposition, infection (especially viral), environmental influences of various geographic regions, and immune dysregulation, such as reduced

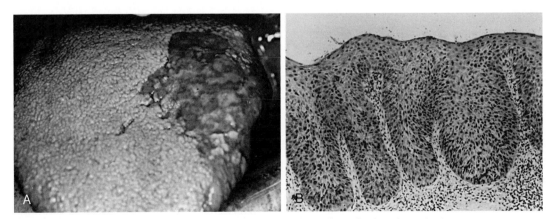

Figure 4–15. *A* and *B*, Erythroplakia of the tongue. Biopsy *(B)* led to a diagnosis of carcinoma *in situ*.

Table 4–2. Features of Kaposi's Sarcoma

PARAMETER	CLASSIC TYPE	ENDEMIC TYPE	IMMUNODEFICIENCY TYPE
Geography	Mediterranean basin	Africa	Metropolitan areas
Prevalence	Rare	Endemic	Relatively common
Age	Older men	Children and adults	Adults
Skin lesions	Lower extremities	Extremities	Any site
Oral lesions	Rare	Rare	Common
Other organs	Occasionally	Occasionally	Frequently
Course	Indolent	Prolonged	Aggressive
Prognosis	Fair	Fair	Poor

immunosurveillance. A newly discovered herpesvirus known as HHV8 or KSHV has been identified in all forms of Kaposi's sarcoma lesions, as well as acquired immunodeficiency syndrome (AIDS)–associated body cavity lymphomas. This virus is believed to have a significant role in the induction and/or maintenance of Kaposi's sarcoma through perturbation of focally released cytokines and growth factors. It is generally regarded as a neoplasm, although much evidence suggests that it is inflammatory in nature, especially in early stages.

Clinical Features. Three different clinical patterns of Kaposi's sarcoma have emerged since it was first described by Kaposi in 1872 (Table 4–2). It was initially seen as a rare skin lesion, predominantly in older men living in the Mediterranean basin. In this classic form, it appears as multifocal reddish-brown nodules primarily in the skin of the lower extremities, although any organ may be affected. Oral lesions are rare in this type. This classic form has a rather long indolent course and only a fair prognosis.

The second pattern of Kaposi's sarcoma was identified in Africa, where it is now considered to be endemic. It is seen typically in the extremities of blacks. The most commonly affected organ is the skin. Oral lesions are rarely seen. The clinical course is prolonged, and the overall prognosis is also only fair.

The third pattern of Kaposi's sarcoma has been seen in patients with immunodeficiency states, organ transplants, and especially AIDS. This type differs from the other two forms in several ways. Skin lesions are not limited to the extremities and may be multifocal. Visceral organs may also be involved. A younger age group is affected. Oral and lymph node lesions are relatively common (Fig. 4–16). The clinical course is relatively rapid and aggressive, and the prognosis is correspondingly poor.

Kaposi's sarcoma, once occurring in about one third of patients with AIDS, is now seen with considerably less frequency in about one fifth of these patients, a shift that may be related to AIDS drug therapy. About half of the AIDS-affected patients with Kaposi's sarcoma develop oral lesions. Of significance is that oral lesions may be the initial site of involvement or the only site. It has been described in most oral regions, although the palate, gingiva, and tongue seem to be the most commonly affected sites. Oral Kaposi's sarcoma ranges from a rather trivial-appearing, flat lesion to a rather ominous, nodular exophytic lesion. It may be single or multifocal. The color is usually red to blue. AIDS-affected patients with oral Kaposi's sarcoma may have other oral problems concomitantly, such as candidiasis, hairy leukoplakia, advancing periodontal disease, and xerostomia.

Histopathology. Early lesions of Kaposi's sarcoma may be rather subtle, being composed of hypercellular foci containing bland-appearing spindle cells, ill-defined vascular channels, and extravasated red blood cells (RBCs). Later, they may superficially resemble pyogenic granulomas (Fig. 4–17). Atypical vascular channels, extravasated RBCs, hemosiderin, and inflammatory cells are characteristic of advanced Kaposi's sarcoma. Macrophages, factor XIIIa–positive dendrocytes, lymphocytes, and mast cells are also seen in oral Kaposi's sarcoma (early and late stages).

Differential Diagnosis. Other clinical considerations would include hemangioma, erythroplakia, melanoma, and pyogenic granuloma. Microscopically, reactive (pyogenic granuloma), congenital (hemangioma), and neoplastic (pericytoma, angiosarcoma) lesions might deserve consideration.

Another remarkable look-alike, known as *bacillary angiomatosis,* mimics Kaposi's sarcoma both clinically and microscopically. The causative organism is *Bartonella henselae* or *B. quintana.* Cats are reservoirs for this organism, and fleas may be vectors. Microscopically, neutrophils and bacterial colonies are seen. This condition is cured with erythromycin or tetracycline therapy. Bacillary an-

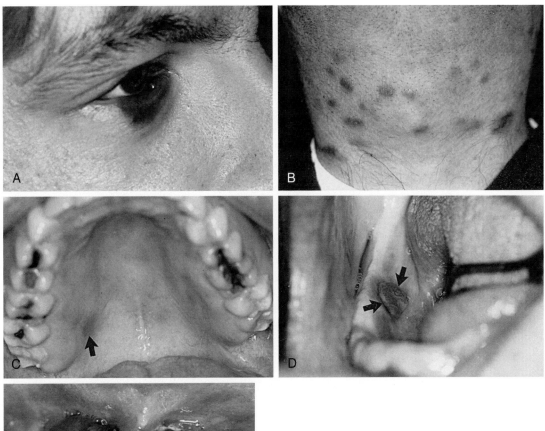

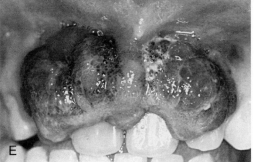

Figure 4–16. *A* to *E*, Kaposi's sarcoma of the skin and mucous membranes.

giomatosis is uncommon in the skin and very rare in oral mucous membranes.

Treatment. Various forms of treatment have been used for Kaposi's sarcoma, but none has been uniformly successful. Surgery has been useful on localized lesions, and low-dose radiation and intralesional chemotherapy have been gaining favor. For larger and multifocal lesions, systemic chemotherapeutic regimens are being used.

Unknown Etiology

GEOGRAPHIC TONGUE

Geographic tongue, or benign migratory glossitis, is described in Chapter 3, but it is mentioned

here because it can on occasion appear as a predominantly red tongue lesion (Fig. 4–18). When the zones of papillary atrophy are relatively prominent and the keratotic margins are relatively subdued, geographic tongue presents as a red lesion. Careful clinical examination should reveal the nature of the lesion. Although this entity should be included in a differential diagnosis of red tongue lesions, it has the same significance as its more typical form.

It should be noted that geographic tongue often occurs in association with *fissured tongue*. Fissured tongue may be seen alone in approximately 5% of the population. It is rare in children and increases in incidence with age. It may also be a component of the *Melkersson-Rosenthal* syndrome. The fissuring, which occurs across the

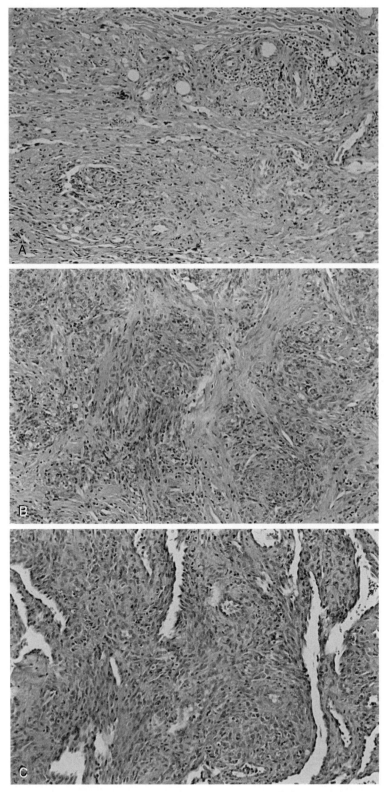

Figure 4–17. Kaposi's sarcoma. *A*, Early (macular) lesion showing subtle hypercellular zones at upper right and lower left. *B*, Moderately advanced lesion with confluent areas of spindle cells. Vascular spaces not yet particularly prominent. *C*, Advanced lesion with abundant spindle cells and atypical vascular spaces.

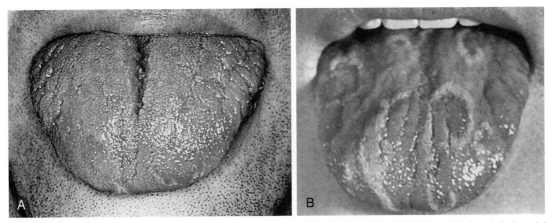

Figure 4–18. *A* and *B*, Geographic tongue occurring in a fissured tongue. Note the dark patches surrounded partially by subtle white keratotic rings in *A*. (*B*, Courtesy of Dr. W. G. Sprague.)

dorsum of the tongue, varies in severity from one patient to another. Fissured tongue is usually asymptomatic, but may become painful if *C. albicans* organisms colonize the base of the fissures.

Metabolic-Endocrine Conditions

VITAMIN B DEFICIENCIES

Etiology. In various areas of the world, especially those with poor socioeconomic conditions, vitamin B deficiencies may be relatively common because of inadequate dietary intake. In the United States, deficiencies of the B vitamins are relatively uncommon.

Vitamin B deficiencies may involve one or several of the water-soluble B complex vitamins. Decreased intake through malnutrition associated with alcoholism, starvation, or fad diets may lead to clinically apparent disease. Decreased absorption because of gastrointestinal disease (e.g., malabsorption syndromes) or increased utilization because of increased demand (e.g., hyperparathyroidism) may also account for deficiencies.

Most of the vitamins classified under the B complex (biotin, nicotinamide, pantothenic acid, and thiamine) are involved in intracellular metabolism of carbohydrates, fats, and proteins. Others (vitamin B_{12} and folic acid) are involved in erythrocyte development. Deficiencies of individual vitamins may produce distinctive clinical pictures. Significant oral changes have been well documented in deficiencies of riboflavin (ariboflavinosis), niacin (pellagra), folic acid (one of the megaloblastic anemias), and vitamin B_{12} (pernicious anemia).

Clinical Features. In general, the oral changes associated with vitamin B deficiencies consist of cheilitis and glossitis (Fig. 4–19). The lips may exhibit cracking and fissuring that is exaggerated at the corners of the mouth, in which case it is called *angular cheilitis.* The tongue becomes reddened, with atrophy of papillae, and patients complain of pain and burning.

In addition to these oral changes, riboflavin deficiency results in keratitis of the eyes and a scaly dermatitis focused on the nasolabial area and genitalia. Niacin deficiency is associated with extraoral problems as well. The "four Ds" of niacin deficiency are dermatitis, diarrhea, dementia, and death. The most striking and consistent feature is a symmetrically distributed dermatitis that eventually shows marked thickening and pigmentary changes. Dementia is in the form of disorientation and forgetfulness. The glossitis in this deficiency may be severe and may extend to other mucosal surfaces.

Folic acid deficiency results in a megaloblastic (enlarged RBC precursors) bone marrow, a macrocytic (enlarged circulating erythrocytes) anemia, and gastrointestinal abnormalities, including diarrhea and the general oral lesions described previously. Vitamin B_{12} deficiency shares many of the signs and symptoms of folic acid deficiency. These are detailed in the following section on anemias.

Diagnosis and Treatment. Diagnosis of B complex deficiencies is based on history, clinical findings, and laboratory data. Replacement therapy should be curative.

PERNICIOUS ANEMIA

Etiology. This is essentially a deficiency of vitamin B_{12} (erythrocyte maturing factor or extrinsic

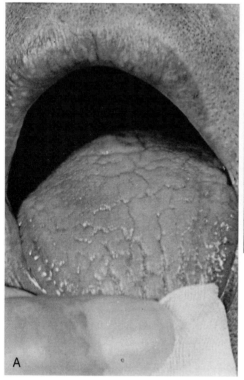
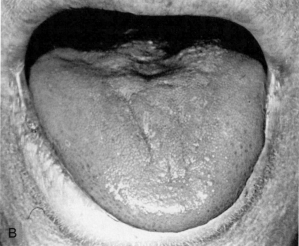

Figure 4–19. Atrophic tongue associated with pernicious anemia *(A)* and vitamin B deficiency *(B)*.

factor), which is necessary for DNA synthesis, especially in rapidly dividing cells, such as those found in bone marrow and the gastrointestinal tract. Pernicious anemia results from the inability to transport vitamin B_{12} across intestinal mucosa because of a relative lack of a gastric substance (intrinsic factor). This intrinsic factor is normally complexed to vitamin B_{12}, making the vitamin available to mucosal cells for absorption. An autoimmune response directed against the intrinsic factor or the gastric mucosa is believed to be a probable mechanism responsible for pernicious anemia. The end result is atrophic gastritis, achlorhydria, neurologic changes, megaloblastic bone marrow, and macrocytic anemia. Additionally, significant oral manifestations may be seen.

Clinical Features. Pernicious anemia affects adults of either gender. The clinical signs of anemia—weakness, pallor, shortness of breath, difficulty in breathing, and increased fatigue on exertion—may be present. Also, in more severe cases, central nervous system manifestations (headache, dizziness, and tinnitus) and gastrointestinal manifestations (nausea, diarrhea, and stomatitis) may be present.

Specific oral complaints center around the tongue. Pain and burning are typical symptoms. The tongue appears more red because of atrophy of the papillae. The resultant smooth, red appear-

ance has been referred to as *Hunter's glossitis* or *Moeller's glossitis.*

Diagnosis. The clinical picture of pernicious anemia can be only presumptive of this disease. Diagnosis is based on laboratory demonstration of a megaloblastic, macrocytic anemia.

Treatment. Parenteral administration of vitamin B_{12} is curative for this condition. An increased risk of the development of gastric carcinoma is associated with the chronic atrophic gastritis that may occur in pernicious anemia.

IRON DEFICIENCY ANEMIA

Etiology. Iron deficiency is the cause of this rather common anemia. The deficiency may be due to inadequate dietary intake, impaired absorption due to a gastrointestinal malady, chronic blood loss due to such problems as excessive menstrual flow, gastrointestinal bleeding, and aspirin ingestion, and increased demand as experienced during childhood and pregnancy.

Clinical Features. This is a relatively prevalent form of anemia that affects predominantly women. In addition to the clinical signs and symptoms associated with anemias in general, iron deficiency anemia may also result in brittle nails and hair and koilonychia (spoon-shaped nails). The tongue may become red, painful, and smooth. Angular cheilitis may also be seen.

In addition to iron deficiency, the Plummer-Vinson syndrome includes dysphagia, atrophy of the upper alimentary tract, and a predisposition to the development of oral cancer.

Diagnosis. Laboratory blood studies show a slight to moderately reduced hematocrit and reduced hemoglobin level. The red blood cells are microcytic and hypochromic. Serum iron level is also low.

Treatment. Recognition of the underlying cause of iron deficiency anemia is necessary to treat this condition effectively. Dietary iron supplements are required to elevate hemoglobin levels and replenish iron stores.

BURNING MOUTH SYNDROME

Patients with burning mouth or burning tongue syndrome usually exhibit no clinically detectable lesions, although symptoms of pain and burning can be intense. This relatively common "nonlesion" clinical problem is included in this section because the symptoms associated with burning mouth also appear in vitamin B deficiency, pernicious anemia, iron deficiency anemia, and chronic atrophic candidiasis. This is a particularly frustrating problem for both patient and clinician, because there is usually no clear-cut cause and no uniformly successful treatment.

Etiology. The etiology of burning mouth syndrome is varied and often difficult to decipher clinically. The symptoms of pain and burning appear to be the result of one of many possible causes. Factors cited as having possible etiologic significance include

1. Microorganisms—especially fungi (C. albicans) and possibly bacteria (staphylococci, streptococci, anaerobes)
2. Xerostomia associated with Sjögren's syndrome, anxiety, and drugs (Table 4–3)
3. Nutritional deficiencies associated primarily with B vitamin complex or iron, and possibly zinc
4. Anemias, namely pernicious anemia and iron deficiency anemia
5. Hormone imbalance, especially hypoestrogenemia associated with postmenopausal changes
6. Neurologic abnormalities, such as depression, cancer phobia, and other psychogenic problems
7. Diabetes mellitus
8. Mechanical trauma, such as an oral habit or chronic denture irritation
9. Idiopathic causes

Table 4–3. Drug Classes Associated with Xerostomia

Anticholinergics
Antidepressants
Antihistamines
Antihypertensives
Antihypoglycemics
Antiparkinsonians
Beta-blockers
Diuretics
Nonsteroidal anti-inflammatories

In some patients, more than one of these may be contributing to the problem of burning mouth syndrome.

Other potential etiologic factors that might be explored are those related to dysgeusia (altered taste), an occasional clinical feature of burning mouth syndrome. Dysgeusia is associated with an equally long list of factors that include zinc deficiency, drugs (especially antibiotics), endocrine abnormalities, Vincent's infection, heavy-metal intoxication, chorda tympani injury, and psychogenic and idiopathic causes (Table 4–4).

The mechanism by which such a varied group of factors causes symptoms of burning mouth syndrome is completely enigmatic. No common thread or underlying defect seems to tie these factors together. It is apparent that burning mouth syndrome is represented in a diverse, complex group of patients. Determination of cause is a difficult and challenging clinical problem that requires careful extensive history taking and, frequently, laboratory support.

Clinical Features. This is a condition that typically affects middle-aged women. Men are affected but generally at a later age than women. Burning mouth syndrome is rare in children and teenagers, very uncommon in young adults, but relatively common in adults older than 40 years.

Symptoms of pain and burning may be accompanied by altered taste and xerostomia. Occasionally, a patient may attribute the initiation of the malady to recent dental work, such as placement

Table 4–4. Factors Associated with Altered Taste (Dysgeusia)

Acute necrotizing gingivitis
Corda tympani injury
Drugs, especially antibiotics
Endocrine diseases
Heavy-metal intoxication
Psychological problems
Zinc deficiency
Idiopathic conditions

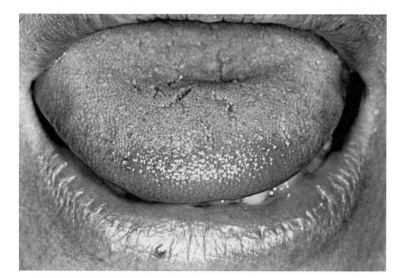

Figure 4–20. Patient with burning tongue. Except for slight redness of the tip, the tongue is normal.

of a new bridge or extraction of a tooth. Symptoms are frequently described as severe and ever present or worsening late in the day and evening. Any and all mucosal regions may be affected, although the tongue is by far the most commonly involved site.

Highly characteristic of the complaint of intense burning mouth or tongue is a completely normal-appearing oral mucosa (Fig. 4–20). Tissue is intact and has the same color as the surrounding tissue, with normal distribution of tongue papillae.

Some laboratory studies that may prove useful are cultures for *C. albicans,* serum tests for Sjögren's syndrome antibodies (SS-A, SS-B), complete blood count, serum iron, total iron-binding capacity, and serum B_{12} and folic acid levels. Whether any or all of these tests should be performed is a consideration to be made on an individual basis, dependent on clinical history and clinical suspicion of chronic candidiasis, Sjögren's syndrome, vitamin deficiency, or anemia.

Histopathology. Because no typical clinical lesion is associated with burning mouth syndrome and because symptoms are more generalized than focal, biopsy is generally not indicated. When an occasional arbitrary site in the area of chief complaint is chosen for biopsy, tissue appears within normal limits in hematoxylin and eosin (H&E) sections. Special stains may reveal the presence of a few *C. albicans* hyphae.

Diagnosis. Diagnosis is based on a detailed history, nondiagnostic clinical examination, laboratory studies, and exclusion of all other possible oral problems. Making the clinical diagnosis of burning mouth syndrome is generally not the difficult aspect of these cases. Rather, it is determining the subtle factor(s) that led to the symptoms that is difficult if not impossible.

Treatment. If a nutritional deficit is the cause, replacement therapy is curative. If a patient wears a prosthetic device, careful inspection of its fit and tissue base should be done. Relining or remaking it may help eliminate chronic irritation. If results of fungal cultures are positive, topical nystatin or clotrimazole therapy should produce satisfactory clinical results. If drugs may be involved, consultation with the patient's physician for an alternative drug may prove beneficial.

Because most patients do not fall neatly into one of these categories in which an identified problem can be rectified, treatment becomes difficult. Hormonal changes, neurologic problems, and idiopathic disease are as difficult to identify as they are to treat. A sensitive, empathic approach should be used when treating patients with this problem. Clinicians should be supportive and offer an explanation of the various facets and frustrations of burning mouth syndrome. No great optimism or easy solution should be offered, because patients may ultimately have to accept the disease and learn to live with the problem.

Other referrals may be useful, if only to exhaust all possibilities and reassure patients. The need for psychologic counseling is often difficult to broach with these patients, but it may be necessary after all logical avenues of investigation have been explored.

Empirical treatment is frequently the approach most clinicians are forced to use for patients with burning mouth syndrome. Even though there may be no evidence of candidiasis, nystatin or clotrimazole may cause a lessening of symptoms. A solution of tetracycline–nystatin–diphenhydramine hydrochloride (Benadryl) or similar remedy may likewise make patients more comfortable. Topical steroids, such as betamethasone (with or without antifungal agent), applied to the area of chief complaint may also be of some benefit. Generally, viscous lidocaine provides only temporary relief of pain, and saliva substitutes are of minimal value in patients suffering from associated xerostomia.

Low-dose tricyclic antidepressants may help some patients. However, they should not be used if xerostomia is a presenting sign, because these drugs may exaggerate this problem. Although incompletely evaluated in the clinical setting, substance P inhibitors (e.g., capsaicin) show some promise.

Infectious Conditions

SCARLET FEVER

Etiology. The characteristic effects of this systemic bacterial infection are the result of an erythrogenic toxin produced by some strains of group A streptococci that causes capillary damage. Other strains of group A streptococci that are unable to elaborate the toxin can cause pharyngitis and all the attendant features of infection but without the red skin rash and oral signs of scarlet fever. Spread of all group A streptococcal infections is generally via droplets from contact with an infected individual and, less likely, a carrier. Crowded living conditions promote the spread of streptococcal infections.

Clinical Features. Children are typically affected, after an incubation period of several days. In addition to the usual symptoms of all group A streptococcal infections—pharyngitis, tonsillitis, fever, lymphadenopathy, malaise, and headache—the child also exhibits a red skin rash that starts on the chest and spreads to other surfaces. The face is flushed except for a zone of circumoral pallor. The palate may show inflammatory changes, and the tongue may become covered with a white coat in which fungiform papillae are enlarged and reddened (strawberry tongue). Later, the coat is lost, leaving a beefy red tongue (red strawberry tongue or raspberry tongue). In untreated, uncomplicated cases, the disease subsides in a matter of days.

Complications of pharyngeal suppuration (abscesses), direct extension to adjacent structures, and metastatic infection may occasionally occur. Nonsuppurative hypersensitivity complications of rheumatic fever and glomerulonephritis are also important potential problems.

Differential Diagnosis. *Staphylococcus aureus* infections, viral infections, and drug eruptions might also be viable considerations in clinical evaluation of children with pharyngitis and an exanthematous skin eruption. Definitive diagnosis is based on history, clinical presentation, and throat culture.

Treatment. Penicillin is the drug of choice for the treatment of group A streptococcal infections. Erythromycin should be used in patients allergic to penicillin. The rationale for antibiotic treatment of this short-lived, self-limited disease is the prevention of complications, especially rheumatic fever and glomerulonephritis.

ATROPHIC CANDIDIASIS

Caused by the fungus *C. albicans,* this form of the disease appears as a red lesion rather than the traditional white lesion usually associated with candidiasis. The fungus is a prevalent intraoral microorganism that can be cultured from the mouths of most normal individuals. When local or systemic conditions change in favor of fungus growth (see Chapter 3), *C. albicans* takes an opportunistic role and causes overt infection.

Acute atrophic candidiasis follows the loss of the white fungal colonies from the surface of the mucosa. The lesion is red and painful. Chronic atrophic candidiasis also appears as a red, painful lesion, typically under a maxillary denture (denture sore mouth) or at the commissures of the mouth (angular cheilitis or perlèche). Detailed discussion of atrophic candidiasis can be found in Chapter 3.

Immunologic Abnormalities

PLASMA CELL GINGIVITIS

Etiology. This highly characteristic condition was first given the name *plasma cell gingivostomatitis* because of the prominent plasma cell infiltrate in the tissues affected and because of the undetermined origin. This condition was subsequently named *allergic gingivostomatitis* because many cases were linked to chewing gum that was believed to be eliciting an allergic reaction. When gum was removed from the diet of affected patients, tissues reverted to normal in a matter of weeks. Similar clinical lesions, however, were noted in patients who did not chew gum, thereby opening to question the original hypothesis. Clinical and microscopic evidence still supports an allergic or hypersensitivity reaction. A possible explanation of the appearance of disease in non–gum chewers might be that it represents a reaction to an ingredient in chewing gum, such as mint or cinnamon flavorings, that might be found in other foods.

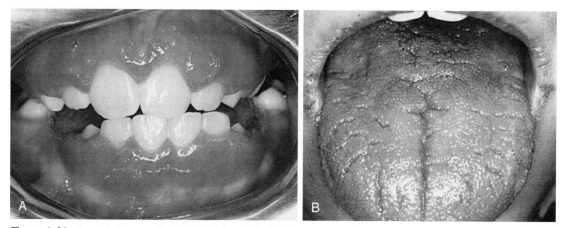

Figure 4–21. *A* and *B*, Plasma cell gingivitis of the attached gingiva, tongue, and commissures.

This peculiar condition is of historical interest because it was relatively prevalent at one time but is rarely encountered today. In the early 1970s, numerous cases, all nearly identical, were seen throughout the United States. Within a few years, the phenomenon all but disappeared. Clinicians speculated that formulas or sources of the offending ingredient(s) were changed, making the product nonallergenic.

Clinical Features. This condition affects adults and occasionally children of either gender. Burning mouth, tongue, or lips is the usual complaint of patients with plasma cell gingivitis. The onset is rather sudden, and the discomfort can wax and wane. This condition should not be classified with burning mouth syndrome, because distinctive clinical changes are present. The attached gingiva is fiery red but not ulcerated; the tongue mucosa is atrophic and red; and the commissures are reddened, cracked, and fissured (Fig. 4–21). Patients have no cervical lymphadenopathy and no systemic complaints.

Histopathology. The affected epithelium is spongiotic and is infiltrated by various types of inflammatory cells (Fig. 4–22). Langerhans cells are also prominent, and apoptotic keratinocytes may occasionally be seen. The lamina propria displays prominent capillaries and is infiltrated by plasma cells of normal morphology.

Differential Diagnosis. The triad of gingivitis, glossitis, and angular cheilitis differentiates this from other oral conditions. If tongue and commissure changes are particularly prominent, vitamin B deficiency or anemia might be included in a differential diagnosis. If gingival changes are particularly prominent, discoid lupus erythematosus, atrophic lichen planus, psoriasis, cicatricial pemphigoid, and contact allergic reaction might be considerations. If gingiva is predominately affected, a newly described condition, foreign body gingivitis, due to implantation of dental abrasives might be considered.

Treatment. Most patients respond rather quickly to the cessation of gum chewing. In non–gum chewers and those gum chewers who do not respond to the elimination of gum, careful dietary history taking is indicated in an attempt to identify an allergic source.

DRUG REACTIONS AND CONTACT ALLERGIES

Allergic reactions to drugs taken systemically or used topically frequently affect the skin but may also affect oral mucous membranes. A wide variety of agents are known to have this capacity, especially in patients who have a predisposition to the development of allergies.

The clinical appearance of allergic response in the skin ranges from red erythematous lesions to an urticarial rash to a vesiculo-ulcerative eruption. The same types of changes may appear in oral mucosa. In the less intense and less destructive injuries, the mucosa exhibits a generalized redness. When the tongue is the primary target, the pattern may be similar to the changes of vitamin B deficiency and anemia. (A detailed discussion on this subject can be found in Chapter 2.)

EXTRAVASCULAR—PETECHIAE AND ECCHYMOSES

Etiology. Soft tissue hemorrhages in the form of petechiae (pinpoint size) or ecchymoses (larger

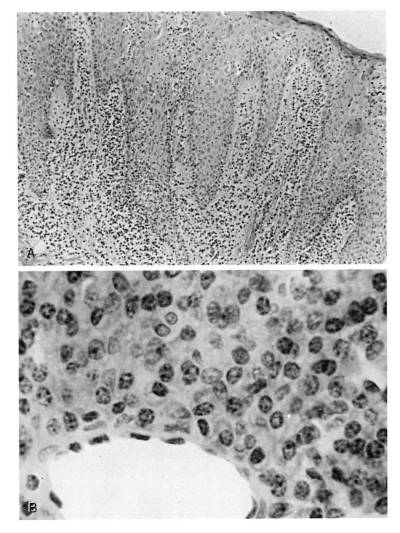

Figure 4–22. *A*, Plasma cell gingivitis showing spongiosis and inflammatory cell response. *B*, Most cells in the connective tissue infiltrate are plasma cells.

than pinpoint size) appear intraorally, generally because of trauma or blood disease (dyscrasia) (Table 4–5). Traumatic injury, if blood vessels are significantly damaged, can result in leakage of blood into surrounding connective tissue, producing red to purple lesions. The types of injury are

many and, among other things, related to cheek biting, coughing, fellatio, trauma from prosthetic appliances, injudicious hygiene procedures, and iatrogenic dental injuries.

In patients with blood dyscrasia, the presenting sign of minor trauma may be oral red to purple macules (Table 4–6). Dental practitioners can therefore have a significant role in the recognition of this abnormality. After ruling out a traumatic

Table 4–5. Blood Dyscrasias That Frequently Have Oral Manifestations

Leukemia
  Monocytic > myelocytic > lymphocytic
  Acute > chronic
Agranulocytosis
Cyclic neutropenia
Infectious mononucleosis
Idiopathic thrombocytopenic purpura
Secondary thrombocytopenic purpura
Hemophilias
Macroglobulinemia

Table 4–6. Oral Manifestations of Blood Dyscrasias

Petechiae, ecchymoses
Gingival enlargement
"Spontaneous" gingival hemorrhage
Prolonged bleeding after oral surgery
Gingivitis refractory to treatment
Loose teeth
Mucosal ulcers

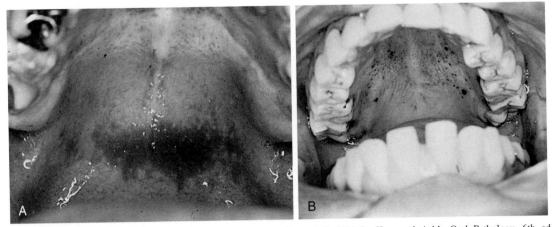

Figure 4–23. *A*, Palatal ecchymosis associated with trauma. (From Ash MM Jr. Kerr and Ash's Oral Pathology, 6th ed. Philadelphia, Lea & Febiger, 1992.) *B*, Petechiae of the palate associated with infectious mononucleosis.

etiology, practitioners should refer patients to an internist or hematologist.

All the various types of leukemia have the potential to produce intraoral lesions. In actual practice, monocytic leukemia (monocyte series) is most often associated with oral manifestations, myelocytic leukemia (granulocyte series) is next, and lymphocytic leukemia (lymphocytes) is least likely to be associated with oral signs. Acute forms of the leukemias are also more likely than chronic forms to be associated with oral lesions.

Platelet and clotting defects make up another large group of blood dyscrasias that may be responsible for petechiae, ecchymoses, and other intraoral manifestations. Platelet problems may be qualitative or quantitative in nature. They may also be of unknown origin (idiopathic thrombocy-

topenic purpura), or they may appear secondary to a wide variety of systemic factors, such as drug ingestion, infection, and immunologic disease. Hemophilia and related disorders in which clotting factors are deficient or defective are predominantly hereditary and are characteristically associated with prolonged bleeding and occasional ecchymoses.

Clinical Features. The color of these lesions varies from red to blue to purple, depending on the age of the lesion and the degree of degradation of the extravasated blood (Fig. 4–23). Soft tissue hemorrhagic lesions usually appear in areas accessible to trauma, such as the buccal mucosa, lateral tongue surface, lips, and junction of the hard and soft palate. In those injuries that are related to uncomplicated trauma, a cause-and-effect relation-

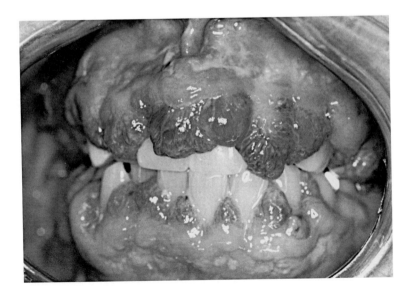

Figure 4–24. Enlargement of the gingiva associated with acute monocytic leukemia.

ship can usually be established after a history has been taken.

The lesions that develop secondary to blood dyscrasias may follow trivial or otherwise insignificant trauma. In addition to petechiae and ecchymoses, other clinical oral signs of blood dyscrasias include gingival enlargement (especially with monocytic leukemia [Fig. 4–24]), gingivitis, "spontaneous" gingival hemorrhage, prolonged bleeding after oral surgery, loose teeth, and mucosal ulcers.

Diagnosis. The inability to otherwise explain the appearance of any of these clinical signs should cause clinicians to suspect one of the blood dyscrasias. Gingivitis that is refractory to standard therapy should be viewed as a potential dyscrasia. The concomitant presence of lymphadenopathy, weight loss, weakness, fever, joint pain, and headache should add to the suspicion of serious systemic disease. Dentists in this situation should see that patients are evaluated by an internist or hematologist.

Bibliography

Chang Y, Cesarman E, Pessin MS, et al. Identification of herpesvirus-like DNA sequences in AIDS-associated Kaposi's sarcoma. Science 266:1865–1869, 1994.

Dictor M, Rambech E, Way D, et al. Human herpesvirus 8 (Kaposi's sarcoma–associated herpesvirus) DNA in Kaposi's sarcoma lesions, AIDS Kaposi's sarcoma cell lines, endothelial Kaposi's sarcoma simulators, and the skin of immunosuppressed patients. Am J Pathol 148:2009–2016, 1996.

Dutree-Meulenberg R, Kozel M, van Jost T. Burning mouth syndrome: a possible role for local contact sensitivity. J Am Acad Dermatol 26:935–940, 1992.

Ensoli B, Gendelman R, Markham P, et al. Synergy between basic fibroblast growth factor and HIV-1 tat protein in induction of Kaposi's sarcoma. Nature 371:674–680, 1994.

Epstein J, Scully C. HIV infection: clinical features and treatment of thirty-three homosexual men with Kaposi's sarcoma. Oral Surg Oral Med Oral Pathol 71:38–41, 1991.

Ficarra G, Berson A, Silverman S, et al. Kaposi's sarcoma of the oral cavity: a study of 134 patients with a review of the pathogenesis, epidemiology, clinical aspects, and treatment. Oral Surg Oral Med Oral Pathol 66:543–550, 1988.

Forbosco A, Criscuolo M, Coukos G. Efficacy of hormone replacement therapy in postmenopausal women with oral discomfort. Oral Surg Oral Med Oral Pathol 73:570–574, 1992.

Gordon SC, Daley TD. Foreign body gingivitis: identification of foreign material by energy-dispersive x-ray microanalysis. Oral Surg Oral Med Oral Pathol 83:571–576, 1997.

Gordon SC, Daley TD. Foreign body gingivitis: clinical and microscopic features of 61 cases. Oral Surg Oral Med Oral Pathol 83:562–570, 1997.

Gorsky M, Silverman S, Chinn H. Clinical characteristics and management outcome in the burning mouth syndrome. Oral Surg Oral Med Oral Pathol 72:192–195, 1991.

Guttmacher AE, Marchuk DA, White RI. Hereditary hemorrhagic teleangiectasia. N Engl J Med 333:918–924, 1995.

Itoiz M, Conti C, Lanfranchi H, et al. Immunohistochemical detection of filaggrin in preneoplastic and neoplastic lesions of the human oral mucosa. Am J Pathol 119:456–461, 1985.

Kaban L, Mulliken J. Vascular anomalies of the maxillofacial region. J Oral Maxillofac Surg 44:203–213, 1986.

Karlis V, Glickman RS, Stern R, Kinney L. Hereditary angioedema. Oral Surg Oral Med Oral Pathol 83:462–464, 1997.

Koehler JE, Glaser CA, Tappero JW. *Rochalimaea henselae* infection: a zoonosis with the domestic cat as reservoir. JAMA 271:531–535, 1994.

Koehler JE, Quinn FD, Berger TG, et al. Isolation of *Rochalimaea* species from cutaneous and osseous lesions of bacillary angiomatosis. 327:1625–1631, 1992.

Lamey P, Hammond A, Allam B, et al. Vitamin status of patients with burning mouth syndrome and the response to replacement therapy. Br Dent J 160:81–84, 1986.

Littner M, Dayan D, Gorsky M, et al. Migratory stomatitis. Oral Surg Oral Med Oral Pathol 63:555–559, 1987.

Lozada F, Silverman S, Migliorati C, et al. Oral manifestations of tumor and opportunistic infections in the acquired immunodeficiency syndrome (AIDS): findings in 53 homosexual men with Kaposi's sarcoma. Oral Surg Oral Med Oral Pathol 56:491–494, 1983.

Lumerman H, Freedman P, Kerpel S, Phelan J. Oral Kaposi's sarcoma: a clinicopathologic study of 23 homosexual and bisexual men from the New York metropolitan area. Oral Surg Oral Med Oral Pathol 65:711–716, 1988.

Maragon P, Ivanyi L. Serum zinc levels in patients with burning mouth syndrome. Oral Surg Oral Med Oral Pathol 71:447–450, 1991.

Miles SA. Pathogenesis of AIDS-related Kaposi's sarcoma. Evidence of a viral etiology. Hematol Oncol Clin North Am 10:1011–1021, 1996.

Morris CB, Gendelamn R, Marrogi AJ, et al. Immunohistochemical detection of Bcl-2 in AIDS-associated and classical Kaposi's sarcoma. Am J Pathol 148:1055–1063, 1996.

Nickoloff B, Griffiths C. Factor XIIIa–expressing dermal dendrocytes in AIDS-associated cutaneous Kaposi's sarcomas. Science 243:1736–1737, 1989.

Qu Z, Liebler JM, Powers MR, et al. Mast cells are a major source of basic fibroblast growth factor in chronic inflammation and cutaneous hemangioma. Am J Pathol 147:564–573, 1995.

Sassoon A, Said J, Nash G, et al. Involucrin in intraepithelial and invasive squamous cell carcinoma. Hum Pathol 16:467–470, 1985.

Sreebny L, Valdini A, Yu A. Xerostomia. Part II: Relationship to normal symptoms, drugs, and diseases. Oral Surg Oral Med Oral Pathol 68:419–427, 1989.

Tourne LPM, Fricton JR. Burning mouth syndrome: critical review and proposed management. Oral Surg Oral Med Oral Pathol 74:158–167, 1992.

Tylenda C, Ship J, Fox P, Baum B. Evaluation of submandibular salivary flow rate in different age groups. J Dent Res 67:1225–1228, 1988.

van der Waal I, Beemster G, van der Kwast W. Median rhomboid glossitis caused by Candida? Oral Surg Oral Med Oral Pathol 47:31–35, 1979.

vander Ploeg H, vander Wal N, Eijkman M, et al. Psychological aspects of patients with burning mouth syndrome. Oral Surg Oral Med Oral Pathol 63:664–668, 1987.

Weiss R, Guillet G, Freedberg I, et al. The use of monoclonal antibody to keratin in human epidermal disease: alterations in immunohistochemical staining pattern. J Invest Dermatol 81:224–230, 1983.

5

Pigmentations of Oral and Perioral Tissues

BENIGN LESIONS OF MELANOCYTE
  ORIGIN
Physiologic Pigmentation
Smoking-Associated Melanosis
Ephelis
Lentigo
Oral Melanotic Macule
NEOPLASMS
Nevi
Melanoma
Neuroectodermal Tumor of Infancy
PIGMENTATIONS CAUSED BY
  EXOGENOUS DEPOSITS
Amalgam Tattoo (Focal Argyrosis)
Heavy-Metal Pigmentations
Drug-Induced Pigmentations

BENIGN LESIONS OF MELANOCYTE ORIGIN

Melanin-producing cells (melanocytes) have their embryologic origin in the neural crest. These cells find their way to epithelial surfaces and reside among basal cells. They exhibit numerous dendritic processes that extend to adjacent keratinocytes, where transfer of pigment occurs (Fig. 5–1). The packaged pigment granules (melanosomes) produced by these melanocytes are ordinarily not retained within the cell itself but rather are delivered to the surrounding keratinocytes and occasionally to the subjacent macrophages. Light, hormones, and genetic constitution influence the amount of pigment produced.

Melanocytes are found throughout the oral mucosa but go unnoticed because of their relatively low level of pigment production and because of their clear, nonstaining cytoplasm on routine preparation. When focally or generally active in pigment production or proliferation, they may be responsible for several different recognized entities in the oral mucous membranes, ranging from physiologic pigmentation to malignant neoplasia.

A relative of the melanocyte, the nevus cell, is responsible for pigmented nevi. Nevus cells, although morphologically different from melanocytes, possess the same enzyme, tyrosinase, which is responsible for conversion of tyrosine to melanin in the melanosome organelle.

Oral melanin pigmentations range from brown to black to blue, depending on the amount of melanin produced and the depth or location of the pigment. Generally, superficial pigmentation is brown, whereas deeper pigmentation is black to blue. Darkening of a preexisting lesion that has not been stimulated by known factors suggests that pigment cells are producing more melanin or invading deeper tissue.

Physiologic Pigmentation

Clinical Features. This type of pigmentation is symmetric and persistent and does not alter normal architecture, such as gingival stippling (Fig. 5–2). This pigmentation may be seen in persons of any age and is without gender predilection. Physiologic pigmentation may be found in any location, although the gingiva is the most commonly affected intraoral tissue. A related type

Table 5–1. Syndromes Associated with Oral and Cutaneous Macular Pigmentation

SYNDROME	FEATURES
Peutz-Jeghers syndrome	Perioral ephelides, intestinal polyposis (not premalignant), autosomal dominant
Addison's disease	Diffuse cutaneous pigmentation, oral ephelides, adrenal cortical insufficiency
Albright's syndrome	Café au lait macules, polyostotic fibrous dysplasia, precocious puberty
Neurofibromatosis	Café au lait macules, oral cutaneous neurofibromas (malignant potential); some inherited as autosomal dominant

146

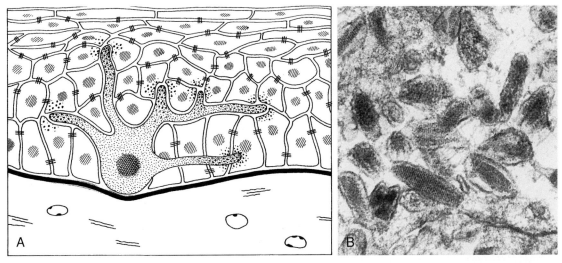

Figure 5–1. *A,* Typical melanocyte showing dendritic morphology and relationship to keratinocytes. Maturing melanosomes are evident in the dendritic processes of the melanocyte. Mature granules can be found in the keratinocytes. *B,* Electron micrograph of maturing melanosomes (premelanosomes) in the dendritic process of a melanocyte. Note the internal lattice structure of the ovoid premelanosomes.

of pigmentation, called *postinflammatory pigmentation,* is occasionally seen after mucosal reaction to injury. In occasional cases of lichen planus of the buccal mucosa, areas surrounding active disease may eventually show mucosal pigmentation (Fig. 5–3).

Histopathology. Physiologic pigmentation is due not to increased numbers of melanocytes but rather to increased melanin production. The melanin is found in surrounding basal keratinocytes and subjacent macrophages (melanophages).

Differential Diagnosis. Clinical differential diagnosis would include smoking-associated melanosis, Peutz-Jeghers syndrome, Addison's disease

(Table 5–1), and melanoma. Although physiologic pigmentation is usually clinically diagnostic, biopsy may be justified if clinical features are atypical.

Smoking-Associated Melanosis

Etiology and Pathogenesis. Abnormal melanin pigmentation of oral mucosa has been linked to cigarette smoking and has been designated smoking-associated melanosis or smoker's melanosis. The pathogenesis is believed to be related

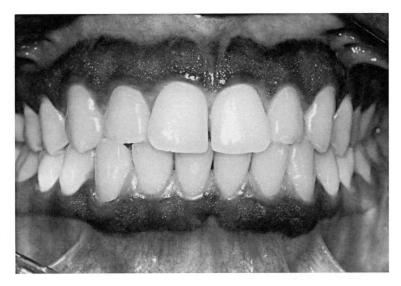

Figure 5–2. Physiologic pigmentation in a young adult male. Note the symmetry and normal gingival stippling. (Courtesy of Dr. A. Plotzke.)

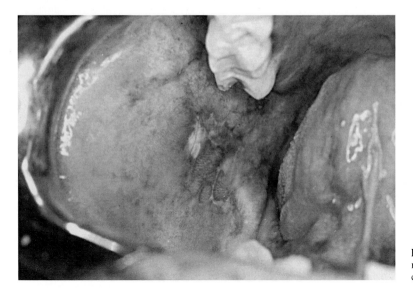

Figure 5–3. Postinflammatory pigmentation in a patient with oral lichen planus.

to a component in tobacco smoke that stimulates melanocytes. Female sex hormones are also believed to be modifiers in this type of pigmentation, because females (especially those taking birth control pills) are more commonly affected than males.

Clinical Features. Anterior labial gingiva is the region most typically affected (Fig. 5–4). Palate and buccal mucosa pigmentation has been associated with pipe smoking. The use of smokeless tobacco has not been linked to oral melanosis. In smoking-associated melanosis, the intensity of pigmentation is time and dose related.

Histopathology. Melanocytes show increased melanin production as evidenced by pigmentation of adjacent basal keratinocytes (Fig. 5–4). The microscopic appearance is essentially similar to that seen in physiologic pigmentation and melanotic macule.

Differential Diagnosis. Other entities to consider before definitive diagnosis is established are physiologic pigmentation, Peutz-Jeghers syndrome, Addison's disease, and melanoma.

Treatment. With cessation of smoking, improvement is expected over the course of months to years. Smoker's melanosis, per se, appears to be of little significance. It may, however, potentially mask other lesions or may be cosmetically objectionable.

Ephelis

Clinical Features. Ephelides, or freckles, are common, small (less than 5 mm in diameter), tan or brown cutaneous macules. These lesions, found on sun-exposed skin, darken with exposure to

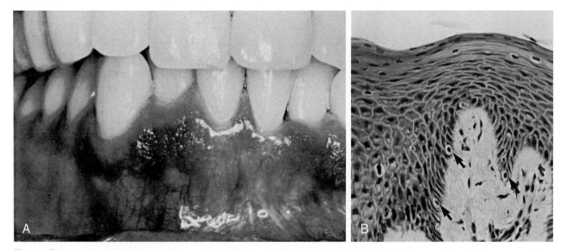

Figure 5–4. A, Smoker's melanosis in a young adult female. Pigmentation faded slowly after cessation of cigarette smoking. (Courtesy of Dr. P. Chiravalli.) B, Biopsy specimen showing normal melanocytes in the basal cell layer *(arrows)*.

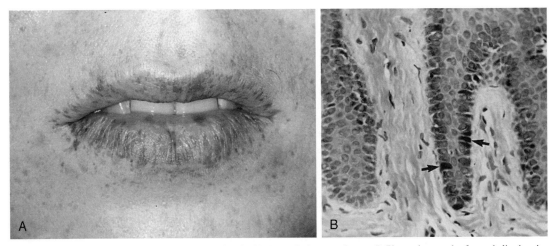

Figure 5–5. *A,* Perioral ephelides (freckles) associated with Peutz-Jeghers syndrome. *B,* Photomicrograph of an ephelis showing melanin deposits in basal keratinocytes *(arrows).*

ultraviolet light and lighten during periods of nonexposure.

When freckles (a subset of melanotic macules) are seen in excess in an oral and perioral distribution, *Peutz-Jeghers syndrome* (Fig. 5–5) and *Addison's disease* (Fig. 5–6) should be considered. Peutz-Jeghers syndrome is a condition that is inherited in an autosomal dominant pattern. In addition to ephelides or melanotic macules, intestinal polyposis is seen. These polyps are regarded as being hamartomatous without, or with very limited, neoplastic potential. They are usually found in the small intestine (jejunum) and may produce signs and symptoms of abdominal pain, rectal bleeding, and diarrhea.

Addison's disease, primary adrenal cortical insufficiency, may result from adrenal gland infection (tuberculosis), autoimmune disease, or idiopathic causes. With reduced cortisol production by the adrenals, pituitary adrenocorticotropic hormone (ACTH) and melanocyte-stimulating hormone (MSH) increase as part of a negative feedback mechanism. Overproduction of both ACTH and MSH results in stimulation of melanocytes, leading to diffuse pigmentation of the skin. Oral freckles and larger melanotic macules occur with the generalized pigmentation. Other presenting signs and symptoms of this syndrome include weakness, weight loss, nausea, vomiting, and hypotension.

Perioral pigmented macules have been described in association with two syndromes. One includes soft tissue myxomas and endocrinopathies *(myxoma syndrome).* Oral, cutaneous, and cardiac

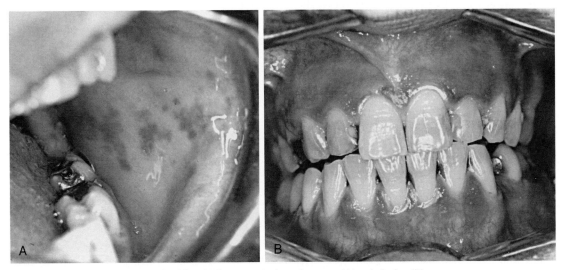

Figure 5–6. Pigmented macules of Addison's disease on the buccal mucosa *(A)* and gingiva *(B).*

myxomas may be seen in this autosomal dominant syndrome. The other, known as *Laugier-Hunziker syndrome* or *phenomenon,* is a rare acquired pigmentary disorder that presents as lip, oral, and finger macules.

Histopathology. Ephelides result from increased melanocyte function or melanin production rather than from increased numbers of melanocytes. Increased amounts of melanin are found in the basal cell layer because of focal melanocyte hyperactivity and melanosome transfer to the basal keratinocytes.

Treatment. There is no treatment indicated for this lesion. Its significance is negligible, unless associated with one of the two syndromes mentioned.

Lentigo

Lentigines, common skin lesions etiologically related to age and ultraviolet light exposure, are rarely seen intraorally. They appear as brown macules, typically in the palate, gingiva, and lips. Clinical differential diagnosis would include oral melanotic macule, amalgam tattoo, and *in situ* melanoma. Microscopically, benign melanocytic hyperplasia is seen in conjunction with elongation of rete ridges, rather than simple increased melanin production as seen in ephelides and oral melanotic macules. Oral lentigines are probably unrelated to melanomas, although some oral melanomas have been described as having a "lentiginous" microscopic pattern.

Oral Melanotic Macule

Clinical Features. Oral melanotic macule (or focal melanosis) is a focal pigmented lesion that

may represent (1) an intraoral freckle, (2) postinflammatory pigmentation, or (3) the macules associated with Peutz-Jeghers syndrome or Addison's disease.

Melanotic macules have been described as occurring predominantly on the vermilion of the lips and gingiva, although they may appear on any mucosal surface (Fig. 5–7). They are asymptomatic and have no malignant potential.

Histopathology. Microscopically, these lesions are characterized by melanin accumulation in basal keratinocytes and normal numbers of melanocytes (Fig. 5–7). Melanophagocytosis is also typically seen.

Differential Diagnosis. These oral pigmentations must be differentiated from early superficial melanomas (Table 5–2). They may be confused with blue nevi or amalgam tattoos. If they are numerous, Peutz-Jeghers syndrome and Addison's disease may be possible clinical considerations.

Treatment. Biopsy may be required to establish definitive diagnosis of this lesion. Otherwise, no treatment is indicated.

NEOPLASMS

Nevi

Etiology. *Nevus* is a general term that may refer to any congenital lesion of various cell types or tissue types. Generally, however, *nevus* (or mole), used without a modifier, refers to the pigmented lesion composed of nevus cells. It is sometimes called, more specifically, *nevocellular nevus, melanocytic nevus,* or *pigmented nevus.*

Nevi are collections of nevus cells that are round or polygonal and are typically seen in a

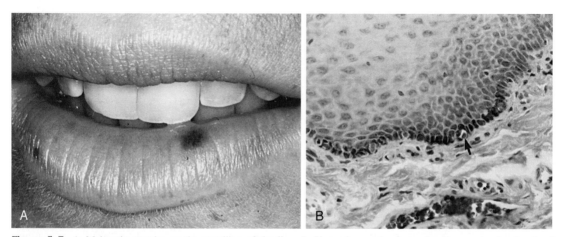

Figure 5–7. *A,* Melanotic macules on the vermilion of the lips. *B,* Photomicrograph of a melanotic macule showing basal keratinocyte pigmentation. Note the melanocyte *(arrow).*

Table 5–2. Clinical Differentiation of Oral Pigmentations from Early Melanoma

LESION	DIFFERENTIATING FEATURES
Focal argyrosis	Uniform slate-gray color, history of dental trauma, macular, no change with time
Physiologic pigment	Symmetric, not recently acquired, uniform color, no obstruction of normal landmarks
Melanotic macule	Uniform color, macular, relatively uniform contour
Melanoma	Recently acquired, variable color, irregular margins, satellite lesions, may be ulcerated or papular

nested pattern. They may be found in epithelium or supporting connective tissue or both. The origin of nevus cells has been postulated to be from cells that migrate from the neural crest to the epithelium and dermis (submucosa) or to be from altered resident melanocytes.

Clinical Features. Nevi of the skin are common acquired papular lesions that usually appear shortly after birth and throughout childhood. Intraoral nevi are relatively rare lesions that may occur at any age. Most oral nevi present as small (<0.5 cm) elevated papules, frequently nonpigmented (20%). The palate is the most commonly affected site (Fig. 5–8). Less frequent sites are the buccal mucosa, labial mucosa, gingiva, alveolar ridge, and vermilion.

Histopathology. Microscopically, several subtypes are recognized (Fig. 5–9). Classification is dependent on location of nevus cells. When cells are located in the epithelial-connective tissue junction, it is called a *junctional nevus;* when located in connective tissue it is called *intradermal nevus* or *intramucosal nevus,* or in a combination of zones a *compound nevus* (Fig. 5–10). A fourth type of nevus, in which cells are spindle shaped and found deep in the connective tissue, is known as the *blue nevus.* Malignant transforma-

tion of an oral benign nevus is highly improbable. Because oral nevi can mimic melanoma clinically, undiagnosed pigmented lesions should undergo biopsy.

In the oral cavity, intramucosal nevi are the most common variety seen, and blue nevi are the second most common. Compound and junctional nevi occur relatively rarely in the oral mucosa. The so-called *dysplastic nevus* that is commonly seen in skin has not been appreciated in oral mucous membranes.

Differential Diagnosis. Other clinical considerations that should be included along with any type of oral nevus are melanotic macule, amalgam tattoo, and melanoma. Lesions of vascular origin might also be considered. These include hematoma, Kaposi's sarcoma, varix, and hemangioma. Diascopy (compression under glass) could be used to rule out the last two lesions, in which the blood is contained within a well-defined vascular system.

Treatment. Because of the infrequency with which oral nevi occur and because of their inability to clinically mimic melanoma, all suspected oral nevi should be excised. Since their size is generally less than 1 cm, excisional biopsy would usually be indicated.

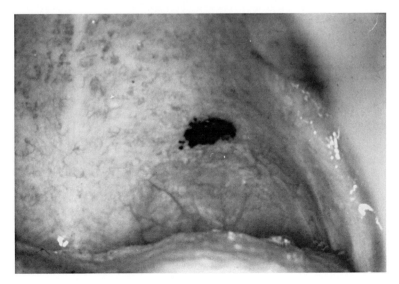

Figure 5–8. Compound nevus of the soft palate.

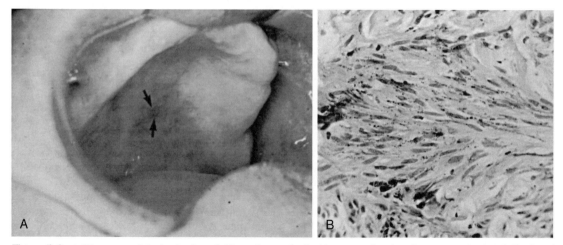

Figure 5–9. *A,* Blue nevus of the hard palate. *B,* Photomicrograph of a blue nevus showing pigment granules in spindle-shaped melanocytes deep in the submucosa.

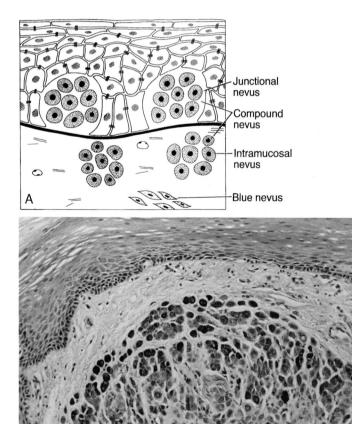

Junctional nevus

Compound nevus

Intramucosal nevus

Blue nevus

Figure 5–10. *A,* Nevus cells showing the location of cells in the various types of nevi. *B,* Biopsy of intramucosal nevus. Pigmentation is most intense near the surface.

Melanoma

Etiology. Melanomas of the skin have been increasing in frequency during the past several years and now represent approximately 2% of all cancers (excluding carcinomas of the skin). Overall, the cancer-related death rate due to melanoma of the skin is about 1 to 2%. Cutaneous melanoma is more common in southern climates than in northern climates and is much more common in whites than in blacks and Asians. For melanomas in the oral mucous membranes, there are no geographic differences, and the racial predilection seen with skin melanomas does not occur. In fact, blacks and Asians appear to be proportionately more frequently affected with this neoplasm in the oral mucosa than are whites.

Predisposing factors for skin lesions include extensive sun exposure (increased risk), dark natural pigmentation (reduced risk), and precursor lesions, such as congenital and dysplastic nevi. Intraorally, preexisting melanosis has been thought to appear before development of some melanomas. This pigmentary defect, however, very likely represents an early growth phase of these lesions. It is now well recognized that some types of melanomas in skin and mucosa may exhibit a prolonged superficial or radial growth phase occurring at the junction of epithelium and connective tissue before they enter an invasive vertical growth phase.

Clinical-Pathologic Features. Melanomas of oral mucosa are much less common than their cutaneous counterparts. Cutaneous melanomas generally occur in a younger population than do mucosal lesions (which usually appear after the age of 50). There is no sex predilection. Cutaneous melanomas occurring in the head and neck region are most often seen in sun-exposed areas. Oral lesions have a strong predilection for the palate and gingiva. Pigmentation patterns that suggest melanoma include different mixtures of color—such as brown, black, blue, and red—asymmetry, and irregular margins.

Recognition of radial and vertical growth phases in melanomas has led to the subclassification of these lesions into several clinical-pathologic entities. Subtypes occurring in the skin are nodular melanoma, superficial spreading melanoma, acral-lentiginous melanoma, and lentigo maligna melanoma. Each of these is now known to exhibit distinctive microscopic features, clinical features, and natural histories. Lesions similar to but not identical to the first three have been identified intraorally. Until more is learned about oral lesions, oral melanomas are best classified into *in situ* and invasive types (Figs. 5–11 to 5–14).

Differential Diagnosis. Intraorally, differential considerations would include amalgam tattoo, physiologic pigmentation, melanotic macule, and Kaposi's sarcoma. History, symmetry, and uniformity and evenness of pigmentation would all be of significant value in differentiating these lesions. Because melanomas may initially have a relatively innocuous appearance, biopsy should be done on any questionable acquired pigmentations.

Treatment and Prognosis. Surgery remains the primary mode of treatment for melanomas.

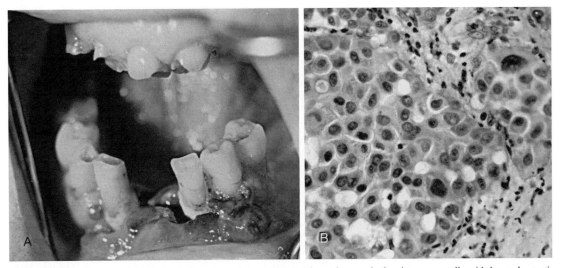

Figure 5–11. *A,* Invasive melanoma of the mandibular gingiva. *B,* Photomicrograph showing tumor cells with hyperchromatic and pleomorphic nuclei.

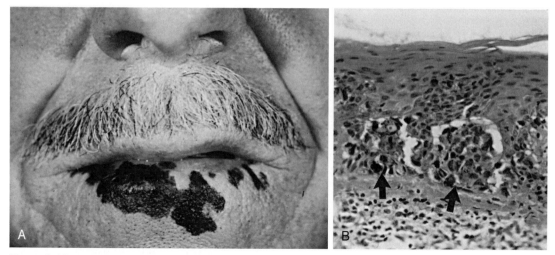

Figure 5–12. *A, In situ* melanoma of 8 years' duration. *B,* Photomicrograph showing nests of malignant melanocytes at the epithelium-connective tissue junction *(arrows).*

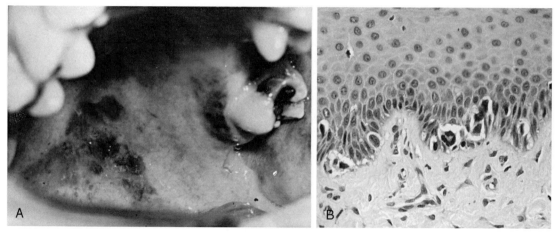

Figure 5–13. *A, In situ* melanoma of the palate. *B,* Malignant cells are found along the basement membrane during the radial growth phase.

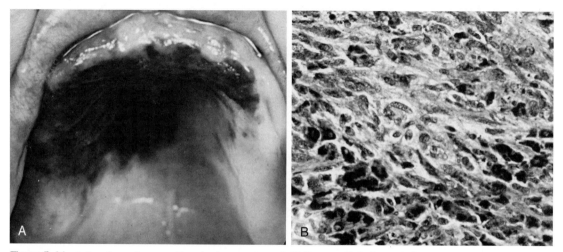

Figure 5–14. *A,* Invasive melanoma with an *in situ* component. *B,* Malignant cells in the vertical growth phase are spindle shaped.

Chemotherapy is often used, and immunotherapy is occasionally used as an adjunct. Radiotherapy has not been fully explored as a primary treatment method, but it may have a supportive role in disease management. Treatment failures of mucosal melanomas are most commonly linked to incomplete excision, resulting in local recurrence and distant metastasis. Regional lymph node metastasis seems to be a less important reason for persistence of disease. The need for wide surgical excision of *in situ* melanomas with a radial growth pattern is apparent from the microscopic appearance of this phenomenon.

Prognosis is based on both histologic subtype and depth of tumor invasion. The latter feature is a well-established prognosticator for skin lesions that has been applied to oral melanomas. Oral lesions have been found to be of considerably greater thickness (and consequently to be more advanced) than skin lesions at the time of biopsy. The overall poor prognosis of oral lesions as compared with skin lesions may therefore be partly related to late recognition of the oral lesions. Another factor is probably the more confining and difficult treatment area of the oral cavity. Oral lesions may also be inherently biologically more aggressive than skin lesions. Until more lesions are subclassified and measured for depth of invasion, these questions will go unanswered. After 5 years, the survival rate for patients with cutaneous melanomas is about 65% and the prognosis for oral lesions is about 20%. Unfortunately, the survival rate for patients with the oral lesions continues to decline after the traditional measure of 5 years.

Neuroectodermal Tumor of Infancy

Etiology. This rare, benign neoplasm is composed of relatively primitive pigment-producing cells. Like melanocytes and nevus cells, these cells have their origin in the neural crest.

Clinical Features. This lesion is found in infants usually younger than 6 months and occurs typically in the maxilla, although the mandible and the skull have been involved. This lesion usually presents as a nonulcerated and occasionally darkly pigmented mass (Fig. 5–15). The latter feature is due to melanin production by tumor cells. Radiographs show an ill-defined lucency that may contain developing teeth.

Histopathology. This neoplasm exhibits an alveolar pattern—that is, nests of tumor cells with small amounts of intervening connective tissue (Fig. 5–16). The variably sized nests of round to oval cells are found within a well-defined connective tissue margin. Cells located centrally within the neoplastic nests are dense and compact; peripheral cells are larger and often contain melanin.

Differential Diagnosis. Few other lesions would present in this age group and in this characteristic location. Malignancies of early childhood, such as neuroblastomas, sarcomas, or "histiocytic" tumors, might be considered. Odontogenic cysts and tumors would not be seriously entertained in a differential diagnosis.

Treatment and Prognosis. This lesion has been treated with surgical excision with good results. A few cases of local recurrence have been

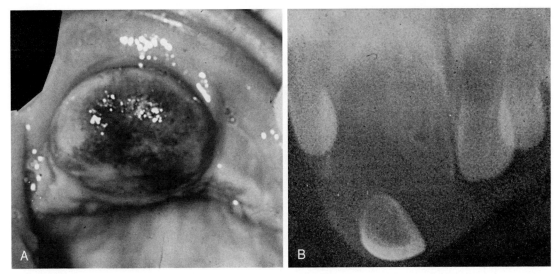

Figure 5–15. *A,* Neuroectodermal tumor of infancy in the maxilla. *B,* Radiograph showing a poorly defined lucency.

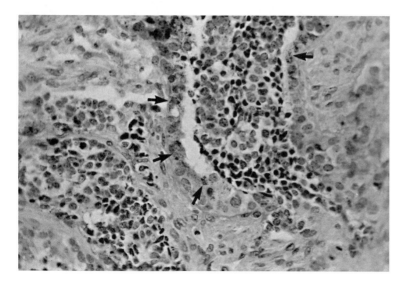

Figure 5–16. Photomicrograph of neuroectodermal tumor showing nests of round tumor cells. Pigment granules can be seen in the peripheral layer of cells *(arrows)*.

recorded, and in at least one documented case, metastasis has followed local excision.

PIGMENTATIONS CAUSED BY EXOGENOUS DEPOSITS

Amalgam Tattoo (Focal Argyrosis)

Etiology. Amalgam tattoo, or focal argyrosis, is an iatrogenic lesion that follows traumatic soft tissue implantation of amalgam particles or a passive transfer by chronic friction of mucosa against an amalgam restoration. This usually follows tooth extraction or preparation of teeth having old amalgam fillings for gold-casting restorations.

Clinical Features. This is the most common pigmentation of oral mucous membranes. These lesions would be expected in the soft tissues con-tiguous with teeth restored with amalgam alloy (Fig. 5–17A). Therefore, the most frequently affected sites are gingiva, buccal mucosa, palate, and tongue. Because amalgam is relatively well tolerated by soft tissues, clinical signs of inflammation are rarely seen. The lesions are macular and gray and do not change appreciably with time. If the amalgam particles are of sufficient size, they may be detected on soft tissue radiographs (Fig. 5–17B).

Histopathology. Microscopically, amalgam particles are typically aligned along collagen fibers and around blood vessels (Fig. 5–18). Few lymphocytes and macrophages are found, except in cases in which particles are relatively large. Multinucleated foreign-body giant cells may also be seen.

Differential Diagnosis. The significance of the amalgam tattoo lies in its clinical similarity to melanin-producing lesions. In a gingival or a pala-

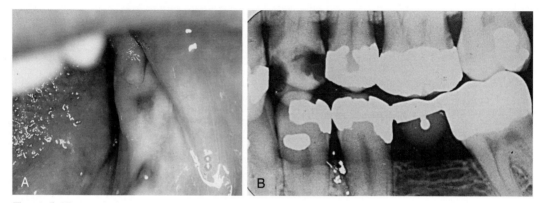

Figure 5–17. *A,* Amalgam tattoo of the alveolar ridge. *B,* Amalgam tattoo with large particles that can be seen in a radiograph.

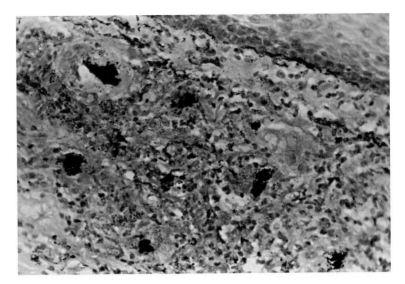

Figure 5–18. Amalgam tattoo showing connective tissue deposits of various-sized amalgam particles. Note deposition along basement membrane (top right).

tal location, separation from nevi and, more important, early melanoma is mandatory, because these are the most common areas for the latter lesions as well. Radiographs, history, and an even, persistent gray appearance all would help separate amalgam tattoo from melanoma. Any questionable lesions should undergo biopsy.

Heavy-Metal Pigmentations

Etiology. Some heavy metals (arsenic, bismuth, platinum, lead, mercury) may be responsible for oral pigmentation. This phenomenon occurs predominantly after occupational exposure to vapors of these metals. Historically, arsenic and bismuth compounds were used to treat diseases such as syphilis, lichen planus, and other dermatoses, providing another method for oral heavy-metal deposition. *Cis*-platinum, the salt of the heavy metal, has antineoplastic activity and is used to treat some malignancies. The side effect of a gingival platinum line has been described.

Clinical Features. These heavy metals may be deposited in both skin and oral mucosa (especially in gingiva). The characteristic color is gray to black, and the distribution is linear when found along the gingival margin. Bismuth and lead staining of gingival tissues are known as bismuth line and lead line (Fig. 5–19), respectively. This is proportional to the amount of gingival inflammation and appears to be the result of the reaction product of the heavy metal with hydrogen sulfide in the inflammatory zones.

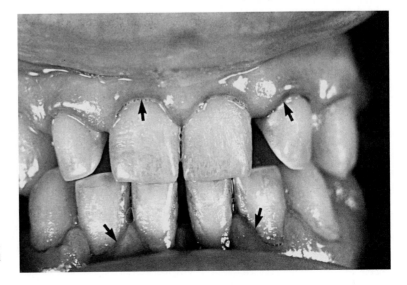

Figure 5–19. Gingival pigmentation (lead line) associated with lead intoxication *(arrows)*.

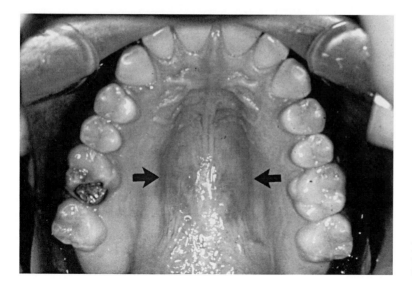

Figure 5–20. Minocycline pigmentation of the palate *(arrows).* (Courtesy of Dr. C. Witkop.)

Significance. The metallic deposits in oral mucosa, per se, are relatively insignificant. The underlying cause must be investigated because of detrimental effects of systemic toxicity. For dental personnel, chronic mercury vapor exposure is now recognized as a significant occupational hazard, if dental amalgam is handled carelessly and without proper precautions. Dental patients, however, are apparently at no risk, because of the relatively short exposure periods that they experience with routine office visits. Toxicity from the restorations themselves is also apparently negligible.

If, in the dental office, the atmospheric air has elevated mercury vapor levels, dental personnel may show elevated body levels of mercury as measured in hair, nails, saliva, and urine. *Chronic mercury intoxication* may produce symptoms of tremors, loss of appetite, nausea, depression, headache, fatigue, weakness, and insomnia. Hazard due to mercury can be eliminated in the dental office

if precautions are observed. The most common recommendations include (1) storage of mercury in sealed containers, (2) coverage of mercury spills with sulfur dust to prevent vaporization, (3) use of hard, seamless floor surfaces instead of carpeting, (4) working in well-ventilated spaces with frequent air filter changes, (5) storage of amalgam scraps under water in a sealed container, (6) use of well-sealed amalgamation capsules, and (7) use of water spray and suction when grinding amalgam.

Drug-Induced Pigmentations

Tetracycline-associated pigmentation may be found after the treatment of acne with prolonged high doses of *minocycline.* Diffuse skin pigmentation may be seen in sun-exposed areas, apparently as a result of increased melanin production, or

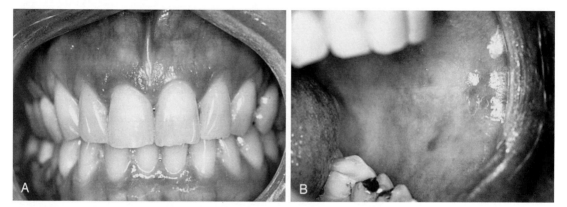

Figure 5–21. *A* and *B,* Cyclophosphamide (Cytoxan)-induced pigmentation of the marginal gingiva and buccal mucosa.

focal pigment deposits may be seen in the legs and periorbital skin, apparently as a result of drug complexes in melanocytes. Pigmentation of the gingiva and palate may be due to deposits in bone and tooth roots (Fig. 5–20).

Other exogenous drugs that may produce pigmentation of oral tissues include *aminoquinolines* (e.g., *chloroquine*), *cyclophosphamide* (Fig. 5–21), *amiodarone,* and *zidovudine (azidothymidine [AZT]).* The last drug, AZT, which is frequently used in the treatment of acquired immunodeficiency syndrome, may cause nail pigmentation, in addition to mucosal pigmentation.

Bibliography

Barker B, Carpenter WM, Daniels TE, et al. Oral mucosal melanomas: the WESTOP Banff workshop proceedings. Oral Surg Oral Med Oral Pathol 83:672–679, 1997.

Batsakis J, Regezi J, Solomon A, Rice D. The pathology of head and neck tumors: mucosal melanomas. Head Neck Surg 4:404–418, 1982.

Berthelsen A, Andersen A, Jensen T, Hansen H. Melanomas of the mucosa in the oral cavity and the upper respiratory passages. Cancer 54:907–912, 1984.

Buchner A, Hansen L. Melanotic macule of the oral mucosa: a clinicopathologic study of 105 cases. Oral Surg Oral Med Oral Pathol 48:244–249, 1979.

Buchner A, Hansen L. Pigmented nevi of the oral mucosa: a clinicopathologic study of 36 new cases and review of 155 cases from the literature. Part I: a clinicopathologic study of 36 new cases. Oral Surg Oral Med Oral Pathol 63:566–572, 1987.

Buchner A, Hansen L. Pigmented nevi of the oral mucosa: a clinicopathologic study of 36 new cases and review of 155 cases from the literature. Part II: analysis of 191 cases. Oral Surg Oral Med Oral Pathol 63:676–682, 1987.

Buchner A, Merrell P, Hansen L, Leider A. Melanocytic hyperplasia of the oral mucosa. Oral Surg Oral Med Oral Pathol 71:58–62, 1991.

Cale AE, Freedman PD, Lumerman H. Pigmentation of the jawbones and teeth secondary to minocycline hydrochloride therapy. J Periodontol 59:112–114, 1989.

Cook C, Lund B, Carney J. Mucocutaneous pigmented spots and oral myxomas: the oral manifestations of the complex of myxomas, spotty pigmentation, and endocrine overactivity. Oral Surg Oral Med Oral Pathol 63:175–183, 1987.

Dehner L, Sibley R, Sauk J Jr, et al. Malignant melanotic neuroectodermal tumor of infancy. Cancer 43:1389–1410, 1979.

Ettinger L, Freeman A. The gingival platinum line. Cancer 44:1882–1884, 1979.

Fitzpatrick JE. New histopathologic findings in drug eruptions. Dermatol Clin 10:19–36, 1992.

Gerbig AW, Hunziker T. Idiopathic lenticular mucocutaneous pigmentation or Laugier-Hunziker syndrome with atypical features. Arch Dermatol 132:844–845, 1996.

Greenberg R, Berger T. Nail and mucocutaneous hyperpigmentation of azidothymidine therapy. J Am Acad Dermatol 22:327–330, 1990.

Odell EW, Hodgson RP, Haskell R. Oral presentation of minocycline-induced black bone disease. Oral Surg Oral Med Oral Pathol 79:459–461, 1995.

Patton LL, Brahim JS, Baker AR. Metastatic malignant melanoma of the oral cavity: a retrospective study. Oral Surg Oral Med Oral Pathol 78:51–56, 1994.

Rapini RP, Goltz LE, Greer RO, et al. Primary malignant melanoma of the oral cavity: a review of 177 cases. Cancer 55:1543–1551, 1985.

Rees T. Oral effects of drug abuse. Crit Rev Oral Biol Med 3:163–184, 1992.

Regezi J, Hayward J, Pickens T. Superficial melanomas of oral mucous membranes. Oral Surg Oral Med Oral Pathol 45:730–740, 1978.

Rustgi AK. Hereditary gastrointestinal polyposis and non-polyposis syndromes. N Engl J Med 331:1694–1702, 1994.

Slootweg P. Heterologous tissue elements in melanotic neuroectodermal tumor of infancy. J Oral Pathol Med 21:90–92, 1992.

Tadini G, D'Orso M, Cusini M, et al. Oral mucosa pigmentation: a new side effect of azidothymidine therapy in patients with acquired immunodeficiency syndrome. Arch Dermatol 127:267–268, 1991.

Tanaka N, Amagasa T, Iwaki H, et al. Oral malignant melanoma in Japan. Oral Surg Oral Med Oral Pathol 78:81–90, 1994.

Veraldi S, Cavicchini S, Benelli C, Gasparini G. Laugier-Hunziker syndrome: a clinical, histopathologic, and ultrastructural study of four cases and review of the literature. J Am Acad Dermatol 25:632–636, 1991.

6

Verrucal-Papillary Lesions

REACTIVE LESIONS
Papillary Hyperplasia
Condyloma Latum
Squamous Papilloma/Oral Warts
Condyloma Acuminatum
Focal Epithelial Hyperplasia
NEOPLASMS
Keratoacanthoma
Verrucous Carcinoma
UNKNOWN ETIOLOGY
Pyostomatitis Vegetans
Verruciform Xanthoma

The oral mucosa may be the site of a class of lesions that may be clinically designated as verrucal-papillary. The majority of verrucal-papillary lesions are benign exophytic growths capable of arising from any portion of the oral mucosa in both keratinized and nonkeratinized areas. A wide range of etiologic factors, including viral, bacterial, fungal, traumatic, and neoplastic, may be implicated in this class of lesions. These lesions range from relatively trivial to potentially life threatening. The range of possibilities in the clinical differential diagnosis can be rather wide, encompassing many etiologically unrelated conditions.

REACTIVE LESIONS

Papillary Hyperplasia

Etiology. Papillary hyperplasia or palatal papillomatosis appears almost exclusively on the hard palate and almost always in association with a removable prosthesis. A definitive physical relationship with the mucosa covered by a removable denture base is seen; this may be noted in 1 in 10 people who wear appliances that cover the hard palatal mucosa.

The precise cause of papillary hyperplasia is not well understood, although it appears to be associated with ill-fitting or loose dentures that predispose to or potentiate growth of *Candida albicans* organisms beneath or at the interface of the denture base material and the mucosa. The

tissue hyperplasia has been related to the presence of the fungal organism in the setting of low-grade chronic trauma.

Clinical Features. The area of mucosa over the palate that tends to be most frequently involved is the vault. Less commonly the alveolar ridge or the palatal incline is affected.

Presentation is characterized by multiple erythematous and edematous papillary projections that are tightly aggregated, producing an overall verrucous granular or cobblestone appearance (Fig. 6–1). The projections may be slender and almost villous, although, in a majority of cases, each projection tends to be rounded and blunted, with narrow spaces on either side. Ulceration is rare, although intense erythema may at times provide an overall appearance of erosion. Focal telangiectatic sites may also be noted on occasion.

Histopathology. On perpendicular cross section, the lesion appears as numerous small fronds or papillary projections covered with intact parakeratotic stratified squamous epithelium (Fig. 6–1). The epithelium is supported by hyperplastic central cores of well-vascularized stromal tissue. The epithelium is hyperplastic and often demonstrates pseudoepitheliomatous features, occasionally severe enough to mimic squamous cell carcinoma. There is no evidence of dysplasia in association with this lesion and no increased risk of malignant transformation.

Differential Diagnosis. The range of possibilities in the differential diagnosis of papillary hyperplasia of the palate is rather narrow, because this particular entity is seldom confused with other forms of pathology. The chief lesion to be separated from papillary hyperplasia is nicotine stomatitis involving the hard palate; however, nicotine stomatitis does not occur on the hard palate of pipe smokers who wear complete maxillary removable appliances. Also, nicotine stomatitis tends to be more keratinized and usually demonstrates the presence of a small dot or punctum in the center of each nodular excrescence, which represents the orifice of the subjacent minor salivary gland duct. Rarely, in *Darier's disease,* the mucosa of the palate may demonstrate numerous papules. Numerous squamous papillomas may occur on the palate; however, these lesions tend to

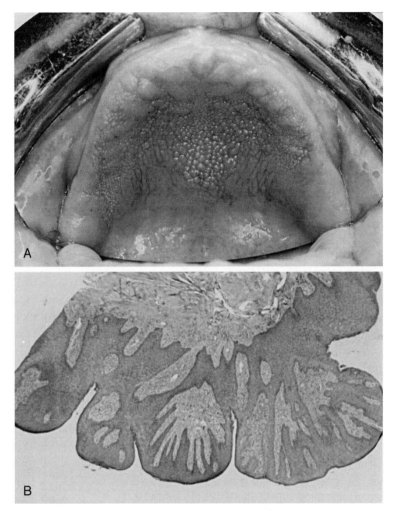

Figure 6–1. *A* and *B,* Papillary hyperplasia of the hard palate.

A

B

be more keratinized with more delicate projections. In the so-called malignant form of *acanthosis nigricans,* oral lesions are papillary in nature and may regress relative to the treatment response of the underlying distant malignancy. Finally, in the multiple hamartoma syndrome (*Cowden's syndrome*), the oral mucosa may exhibit numerous papillary mucosal nodules. These nodules, composed of benign fibroepithelial proliferations, may impart a cobblestone appearance, but usually to the tongue, buccal mucosa, and gingiva.

Treatment and Prognosis. Surgical removal is indicated before reconstructing a denture for the patient. The actual surgical method is often a matter of individual preference and may include curettage, cryosurgery, electrosurgery, mucoabrasion, or laser ablation.

Removal of appliances at bedtime and soaking in an antifungal medium, and maintenance of good oral hygiene coupled with topical antifungal therapy may significantly reduce the intensity of le-

sions. In mild cases, use of soft tissue conditioning agents and liners, with frequent changing of lining material, can produce sufficient resolution to preclude surgery. Topical antifungal therapy may also help reduce the intensity of the lesion, although when used alone it will not effect a cure.

Condyloma Latum

Condyloma latum is one of the many and variable expressions of secondary syphilis. As with all forms of syphilis, cutaneous, mucosal, and systemic lesions that mimic other conditions or diseases can be seen. Characteristic of condyloma latum is the presence of exophytic, sometimes friable, papillary to polypoid lesions within the oral cavity. Condyloma latum contains abundant microorganisms *(Treponema pallidum),* making it a potential source of infection.

Condyloma latum usually appears on the skin,

especially in the perianal and genital areas. Lesions may also be noted within the oral cavity. Here the tissue is formed into a soft, red, often mushroom-like mass with a generally smooth, lobulated surface (Fig. 6–2).

Microscopically, the overlying epithelium demonstrates significant acanthosis, along with intracellular and intercellular edema and transmigration of neutrophils. A perivascular plasma cell infiltrate is common within the lamina propria in the absence of a true vasculitis.

Patients require systemic administration of antibiotics to eliminate the underlying bacteremia. The oral lesions generally regress as the systemic disease is brought under control.

Squamous Papilloma/Oral Warts

Oral squamous papilloma is used as a generic term to include papillary and verrucal growths composed of benign epithelium and minor amounts of supporting connective tissue.

Oral squamous papilloma (including the vermilion portion of the lip) is the most common papillary lesion of the oral mucosa and makes up approximately 2.5% of all oral lesions. Whether all intraoral squamous papillomas are related etiologically to classic cutaneous verruca vulgaris is unknown. However, many oral squamous papillomas have been shown to be associated with the same human papillomavirus (HPV) subtype that causes cutaneous warts (Table 6–1). Other oral papillomas have been associated with different HPV subtypes. Whether all oral papillomas are of

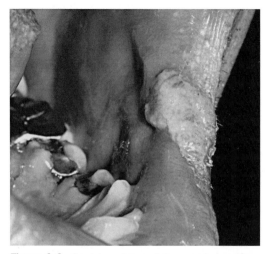

Figure 6–2. Condyloma latum of the commissure. (Courtesy of Dr. C. G. Taylor.)

Table 6–1. Lesions Associated with Human Papillomavirus

LOCATION/DIAGNOSIS	HPV SUBTYPE
Oral squamous papilloma (including oral warts)	2, 6, 11, 57
Cutaneous verruca vulgaris	2, 4, 40
Flat warts	3, 10
Condyloma acuminatum	6, 11
Laryngeal papillomas	11
Conjunctival papillomas	11
Focal epithelial hyperplasia	13, 32
Squamous dysplasia/neoplasia	16, 18

viral cause is open to question. It has been shown that the class of HPVs is very large (more than 100 subtypes) and that individually these viruses are associated with many conditions of squamous epithelium. For example, HPV subtypes 2 and 4 have been demonstrated within cutaneous warts by DNA hybridization techniques and by ultrastructural analysis; flat warts of the skin have been associated with HPV subtypes 3 and 10. HPV subtype 11 has been found within papillomas of the sinonasal tract and the oral cavity. HPV subtypes 16 and 18 have been related to neoplastic changes of squamous epithelium.

Etiology. The putative etiologic agent of papillomas of the upper aerodigestive tract is a member of the papovavirus group, currently designated HPV. This is a DNA virus containing a single molecule of double-stranded DNA. The viruses themselves are nonenveloped icosahedral particles ranging from 45 to 55 nm in diameter with 72 capsomeres in a skewed arrangement. Various species are antigenically distinct, with some common antigenic determinants shared by many such species. Replication of HPV occurs within the nuclei of epithelial cells as a result of stimulation of cellular DNA synthesis (Fig. 6–3). The viral genome is expressed in both early and late stages with the host histone proteins being incorporated into the virions. If progeny production is blocked, persistent infection may result. However, if intact viruses are produced, new infective particles can be released with or without cell death.

Clinical Features. Oral squamous papillomas may be found on the vermilion portion of the lips and any intraoral mucosal site, with predilection for the hard and the soft palates and the uvula (Fig. 6–4). The latter three sites account for approximately one third of the lesions found. The lesions generally measure less than 1 cm in greatest dimension and appear as exophytic granular to cauliflower-like surface alterations. The lesions generally are solitary in their presentation, al-

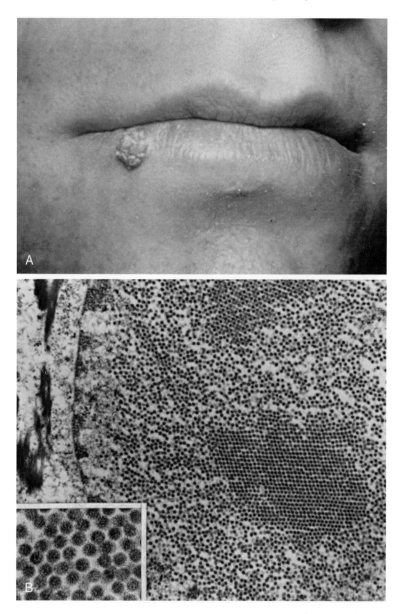

Figure 6–3. *A,* Squamous papilloma (wart) of the vermilion. *B,* Electron micrograph of human papillomavirus in the nucleus of an epithelial cell ($\times 33,000$; inset, $\times 100,000$).

though several lesions may be noted on occasion. The lesions are generally asymptomatic.

Histopathology. Oral squamous papillomas represent an exaggerated growth of normal squamous epithelium. Extensions of epithelium, supported by a well-vascularized connective tissue stroma, project from the surface of the epithelium (Fig. 6–5). The histologic architecture may mimic the pattern of the cutaneous wart (Fig. 6–6). Koilocytosis of upper-level epithelial cells may be found.

Some oral papillomas in patients with acquired immunodeficiency syndrome exhibit microscopic changes that are dysplastic in appearance (Fig. 6–7). The outcome or natural history of these

dysplastic warts is unknown. Various HPV subtypes can be demonstrated in these lesions.

Differential Diagnosis. The differential diagnosis of the oral squamous cell papilloma, when solitary, includes verruciform xanthoma, papillary hyperplasia, and condyloma acuminatum. The verruciform xanthoma may resemble the squamous papilloma, although this lesion has a distinct predilection for the gingiva and the alveolar ridge. A cause-and-effect relationship (e.g., lesion appearing under an ill-fitting denture) should be evident for inflammatory papillary hyperplasia. The condyloma would be larger than the papilloma and would have a broader base.

Treatment and Prognosis. Although many

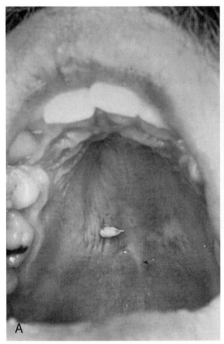

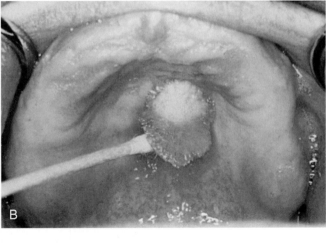

Figure 6–4. *A* and *B,* Squamous papillomas of the palate.

oral squamous papillomas appear to be virally induced, the infectivity of the HPV must be of a very low order. Route of transmission of the virus is unknown for oral lesions, although direct contact would be favored.

Surgical removal is the treatment of choice by either routine excision or laser ablation. Recurrence is uncommon, except for lesions in patients infected with human immunodeficiency virus (HIV).

Condyloma Acuminatum

Condyloma acuminatum is an infectious lesion that is characteristically located in the anogenital

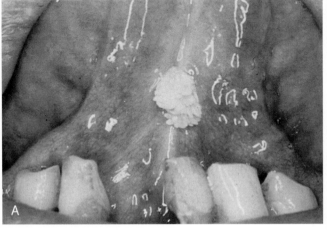

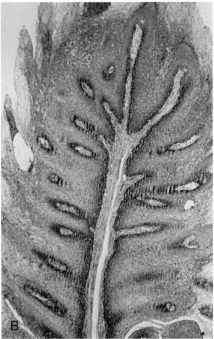

Figure 6–5. *A,* Squamous papilloma of the lingual frenum. *B,* Photomicrograph showing benign epithelium supported by fibrovascular cores.

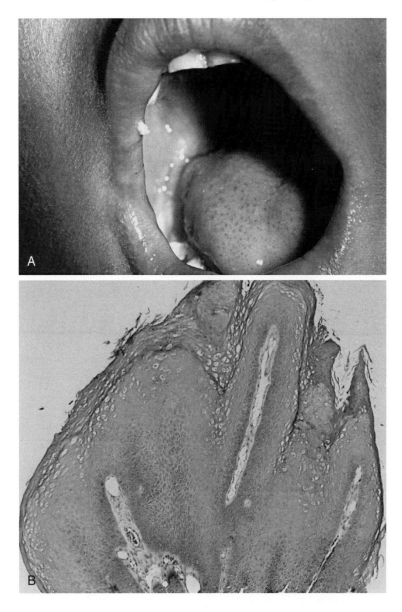

Figure 6–6. *A* and *B,* Oral verruca vulgaris. Note the columns of keratin and occasional clear cells (koilocytes) *(B).*

region but may also involve the oral mucosa. Common to these sites is a warm, moist squamous epithelial surface. An increasing frequency of this lesion has been noted in HIV-infected patients, reflecting an aspect of opportunistic infection.

Etiology and Pathogenesis. Condyloma acuminatum is a verrucous or a papillary growth that has been etiologically related to HPV subtypes 6 and 11. The maturation of the various subtypes of HPV within oral and genital mucosal cells is essentially the same. The keratinized cells act as the hosts for the virus, with replication linked to the process of keratinization.

Clinical Features. Characteristic of early condyloma acuminatum formation is a group of nu-

merous pink nodules that grow and ultimately coalesce. The result is a soft, broadbased, exophytic papillary growth that may be keratinized or nonkeratinized (Fig. 6–8).

One to 3 months after viral implantation—presumably as a result of orogenital contact with an infected partner—the disease becomes apparent. The lesions at times may be rather extensive, but they are generally self-limiting. The risk of autoinoculation is possible, thus offering a rationale for complete elimination of the lesions.

Histopathology. Papillary projections extending from the base of each lesion are covered by stratified squamous epithelium that is often parakeratotic but at times may be nonkeratinized

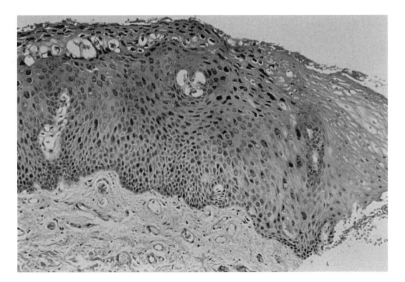

Figure 6–7. Dysplastic wart in an HIV-positive patient. Normal buccal mucosa mucosa epithelium to the right.

(Fig. 6–8). Upper-level epithelial cells demonstrate nuclei that are pyknotic and crenated, often surrounded by an edematous or optically clear zone forming the so-called koilocytic cell. This cell is thought to be indicative of a virally altered state. The epithelial layer itself is hyperplastic without evidence of dysplastic change. The underlying stroma is well vascularized and may contain a trace of chronic inflammatory cells.

Differential Diagnosis. Condyloma acumina-

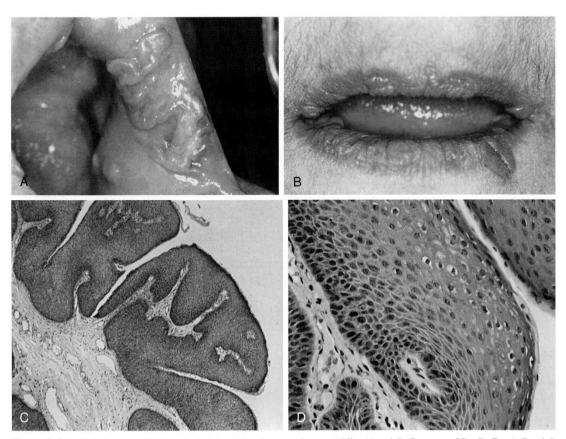

Figure 6–8. *A* and *B*, Condyloma acuminatum involving the commissure and lip. (*A* and *B*, Courtesy of Dr. D. Fear.) *C* and *D*, Papillary folds of condyloma acuminatum.

tum may resemble focal epithelial hyperplasia in some cases. Multiple intraoral warts (verruca vulgaris) may be a consideration, indeed representing the same type of infection. There are no universally accepted microscopic features that are capable of delineating condyloma acuminatum from verruca vulgaris. *In situ* DNA hybridization studies may be required to classify these lesions accurately.

Treatment and Prognosis. Treatment for these lesions is generally surgical excision, which may be cryosurgery, scalpel excision, electrodesiccation, or laser ablation. Recurrences are common, perhaps related to the surrounding normal-appearing tissue that may be harboring the infectious agent.

Focal Epithelial Hyperplasia

Focal epithelial hyperplasia (Heck's disease) was identified as a distinct entity in 1965. Early studies described lesions in Native Americans, in both the United States and Brazil, and in Eskimos. More recent studies have also identified lesions in other populations and ethnic groups from South Africa, Mexico, and Central America.

Etiology and Pathogenesis. Factors ranging from local low-grade irritation to vitamin deficiencies have been proposed as the cause of this condition. Convincing evidence, however, has been presented that HPV subtype 13 (and possibly 32) has an important etiologic role. Suggestions that genetic factors are involved have been made but not substantiated.

Clinical Features. This condition is characterized by the presence of numerous nodular soft tissue masses distributed over the mucosal surfaces, especially the buccal mucosa, the labial mucosa, and the tongue (Fig. 6–9). Lesions may appear as discrete or clustered papules, often similar in color to the surrounding mucosa. If found in areas of occlusal trauma, they may appear whitish because of keratosis. The lesions are asymptomatic and are often discovered incidentally. Initially described in children, this condition is now known to affect patients in a wide age range. An equal gender distribution has been noted.

Histopathology. Acanthosis and parakeratosis are consistent findings (Fig. 6–9). Prominent clubbing and fusion of epithelial ridges is also seen. Enlarged ballooning cells with abnormal nuclear chromatin patterns are often seen within the spinous layer. More superficial elements demonstrate cytoplasmic granular changes and nuclear fragmentation. Cells immediately beneath the surface

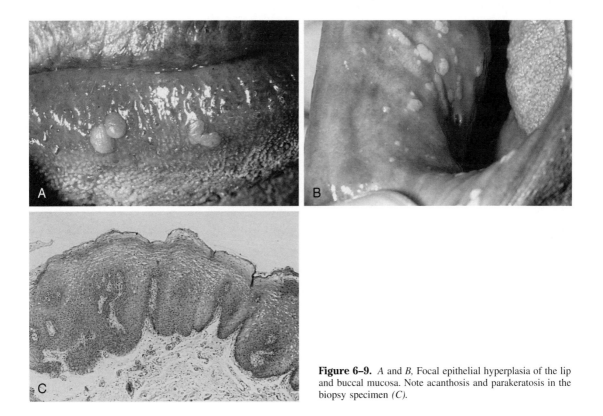

Figure 6–9. *A* and *B,* Focal epithelial hyperplasia of the lip and buccal mucosa. Note acanthosis and parakeratosis in the biopsy specimen *(C).*

often show pyknotic nuclei with a surrounding clear zone.

Ultrastructurally, crystalline arrangements of virus-like particles may be noted. Such particles measure approximately 50 nm in diameter, within the superficial spinous cells. Viruses may be found within the nucleus as well as the cytoplasm of spinous layer cells.

Differential Diagnosis. A differential diagnosis would include verruca vulgaris and multiple squamous papillomas. The oral mucosal lesions of Cowden's (multiple hamartoma) syndrome may present similarly and should be ruled out. Additionally, oral manifestations of Crohn's disease and pyostomatitis vegetans might also be considered.

Treatment. No particular treatment is indicated, especially with widespread involvement. Surgical removal may be used if few lesions are present. Of significance is that spontaneous regres-

sion has been noted in many cases, perhaps an expression of viral recognition and cell-mediated immunity.

NEOPLASMS

Keratoacanthoma

Etiology. The keratoacanthoma is a benign lesion of unknown cause that occurs chiefly on sun-exposed skin and, far less commonly, at the mucocutaneous junction. Rarely has this lesion been reported to arise on mucous membranes. In skin, the keratoacanthoma originates within the pilosebaceous apparatus, which explains its predominance in skin. It has been suggested that ectopic sebaceous glands may represent the site of origin intraorally. Virus-like intranuclear inclusions have been described in keratoacanthoma.

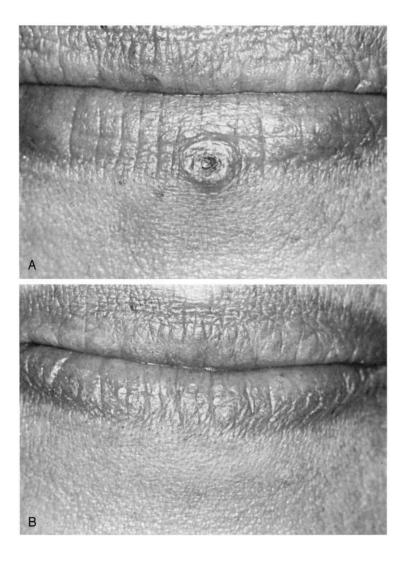

Figure 6–10. *A,* Keratoacanthoma of the lower lip. *B,* Same patient several weeks later showing spontaneous regression of the lesion.

However, attempts to produce such lesions in experimental animals by inoculation of tumor tissue have been unsuccessful. In addition to sunlight and viruses, suspected etiologic agents include chemical carcinogens, trauma, and disordered cellular immunity.

Clinical Features. Keratoacanthoma may be solitary or multiple (Fig. 6–10). The lesion usually begins as a small red macule that soon becomes a firm papule with a fine scale over its highest point. Rapid enlargement of the papule occurs over approximately 4 to 8 weeks, resulting ultimately in a hemispheric, firm, elevated, asymptomatic nodule. When fully developed, the keratoacanthoma contains a core of keratin surrounded by a concentric collar of raised skin or mucosa. A peripheral rim of erythema at the lesion base may parallel the raised margin.

If the lesion is not removed, spontaneous regression occurs. The central keratin mass is exfoliated, leaving a saucer-shaped lesion that heals with scar formation.

Histopathology. Keratoacanthoma is characterized by a central keratin plug with an overhanging lip or a marginal buttress of epithelium (Fig. 6–11). Marked pseudoepitheliomatous hyperplasia is evident, along with an intense mixed inflammatory infiltrate.

Of great importance is the histologic similarity between the keratoacanthoma and a well-differentiated squamous cell carcinoma. Numerous histologic criteria such as high level of differentiation, formation of keratin masses, smooth symmetric infiltration, and abrupt epithelial changes at lateral margins have been used to distinguish keratoacanthoma from carcinoma. Analysis of DNA indices and proliferative levels by flow cytometry of both well-differentiated squamous cell carcinomas and

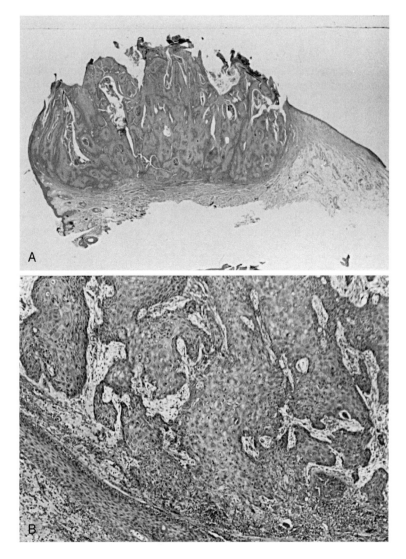

Figure 6–11. *A,* Low magnification of a keratoacanthoma showing its cup-shaped outline and central keratin plug. *B,* The base of a keratoacanthoma exhibiting epithelial proliferation similar to that seen in squamous cell carcinoma.

keratoacanthomas fails to separate the two lesions. Some investigators believe that keratoacanthoma should be regarded as a well-differentiated carcinoma.

Differential Diagnosis. The primary entity to be distinguished from solitary keratoacanthoma is squamous cell carcinoma, from both a clinical and a microscopic perspective. Squamous cell carcinomas have a relatively slow growth rate, are of irregular shape, and generally begin later in life. On the lip, other conditions to be differentiated include molluscum contagiosum, solar keratosis, and verruca vulgaris. Most of these entities, however, can be easily excluded on the basis of histologic examination of the biopsy specimen.

Treatment and Prognosis. At the least, a very careful follow-up is required in all cases because of the difficulties in diagnosis and distinction from squamous cell carcinoma. Any dubious lesion should be treated, because there are no absolutely reliable diagnostic, clinical, or histologic criteria to differentiate these two lesions. Additionally, during the early phase of this lesion, prediction of its ultimate size may be impossible.

The solitary keratoacanthoma may be removed by surgical excision or by thorough curettage of the base; both methods are equally effective. No recurrence is expected. In cases in which no treatment is accomplished, spontaneous involution, often with scar, is seen.

Verrucous Carcinoma

Since the original description of verrucous carcinoma as a subset of well-differentiated squamous cell carcinoma in 1948, significant confusion has developed regarding diagnostic criteria. A lesion designated as verrucous hyperplasia has been defined in the oral mucosa, adding to the confusion surrounding these microscopically bland verrucal growths.

Etiology. Verrucous carcinoma of oral mucous membranes is most closely associated with use of tobacco in various forms, especially smokeless tobacco. A role for HPV in either a primary or an ancillary relationship is suspected. Identification of intratumor HPV DNA adds support for a role of this virus in tumor development.

Clinical Features. This form of carcinoma accounts for 5% of all intraoral squamous cell carcinomas. The buccal mucosa accounts for more than half of all cases, and the gingiva is the location for nearly one third (Table 6–2). The mandibular gingiva shows a slight predominance over the maxillary gingiva. There is a distinct male pre-

Table 6–2. Intraoral Sites of Verrucous Carcinoma

SITE	NUMBER
Buccal mucosa	101
Gingiva	49
Tongue	12
Floor of mouth	7
Palate	7

From Batsakis JG, Hybels R, Crissman JD, Rice DH. The pathology of head and neck tumors, part 15. Verrucous carcinoma. Head Neck Surg 5:29–38, 1982. Copyright © 1982 John Wiley & Sons, Inc. Reprinted by permission of John Wiley & Sons, Inc.

dominance, and most individuals are over 50 years of age.

Early lesions, which may initially be interpreted as verrucous hyperplasia, are relatively superficial and tend to appear white clinically. These lesions may arise in leukoplakia. In time, the lesion borders become irregular and indurated. As verrucous carcinoma develops, the lesion becomes exophytic with a whitish to gray shaggy surface (Fig. 6–12). Although not highly infiltrative, the lesion pushes into surrounding tissues. When it involves the gingival tissues, it becomes fixed to the underlying periosteum. If it is untreated, gradual invasion of periosteum and destruction of bone occur (Fig. 6–13).

Histopathology. At low magnification, surface papillary fronds are covered by a markedly acanthotic and highly keratinized epithelial surface (Fig. 6–14). Bulbous, well-differentiated epithelial masses extend into the submucosa, with margins that are blunted and pushing. Adjacent to the pushing margins of the carcinoma is a lymphocytic infiltrate. Focal areas of acute inflammation surrounding foci of well-formed keratin are at times seen.

Of importance is the absence of significant cellular atypia and a deceptively benign microscopic pattern. Diagnosis can be made only by providing a biopsy specimen of sufficient size to include the full thickness of the epithelial component as well as the supporting connective tissue.

Differential Diagnosis. In well-developed cases of verrucous carcinoma, the clinical-pathologic diagnosis is relatively straightforward. However, in less than obvious situations, leukoplakia might be a clinical consideration. Also to be included would be papillary squamous carcinoma, which may be distinguished from verrucous carcinoma by its more infiltrative nature, its greater degree of cytologic atypia, and its more rapid growth. Verrucous carcinoma may develop from preexisting (and usually multiple) leukoplakia, representing part of

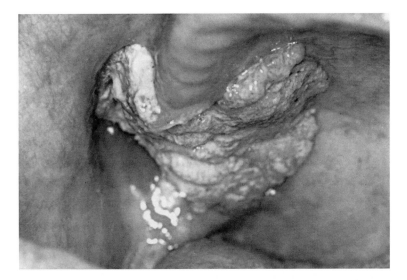

Figure 6–12. Verrucous carcinoma of the maxillary alveolar ridge and palate.

the spectrum of *proliferative verrucous leukoplakia.*

Treatment and Prognosis. Surgical methods are generally used as the primary form of therapy in most cases of verrucous carcinoma. This is chiefly because of early reports of dedifferentiation occurring in verrucous carcinoma after radiotherapy. Literature, however, suggests that transformation to squamous cell carcinoma occurs far less frequently than had been reported. Aggressive radiotherapy early or in combination with surgery may be a viable alternative treatment method.

Verrucous carcinoma rarely metastasizes, though it is locally destructive. In advanced cases in which the maxilla or the mandible exhibits significant destruction, resection may be necessary.

The prognosis for verrucous carcinoma is excellent, primarily because of its high level of differentiation and rarity of metastatic spread. Local recurrence, however, remains a distinct possibility if inadequate treatment is rendered.

UNKNOWN ETIOLOGY

Pyostomatitis Vegetans

Originally described in 1949, this benign chronic and pustular form of mucocutaneous disease is most often seen in association with inflammatory bowel disease. In two of the three original patients with oral disease, the lesions were confined to the oral mucosa. The cause of pyostomatitis vegetans is unknown, although it may be seen in association with ulcerative colitis, spastic

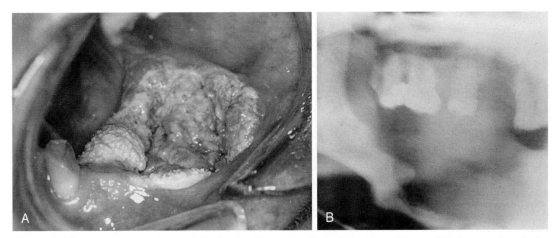

Figure 6–13. *A,* Verrucous carcinoma of the alveolar ridge and vestibule. *B,* Invasion of the mandible by a neoplasm in the same patient.

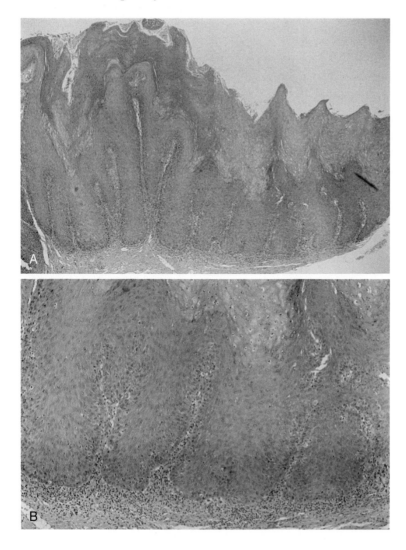

Figure 6–14. *A*, Verrucous carcinoma. *B*, Base of the lesion showing well-differentiated blunt margins. Specimen from a patient with proliferative verrucous leukoplakia.

colitis, chronic diarrhea, and Crohn's disease. More than 25% of cases are not associated with gastrointestinal disturbances.

Clinical Features. Early in the evolution of pyostomatitis vegetans, the oral mucosa (especially buccal mucosa) appears erythematous and edematous, often thrown into deep folds. Numerous tiny yellow pustules, ranging from 2 to 3 mm in diameter, and small vegetating papillary projections may be seen over the surface of friable mucosa. Oral mucosal involvement may include the gingiva, hard and soft palates, buccal and labial mucosa, lateral and ventral aspects of the tongue, and floor of the mouth. Males are affected nearly twice as often as females, and the age range is generally between the third and sixth decades, with an average age of 34 years. Laboratory values are generally within normal limits, although in many patients peripheral eosinophilia or anemia may be noted.

Histopathology. The oral mucosa demonstrates hyperkeratosis and pronounced acanthosis, often with a papillary surface or with pseudoepitheliomatous hyperplasia. A pronounced inflammatory infiltrate composed of neutrophils and eosinophils is a constant finding. Superficial abscesses may be seen within the lamina propria, with extension into the parabasal regions of the overlying epithelium. Ulceration and superficial epithelial necrosis may also be noted.

Treatment and Prognosis. The management of this entity relates to controlling the associated bowel disease. Topical agents, such as corticosteroids, may be used intraorally. Additionally, antibiotics, multivitamins, and nutritional supplements may be given; however, all are associated with variable results. Remission of oral lesions reflects inadequate control of the underlying bowel disease and serves as a specific mucosal marker for the process.

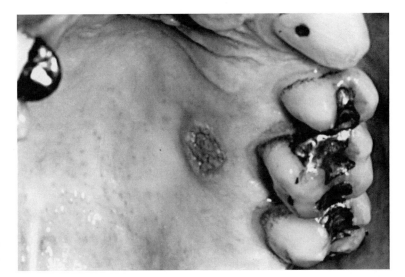

Figure 6–15. Verruciform xanthoma of the palate. (Courtesy of Dr. C. Allen.)

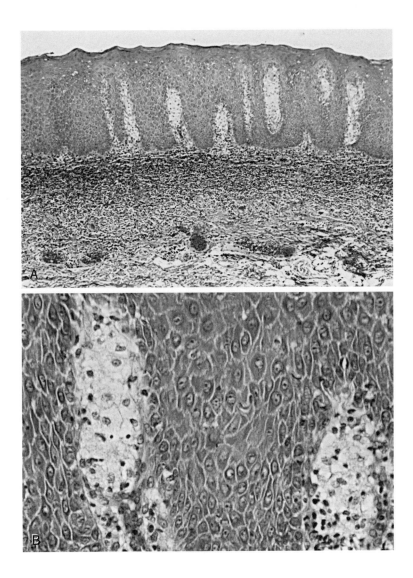

Figure 6–16. *A* and *B,* Verruciform xanthoma. Note the pale xanthoma cells in the lamina propria.

Verruciform Xanthoma

Verruciform xanthoma is an uncommon, benign oral mucosal lesion that occasionally may be found on the skin. The cause is unknown.

Clinical Features. Clinically, verruciform xanthoma is well circumscribed, with a granular to papillary surface (Fig. 6–15). Size ranges from 2 mm to over 2 cm. Either an exophytic or a depressed surface is present, and the lesion may occasionally be ulcerated. The level of keratinization of the surface influences its color, which ranges from white to red.

The majority of cases have been reported in whites; there is no gender predilection. The average patient age is 45 years, with a few cases reported within the first and second decades. The lesions are usually discovered incidentally.

Histopathology. Lesion architecture is flat or slightly raised with a papillomatous or verrucous surface composed of parakeratinized epithelial cells (Fig. 6–16). Uniformly invaginated crypts alternate with papillary extensions. Elongated epithelial ridges extend into the lamina propria at a uniform depth. The epithelial component is normal, with no evidence of dysplasia or atypia.

Numerous foam or xanthoma cells are found within the lamina propria or connective tissue papillae. Characteristic of the foam cells is a granular to flocculent cytoplasm that may contain periodic acid–Schiff (PAS)–positive, diastase-resistant granules or lipid droplets, or both. Ultrastructurally, the foam cells are best characterized as macrophages.

Differential Diagnosis. A differential diagnosis for this entity includes squamous papilloma, papillary squamous carcinoma, and condyloma acuminatum.

Treatment. The treatment is conservative excision. No recurrences have been reported.

Bibliography

Papillary Hyperplasia

Chang F, Syrjanen S, Kellokoski J, Syrjanen K. Human papillomavirus (HPV) infections and their associations with oral disease. J Oral Pathol 20:305–307, 1991.

Kozlowski L, Nigra T. Esophageal acanthosis nigricans in association with adenocarcinoma from an unknown primary site. J Am Acad Dermatol 26:348–351, 1992.

Nomachi K, Mori M, Matsuda N. Improvement of oral lesions associated with malignant acanthosis nigricans after treatment of lung cancer. Oral Surg Oral Med Oral Pathol 68:74–79, 1989.

Swart JGN, Lekkas C, Allard RHB. Oral manifestations in Cowden syndrome. Oral Surg Oral Med Oral Pathol 59:264–268, 1985.

Tyler MT, Ficarra G, Silverman S, et al. Malignant acanthosis nigricans with florid papillary oral lesions. Oral Surg Oral Med Oral Pathol 81:445–449, 1996.

Young S, Min K. In situ DNA hybridization analysis of oral papillomas, leukoplakias, and carcinomas for human papillomavirus. Oral Surg Oral Med Oral Pathol 71:726–729, 1991.

Condyloma Latum

De Swaan B, Tjiam KH, Vuzevski VD, et al. Solitary oral condyloma lata in a patient with secondary syphilis. Sex Transm Dis 12:238–240, 1985.

Manton SL, Egglestone SI, Alexander I, et al. Oral presentation of secondary syphilis. Br Dent J 160:237–238, 1986.

Squamous Papilloma/Oral Verruca Vulgaris

Broich G, Saskai I. Electronmicroscopic demonstration of HPV in oral warts. Microbiologica 13:27–34, 1990.

de Villiers EM, Hirsch-Benham A, von-Knebel-Doeberitz C, et al. Two newly identified human papillomavirus types (HPV 40 and 57) isolated from oral mucosal lesions. Virology 171:248–253, 1989.

Eversole LR, Laipis P. Oral squamous papillomas: detection of HPV DNA by in situ hybridization. Oral Surg Oral Med Oral Pathol 65:545–550, 1988.

Eversole LR, Laipis PJ, Green TL. Human papillomavirus type 2 DNA in oral and labial verruca vulgaris. J Cutan Pathol 14:319–325, 1987.

Kellokoski J, Syrjanen S, Syrjanen K, Yiskoski M. Oral mucosal changes in women with genital HPV infection. J Oral Pathol Med 19:142–148, 1990.

McNab J, Walkinshaw S, Cordiner J, et al. Human papillomavirus in clinically and histologically normal tissue of patients with genital cancer. N Engl J Med 315:1052–1058, 1986.

Regezi JA, Greenspan D, Greenspan JS, et al. HPV-associated epithelial atypia in oral warts in HIV+ patients. J Cutan Pathol 21:217–223, 1994.

Zeuss M, Miller C, White D. In situ hybridization analysis of human papilloma virus DNA in oral mucosal lesions. Oral Surg Oral Med Oral Pathol 71:714–720, 1991.

Condyloma Acuminatum

Barone R, Ficarra G, Gaglioti D, et al. Prevalence of oral lesions among HIV-infected intravenous drug abusers and other risk groups. Oral Surg Oral Med Oral Pathol 69:169–173, 1990.

Silverman S Jr, Migliorati CA, Lazada-Nur F, et al. Oral findings in people with or at high-risk for AIDS: a study of 375 homosexual males. J Am Dent Assoc 112:187–192, 1986.

Zunt S, Tomich CE. Oral condyloma acuminatum. J Dermatol Surg Oncol 15:591–594, 1989.

Focal Epithelial Hyperplasia

Garlick JA, Calderon S, Buchner A, Mitrani-Rosenbaum S. Detection of human papillomavirus (HPV) DNA in focal epithelial hyperplasia. J Oral Pathol Med 18:172–177, 1989.

Padayachee A, van Wyk CW. Human papillomavirus (HPV) DNA in focal epithelial hyperplasia by in situ hybridization. J Oral Pathol Med 20:210–214, 1991.

Pfister H, Hettich I, Runne V, et al. Characterization of human papilloma virus type 14 from focal epithelial hyperplasia (Heck) lesions. J Virol 47:363–366, 1983.

Keratoacanthoma

Lawrence N, Reed RJ. Actinic keratoacanthoma speculations on the nature of the lesion and the role of cellular immunity in its evolution. Am J Dermatopathol 12:517–533, 1990.

Randall MB, Geisinger RR, Kute TE, et al. DNA content and proliferative index in cutaneous squamous cell carcinoma and keratoacanthoma. Am J Clin Pathol 93:159–262, 1990.

Street ML, White JW, Gibson LE. Multiple keratoacanthomas treated with oral retinoids. J Am Acad Dermatol 23:862–866, 1990.

Verrucous Carcinoma

Greer RO Jr, Eversole LR, Crosby LK. Detection of human papillomavirus genome DNA in oral epithelial dysplasias, oral smokeless tobacco-associated leukoplakias and epithelial malignancies. J Oral Maxillofac Surg 48:1201–1209, 1990.

Hansen LS, Olson JA, Silverman S Jr. Proliferative verrucous leukoplakia. A long-term study of 30 patients. Oral Surg Oral Med Oral Pathol 60:285–298, 1985.

Kamath VV, Varma RR, Gadewar DR, Muralldahr M. Oral verrucous carcinoma: an analysis of 37 cases. J Craniomaxillary Surg 17:309–314, 1989.

McDonald JS, Crissman JD, Gluckman JL. Verrucous carcinoma of the oral cavity. Head Neck Surg 5:22–28, 1982.

Palefsky JM, Silverman S, Abdel-Salaam M, et al. Association between proliferative verrucous leukoplakia and infection with human papillomavirus type 16. J Oral Pathol Med 24:193–197, 1995.

Vidyasagar MS, Fernandes DJ, Kasturi P, et al. Radiotherapy and verrucous carcinoma of the oral cavity. Acta Oncol 31:43–47, 1992.

Pyostomatitis Vegetans

Ballo PS, Camisa C, Allen CM. Pyostomatitis vegetans: report of a case and review of the literature. J Am Acad Dermatol 21:381–387, 1989.

Hansen LS, Silverman S Jr, Daniels TE. The differential diagnosis of pyostomatitis vegetans and its relations to bowel disease. Oral Surg Oral Med Oral Pathol 55:363–373, 1983.

Healy CM, Farthing PM, Williams DM, Thornhill MH. Pyostomatitis vegetans and associated systemic disease. Oral Surg Oral Med Oral Pathol 78:323–328, 1994.

Neville BW, Laden SA, Smith SE, et al. Pyostomatitis vegetans: Am J Dermatopathol 7:69–77, 1985.

Thornhill M, Zakrzawska J, Gilkes J. Pyostomatitis vegetans: report of 3 cases and review of the literature. J Oral Pathol Med 21:128–133, 1992.

Van Hale HM, Rogers RS III, Zone JJ, et al. Pyostomatitis vegetans. A marker for inflammatory disease of the gut. Arch Dermatol 121:94–98, 1985.

Verruciform Xanthoma

Neville B. The verruciform xanthoma. A review and report of eight new cases. Am J Dermatopathol 8:247–253, 1986.

Nowparast B, Howell FV, Rick GM. Verruciform xanthoma. A clinicopathologic review and report of 54 cases. Oral Surg 51:619–625, 1981.

Rowden D, Lovas G, Shafer W, et al. Langerhans cells in verruciform xanthomas: an immunoperoxidase study of ten oral cases. J Oral Pathol 15:48–53, 1986.

Santa Cruz DJ, Martin SA. Verruciform xanthoma of the vulva. Report of two cases. Am J Clin Pathol 71:224–228, 1979.

Travis WD, Davis GE, Tsokos M, et al. Multifocal verruciform xanthoma of the upper aerodigestive tract in a child with systemic lipid storage disease. Am J Surg Pathol 13:309–316, 1989.

Van der Waal I, Kerstens HCJ, Hens CJJ. Verruciform xanthoma of the oral mucosa. J Oral Maxillofac Surg 43:623–626, 1985.

7

Connective Tissue Lesions

FIBROUS CONNECTIVE TISSUE LESIONS

Reactive Hyperplasias

This is a group of fibrous connective tissue lesions that commonly occur in oral mucosa secondary to injury. The group represents a chronic process in which overexuberant repair (granulation tissue and scar) follows injury. As a group, these lesions present as submucosal masses that may become secondarily ulcerated when traumatized during mastication. Their color ranges from lighter than the surrounding tissue (because of a relative increase in collagen) to red (because of an abundance of well-vascularized granulation tissue). Because nerve does not proliferate with the reactive hyperplastic tissue, these lesions are painless. The reason for the overexuberant repair is unknown. Treatment is generally surgical excision and removal of the irritating factor(s).

Although these are all pathogenically related lesions, different names or subdivisions have been devised because of variations in anatomic site, clinical appearance, or microscopic picture. Those lesions that present as prominent red masses are discussed in Chapter 4.

PYOGENIC GRANULOMA AND PERIPHERAL GIANT CELL GRANULOMA

These conditions are discussed in detail in Chapter 4.

PERIPHERAL FIBROMA

Clinical Features. By definition, this reactive hyperplastic mass occurs in the gingiva and may be derived from connective tissue of the submucosa or the periodontal ligament (Fig. 7–1). Some lesions may represent a "mature" pyogenic granuloma in which the granulation tissue has been largely replaced by collagen. It may occur at any age, although it does have a predilection for young

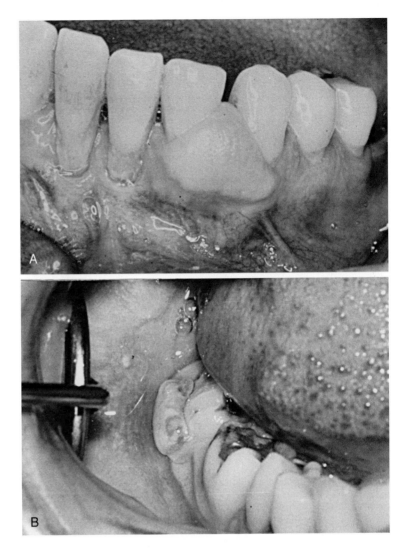

Figure 7–1. *A,* Peripheral fibroma. *B,* Peripheral fibroma with ossification.

adults. Females develop these lesions more commonly than do males, and the gingiva anterior to the permanent molars is most frequently affected.

The peripheral fibroma presents clinically as either a pedunculated or a sessile mass that is similar in color to the surrounding connective tissue. Ulceration may be noted over the summit of the lesion. It rarely causes erosion of subjacent alveolar bone.

Histopathology. The peripheral fibroma is a focal fibrous hyperplasia that may also be called *hyperplastic scar.* It is highly collagenous and relatively avascular and may contain a mild to moderate chronic inflammatory cell infiltrate. This is basically the gingival counterpart to the traumatic fibroma occurring in other mucosal regions.

Microscopically, several subtypes of this lesion have been identified. These are essentially of academic interest, because biologic behavior and treatment of these microscopic variants are the same.

The *peripheral ossifying fibroma* is a gingival mass in which calcified islands, presumed to be metaplastic bone, are seen (Fig. 7–2). The bone is found within a nonencapsulated proliferation of plump, benign fibroblasts. Chronic inflammatory cells tend to be seen around the periphery of the lesion. The surface is often ulcerated.

The *peripheral odontogenic fibroma* is a gingival mass composed of well-vascularized, nonencapsulated fibrous connective tissue. The distinguishing feature of this variant is the presence of strands of odontogenic epithelium, often abundant, throughout the connective tissue (Fig. 7–3). The lesion is usually nonulcerated.

The so-called *giant cell fibroma* (Fig. 7–4) is a focal fibrous hyperplasia in which connective tissue cells, many of which are multinucleated, as-

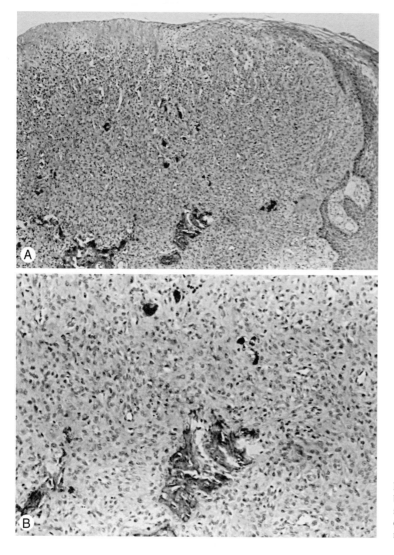

Figure 7–2. Peripheral ossifying fibroma. *A,* Low magnification showing surface ulceration. *B,* High magnification of fibroblastic matrix with islands of new bone.

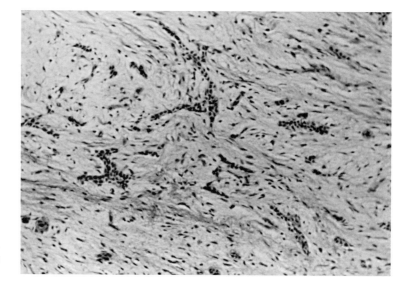

Figure 7–3. Peripheral odontogenic fibroma. Note the numerous strands of odontogenic epithelium.

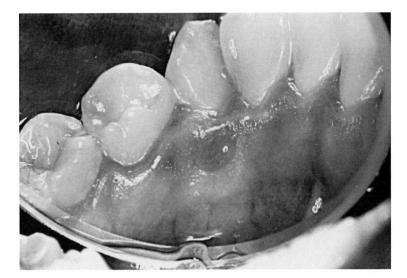

Figure 7–4. Peripheral fibroma (retrocuspid papilla).

sume a stellate shape (Fig. 7–5). Immunohisto-chemical studies have shown that most of these cells are fibroblasts (few factor XIIIa-positive den-drocytes are also typically present). These same peculiar cells can also be found in focal fibrous hyperplastic lesions throughout the oral mucosa and occasionally on the skin (fibrous papule). One form of this type of lesion is known as *retrocuspid papilla* of the mandible (Figs. 7–4 and 7–5).

Differential Diagnosis. Clinically, these lesions are usually not confused with anything else. There may, however, be some overlap with pyogenic granuloma and, rarely, peripheral giant cell granuloma, when these two lesions do not have a prominent vascular component.

Treatment. Peripheral fibroma should be treated by local excision that should include the periodontal ligament, if involved. Also, any identifiable etiologic agent, such as calculus or other foreign material, should be removed. Recurrence may occasionally be associated with the microscopic subtype peripheral ossifying fibroma. Reexcision to periosteum or periodontal ligament should prevent further recurrence.

GENERALIZED GINGIVAL HYPERPLASIA

Etiology. In this form of gingival enlargement, overgrowth may vary from mild enlargement of interdental papillae to such severe uniform enlargement that the crowns of the teeth may be covered by hyperplastic tissue. Uniform or generalized gingival fibrous connective tissue hyperplasia may be due to one of several etiologic factors. Most cases are nonspecific and are a result of an unusual hyperplastic tissue response to chronic inflammation associated with local factors such as plaque, calculus, or bacteria (Fig. 7–6). Why only some patients have a propensity for the development of connective tissue hyperplasia in response to local factors is unknown.

Other conditions such as hormonal changes and drugs can significantly potentiate or exaggerate the effects of local factors on gingival connective tissue. Hormonal changes occurring during pregnancy and puberty have long been known to be associated with generalized gingival hyperplasia. The hyperresponsiveness during pregnancy has led to the infrequently used and inappropriate term *pregnancy gingivitis.* Altered hormonal conditions act in concert with local irritants to produce the hyperplastic response. It is questionable whether significant gingival enlargement during periods of hormonal imbalance would occur in individuals with scrupulous oral hygiene.

Phenytoin (Dilantin), the drug used in the control of seizure disorders, is a well-known etiologic factor in generalized gingival enlargement (Fig. 7–7). The extent or severity of so-called *Dilantin hyperplasia* is dependent on the presence of local factors. The effect of time and dose of drug on gingival tissue is not clear. The reported prevalence of this condition has ranged from 0 to 80%, depending on the investigator's clinical criteria and the number of patients observed. A 50% figure is generally accepted as the probable prevalence. In any event, the fact that not all patients taking Dilantin develop gingival hyperplasia indicates that some patients are predisposed to the development of this condition. It has only rarely been described in edentulous patients and in children before tooth eruption. The mechanism by

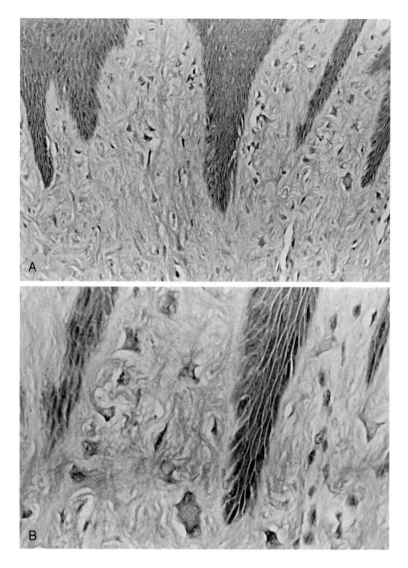

Figure 7–5. *A* and *B*, Peripheral fibroma, giant cell type. Note the stellate and multinucleated fibroblasts.

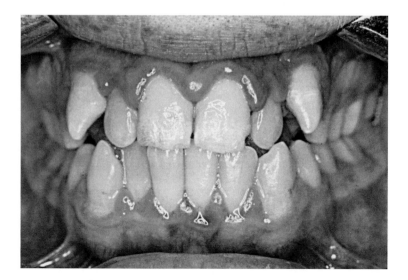

Figure 7–6. Generalized gingival hyperplasia due to reaction to local factors.

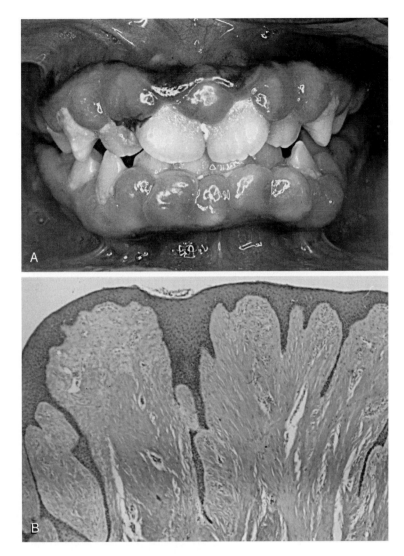

Figure 7–7. *A* and *B*. Generalized gingival hyperplasia, phenytoin (Dilantin) induced. Note the dense collagen making up the bulk of the enlargement.

which the drug causes fibrous hyperplasia is unclear, although the drug appears to have a regulating effect on fibroblast metabolism or growth rate. All fibroblasts are thought to be susceptible to the drug to some degree. The exaggerated response of gingival fibroblasts is probably related to the influence of concomitant inflammation.

A side effect of another drug, *cyclosporine,* has more recently been linked to fibrous hyperplasia of the gingiva. Cyclosporine is an immunosuppressive drug that is used to suppress T lymphocyte function in transplant recipients and in patients with various autoimmune diseases. Not all patients are affected (10 to 70%) and local factors have a synergistic role. Unlike Dilantin hyperplasia, cyclosporine-induced hyperplasia has been reported to be a reversible process following cessation of drug use.

Nifedipine and other calcium channel blockers for treatment of angina and arrhythmias are known to contribute to gingival hyperplasia. The process mimics phenytoin-related hyperplasia but appears to be reversible.

Gingival enlargement is also known to occur in patients with leukemia, especially those with the monocytic type. This is believed to be the result of infiltration of the gingival soft tissues by malignant white blood cells (Fig. 7–8). This may also be due, totally or in part, to reactive fibrous hyperplasia caused by local factors (Fig. 7–9). Because of the bleeding tendency associated with leukemia, patients may be reluctant to practice correct oral hygiene, resulting in accumulation of plaque and debris. This accumulation may provide the inflammatory stimulus for connective tissue hyperplasia.

Another form of gingival enlargement, appearing early in childhood, is known as *idiopathic*

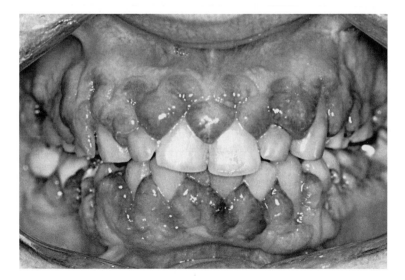

Figure 7–8. Gingival hyperplasia resulting from leukemic infiltrates in monocytic leukemia.

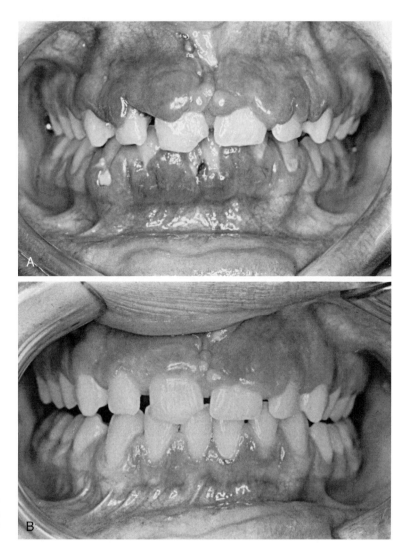

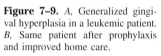

Figure 7–9. *A*, Generalized gingival hyperplasia in a leukemic patient. *B*, Same patient after prophylaxis and improved home care.

hyperplasia or *hereditary gingival fibromatosis* (Fig. 7–10). In this rarely seen condition, some patients have a hereditary predisposition, whereas others have no apparent genetic link. It may appear as an isolated entity or it may be part of one of several syndromes (Zimmerman-Laband, Cross', Rutherfurd's, Murray-Puretic-Drescher, Cowden's).

Clinical Features. The clinical feature common to the variously caused gingival hyperplasias is an increase in the bulk of the free and attached gingiva, especially the interdental papillae. Stippling is lost, and gingival margins become rolled and blunted. Consistency ranges from soft and spongy to firm and dense, depending directly on the degree of fibroplasia. A range of color from red-blue to lighter than surrounding tissue is also seen; this depends on the severity of the inflammatory response as well. Generally, the hyperplasias associated with nonspecific local factors and hormonal changes appear more inflamed clinically than the drug-induced and the idiopathic forms. The idiopathic type is particularly dense and fibrous, with relatively little inflammatory change.

Histopathology. The microscopic picture of gingival hyperplasia is one in which abundant collagen deposition dominates. Fibroblasts are increased in number, and various degrees of chronic inflammation are seen. In some cases, especially those in which hormonal changes are important, capillaries may be increased and prominent. The overlying epithelium usually exhibits some hyperplasia. In leukemic enlargements, atypical and immature white blood cells, representing a malignant infiltrate, may be found.

Treatment. In all forms of generalized gingival hyperplasia, attentive oral hygiene is necessary to minimize the effects of inflammation on fibrous proliferation and the effects of systemic factors. Gingivoplasty or gingivectomy may be required but should be done in combination with prophylaxis and oral hygiene instruction.

TRAUMATIC FIBROMA

Etiology. Traumatic fibroma, also known as *irritation fibroma, focal fibrous hyperplasia,* and *hyperplastic scar,* is a reactive lesion caused usually by chronic trauma to oral mucous membranes. Overexuberant fibrous connective tissue repair results in a clinically evident submucosal mass.

Clinical Features. There is no gender or racial predilection for the development of this intraoral lesion. It is a very common reactive hyperplasia that is typically found in frequently traumatized areas, such as the buccal mucosa, lateral border of the tongue, and lower lip (Fig. 7–11). It is a painless, broad-based swelling that is lighter than the surrounding tissue, because of its relative lack of vascular channels. The surface may occasionally be traumatically ulcerated, particularly in larger lesions. Traumatic fibromas have limited growth potential, usually not exceeding 1 cm in diameter and rarely greater than 2 cm.

Multiple traumatic fibroma-like lesions may be part of a rare autosomal dominant syndrome known as *Cowden's syndrome* or *multiple hamartoma syndrome.* Many organ systems, such as the mucosa, skin, breast, thyroid, and colon, may be affected. Frequently encountered abnormalities include numerous oral fibromas and papillomas; cutaneous papules, keratoses, and trichilemmomas;

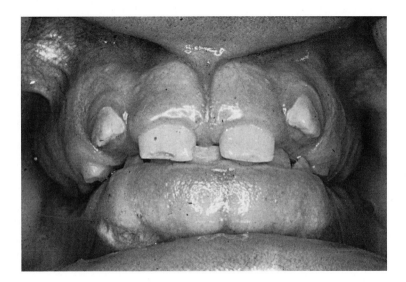

Figure 7–10. Generalized gingival hyperplasia, idiopathic type.

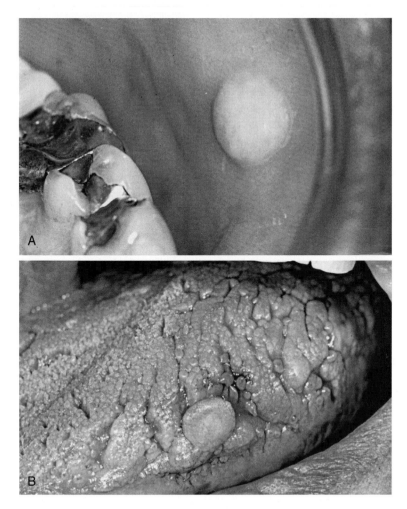

Figure 7–11. *A* and *B*, Traumatic fibromas.

benign and malignant neoplasms of the breast and thyroid; and colonic polyps.

Histopathology. Collagen overproduction is the basic process that dominates the microscopy of this lesion (Fig. 7–12). Fibroblasts are mature and widely scattered in a dense collagen matrix. Sparse chronic inflammatory cells may be seen, usually in a perivascular distribution. Overlying epithelium is often thinned and hyperkeratotic, because of chronic low-grade friction.

Differential Diagnosis. This is a relatively trivial lesion that should be removed to rule out other pathologic processes. Depending on location, several other entities might be included in a clinical differential diagnosis of small, asymptomatic submucosal masses. Neurofibroma, neurilemoma, and granular cell tumor would be possibilities for masses in the tongue. In the lower lip and buccal mucosa, lipoma, mucocele, and salivary gland tumors might be considered. Although rare, benign neoplasms of mesenchymal origin could present as submucosal masses not unlike the traumatic fibroma.

Treatment. Simple surgical excision is usually effective. Infrequently, recurrences may be caused by continued trauma to the involved area. These lesions have no malignant potential.

DENTURE-INDUCED FIBROUS HYPERPLASIA

Etiology. This fibrous hyperplasia of oral mucosa is related to the chronic trauma produced by an ill-fitting denture. It is essentially the same process that leads to the traumatic fibroma, except that a denture is specifically identified as the causative agent. This lesion has also been designated by the outdated synonyms *inflammatory hyperplasia, denture hyperplasia,* and *epulis fissuratum.*

Clinical Features. Denture-induced fibrous hyperplasia is a common lesion that occurs in the vestibular mucosa where the denture flange contacts tissue (Figs. 7–13 and 7–14). As the bony ridges of the mandible and the maxilla resorb with long-term denture use, the flanges gradually

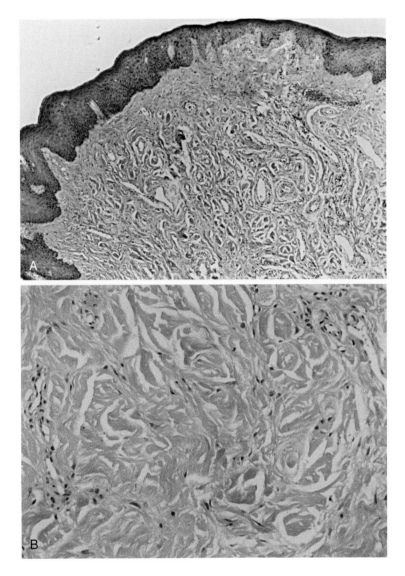

Figure 7–12. *A* and *B,* Traumatic fibroma. Lesion is composed of dense collagen.

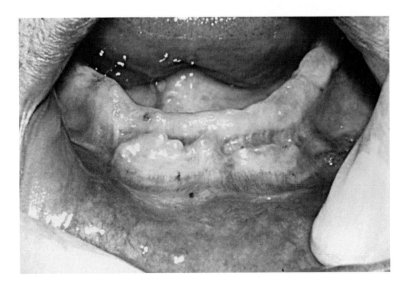

Figure 7–13. Denture-induced fibrous hyperplasia of the anterior vestibule.

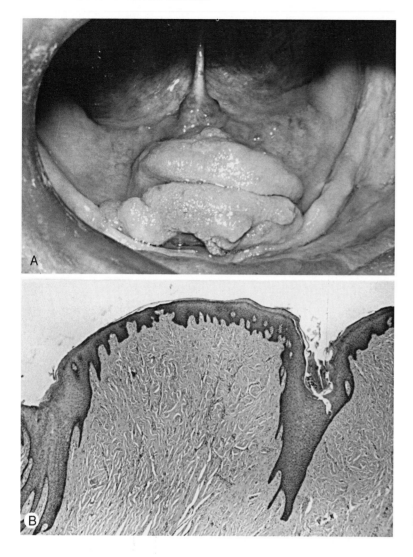

Figure 7–14. *A,* Denture-induced fibrous hyperplasia. *B,* Micrograph showing folds of dense collagen.

extend farther into the vestibule. There, chronic irritation and trauma may incite an overexuberant fibrous connective tissue reparative response. The result is the appearance of painless folds of fibrous tissue surrounding the overextended denture flange.

Treatment. Some reduction in size of the lesion may follow prolonged removal of the denture. However, because the hyperplastic scar is relatively permanent, surgical excision is usually required. Construction of a new denture or relining of the old one is also required to prevent recurrences.

Neoplasms

MYXOMA

Clinical Features. The oral soft tissue myxoma is a rare lesion that presents as a slow-growing, asymptomatic submucosal mass. There appears to be no gender predilection, and the lesion may occur at any age. Myxomas have been reported in all oral locations, although the palate is most frequently affected.

Oral myxomas have been reported in an autosomal dominantly inherited syndrome consisting of myxomas, spotty mucocutaneous pigmentation (similar to Peutz-Jeghers syndrome), and endocrine abnormalities. Of greatest significance is the occurrence of cardiac myxoma, which may be life threatening because of its growth potential in this vital organ. Young patients with a diagnosed oral myxoma should be considered at risk for the syndrome if they have numerous or recurrent lesions and perioral pigmentation.

Histopathology. Oral myxomas are not encapsulated and may exhibit infiltration into surrounding soft tissue. Dispersed stellate and spindle-shaped fibroblasts are found in a loose myxoid

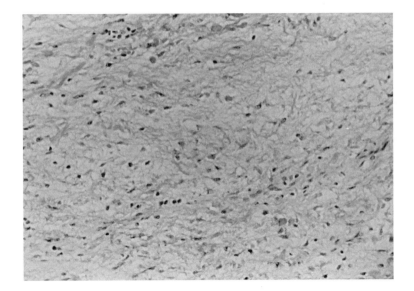

Figure 7–15. Soft tissue myxoma.

stroma (Fig. 7–15). With the use of special stains, collagen fibers appear relatively sparse and reticulin fibers are apparent. Inflammatory cells are generally not seen within the tumor mass.

Differential Diagnosis. As an asymptomatic uninflamed mass of mucous membrane, myxomas are usually regarded clinically as mucoceles or traumatic fibromas. Ordinarily, myxomas would not be included in a differential diagnosis of soft submucosal masses, because of their rarity.

Microscopically, soft tissue myxomas may be confused with several other myxoid lesions. Included in a microscopic differential diagnosis would be nerve sheath myxoma and oral focal mucinosis (Table 7–1). Secondary considerations might also be given to myxoid lipoma, mucocele, and myxomatous change in a fibrous lesion or neurofibroma.

Nerve sheath myxoma arises from the endoneurium of a peripheral nerve. It typically exhibits lobulated mucoid tissue containing stellate and spindle-shaped cells. Condensed connective tissue, representing perineurium, surrounds the lesion. With special stains, a fine reticulin network is seen throughout. Mast cells are characteristically present in this lesion.

Oral focal mucinosis represents the mucosal counterpart of cutaneous focal mucinosis. The lesion appears as a well-circumscribed area of myxomatous connective tissue in the submucosa or the dermis. It contains no mast cells and no reticulin network except that which surrounds supporting blood vessels.

Treatment. The treatment of choice for oral soft tissue myxoma as well as other myxoid lesions is surgical excision. Recurrence is not uncommon for myxomas but is unexpected for nerve sheath myxoma and focal mucinosis. All are benign processes and require conservative therapy only.

NASOPHARYNGEAL ANGIOFIBROMA

Clinical Features. Nasopharyngeal angiofibroma is also known as *juvenile nasopharyngeal angiofibroma* because of its almost exclusive occurrence in the second decade of life. It is an uncommon to rare neoplasm that nearly always affects males. It characteristically produces a mass in the nasopharynx that leads to obstruction or epistaxis that may, on occasion, be severe. Rarely, this lesion may present intraorally, causing palatal expansion that appears blue owing to the intense vascularity of the lesion. This lesion can generally

Table 7–1. Microscopic Differentiation of Oral Myxoid Lesions

LESION	MAST CELLS	RETICULIN FIBER	PATTERN	PERIPHERY
Soft tissue myxoma	No	Yes	Diffuse, uniform	Blending, infiltration
Nerve sheath myxoma	Yes	Yes	Lobular	Condensed fibrous tissue
Focal mucinosis	No	No	Uniform	Well circumscribed

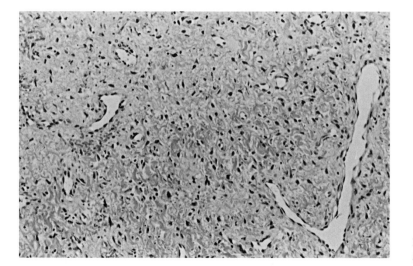

Figure 7–16. Nasopharyngeal angiofibroma.

be described as benign and slow growing but unencapsulated and locally invasive. On occasion, it may exhibit aggressive clinical behavior in which there is direct extension into the bones of the midface and the skull base.

Histopathology. Microscopically, nasopharyngeal angiofibroma has the appearance of a mature, well-collagenized lesion containing cleft-like vascular channels (Fig. 7–16). The fibroblasts have a uniform benign appearance. The vascular channels vary in size and are lined by endothelium that may occasionally be rimmed by smooth muscle cells.

Differential Diagnosis. The presentation of a submucosal bluish mass in the palate should suggest several clinical possibilities. Hemangioma, lymphoma, salivary gland tumor, and mucus extravasation phenomenon would be likely candidates in a differential diagnosis. Nasopharyngeal angiofibroma should be included if the patient also has symptoms involving the nasal cavity. Biopsy of a lesion that is believed to be an angiofibroma should be done with caution and in a hospital setting, because of the potential for excessive bleeding.

Treatment. Although numerous forms of treat-ment, such as radiation, exogenous hormone administration, sclerosant therapy, and embolization, have been used for nasopharyngeal angiofibroma, surgery remains the preferred form of therapy. Recurrences are common (up to 50% of cases) and are due to incomplete excision, the invasive nature of the lesion, and the surgically difficult anatomic location.

NODULAR FASCIITIS

Clinical Features. Nodular fasciitis, also known as *pseudosarcomatous fasciitis,* is a well-recognized entity representing a reactive fibrous connective tissue growth (Table 7–2). This, along with a closely related lesion of muscle known as *proliferative myositis,* could be considered subsets of generic *inflammatory pseudotumors.* The cause of this proliferation is unknown, although trauma is believed to be important in many cases because of the location of lesions over bony prominences such as the angle of the mandible and zygoma. The lesion typically presents as a firm mass in the dermis or the submucosa (Fig. 7–17). It exhibits

Table 7–2. Comparative Clinical Features of Nodular Fasciitis and Fibromatosis

FEATURE	NODULAR FASCIITIS	FIBROMATOSIS
Tumor type	Reactive	Benign aggressive
Age affected	Young adults, adults	Children, young adults
Symptoms	Often	Infrequently
Areas affected	Trunk and extremities (head and neck 10%)	Shoulder and trunk (head and neck 10%)
Growth rate	Rapid	Moderate
Periphery	Often circumscribed	Infiltrative
Recurrence	Rarely	Frequently
Treatment	Conservative surgery	Aggressive surgery

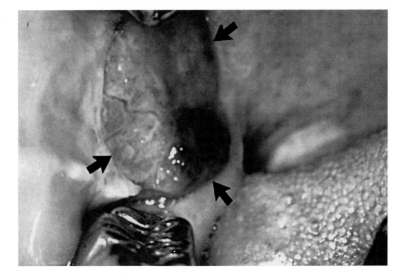

Figure 7–17. Nodular fasciitis *(arrows)* of the buccal mucosa.

such rapid growth clinically that malignancy may be suspected. Pain or tenderness often accompanies the process. There is no gender predilection, and young adults and adults are usually affected. The trunk and extremities are the areas most commonly involved, with about 10% of cases appearing in the head and neck, usually in the skin of the face and the parotid sheath.

Histopathology. As the name implies, this lesion exhibits a nodular growth pattern (Fig. 7–18). It is often well circumscribed but may show some infiltrative tendency. Plump fibroblasts with vesicular nuclei are seen in a haphazard to a storiform or a cartwheel arrangement. Myxoid areas are often found. Multinucleated giant cells are occasionally present and may originate from adjacent muscle or from fusion of macrophage-histiocytes (tumor giant cells). Mitotic figures may be frequent but are morphologically normal in appearance. Capillaries in the tumor are immature, with prominent endothelial cells, and are arranged in a radial or a parallel fashion. Inflammatory cells and extravasated red blood cells are also microscopic features of nodular fasciitis.

Several subtypes of nodular fasciitis have been reported as representing variations on the typical microscopic picture. These include proliferative fasciitis, parosteal fasciitis, and intravascular fasciitis. The terms *myxoid, cellular,* and *fibrous* have also been used to describe these lesions when one of these characteristics is present.

Proliferative myositis, the analogous lesion occurring within muscle, is a reactive lesion, which usually occurs in the trunk and rarely in the head and the neck (sternocleidomastoid muscle), parallels the clinical course of nodular fasciitis. It does, however, appear in an older age group.

Differential Diagnosis. Diagnostic problems relative to nodular fasciitis occur because many of its microscopic features are shared by other fibrous proliferations, such as fibromatosis, fibrous histiocytoma, and fibrosarcoma (Table 7–3). Fibromatosis is more infiltrative than nodular fasciitis and may exhibit a fascicular growth pattern. It also produces more collagen, is generally less cellular, and has fewer mitotic figures. Fibrous histiocytoma has a dual population of fibroblasts and macrophages, and it may not be as well cir-

Table 7–3. Comparative Microscopic Features of Fibrous Proliferations

FEATURE	NODULAR FASCIITIS	FIBRO-MATOSIS	BENIGN FIBROUS HISTIOCYTOMA	FIBROSARCOMA
Periphery	Often circumscribed	Infiltrative	Occasionally circumscribed	Infiltrative
Growth pattern	Nodular, haphazard to storiform	Fascicular	Storiform	"Herringbone"
Mitoses	Frequent, normal	Few, normal	Few, normal	Few to many, abnormal
Cellular atypia	No	No	No	No
Inflammatory cells	Yes	No	No	No
Extravasated RBCs	Yes	No	No	No
Tumor giant cells	Occasionally	No	Frequently	Infrequently
Macrophages	Occasionally	No	Yes	No

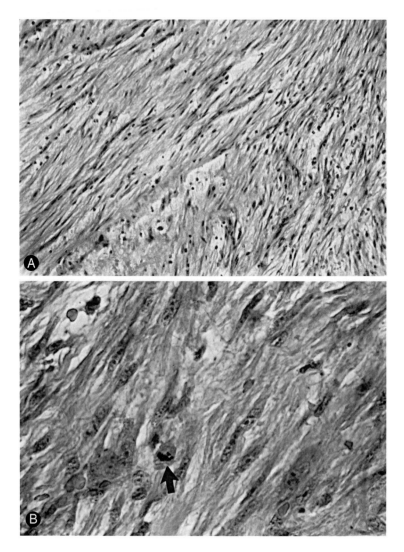

Figure 7–18. *A* and *B,* Nodular fasciitis. Note the inflammatory cells *(A)* and mitotic figure *(B, arrow)*

cumscribed as nodular fasciitis. Fibrosarcoma is infiltrative and exhibits a herringbone pattern. Nuclei are pleomorphic and hyperchromatic, and mitoses are more abundant and atypical.

Treatment. Conservative surgical excision is the treatment of choice for nodular fasciitis. Recurrences are rarely encountered.

FIBROMATOSIS

Clinical Features. Fibromatosis, also known as extra-abdominal desmoid, is a benign fibrous proliferation that may be a troublesome clinical problem because of often aggressive behavior and its tendency for recurrence (see Table 7–2). It is typically seen in children and young adults, with approximately equal gender distribution. This lesion is most commonly found in the shoulder area and trunk, with about 10% of cases appearing in the soft tissues of the head and neck. The mandible and contiguous soft tissues are most frequently involved intraorally. It is slower growing than nodular fasciitis and less likely to be symptomatic.

Histopathology. Fibromatosis is a nonencapsulated infiltrative lesion with a fascicular growth pattern (Fig. 7–19). The lesion is composed of highly differentiated connective tissue containing uniform compact fibroblasts, often surrounded by abundant collagen. Nuclei are not atypical, and mitotic figures are infrequent. When muscle invasion occurs, giant cells of muscle origin may be seen. Slit-like vascular spaces are usually seen as well. Overall, the bland microscopic appearance of this lesion belies its locally aggressive growth (Table 7–3).

A rare histologic subtype known as *infantile myofibromatosis* has been described in oral soft

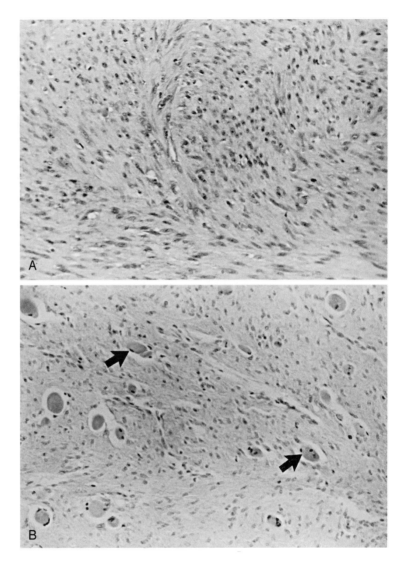

Figure 7–19. *A* and *B,* Two cases of fibromatosis showing the range of cellularity in this lesion. Note the residual muscle in *B (arrows).*

tissues and bone. It may be solitary or multifocal and is seen in infants and children. It is a benign spindle cell proliferation of myofibroblasts with low recurrence potential.

Treatment. Recurrence rates in the range of 20 to 60% have been reported for fibromatoses. Because of this and because of the locally destructive nature of fibromatosis, an aggressive surgical approach is recommended.

FIBROSARCOMA

Clinical Features. Fibrosarcoma is a rare soft tissue and bony malignancy of the head and neck. When occurring in bone, the lesion may theoretically arise from periosteum, endosteum, or periodontal ligament.

A tumescence resulting from proliferation of

malignant fibroblasts appears at the site of origin (Fig. 7–20). Secondary ulceration may be seen as the lesion enlarges. Young adults are most commonly affected. This is an infiltrative neoplasm that is more of a locally destructive problem than a metastatic problem.

Histopathology. Microscopically, fibrosarcoma exhibits malignant-appearing fibroblasts, typically in a herringbone or interlacing fascicular pattern (Fig. 7–21). Collagen may be sparse, and mitotic figures frequent. Cell differentiation from one tumor to another may be quite variable. The periphery of this lesion is ill defined, because the neoplasm freely invades surrounding tissue.

Treatment. Wide surgical excision is generally advocated for fibrosarcoma, because of the difficulty in controlling local growth. Although recurrence is not uncommon, metastasis is infrequent. Bone lesions are more likely to metastasize via

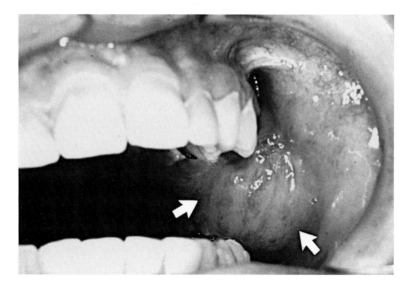

Figure 7–20. Fibrosarcoma of the buccal mucosa *(arrows).*

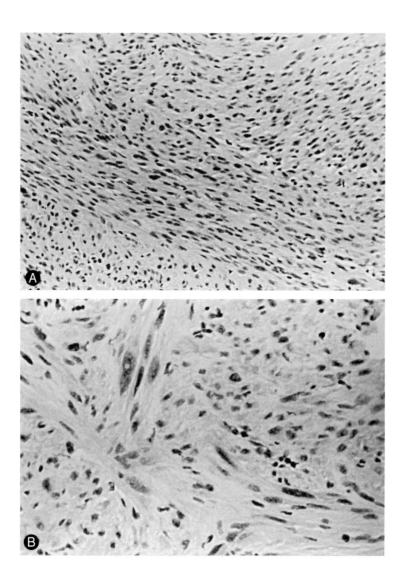

Figure 7–21. *A* and *B*, Fibrosarcoma of oral soft tissues. Moderate nuclear pleomorphism is evident in *B*.

Table 7–4. Classification of Fibrous Histiocytomas

Benign
  Benign fibrous histiocytoma (oral)
  Dermatofibroma (skin)
  Giant cell tumor of tendon sheath
  Xanthogranuloma
  Atypical fibroxanthoma (skin)
Malignant
  Dermatofibrosarcoma protuberans (skin)
  Malignant fibrous histiocytoma
    Storiform-pleomorphic
    Myxoid
    Giant cell
    Inflammatory
    Angiomatoid

the bloodstream than are soft tissue lesions. The overall 5-year survival rate ranges between 30 and 50%. Generally, patients with soft tissue lesions fare better than patients with primary lesions of bone. Also, those with well-differentiated lesions have a better prognosis than do those with poorly differentiated lesions.

BENIGN FIBROUS HISTIOCYTOMA

Fibrous histiocytoma is a generic term that encompasses benign neoplasms consisting of a dual population of fibroblasts and macrophages (Table 7–4). Although the precise histogenesis remains in dispute, immunohistochemical evidence has favored a fibroblast cell of origin over a macrophage origin.

Clinical Features. Benign fibrous histiocytoma is a rare oral neoplasm that may affect either soft tissue or bone. It is a lesion of adults, typically noted in the fifth decade. It presents as a mass that may be ulcerated and is usually painless (Fig. 7–22). Intrabony lesions present as radiolucencies, often with ill-defined margins. They are often initially interpreted as osteomyelitis on radiographic examination.

Histopathology. The dual population of fibroblasts and macrophages must be present before a diagnosis of benign fibrous histiocytoma can be considered (Fig. 7–23). The cellular proliferation is typically in a storiform pattern that is often circumscribed peripherally. Tumor giant cells may be seen. There is no cellular atypia, and mitotic figures are infrequent and normal (see Table 7–3).

Treatment. Surgical excision is the treatment of choice for benign fibrous histiocytoma. Recurrence is not usual.

MALIGNANT FIBROUS HISTIOCYTOMA

Clinical Features. Malignant fibrous histiocytoma is an infrequently reported lesion in the head and neck, although it is the most common adult

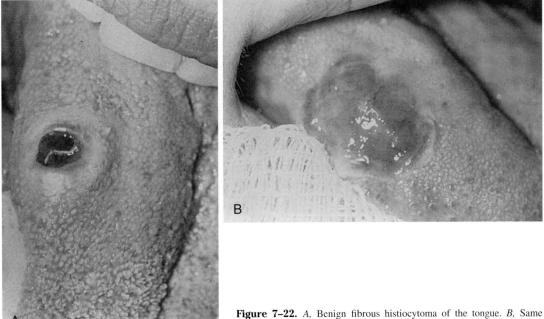

Figure 7–22. *A,* Benign fibrous histiocytoma of the tongue. *B,* Same lesion after a 2-week observation period.

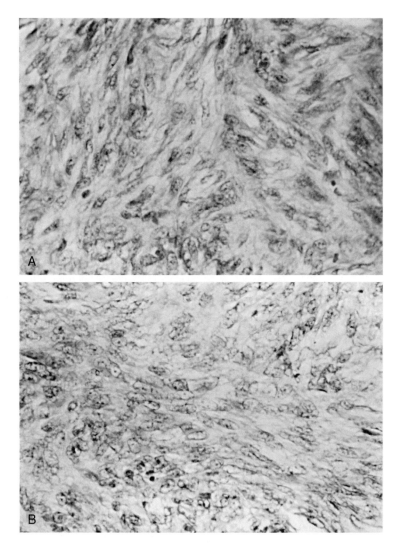

Figure 7–23. *A* and *B,* Benign fibrous histiocytomas.

soft tissue sarcoma in the rest of the body. It may also occur in bone, where it follows a more aggressive course than in soft tissue. Biologically, it has significant recurrence and metastatic potential that is dependent, in part, on clinical factors such as anatomic site, superficial or deep location, and size.

Overall, malignant fibrous histiocytomas occur in late adult life and are rare in children. Males are affected more frequently than females. The extremities and retroperitoneum are favored sites.

In the extremities, these tumors typically present as painless masses. In the retroperitoneum, signs and symptoms of malaise, anorexia, weight loss, and hyperpyrexia may accompany tumor growth. In the head and neck, these neoplasms present usually as a mass. Other accompanying signs and symptoms are dependent on specific location in the head and neck. Pain, facial paraly-

sis, epistaxis, rhinorrhea, hemoptysis, and dysphagia may occur.

Malignant fibrous histiocytomas have been reported in the mandible and the maxilla. These lesions cause radiolucencies with poorly defined margins and may have a moth-eaten appearance. Cortical expansion may be seen, and pathologic fracture may occur with larger lesions.

Intraoral soft tissue lesions appear to have no site predilection. Although only a small number have been reported, almost all regions have been affected.

Histopathology. Basic to all malignant fibrous histiocytomas is the proliferation of fibroblasts, macrophages, and giant cells (Fig. 7–24). Abnormal and frequent mitotic figures, necrosis, and extensive cellular atypia may be seen. In some lesions, a storiform pattern may dominate the microscopic picture; in others, myxoid zones, giant

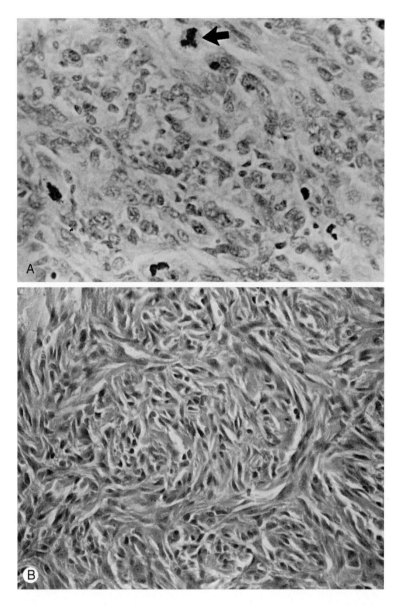

Figure 7–24. *A* and *B,* Malignant fibrous histiocytomas. Note the tripolar mitotic figure in *A (arrow)* and hypercellularity in *B.*

cells, acute inflammatory cells, xanthoma cells, or blood vessels may be prominent (see Table 7–4). The recognition of these different microscopic features has led to subclassification into storiform-pleomorphic (most common), myxoid, giant cell, inflammatory, and angiomatoid types. Data relative to prediction of behavior from each histologic subtype are conflicting.

Treatment. Wide surgical excision is the usual treatment. Radiation or chemotherapy apparently offers limited additional benefit, although these methods have not been fully explored.

Location of the neoplasm is an important factor for prognosis. Lesions located in deeper soft tissues generally have exhibited a more aggressive clinical course. Intraosseous neoplasms exhibit a worse prognosis than soft tissue lesions. As the size of the lesion increases, the metastatic potential increases. The presence of an inflammatory cell host response improves the prognosis. Survival is variable and is dependent in large part on the factors discussed here.

The 5-year survival rate ranges from 20 to 60%. Patients with oral lesions generally fare somewhat worse than others. Recurrence and metastatic rates are about 40%.

VASCULAR LESIONS

Reactive Lesions

VENOUS VARIX

This condition is discussed in detail in Chapter 4.

Congenital Lesions

HEMANGIOMA

This condition is discussed in detail in Chapter 4.

LYMPHANGIOMA

Etiology. Lymphangiomas are generally regarded as congenital lesions rather than as neoplasms. Often present at or around the time of birth, they usually appear within the first 2 decades of life. Involution over time is not usual with these lesions, in contrast to congenital hemangiomas.

Clinical Features. Lymphangiomas present as painless, nodular, vesicle-like swellings when superficial or as a submucosal mass if located deeper (Fig. 7–25). The color ranges from lighter than the surrounding tissue to red-blue when capillaries are part of the congenital malformation. On palpation, the lesions may produce a crepitant sound as lymphatic fluid is pushed from one area to another.

The tongue is the most common intraoral site, and the lesions may be responsible for macroglossia when diffusely distributed throughout the submucosa. Lymphangioma of the lip may cause a macrocheilia. Lymphangioma of the neck is known as *cystic hygroma, hygroma colli,* or *cavernous lymphangioma.* This diffuse soft tissue swelling may be life threatening, because it in-

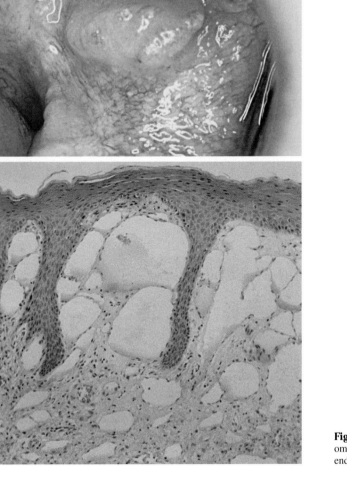

Figure 7–25. *A* and *B,* Lymphangioma of the buccal mucosa. Note the endothelium-lined spaces in *B.*

volves vital structures of the neck. Respiratory distress, intralesional hemorrhage, and disfigurement all are potential sequelae to cystic hygroma.

Histopathology. Endothelium-lined lymphatic channels are diffusely distributed in the submucosa. The channels contain eosinophilic lymph that occasionally includes red blood cells, especially in mixed lymphatic and capillary proliferations. There is no capsule. A characteristic feature is the location of lymphatic channels directly adjacent to overlying epithelium, without any apparent intervening connective tissue.

Differential Diagnosis. Clinically, the lymphangioma may occasionally appear similar to hemangioma when it has a significant capillary component. When small, the lesions may be confused with mucoceles. Superficial lesions should not be confused with vesiculo-bullous eruptions, because lesions associated with the latter are short lived and often painful and inflamed.

Treatment. Lymphangiomas are usually surgically removed, but because of their lack of encapsulation, recurrences are common. Large lymphangiomas, such as cystic hygromas, may require staged surgical procedures to gain control of the lesion. Sclerosant therapy and radiation have been used with limited success, and they are not generally recommended as standard therapy.

Neoplasms

HEMANGIOPERICYTOMA

The hemangiopericytoma is a rare neoplasm that is derived from the pericyte. This cell is normally found surrounding capillaries and venules, between the basement membrane and endothelium. The cell probably has a contractile property and serves as an endothelial reserve cell. The neoplasm that arises from this cell may appear as a mass in any location of the body across a wide age spectrum. No distinguishing clinical signs would suggest a diagnosis of hemangiopericytoma (Fig. 7–26).

Microscopically, the neoplasm is characterized by proliferation of well-differentiated, oval to spindle-shaped mesenchymal cells separated by small, slit-like vascular channels (Fig. 7–27). The vessels are thin walled and may exhibit staghorn profiles.

The biologic behavior of the hemangiopericytoma is unpredictable, exhibiting on occasion a benign course and on other occasions an aggressive metastatic course. Unfortunately, there are no reliable histologic criteria that can be used to predict the clinical course, although necrosis, numerous mitotic figures, and hypercellularity may be suggestive of a more aggressive lesion. The treatment of choice is wide surgical excision. Recurrence and metastases are not uncommon.

ANGIOSARCOMA

Angiosarcoma is a rare neoplasm of endothelial cell origin. A distinct clinical pathologic variant of angiosarcoma is Kaposi's sarcoma.

The scalp is the usual location for angiosarcomas, although occasional lesions have been reported in the maxillary sinus and the oral cavity (Fig. 7–28). The lesion consists of an unencapsulated proliferation of anaplastic endothelial cells enclosing irregular luminal spaces. It has an aggressive clinical course and a poor prognosis.

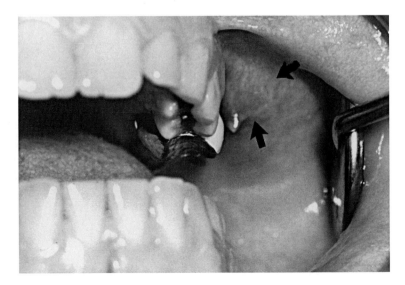

Figure 7–26. Hemangiopericytoma of the buccal mucosa *(arrows)*.

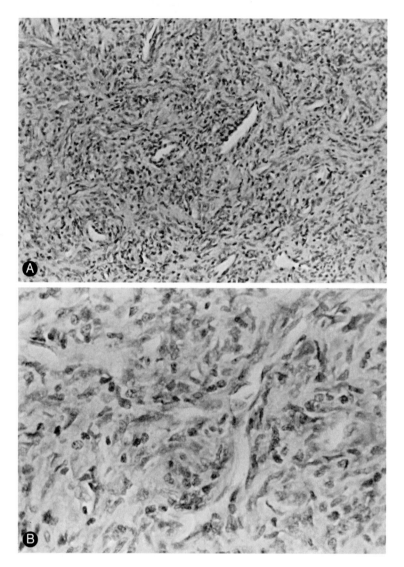

Figure 7–27. *A* and *B*, Hemangiopericytoma showing numerous capillary spaces.

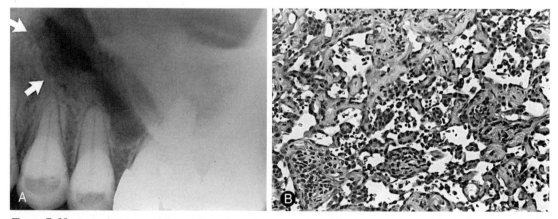

Figure 7–28. *A*, Angiosarcoma of the maxillary sinus. Note the erosion of the sinus wall *(arrows)*. *B*, Angiosarcoma showing anaplastic endothelial cells lining irregular vascular spaces.

KAPOSI'S SARCOMA

This condition is discussed in detail in Chapter 4.

NEURAL LESIONS

Reactive Lesions

TRAUMATIC NEUROMA

Etiology. As the name suggests, neural lesions are caused by trauma to a peripheral nerve. In the oral cavity, the injury may be in the form of trauma from a surgical procedure such as a tooth extraction, from a local anesthetic injection, or from an accident. Transection of a sensory nerve can result in inflammation and scarring in the area of injury. As the proximal nerve segment proliferates in an attempt to regenerate into the distal segment, it becomes entangled and trapped in the developing scar, resulting in a composite mass of fibrous tissue, Schwann cells, and axons. This may be regarded as another type of reactive hyperplasia.

Clinical Features. About half the patients with oral traumatic neuromas have associated pain. The type of pain varies from one patient to another and ranges from occasional tenderness to constant severe pain. Radiating facial pain may occasionally be caused by a traumatic neuroma. Injection of local anesthesia into the area of tumescence relieves the pain.

The lesions occur in a wide age range, although most are seen in adults. The mental foramen is the most common location, followed by extraction sites in the anterior maxilla and the posterior mandible (Fig. 7–29). Lower lip, tongue, buccal mu-

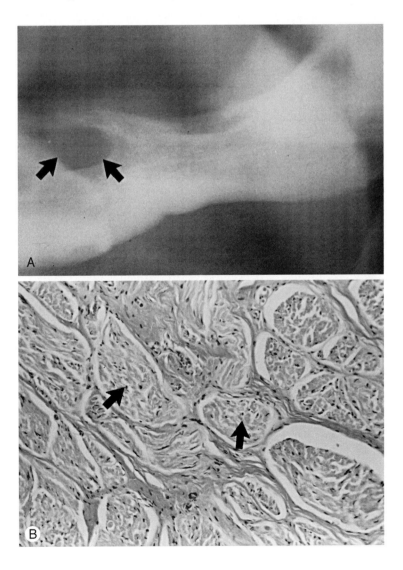

Figure 7–29. *A*, Traumatic neuroma in the mental nerve area *(arrows)*. *B*, Micrograph showing proliferating nerve *(arrows)* and scar.

cosa, and palate are also relatively common locations.

Histopathology. Microscopically, bundles of nerves in haphazard or tortuous arrangement are found admixed with dense collagenous fibrous tissue. A chronic inflammatory cell infiltrate may be seen in a minority of cases, particularly those that are symptomatic.

Diagnosis. Clinical diagnosis may be difficult if patients present with atypical facial pain. Excisional biopsy of a suspected mass or radiolucency will ultimately be required to prove the clinical impression. Traumatic neuroma should be included in a clinical differential diagnosis of any small mass that is spontaneously painful or painful when compressed. Acute infection may cause similar symptoms, but other clinical signs of inflammation should separate this process from traumatic neuroma.

Treatment. Even though surgical transection of a peripheral nerve may have caused the lesion, surgical excision is the treatment of choice. Recurrence is infrequent.

Neoplasms

GRANULAR CELL TUMORS

Etiology and Histogenesis. The granular cell tumor, formerly known as *granular cell myoblastoma,* is an uncommon benign tumor of unknown cause. The unique granular cells that make up the lesion are believed to be of neural (Schwann cell) origin based predominantly on immunohistochemical studies. Origins from skeletal muscle, macro-phages, undifferentiated mesenchymal cells, and pericytes all have been suggested but incompletely supported.

A related lesion known as *congenital gingival granular cell tumor* (congenital epulis) is composed of cells that are light microscopically identical to those of the granular cell tumor. Slight differences have been noted ultrastructurally and immunohistochemically, however. In the cells making up the congenital gingival granular cell tumor, so-called angulate bodies are not found ultrastructurally, and S-100 protein is absent immunohistochemically. These findings suggest that the congenital gingival tumor has a different histogenesis from the granular cell tumor. It has been suggested that rather than having a neural origin, the congenital gingival tumor may be derived from the pericyte or a related cell with potential smooth muscle differentiation.

Granular cell lesions may also be found in other tissues and diverse sites such as the jaw (e.g., granular cell ameloblastoma), skin, gastrointestinal tract, and respiratory tract. Because histologic and ultrastructural similarities are seen in the granular cells of all these lesions, it is suggested that granular cells represent a common morphologic expression of a degenerative process.

Clinical Features. Granular cell tumors appear in a range of patients from children to the elderly, with the mean usually in middle adult life (Table 7–5). Some studies have shown a predilection for females; others have shown near-equal gender distribution. In the head and neck, the tongue is by far the most common location for granular cell tumors (Fig. 7–30). However, any oral location may be affected.

Table 7–5. Comparative Features of Oral Granular Cell Lesions

FEATURE	GRANULAR CELL TUMOR	CONGENITAL GINGIVAL GRANULAR CELL TUMOR
Age	All	Infants
Gender	Females $\geqq$ males	Females $>$ males
Location	Oral mucosa, skin, other	Gingiva only
Light microscopy		
Granular cells	Yes	Yes
Pseudoepitheliomatous hyperplasia	Yes, frequently	No
Ultrastructure		
Autophagic vacuoles	Yes	Yes
Angulate bodies	Yes	No
Smooth muscle features	No	Yes
Immunohistochemical		
S-100	Positive	Negative
Carcinoembryonic antigen	Positive	Positive
HLA-DR	Positive	Positive
Antichymotrypsin	Negative	Negative
Muscle actin	Negative	Negative
CD57	Positive	—
Collagen IV	Positive	—

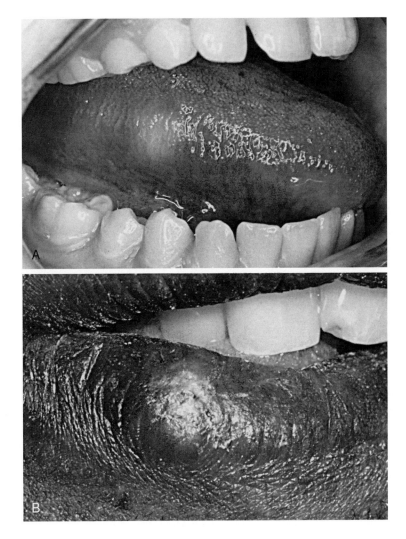

Figure 7–30. *A* and *B*, Granular cell tumors of the tongue and lip. (Courtesy of Dr. W. Jerome.)

Presentation is typically as an uninflamed asymptomatic mass less than 2 cm in diameter. The overlying epithelium is intact. Multiple lesions have occasionally been described.

The congenital gingival granular cell tumor appears on the gingiva (usually anterior) of newborns (Fig. 7–31). It presents as a noninflamed, pedunculated or broad-based mass. The maxillary gingiva is more often involved than the mandibular gingiva, and females are affected more than males. The lesion does not recur, and spontaneous regressions have been reported.

Histopathology. The clinical tumescence of granular cell tumors is due to the presence of unencapsulated sheets of large polygonal cells with pale granular or grainy cytoplasm (Figs. 7–32 and 7–33). The nuclei are small, compact, and morphologically benign. Mitotic figures are rare. Pseudoepitheliomatous hyperplasia of the overlying oral epithelium is seen in about half the cases.

This may be such a prominent feature that subjacent granular cells are overlooked, resulting in an overdiagnosis of squamous cell carcinoma. The pseudoepitheliomatous hyperplasia of granular cell tumor represents a completely benign process; it is not known to have malignant potential. The absence of a chronic inflammatory cell infiltrate, which would be typically seen in well-differentiated squamous cell carcinomas, indicates that the epithelial changes are hyperplastic rather than neoplastic.

The cells of the congenital gingival granular cell tumor appear identical to those of the granular cell tumor. Seen with the light microscope, the only difference between the two lesions is that the former does not exhibit overlying pseudoepitheliomatous hyperplasia.

Ultrastructurally, granular cells of both the granular cell tumor and the congenital gingival counterpart contain autophagic vacuoles (Fig. 7–34).

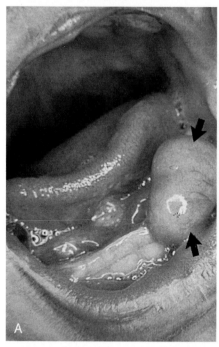

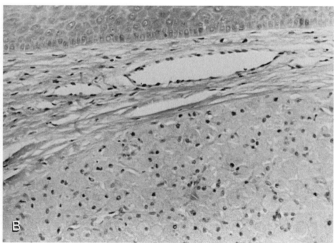

Figure 7–31. *A,* Congenital gingival granular cell tumor *(arrows). B,* Micrograph showing granular cells below and nonpapillated epithelium above.

One of the consistent differences noted has been the absence of angulate bodies in the gingival lesion. Also, in some gingival lesions, the presence of microfilaments with fusiform dense bodies, pinocytotic vesicles, and basement membrane has been noted.

Immunohistochemically, both lesions contain carcinoembryonic and HLA-DR antigens. Granular cell tumors express neural-associated antigens, S-100 protein, CD57, and collagen IV. Both granular cell tumor and congenital granular cell tumor are negative for α-1-antichymotrypsin and muscle actin.

Differential Diagnosis. Clinically, the granular cell tumor might be confused with other connective tissue lesions. Neurofibroma and schwannoma would be prime considerations for tongue lesions. Salivary gland tumors, lipoma, and other benign mesenchymal neoplasms may present intraorally as asymptomatic lumps similar to granular cell tumor. Traumatic fibroma is a common reactive lesion that should be included in a differential diagnosis. Biopsy is the only way to achieve a definitive diagnosis.

The congenital gingival granular cell tumor is clinically distinctive because of the age of the patient and the location in which the mass is seen. Other submucosal masses that occur in the gingiva of infants, such as gingival cyst and neuroectodermal tumor of infancy, are more deeply seated and broad based.

Treatment. Granular cell tumors are surgically

Table 7–6. Comparative Features of Neural Tumors

FEATURE	SCHWANNOMA	NEUROFIBROMA	MUCOSAL NEUROMA	PALISADED ENCAPSULATED NEUROMA
Cell of origin	Schwann cell	Schwann cell or perineural fibroblast	Nerve tissue ?Hamartoma	Schwann cell
Age	Any	Any	Children, young adults	Adults
Location	Any, especially tongue	Any, tongue, buccal mucosa, vestibule	Tongue, lip, buccal mucosa	Palate, lip
Number	Usually solitary	Solitary to multiple	Multiple	Solitary
Bone lesions?	Occasionally	Frequently	No	No
Part of neurofibromatosis?	Rarely	Typical	No	No
Malignant change?	Rarely	Frequently	No	No
Part of MEN III?	No	No	Typical	No

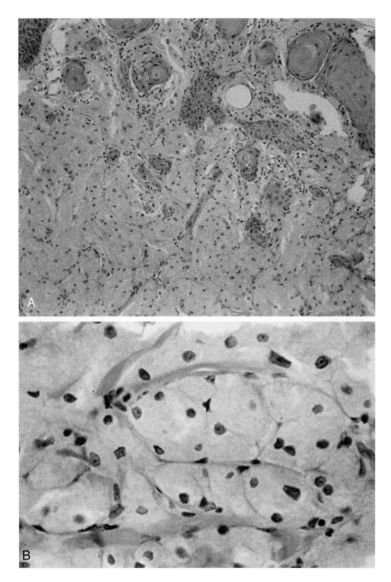

Figure 7–32. *A,* Granular cell tumor cells with overlying pseudoepitheliomatous hyperplasia. *B,* High magnification of granular cells.

excised, and recurrence is not expected. Spontaneous regression has been noted but is apparently a rare event.

SCHWANNOMA

Etiology. The schwannoma or *neurilemoma* is a benign neoplasm with no known cause or stimulus. It is derived from proliferation of Schwann cells (neural crest origin) of the neurilemma that surrounds peripheral nerves. As the lesion grows, the nerve is pushed aside and does not become enmeshed within the tumor.

Clinical Features. This is an encapsulated submucosal mass that presents typically as an asymptomatic lump in patients of any age (Table 7–6).

The tongue is the favored location, although lesions have been described in the palate, floor of the mouth, buccal mucosa, gingiva, lips, vestibule, and jaws. Bony lesions produce a radiolucent pattern and may also cause pain or paresthesia. The schwannoma is usually slow growing but may undergo a sudden increase in size, thought in some cases to be due to intralesional hemorrhage. Of considerable clinical significance is the fact that solitary schwannomas are not seen in the syndrome neurofibromatosis. If numerous, however, they may rarely be part of this syndrome. Another important clinical feature is the extremely low rate of malignant transformation associated with schwannoma as compared with the relatively high rate associated with neurofibroma in neurofibromatosis.

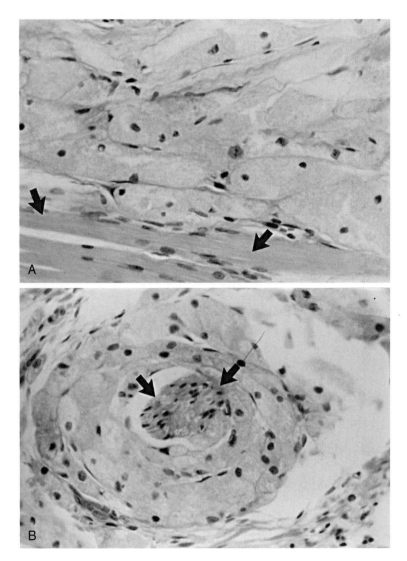

Figure 7–33. Granular cell tumor cells intimately associated with muscle *(A, arrows)* and nerve *(B, arrows).*

Histopathology. The microscopic features of schwannoma are usually highly characteristic, making diagnosis relatively easy (Fig. 7–35). Spindle cells that assume two different patterns are surrounded by a capsule. In one pattern, so-called Antoni A areas consist of spindle cells organized in palisaded whorls and waves. These cells frequently surround an acellular eosinophilic zone (Verocay body). Ultrastructurally, the acellular zone has been shown to be composed of inter-digitated cytoplasmic processes and reduplicated basement membrane. The other pattern is the so-called Antoni B tissue, consisting of spindle cells haphazardly distributed in a light fibrillar matrix.

A microscopic variant known as *ancient schwannoma* has been described. This unusual designation was coined to reflect what was believed to be degenerative changes in a long-standing schwannoma. In this variant, fibrosis, in-flammatory cells, and hemorrhage may be seen. Some nuclear atypia may also be present. The clinical and behavioral characteristics are believed to be the same as those for schwannoma.

Differential Diagnosis. Schwannoma has no distinctive features that allow identification of this lesion on clinical grounds. Intraorally, differential diagnosis would include other benign mesenchymal neoplasms, salivary gland tumors, and traumatic fibroma.

Treatment. Schwannomas are surgically excised, and recurrence is unlikely. Prognosis is excellent.

NEUROFIBROMA

Etiology. Neurofibromas may appear as solitary lesions or as multiple lesions as part of the

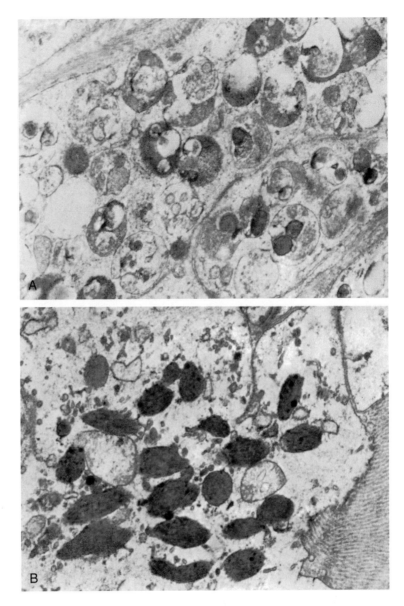

Figure 7–34. Electron micrographs of autophagic vacuoles *(A)* and angulate bodies *(B)* found in granular cells of the granular cell tumor.

syndrome *neurofibromatosis (von Recklinghausen's disease of skin)*. The cause of solitary neurofibroma is unknown. Neurofibromatosis, on the other hand, is inherited as an autosomal dominant trait. It has variable expressivity and often (50% of cases) appears after spontaneous mutation. Two subsets have recently been defined: one associated with the NF1 gene and the other with the NF2 gene.

The cell of origin of the neurofibroma is not clearly established. Most investigators believe it is the Schwann cell; others believe that the perineural fibroblast is responsible.

Clinical Features. The solitary neurofibroma presents at any age as an uninflamed asymptomatic, submucosal mass (Table 7–6). The tongue,

buccal mucosa, and vestibule are the oral regions most commonly affected.

Oral lesions are typically associated with neurofibromatosis 1. This condition includes multiple neurofibromas, cutaneous café au lait macules, bone abnormalities, central nervous system changes, and other stigmata. The neurofibromas range clinically from discrete superficial nodules to deep, diffuse masses (Fig. 7–36). Lesions may be so numerous and prominent that they become cosmetically significant. Intraoral neurofibromas may be seen in as many as 25% of patients with neurofibromatosis. When other oral stigmata such as enlarged fungiform papillae and bone abnormalities are included, oral manifestations may be seen in as many as 70% of neurofibromatosis

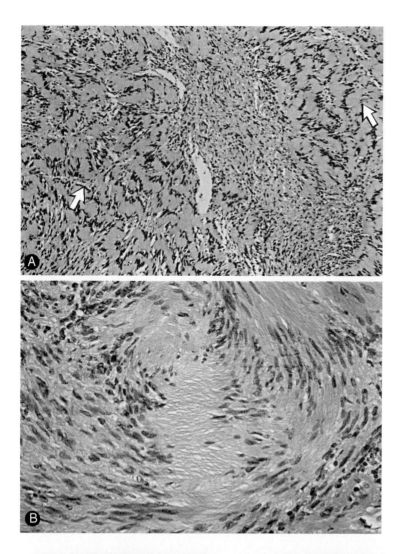

Figure 7-35. *A*, Micrograph of schwannoma showing areas of so-called Antoni A tissue *(arrows)* and so-called Antoni B tissue between (center). *B*, Note the acellular foci in the Antoni A tissue.

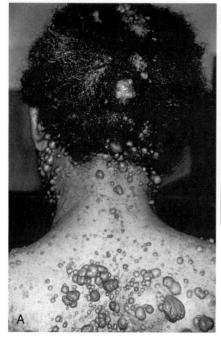

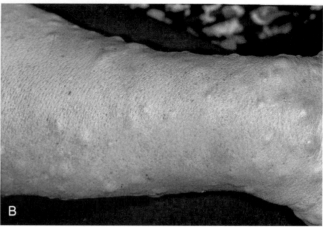

Figure 7-36. *A*, Neurofibromatosis. (Courtesy of Dr. R. Wesley.) *B*, Neurofibromas of the arm.

patients (Fig. 7–37). Malignant degeneration of neurofibromas into neurogenic sarcoma is seen in 5 to 15% of patients with this syndrome.

The presence of six or more café au lait macules greater than 1.5 cm in diameter is generally regarded as being suggestive of neurofibromatosis. Axillary freckling (Crowe's sign) and iris freckling (Lisch spots) are also commonly seen pigmentary abnormalities.

Bone changes may be seen in half or more of patients with neurofibromatosis. The changes may be in the form of cortical erosion from adjacent soft tissue tumors or medullary resorption from intraosseous lesions. In the mandible, lesions most commonly arise from the mandibular nerve and may result in pain or paresthesia. In such cases of mandibular involvement, an accompanying radiographic sign may be the formation of a flaring of the inferior alveolar foramen, the so-called blun-

derbuss foramen. Involvement of the spine is frequently seen and may result in kyphoscoliosis, which may eventually cause spinal cord compression and paralysis. Some intrabony lesions are believed to be the result of mesodermal dysplasia.

Neurologic abnormalities in neurofibromatosis may result from cranial nerve involvement. Acoustic neuromas, often bilateral, are not uncommon lesions, and they may lead to deafness, dizziness, and headache. Trigeminal nerve involvement may cause facial pain or paresthesia. Other neurologic abnormalities include gliomas, meningiomas, mental retardation, and seizures.

Histopathology. Solitary and multiple neurofibromas have the same microscopic features. They contain spindle-shaped cells, with fusiform or wavy nuclei found in a delicate connective tissue matrix; this matrix may be notably myxoid in character (Fig. 7–38). These lesions may be

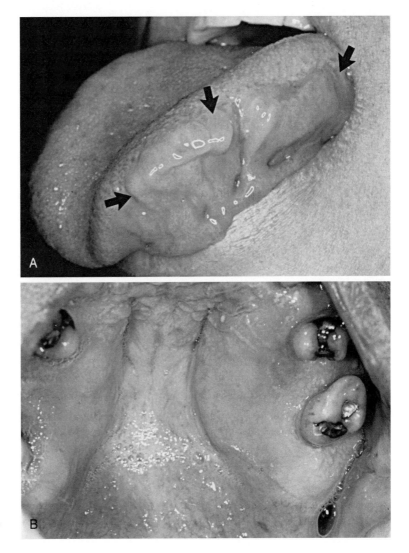

Figure 7–37. Neurofibromas of the tongue *(A)* and left hard palate *(B).*

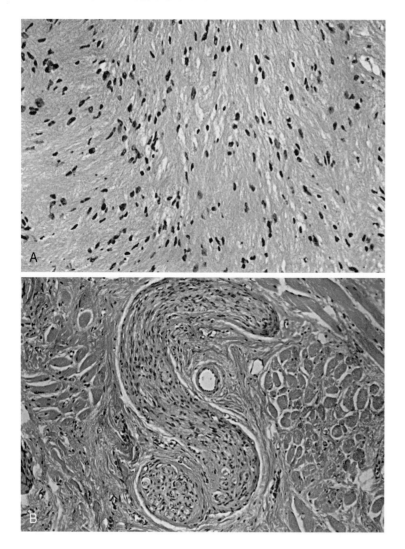

Figure 7–38. Two histologic patterns of neurofibroma. *A,* Typical neurofibroma. *B,* Plexiform neurofibroma.

well circumscribed or may blend into surrounding connective tissue. Mast cells are characteristically scattered throughout the lesion. A histologic subtype known as *plexiform neurofibroma* is regarded as being highly characteristic of neurofibromatosis. In this variety, extensive interlacing masses of nerve tissue are supported by a collagen matrix. Small axons may be seen among the proliferating Schwann cells and perineural cells.

Differential Diagnosis. A solitary nodular neurofibroma should be considered in a clinical differential diagnosis with other submucosal masses of connective tissue origin such as traumatic fibroma, granular cell tumor, and lipoma. Biopsy is the only way to separate these lesions definitively. A diffuse neurofibroma resulting in macroglossia may require differentiation from lymphangioma and possibly amyloidosis.

Treatment. Solitary neurofibromas are treated by surgical excision and have little chance of

recurrence. Multiple, lesions of neurofibromatosis may be treated in the same way but may be so numerous that this becomes impractical. In this case, the importance of lesions is the high risk of malignant transformation. Cosmetic factors are also significant. The prognosis for a patient who has had neurosarcomatous change of a preexisting lesion is poor.

MUCOSAL NEUROMAS OF MULTIPLE ENDOCRINE NEOPLASIA SYNDROME, TYPE III

Etiology. Multiple endocrine neoplasia syndrome, type III (MEN III), of which mucosal neuromas are a prominent part, is inherited as an autosomal dominant trait. The clinical stigmata of this syndrome are related to a defect in neuroectodermal tissue.

Clinical Features. MEN III consists of medullary carcinoma of the thyroid, pheochromocytoma of the adrenal, and mucosal neuromas (Table 7–6). Café au lait macules and neurofibromas of the skin may also be seen in this condition. MEN I and II are related to MEN III in that patients with types I and II syndromes have neoplasms of various endocrine organs, but they do not have the oral manifestation of mucosal neuromas.

The mucosal neuromas of MEN III usually appear early in life as small discrete nodules on the conjunctiva, labia, larynx, or oral cavity (Fig. 7–39). The oral lesions are seen on the tongue, lips, and buccal mucosa.

Histopathology. Mucosal neuromas are composed of serpiginous bands of nerve tissue surrounded by normal connective tissue. Axons have been found in the proliferating nerve tissue. The microscopic appearance has suggested to some that these lesions may be hamartomatous rather than neoplastic.

Differential Diagnosis. The soft tissue masses of mucosal neuromas may share clinical features with neurofibromatosis or multiple papillomas. There may also be some similarity to the mucosal presentation seen in amyloidosis and hyalinosis cutis et mucosae (lipoid proteinosis). Because the endocrine neoplasia associated with this syndrome is often manifested very early in life, biopsy should be performed to establish diagnosis.

Treatment. Mucosal neuromas are surgically excised and are not expected to recur. The neuromas themselves are relatively trivial, but they are of considerable significance because they may be the first sign of this potentially fatal syndrome. The medullary carcinoma of the thyroid is a progressive malignancy that invades locally and has the ability to metastasize to local lymph nodes and distant organs. The 5-year survival rate of this malignancy is about 50%. Pheochromocytoma is a benign neoplasm that produces catecholamines that may cause significant hypertension and other cardiovascular abnormalities. Early detection of the mucosal neuromas is therefore of utmost importance in follow-up screening of these patients.

PALISADED ENCAPSULATED NEUROMA

Palisaded encapsulated neuroma is another oral tumor of neural origin. It is not associated with neurofibromatosis or MEN III. It occurs typically in the palate and occasionally the lips. This dome-shaped nodule is encapsulated and exhibits a fascicular microscopic pattern with some suggestion of nuclear palisading. The tumor is composed of S-100–positive cells (Schwann cells) and some axons. After surgical removal, recurrence is unexpected.

NEUROGENIC SARCOMA

Neurogenic sarcoma is a rare malignancy that develops either from a preexisting lesion of neurofibromatosis or *de novo*. The cell of origin is believed to be the Schwann cell and possibly other nerve sheath cells.

In soft tissues, this neoplasm appears as an expansile mass that is usually asymptomatic. In bone, where it is believed to arise most often from a mandibular nerve, it presents as a dilatation of the mandibular canal or as a diffuse lucency. Pain or paresthesia may accompany the lesion in bone; this is also the case for other malignancies within the mandible or maxilla.

Microscopically, neurogenic sarcoma can be

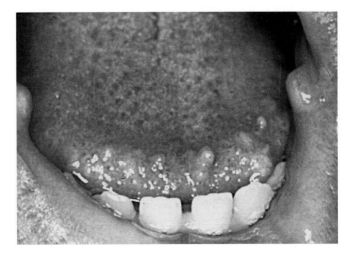

Figure 7–39. Mucosal neuromas of MEN III syndrome. (Courtesy of Dr. R. M. Courtney.)

seen arising from a neurofibroma or from a nerve trunk. The lesion is very cellular and is composed of abundant spindle cells with variable numbers of abnormal mitotic figures. Streaming and palisading of nuclei are often seen, and nuclear pleomorphism may also be prominent (Fig. 7–40). Microscopic separation of this lesion from fibrosarcoma and leiomyosarcoma may be difficult, making electron microscopy and immunohistochemistry important diagnostic adjuncts.

The primary method of treatment is wide surgical excision. However, recurrence is common, and metastases are frequently seen. Prognosis varies from fair to good, depending on clinical circumstances.

OLFACTORY NEUROBLASTOMA

This malignancy, also known as *esthesioneuroblastoma,* is a rare lesion that arises from olfactory tissue in the superior portion of the nasal cavity. This lesion, typically occurring in young adults, may cause epistaxis, rhinorrhea, or nasal obstruction, or it may present as polyps in the roof of the nasal cavity. It may also result in a nasopharyngeal mass or an invasive maxillary sinus lesion.

Microscopically, this lesion consists of small, undifferentiated, round cells with little visible cytoplasm (Fig. 7–41). Compartmentalization and pseudorosette and rosette formation are often seen. Immunohistochemistry study for chromogranin or synaptophysis can be used to confirm the light microscopic diagnosis. Microscopic differential diagnosis would include lymphoma, embryonal rhabdomyosarcoma, Ewing's sarcoma, and undifferentiated carcinoma.

Surgery or radiation is used to treat esthesioneuroblastoma. Recurrences are not uncommon, ap-

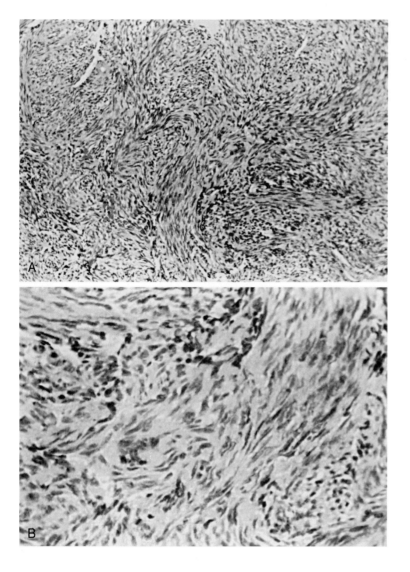

Figure 7–40. *A* and *B,* Neurogenic sarcoma showing high cellularity and slight pleomorphism.

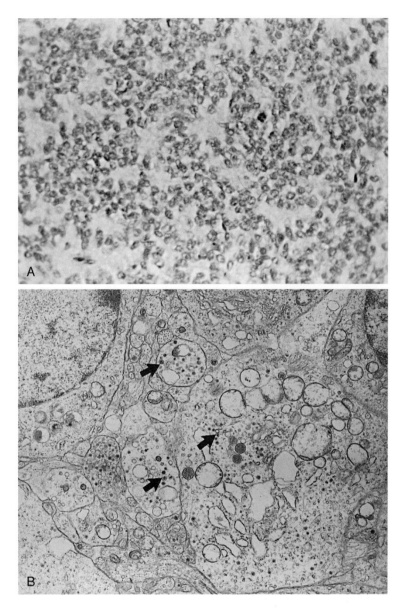

Figure 7–41. *A* and *B,* Esthesioneuroblastoma. Electron micrograph *(B)* shows numerous cytoplasmic neurosecretory granules *(arrows).*

pearing in about half the patients. Metastases, usually to local nodes or lung, are infrequent.

LESIONS OF MUSCLE AND FAT

Reactive Lesions

MYOSITIS OSSIFICANS

This is an uncommon reactive lesion of skeletal muscle. It may appear in the muscles of the head and neck. As the name implies, the condition is an intramuscular inflammatory process in which ossification occurs. The reason for the appearance of bone in the muscle reparative process has not been fully explained.

Muscle ossification may be seen in either of two forms: as a progressive systemic disease (myositis ossificans progressiva) of unknown cause or as a focal single-muscle disorder (traumatic myositis ossificans) of traumatic origin. In the latter form, acute or chronic trauma may be responsible for the muscular change. The masseter and the sternocleidomastoid muscles are most commonly affected within the head and neck region. As the lesion matures, soft tissue radiographs show a delicate feathery opacification. The actively proliferating osteoblasts have occasionally been confused with osteosarcoma microscopically. Maturation and organization of the osseous tissue peripheral to the central cellular zone is believed to be an important diagnostic feature of myositis ossificans. The lesion is treated with surgical excision.

Neoplasms

LEIOMYOMA AND LEIOMYOSARCOMA

Smooth muscle neoplasms, in general, are relatively common. They may arise anywhere in the body from muscle cells or their precursors in the media of blood vessels, in the muscularis layer of the gut, and in the body of the uterus. In the oral cavity, these neoplasms are rarely encountered.

Oral *leiomyomas* present as slow-growing, asymptomatic submucosal masses, usually in the tongue, hard palate, or buccal mucosa. They may be seen at any age and are usually discovered when they are 1 to 2 cm in diameter.

Microscopic diagnosis may occasionally be difficult because the spindle cell proliferation has many similarities with neurofibroma, schwannoma, and fibromatosis (Fig. 7–42). Special stains that identify collagen may be helpful in distinguishing these lesions. Immunohistochemical demonstration of myofilament proteins (e.g., smooth muscle actin) can confirm the diagnosis. A microscopic subtype known as *vascular leiomyoma* has numerous thick-walled vessels associated with well-differentiated smooth muscle cells. Leiomyomas are surgically excised, and recurrence is unexpected.

Oral *leiomyosarcomas* have been reported in all age groups and most intraoral regions. Microscopic diagnosis is a considerable challenge because of similarities to other spindle cell sarcomas. As with the benign neoplasms, immunohistochemistry can be a valuable diagnostic tool. This malignancy is usually treated with wide surgical excision. Metastasis to lymph nodes or lung is not uncommon.

RHABDOMYOMA AND RHABDOMYOSARCOMA

Rhabdomyomas are rare lesions, but they have a predilection for the soft tissues of the head and neck. The oral sites most frequently reported are the floor of the mouth, soft palate, tongue, and buccal mucosa. The mean age of patients is about 50 years, and the age range extends from children to older adults. Presentation is as an asymptomatic, well-defined submucosal mass.

Two microscopic variants are recognized. In the adult type, the neoplastic cells closely mimic their normal counterpart (Fig. 7–43); in the fetal type, the neoplastic cells are elongated and less differentiated and exhibit fewer cross-striations. The latter type may be confused with rhabdomyosarcoma. Treatment is excision, and recurrence is unlikely.

Rhabdomyosarcomas are subdivided into pleomorphic, embryonal, and alveolar types, depending on microscopic appearance. The pleomorphic type, the most well differentiated, contains strap or spindle cells that often exhibit cross-striations. The embryonal type consists of primitive round cells in which striations are rarely

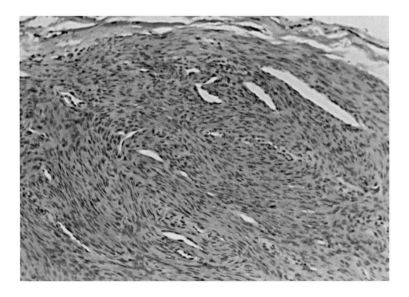

Figure 7–42. Leiomyoma of oral soft tissues. Note the capsule (top).

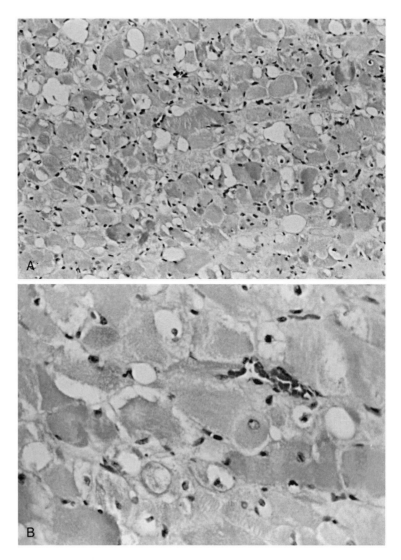

Figure 7–43. *A,* Rhabdomyoma, adult type. Note the resemblance to normal muscle (*B*).

found. The alveolar variant is also composed of round cells but in a compartmentalized pattern.

Rhabdomyosarcoma, when it occurs in the head and neck, is primarily found in children. When occurring outside the head and neck, it is seen typically in adults. Rhabdomyosarcoma presents as a rapidly growing mass, which, if there is jaw involvement, may cause pain or paresthesia. The most commonly affected oral sites are the tongue and soft palate (Fig. 7–44). The embryonal type of rhabdomyosarcoma is the variety most commonly seen in the head and neck. Because of the relatively undifferentiated nature of this microscopic subtype, immunohistochemistry is typically used to support light microscopic interpretations (Fig. 7–45).

The combination of surgery, radiation, and chemotherapy has been shown to produce far better clinical results than any one of these treatment methods alone. Survival rates have increased from less than 10% to better than 70% with this more aggressive treatment approach.

LIPOMA AND LIPOSARCOMA

Lipomas are uncommon neoplasms of the oral cavity that may occur in any region. Buccal mucosa, tongue, and floor of the mouth are among the more common locations (Fig. 7–46). Clinical presentation is typically as an asymptomatic, yellowish submucosal mass. The overlying epithelium is intact, and superficial blood vessels are usually evident over the tumor. Other benign connective tissue lesions such as granular cell tumor, neurofibroma, traumatic fibroma, and salivary gland lesions (mucocele and mixed tumor) might be included in a differential diagnosis.

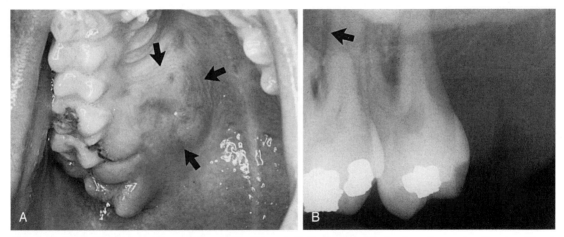

Figure 7–44. *A* Rhabdomyosarcoma of the maxilla *(arrows). B,* Radiograph showing bone loss and uniformly widened periodontal membrane space *(arrow).*

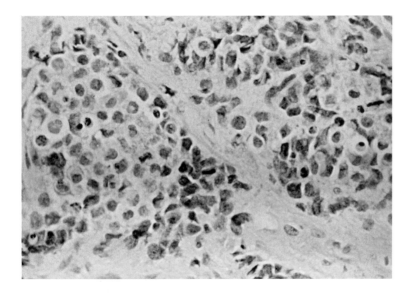

Figure 7–45. Rhabdomyosarcoma, embryonal type.

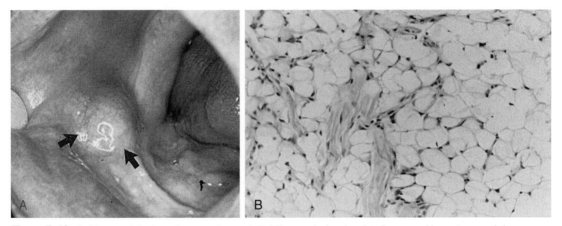

Figure 7–46. *A,* Lipoma of the buccal mucosa *(arrows). B,* Micrograph showing the close resemblance to normal tissue.

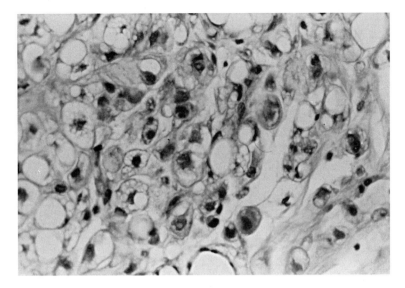

Figure 7–47. Liposarcoma of the oral soft tissues.

Numerous microscopic subtypes have been described, but they are primarily of academic interest. All types have adipocytes of various degrees of maturity. The usual simple lipoma consists of a well-circumscribed, lobulated mass of mature fat cells. The lesions are excised and are not expected to recur.

Liposarcoma is rarely encountered in soft tissues of the head and neck. It is a lesion of adulthood and may potentially occur in any site. It is generally slow growing and thus may be mistaken for a benign process. Considerable microscopic variation in these malignancies has led to subclassification into at least four types (well-differentiated, myxoid, round cell, pleomorphic) (Fig. 7–47). The degree of tumor cell differentiation coupled with identification of microscopic subtype is an important factor in predicting clinical behavior. These neoplasms may be treated with surgery or radiation, and prognosis is fair to good.

Bibliography

Fibrous Connective Tissue Lesions

Bras J, Batsakis J, Luna M. Malignant fibrous histiocytoma of the oral soft tissues. Oral Surg Oral Med Oral Pathol 64:57–67, 1987.

Brown R, Sein P, Corio R, Bottomley W. Nitrendipine-induced gingival hyperplasia. Oral Surg Oral Med Oral Pathol 70:593–596, 1990.

Cook C, Lund B, Carney J. Mucocutaneous pigmented spots and oral myxomas: the oral manifestations of the complex of myxomas, spotty pigmentation, and endocrine overactivity. Oral Surg Oral Med Oral Pathol 63:175–183, 1987.

Daley T, Wysocki G, Day C. Clinical and pharmacologic correlations in cyclosporine-induced gingival hyperplasia. Oral Surg Oral Med Oral Pathol 62:417–421, 1986.

Dent CD, DeBoom GW, Hamlin ML. Proliferative myositis of the head and neck. Oral Surg Oral Med Oral Pathol 78:354–358, 1994.

de Villiers-Slabbert H, Altini M. Peripleral odontogenic fibroma: a clinicopathologic study. Oral Surg Oral Med Oral Pathol 71:86–90, 1991.

Fowler CB, Hartman KS, Brannon RB. Fibromatosis of the oral and paraoral region. Oral Surg Oral Med Oral Pathol 77:373–386, 1994.

Handlers J, Abrams A, Melrose R, et al. Fibrosarcoma of the mandible presenting as a periodontal problem. J Oral Pathol 14:351–356, 1985.

Harel-Raviv M, Eckler M, Lalani K, et al. Nifedipine-induced gingival hyperplasia. Oral Surg Oral Med Oral Pathol 79:715–722, 1995.

Kabot T, Goldman M, Bergman S, et al. Juvenile nasopharyngeal angiofibroma: an unusual presentation in the oral cavity. Oral Surg Oral Med Oral Pathol 59:453–457, 1985.

Melrose R, Abrams A. Juvenile fibromatosis affecting the jaws. Oral Surg Oral Med Oral Pathol 49:317–324, 1980.

Odell E, Lock C, Lombardi T. Phenotypic characterization of stellate and giant cells in giant cell fibroma by immunocytochemistry. J Oral Pathol Med 23:284–287, 1994.

Orlowski W, Freedman P, Lumerman H. Proliferative myositis of the masseter muscle. Cancer 52:904–908, 1983.

Regezi J, Zarbo R, Tomich C, et al. Immunoprofile of benign and malignant fibrohistiocytic tumors. J Oral Pathol 16:260–265, 1987.

Sciubba J, Niebloom T. Juvenile hyaline fibromatosis (Murray-Puretic-Drescher syndrome): oral and systemic findings in siblings. Oral Surg Oral Med Oral Pathol 62:397–409, 1986.

Seymonr RA, Jacobs DJ. Cyclosporine and the gingival tissues. J Clin Periodontol 19:1–11, 1992.

Thompson S, Shear M. Fibrous histiocytomas of the oral and maxillofacial regions. J Oral Pathol 13:282–294, 1984.

Vally I, Altini M. Fibromatosis of the oral and paraoral soft tissues and jaws. Oral Surg Oral Med Oral Pathol 69:191–198, 1990.

Vigneswaran N, Boyd D, Waldron C. Solitary infantile myofibromatosis of the mandible. Oral Surg Oral Med Oral Pathol 73:84–88, 1992.

Werning J. Nodular fasciitis of the orofacial region. Oral Surg Oral Med Oral Pathol 48:441–446, 1979.

Neural Lesions

Chauvin P, Wysocki G, Daley T, Pringle G. Palisaded encapsulated neuroma of oral mucosa. Oral Surg Oral Med Oral Pathol 73:71–74, 1992.

Chrysomali E, Papanicolaou S, Dekker NP, Regezi JA. Benign neural tumors of the oral cavity: a comparative immunohistochemical study. Oral Surg Oral Med Oral Pathol 84:381–390, 1997.

Gutmann DH, Aylsworth A, Carey JC, et al. The diagnostic evaluation and multidisciplinary management of neurofibromatosis 1 and neurofibromatosis 2. JAMA 278:51–57, 1997.

Khansur T, Balducci L, Tavassoli M. Granular cell tumor. Cancer 60:220–222, 1987.

Mills S, Frierson H. Olfactory neuroblastoma. A clinicopathologic study of 21 cases. Am J Surg Pathol 9:317–327, 1985.

Monteil R, Loubiere R, Charbit Y, et al. Gingival granular cell tumor of the newborn: immunoperoxidase investigation with anti-S-100 antiserum. Oral Surg Oral Med Oral Pathol 64:78–81, 1987.

Regezi J, Zarbo R, Courtney R, Crissman J. Immunoreactivity of granular cell lesions of skin, mucosa and jaw. Cancer 64:1455–1460, 1989.

Rubenstein A. Neurofibromatosis: a review of the clinical problem. Ann N Y Acad Sci 486:1–13, 1986.

Sciubba J, D'Amico E, Attie J. The occurrence of multiple endocrine neoplasia, Type IIB, in two children of an affected mother. J Oral Pathol 16:310–316, 1987.

Shapiro S, Abramovitch K, Van Dis M, et al. Neurofibromatosis: oral and radiographic manifestations. Oral Surg Oral Med Oral Pathol 58:493–498, 1984.

Zarbo R, Lloyd R, Beals T, et al. Congenital gingival granular cell tumor with smooth muscle cytodifferentiation. Oral Surg Oral Med Oral Pathol 56:512–520, 1983.

Lesions of Muscle and Fat

Bras J, Batsakis J, Luna M. Rhabdomyosarcoma of the oral soft tissues. Oral Surg Oral Med Oral Pathol 64:585–596, 1987.

Geiger S, Czernobilsky B, Marshak G. Embryonal rhabdomyosarcoma: immunohistochemical characterization. Oral Surg Oral Med Oral Pathol 60:517–523, 1985.

McMillan M, Ferguson J, Kardos T. Mandibular vascular leiomyoma. Oral Surg Oral Med Oral Pathol 62:427–433, 1985.

8

Salivary Gland Diseases

REACTIVE LESIONS (NONINFECTIOUS)

Mucocele is a clinical term that includes mucus extravasation phenomenon and mucus retention cyst. Because each has a distinctive pathogenesis and microscopy, they are justifiably considered separately.

Mucus Extravasation

Etiology and Pathogenesis. The etiology of mucus extravasation phenomenon is related to mechanical trauma to the minor salivary gland excretory duct, resulting in its transection or severance (Fig. 8–1). After this, there is spillage or extravasation of mucus into the surrounding connective tissue stroma, where it induces a secondary inflammatory reaction consisting initially of neutrophils followed by macrophages. A granulation tissue response ensues, resulting in the formation of a wall around the mucin pool. The adjacent salivary gland tissue undergoes a nonspecific inflammatory change secondary to mucus retention. Ultimately, scarring occurs in and around the gland.

A variant of the extravasation-type mucocele is *superficial mucocele*. Rather than arising from traumatic duct rupture, this form of mucocele is believed to arise as a result of increased pressure in the ductal component situated within the overlying epithelium.

Clinical Features. Although the lower lip is the most frequent site of mucus extravasation phenomenon (Fig. 8–2), the buccal mucosa, ventral surface of the tongue (where the glands of Blandin-Nuhn are located), floor of the mouth, and retromolar region are often affected. Lesions are infrequently found in other intraoral regions where salivary glands are located (Fig. 8–3), probably because of the relative absence of trauma to these areas.

These lesions are usually painless and smooth surfaced, with an overall bluish hue or translucency associated with a more superficial location.

217

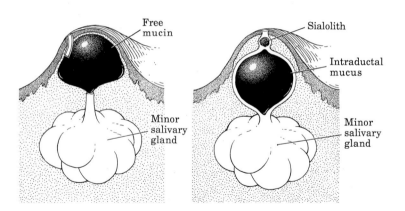

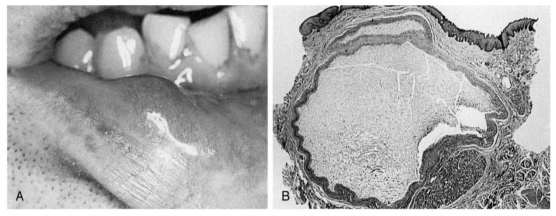

Figure 8–1. *Left*, Mucus extravasation phenomenon—note the severed duct at upper left. *Right*, Mucus retention cyst.

Figure 8–2. *A* and *B*, Mucocele (mucus extravasation phenomenon). Note the mucin pool surrounded by granulation tissue in *B*.

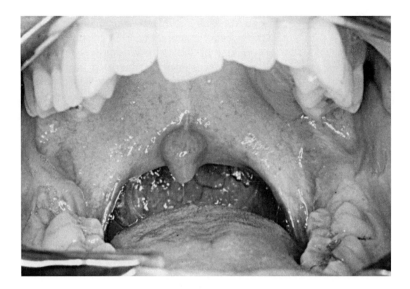

Figure 8–3. Mucocele (mucus extravasation phenomenon) of the soft palate.

They range from a few millimeters to a few centimeters in diameter. Adolescents and children are most commonly affected, with nearly half of reported cases presenting before 21 years of age and more than one fourth between the ages of 11 and 20 years.

The clinical swelling associated with the extravasated mucin may decrease in size, because of rupture of the lesion or because of resorption of pooled mucin. Further production of mucin leads to return of the lesion. Maximum size is usually reached within several days after injury, and a viscous material is found if aspiration is attempted.

In *superficial mucoceles,* focal subepithelial accumulation of mucin is seen (Fig. 8–4). These lesions are asymptomatic and numerous, occurring most commonly in the retromolar area, soft palate, and posterior buccal mucosa. Their clinical appearance suggests a vesiculobullous disease, but the lesions persist for an extended time. Other than being a diagnostic challenge, they are of little significance.

Histopathology. Generally, a well-circumscribed cavity lined by granulation tissue contains free mucin (Fig. 8–5). The mucin and granulation tissue are infiltrated by large numbers of neutrophils, macrophages, lymphocytes, and occasionally plasma cells. The adjacent salivary gland whose duct was transected shows ductal dilatation, scar, chronic inflammatory cells, and acinar degeneration. (Fig. 8–6).

Differential Diagnosis. Although a history of a traumatic event followed by rapid development of a bluish translucency of the lower lip is characteristic of mucus extravasation phenomenon, other lesions might be considered when a typical history is absent. These include salivary gland neoplasm (especially mucoepidermoid carcinoma), vascular

malformation, venous varix, and soft tissue neoplasm such as neurofibroma or lipoma. If a mucocele appears in the alveolar mucosa, an eruption cyst or gingival cyst should be included in the differential diagnosis.

Treatment and Prognosis. The treatment of mucus extravasation phenomenon is surgical excision. Aspiration of the fluid content usually provides no lasting clinical benefit. Removal of the associated minor salivary glands along with the pooled mucus is necessary to prevent recurrence.

No treatment is necessary for a superficial mucocele.

Mucus Retention Cyst

Etiology and Pathogenesis. Mucus retention cyst results from obstruction of salivary flow because of a sialolith, periductal scar, or impinging tumor. The retained mucin is surrounded by ductal epithelium, giving the lesion a cyst-like appearance microscopically.

Clinical Features. Mucus retention cyst is less common than mucus extravasational phenomenon. It usually appears in an older age group, and it rarely occurs in the lower lip. Instead, it is found in the upper lip, palate, cheek, and floor of the mouth, as well as in the maxillary sinus (Fig. 8–7).

Mucus retention cyst presents as an asymptomatic swelling, usually without antecedent trauma. The lesions vary in size from 3 to 10 mm and, on palpation, are mobile, nontender, and generally without peripheral inflammatory change. The overlying mucosa is intact and of normal color. Lesions situated deeper tend to be firmer and more diffuse in their presentation.

Histopathology. The cystic cavity of the mucus retention cyst is lined by ductal epithelial

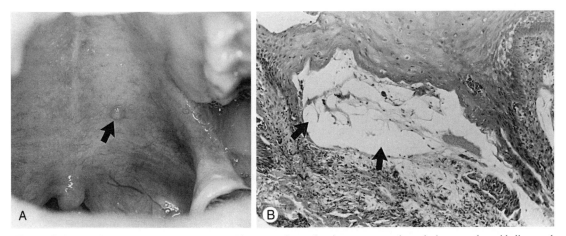

Figure 8–4. *A,* Superficial mucocele *(arrow). B,* Biopsy specimen showing extravasated mucin between the epithelium and connective tissue *(arrows).*

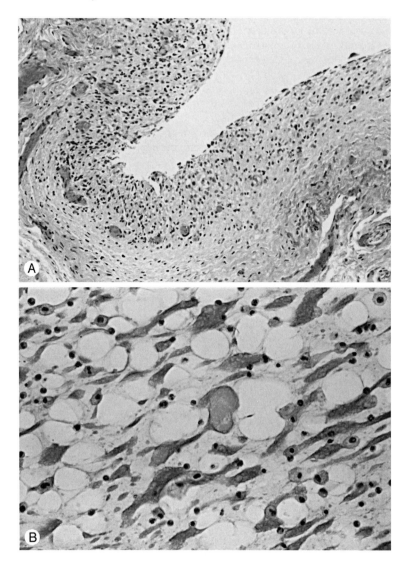

Figure 8–5. Mucus extravasation phenomenon. *A,* Granulation tissue sac surrounding mucin space. *B,* Free mucin containing the usual inflammatory cells, macrophages, and neutrophils.

cells. The type of lining formed by the epithelial cells ranges from pseudostratified to a double layer of columnar or cuboidal cells (Fig. 8–8). The cyst lumen contains mucus plugs or sialoliths (Fig. 8–8*B*). The supportive connective tissue forming the remainder of the cyst is minimally inflammed.

Differential Diagnosis. Salivary gland neoplasms, mucus extravasation phenomenon, and benign connective tissue neoplasms should be included in a clinical differential diagnosis.

Treatment and Prognosis. Removal of the mucus retention cyst and the associated lobules of minor salivary gland elements is indicated. Removal of any glandular elements projecting into the surgical bed is encouraged in order to avoid postoperative mucus extravasation phenomenon. Prognosis is excellent. No recurrence of the cystic element is expected if the associated gland is removed.

Ranula

Ranula, a clinical term that includes mucus extravasation phenomenon and mucus retention cyst, occurs specifically in the floor of the mouth. The ranula is associated with the sublingual salivary glands or the submandibular glands.

Etiology and Pathogenesis. Trauma and ductal obstruction are responsible for ranulas. Obstruction is usually due to a salivary stone or sialolith that may be found anywhere in the ductal system from the gland parenchyma to the excretory duct orifice. *Sialoliths* represent precipitation of calcium salts (predominantly calcium carbonate and

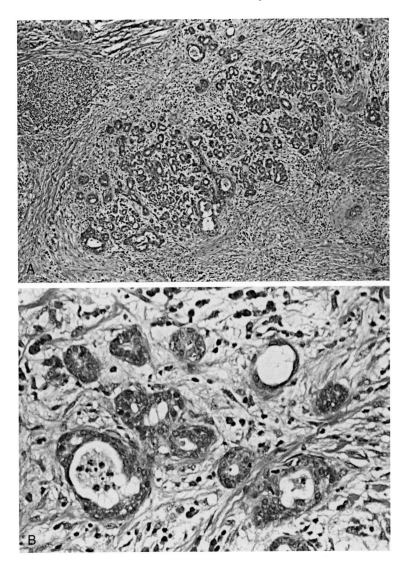

Figure 8–6. *A* and *B,* Nonspecific inflammatory changes in a minor salivary gland. Note fibrosis, inflammatory cells, and acinic atrophy.

calcium phosphate) around a central nidus of cellular debris or inspissated mucin. Floor of mouth trauma may be accidental or surgical. The damage exudes mucus into the surrounding interstitial tissue, inciting an inflammatory reaction.

Clinical Features. Ranula usually presents as a fluctuant, unilateral, soft tissue mass in the floor of the mouth (Fig. 8–9). It typically has a bluish appearance that has been compared to a frog's belly, hence the term *ranula.* A wide variation in size has been noted. When it is significantly large, it can produce medial and superior deviation of the tongue. It may also cross the midline, if the extravasation process dissects through the underlying soft tissue. When the lesion is deeper in the connective tissue, the typical bluish translucent character may not be evident.

In cases due to blockage by sialoliths (Fig. 8–10), radiographs (especially occlusal) may demonstrate the stones. The deep or so-called *plunging ranula* develops as a result of mucus extravasation (herniation) through the mylohyoid muscle and along the fascial planes of the neck (Fig. 8–11). On rare occasions, it may progress into the mediastinum.

Histopathology. Depending on pathogenesis, microscopy of the ranula is the same as for mucus extravasation phenomenon or mucus retention cyst. The majority of the extravasation specimens are characterized by thick mucoserous fluid surrounded by granulation tissue. The retention mucocele features a lining derived from duct epithelium. A concentrically layered, acellular, calcified salivary stone (sialolith) may also be seen within the ductal system.

Differential Diagnosis. Clinical differential di-

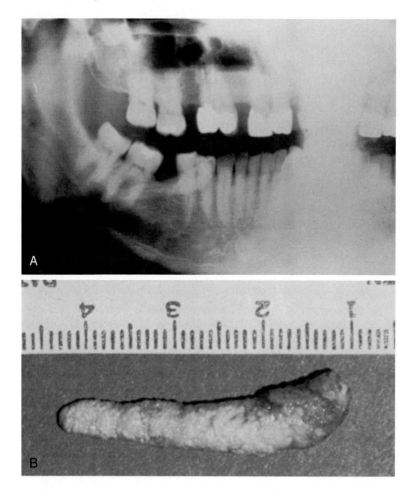

Figure 8–7. *A* and *B*, Sialolithiasis of the submandibular gland. Duct stone *(B)* can be seen superimposed on the bicuspid-molar area.

agnosis of floor of the mouth swellings should include salivary gland tumors, benign mesenchymal neoplasms, and dermoid cyst. Lesion texture should help separate ranula from the others. For plunging ranulas, thymic cysts, and cystic hygroma might be considered.

Treatment. For extravasation-type lesions, surgery is the preferred therapy. Marsupialization may be performed before a definitive excision in an attempt to reduce the overall size of the lesion through natural decompression. Excision of the involved gland is generally performed as well.

In the case of sialolithiasis, the stone is either surgically removed or milked through the duct orifice. If a duct is surgically entered, special precautions are used to aid the healing process so that duct scarring is minimized. Constriction of the duct through excessive scar formation could result in recurrence.

Mucocele of the Maxillary Sinus

Mucocele of the maxillary sinus is defined as obstruction of the ostium. It is separated from pseudocyst and retention cyst of the maxillary sinus because of differences in etiology and biologic behavior.

Etiology and Pathogenesis. The exact cause of paranasal sinus mucoceles is uncertain. However, it is generally believed to be due to blockage or obstruction at a sinus outlet that results in retention of mucus within the sinus cavity. Other factors that may be involved include chronic inflammatory disease producing mucosal thickening, osseous trauma, and tumors located near the ostium. Also, cystic fibrosis may be an important factor in the development of sinus mucoceles in children.

Clinical Features. Paranasal sinus mucoceles are relatively common lesions, usually occurring in people between ages 13 and 80 years. Approximately 65% of mucoceles are found in the frontal sinus and 10% in the maxillary sinus.

With the maxillary lesions, slow expansion may lead to obstruction of the ostium and, in time, erosion of the normal anatomic boundaries of the sinus. If infection supervenes, an acute inflammatory mass (pyocele) may form.

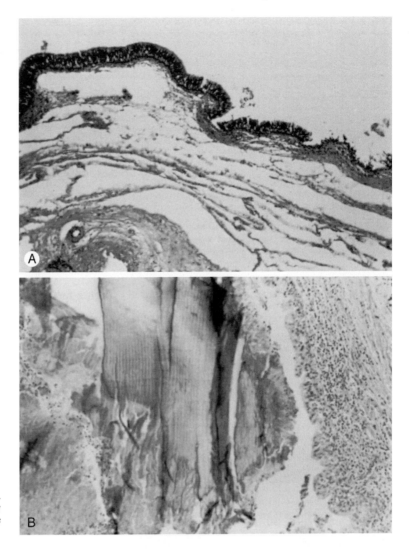

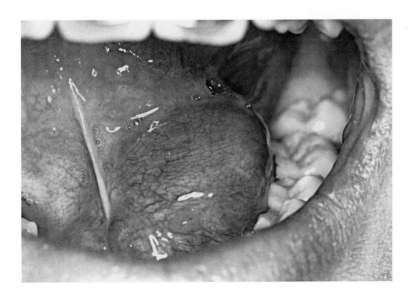

Figure 8–8. Mucus retention cyst. *A,* Lumen space (above) is lined by ductal epithelium. *B,* Salivary stone (left) fills the excretory duct (right).

Figure 8–9. Ranula on the floor of the mouth.

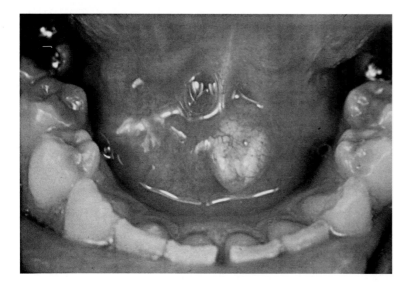

Figure 8–10. Sialolith near the orifice of the submandibular duct.

The radiographic findings show clouding of the sinus because of a soft tissue mass. The involved sinus becomes opacified by entrapped secretions that replace the entire air space if they are not treated. Gradually, decalcification associated with the mucoperiosteal margin produces loss of the

normal osseous borders; the end result is a destructive, smooth, expanded mass surrounded by a zone of sclerosing osteitis. A small percentage of sinus mucoceles contain visible dystrophic calcifications within their walls. Computed tomography is helpful in evaluating the character and extent of these lesions.

Histopathology. The lining of the sinus mucocele is variable. Some linings demonstrate goblet and mucous cell hyperplasia, whereas others show a cuboidal-type epithelium that forms secondary to pressure atrophy. Mucus may escape or herniate into the underlying lamina propria, producing a concomitant inflammatory reaction. The contents of the mucocele itself may vary from thick and mucoid to firm and gelatinous. This material may also solidify within the connective tissue supportive elements and produce, in a small minority of cases, a so-called mucus impaction tumor.

Differential Diagnosis. Inflammatory processes of odontogenic origin must be distinguished from the antral or sinus mucocele. Large odontogenic cysts that become infected are capable of producing a similar clinical and radiographic presentation. Primary neoplasia of the maxillary sinus must likewise be considered, especially in view of the occasional destructive nature of the mucocele.

Treatment and Prognosis. Management of the maxillary sinus mucocele is surgical. In contrast to retention cysts of the maxillary sinus, the mucocele must be managed by thorough curettage and débridement of the sinus cavity. Surgical approaches vary from nasal antrostomy to a more definitive Caldwell-Luc procedure, which allows for removal of the antral contents. With adequate surgical management, the overall prognosis is excellent.

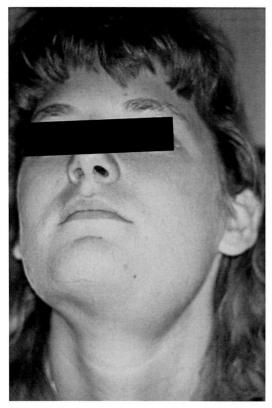

Figure 8–11. Plunging ranula.

Maxillary Sinus Retention Cyst and Pseudocyst

Retention cysts and pseudocysts involving the lining of the maxillary antrum are common findings in panoramic radiographs. These lesions are discovered incidentally and are of little clinical significance.

Etiology and Pathogenesis. Retention cysts seem to arise from blockage of an antral seromucous gland, resulting in a ductal epithelium-lined cystic structure filled with mucin. Pseudocysts are inflammatory in origin and result from fluid accumulation within the sinus membrane. They may be related to infection or allergy. Bacterial toxins, anoxia, or other factors presumably cause leakage of protein into surrounding soft tissue, thus raising the extravascular osmotic pressure with subsequent fluid increase.

Clinical Features. The great majority of these lesions are asymptomatic, although slight tenderness or buccal expansion may occasionally be noted in the region of the mucobuccal fold.

In panoramic and periapical radiographs, retention cysts and pseudocysts of the maxillary sinus are hemispheric, homogeneous, and well delineated (Fig. 8–12). Unlike the antral mucocele, they spare bony structures and landmarks. They usually demonstrate an attachment to the floor of the antrum, with size being a function of the anatomic space rather than of duration. Infrequently these lesions may appear bilaterally.

Histopathology. The pathogenesis of the two forms of antral cysts is reflected in the histologic appearance. The retention cyst is lined by pseudostratified columnar epithelium with occasional mucous cells interspersed. The supportive elements are minimally inflamed. The pseudocyst shows no evidence of an epithelial lining but rather pools of mucoid material surrounded by slightly compressed connective tissue.

Differential Diagnosis. Clinical differential diagnosis of cysts and pseudocysts arising within the mucosa of the maxillary sinus might include polyps, hyperplasia of the sinus lining secondary to odontogenic infection, maxillary sinusitis, and neoplasms arising within the soft tissues of the antral lining.

Treatment. Antral retention cysts and pseudocysts are generally left untreated, because they are limited in growth and are not destructive. Periodic observation is all that is required, after informing the patient of the presence of the lesion.

Necrotizing Sialometaplasia

Necrotizing sialometaplasia is a benign condition that typically affects the palate but may be found in any site containing salivary glands. Recognition of this entity is important because it mimics a malignancy both clinically and microscopically. Unnecessary surgery has been performed because of an erroneous preoperative diagnosis of squamous cell carcinoma or mucoepidermoid carcinoma.

Etiology and Pathogenesis. The initiating event of necrotizing sialometaplasia is believed to be related to ischemia, secondary to alteration of local blood supply. Infarction of the salivary gland follows. Acinar cells become necrotic, although ductal preservation is usually noted within the infarcted lobules. Squamous metaplasia of ductal remnants eventually appears.

This condition is believed to be due to local trauma, including surgical manipulation, and local

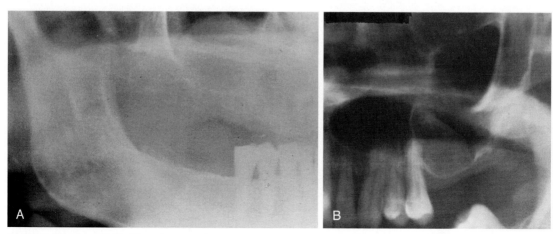

Figure 8–12. *A* and *B*, Maxillary sinus retention cysts.

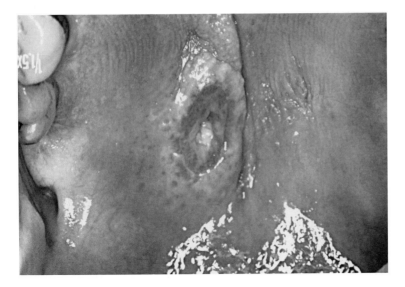

Figure 8–13. Necrotizing sialo-metaplasia.

anesthesia in the area. Patients often have no history of a prior traumatic event.

Clinical Features. Intraorally, necrotizing sialometaplasia is characterized by a seemingly spontaneous appearance, most commonly at the junction of the hard and soft palates (Fig. 8–13). Early in its evolution, the lesion may be noted as a tender swelling, often with a dusky erythema of the overlying mucosa. Subsequently, the mucosa breaks down, with the formation of a sharply demarcated deep ulcer with a yellowish-gray lobular base. In the palate, the lesion may be unilateral or bilateral, with individual lesions ranging from 1 to 3 cm in diameter. Pain is generally dispropor-

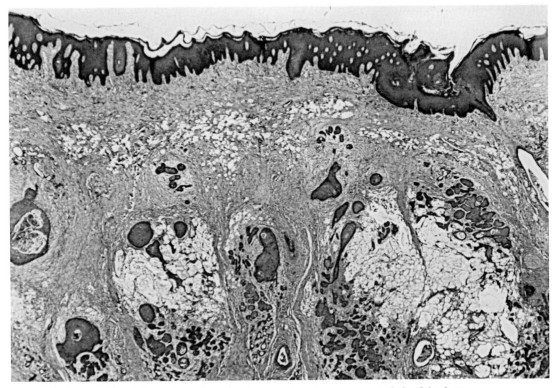

Figure 8–14. Necrotizing sialometaplasia. Note the acinar necrosis and squamous metaplasia of the ducts.

tionately slight compared with the size of the lesion. Healing is generally protracted, taking from 6 to 10 weeks.

Histopathology. The microscopic features of necrotizing sialometaplasia are consistent and unique. The overlying mucosa is ulcerated in the early phases. Lobular necrosis of the salivary glands and prominent squamous metaplasia of salivary duct epithelium are typically seen (Figs. 8–14 and 8–15). The recognition of necrosis and the preservation of lobular architecture serve to distinguish this process from neoplasia. The characteristic squamous metaplasia of ducts may be misinterpreted as squamous cell carcinoma. When this metaplasia is seen in the presence of residual viable salivary gland, the lesion may be mistaken for mucoepidermoid carcinoma.

Differential Diagnosis. Clinically, squamous cell carcinoma or malignant minor salivary gland neoplasms must be ruled out. Syphilitic gummas and deep fungal infections must likewise be ruled out, as they may present as punched-out lesions of the palate. In medically compromised patients, such as those with poorly controlled diabetes, opportunistic fungal infections may cause a similar clinical picture.

Treatment and Prognosis. This condition is a benign, self-limiting process that does not require specific treatment. However, incisional biopsy should be performed to establish a definitive diagnosis. Healing takes place over several weeks by secondary intention. Patient reassurance and wound irrigation, and occasional use of analgesics are the only management steps necessary. Recurrence is not expected, and no functional impairment is anticipated subsequent to healing.

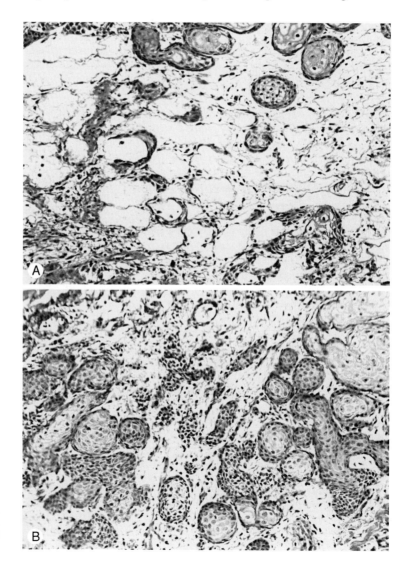

Figure 8–15. Necrotizing sialometaplasia showing necrotic acini *(A)* and squamous metaplasia of the ducts *(B).*

Radiation-Induced Salivary Gland Pathology

Head and neck cancer victims who have received tumoricidal levels of radiation develop a wide range of immediate, intermediate, and long-term changes of many tissues in the path of irradiation. Salivary glands show changes in volume, viscosity, ionic concentration, and pH as well as alterations of inorganic and organic components. Such changes predispose individuals to increased caries rates and periodontal disease. The effect of irradiation on teeth is indirect and results primarily from depression of salivary gland function and subsequent xerostomia.

Radiosensitivity varies from tissue to tissue, but the effect on cells is generally greater when mitotic activity of a cell group is high, when the mitotic process is prolonged, and when differentiation or function is not highly established. One important cell type that is susceptible to therapeutic irradiation is the endothelial cell. Changes including swelling, degeneration, necrosis, and lumen narrowing ultimately lead to circulatory impedance and obstruction.

Irradiation of salivary glands can cause acute salivary flow rate diminution by rapidly destroying serous acinar cells. Mucous cells, being more resistant than serous cells, are affected later. Ductal cells tend to persist longer than all other glandular epithelial cells. Minor salivary glands suffer changes similar to major glands. During radiotherapy and for a few months after treatment, some recovery of glandular function may be evident; however, the process of degeneration proceeds slowly, secondary to alteration of fine vasculature and fibrosis of interstitial tissues. Xerostomia is the clinical result.

Clinical Features. Almost all patients whose salivary glands are exposed to 6000 cGy or more of irradiation develop severe xerostomia (Table 8–1). Not only does the volume of saliva diminish drastically, but qualitative changes in viscosity, pH, immunoglobulin concentration, and electrolytes also occur. From this comes a significant

Table 8–1. Differential Diagnosis of Xerostomia

Sjögren's syndrome
Emotional and anxiety states
Anemia
Negative fluid balance
Polyuria states
Selected nutritional or hormonal deficiencies
Drugs or medications with anticholinergic effect
Acquired immunodeficiency syndrome (AIDS)
Therapeutic radiation through salivary glands

shift in the oral microflora, with an increase in the proportion of cariogenic bacteria. The result is the potential for rapidly progressive dental caries in addition to an increased incidence and severity of periodontal disease. The alteration in the physical nature of salivary fluid may produce difficulties in deglutition. Restitution of salivary gland function is usually not possible, although pilocarpine and other sialogogues may be of some benefit to some patients during and after radiation therapy.

Histopathology. Early changes noted in the serous acinar tissue include neutrophil and eosinophil cellular infiltrates within the glandular interstitium. Degenerative changes appear initially within the serous acini, consisting of nuclear pyknosis, cytoplasmic vacuolation, and loss of zymogen granules. At this early stage, mucous glands show little alteration.

Ultimately, the parenchyma decreases in bulk, with the glands becoming smaller and adhering to surrounding soft tissues. Fibrosis within the interstitial and interlobular elements progresses, with continued and concomitant degeneration of acinar tissue. Variable levels of regeneration may take place, depending on the design of the fields of therapy, total dose, and age of the patient.

Treatment and Prognosis. In many patients, return of salivary function is not significant. Consequently, the risk of periodontal disease and rampant caries is high and persists indefinitely: Ideally, a program of prevention should be initiated before radiotherapy and carried out through the lifetime of the patient. Use of a fluoride-containing topical preparation is the mainstay of ongoing caries management. Additionally, patients should receive frequent dental prophylaxis and maintain high levels of oral hygiene. Saliva substitutes are of some benefit for symptomatic relief of xerostomia. The ominous possibility of osteoradionecrosis developing in irradiated patients must always be kept in mind.

Adenomatoid Hyperplasia

Clinical Presentation. The palate is the chief site of involvement of this salivary gland hyperplasia (Fig. 8–16). There is a male predominance, and age ranges from from 24 to 63 years. The clinical presentation is a unilateral swelling of the hard and/or soft palate. This lesion is asymptomatic, broad based, and covered with intact mucosa of normal color and quality.

Histopathology. Lobules of hyperplastic mucous glands extend beyond the submucosa and into the lamina propria. Individual acinar clusters are more numerous and larger than normal. Ducts

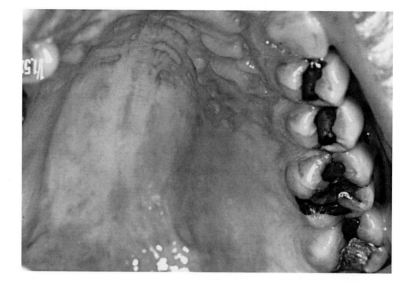

Figure 8–16. Adenomatoid hyperplasia, left hard palate.

exhibit a slight increase in relative prominence. The cytologic and morphologic features of acinar and ductal elements are within normal limits. There is generally no significant inflammatory cell infiltrate.

Differential Diagnosis. Clinical differential diagnosis would include salivary neoplasms, including benign mixed tumor, lymphoma, and extension of nasopharyngeal or sinonasal disease into the oral cavity. Periapical inflammatory disease should be excluded.

Treatment and Prognosis. Subsequent to identification by means of an incisional biopsy, no treatment is necessary, given the purely benign nature of this process. There appears to be no neoplastic potential.

INFECTIOUS CONDITIONS

Viral Diseases

MUMPS

Mumps is an infectious, acute viral sialadenitis primarily affecting the parotid glands. Considered the most common of all salivary gland diseases, it has a year-round endemic pattern, although seasonal peaks are noted in the late winter and spring months.

Etiology and Pathogenesis. The causative agent in mumps is a paramyxovirus. A 2- to 3-week incubation period precedes clinical symptoms. Transmission is by direct contact with salivary droplets.

Clinical Features. Patients develop fever, malaise, headache, and chills in addition to preauricu-

lar pain. Salivary glands, usually the parotid, demonstrate a 70% incidence of bilateral infection. The parotid swelling tends to be asymmetric at the outset, reaching maximum proportion within 2 to 3 days. Perceptible diminution of swelling is noted approximately 10 days after the onset of symptoms. The disease affects males and females equally, especially young adults and children.

Potentially serious complications can occur in adults, who may develop orchitis or oophoritis, which can occasionally result in sterility. Mumps is a systemic infection, as evidenced by the widespread involvement of glandular and other tissues in the body, including liver, pancreas, kidney, and nervous system.

Severe local pain is often noted, especially on movement of the jaws in talking and chewing. Stensen's duct may become partially occluded as the gland swells, with sharp pain secondary to the stimulation of the secretory mechanism by food or drink. This is a variable sign, because not all cases are associated with partial duct obstruction. Papillae at the orifice of Stensen's duct or Wharton's duct may be reddened and enlarged, but this also is not a common or consistent finding.

Differential Diagnosis. Bacterial infections may be considerations in a clinical differential diagnosis. Acute bacterial infection in the form of suppurative parotitis presents with marked tenderness, redness of the skin overlying the glands, and suppuration from the ductal opening. Salivary calculi with obstructive features can also produce similar symptoms. The salivary glands may be enlarged in conditions such as sarcoidosis, lymphoma, benign lymphoepithelial lesion, and certain metabolic diseases, but in these conditions the acute signs and symptoms of mumps are not seen.

Neoplastic states usually present in a unilateral fashion, with few, if any, symptoms.

Treatment and Prognosis. Management relates to symptomatic therapy and bed rest. Analgesics often form the mainstay of treatment. In severe cases, corticosteroids have been prescribed, with variable success.

Complete recovery is generally the rule, although fatalities have been associated with viral encephalitis, myocarditis, and nephritis. Nerve deafness and bilateral testicular atrophy have been noted but are uncommon.

Prevention of the disease is now possible using a live attenuated vaccine that induces a noncommunicable, subclinical infection. Antibody conversion occurs in approximately 90% of susceptible individuals, and immunity is lifelong.

Although mumps is the most common form of viral sialadenitis, it is important to note that parotitis may also be caused by other viral agents, including Coxsackie A virus, echovirus, choriomeningitis virus, cytomegalovirus, and parainfluenza virus types I and II.

CYTOMEGALIC SIALADENITIS

Cytomegalovirus infection of salivary glands, or so-called cytomegalic inclusion disease, formerly was a rare condition that usually affected neonates because of a transplacental infection. It is also now encountered in adults who are in an immunosuppressed state.

Fetal infections may cause debilitation, developmental retardation, and premature birth. Clinically, this disease is characterized by fever, salivary gland enlargement, hepatosplenomegaly, and lymphocytosis. Immunologic abnormalities may also be induced during the infectious period.

Cases of cytomegalovirus infection have been noted in adults who are functionally myelosuppressed owing to leukemia or immunosuppressive medication. Cytomegalovirus has also been cultured from parotid secretion as well as from whole saliva in individuals with human immunodeficiency virus (HIV) infection. The role of this virus, if found in the base of oral ulcers in these patients, is undetermined.

Bacterial Sialadenitis

Etiology and Pathogenesis. Bacterial infections of salivary glands may be subdivided into acute and chronic forms. Regardless of cause, the involved gland becomes enlarged and painful; disruption of salivary flow is a frequent phenomenon.

Acute bacterial infections of the major salivary glands are not uncommon in clinical practice. A reduction in salivary flow is the primary predisposing factor. Such reduction in flow may be noted subsequent to dehydration and debilitation. Numerous drugs associated with decreased salivary flow rate likewise contribute to infections of the major salivary glands, especially the parotid. Other possible causes include trauma to the duct system and hematogenous spread of infection from other areas.

The most commonly isolated organism in acute parotitis is penicillin-resistant *Staphylococcus aureus*. Also implicated in this form of parotitis are *Streptococcus viridans* and *Streptococcus pneumoniae* as the primary infecting organisms. It is of interest to note the marked reduction in the overall incidence of acute parotitis after the introduction of antibiotic preparations. As resistant strains of bacteria have appeared, the prevalence of acute parotitis has increased.

Clinical Features. Clinical features are chiefly characterized by the presence of a painful swelling, low-grade fever, malaise, and headache. Laboratory studies disclose an elevated erythrocyte sedimentation rate and leukocytosis, often with a characteristic shift to the left. The involved gland is extremely tender, with the patient often demonstrating guarding during examination. Trismus is often noted, and purulence at the duct orifice may be produced by gentle pressure on the involved gland or duct.

If the infection is not eliminated early, suppuration may extend beyond the limiting capsule of the parotid gland. Extension into surrounding tissues along fascial planes in the neck or extension posteriorly into the external auditory canal may follow.

Treatment and Prognosis. The primary role of the clinician is to eliminate the causative organism, coupled with rehydration of the patient and drainage of purulence, if present. Culture and sensitivity testing of the exudate at the orifice of the duct is the first step in antibiotic management. After a culture is obtained, all patients should be empirically placed on a penicillinase-resistant antibiotic such as semisynthetic penicillin. Along with rehydration and attempts at establishing and encouraging salivary flow, moist compresses, analgesics, and rest are in order. Medications containing parasympathomimetic agents should be reduced or eliminated.

Biopsy and retrograde sialography should be avoided. The former may cause sinus tract formation, and the latter may allow infection to proceed beyond the boundaries of the gland into surrounding soft tissues. With prompt and effective treatment, recurrence is generally avoided. In cases of recurrent parotitis, considerable destructive glandular changes can be seen.

In the so-called *juvenile variant of parotitis,* intermittent unilateral or bilateral painful swelling is accompanied by fever and malaise. The initial attack usually occurs in individuals between ages 2 and 6 years, with numerous recurrences thereafter. Gross destruction of the parenchymal and ductal elements may be noted on sialographic examination. Absence of secretory acinar components and a damaged ductal system with numerous punctate globular spaces may be seen. Spontaneous regeneration of parotid salivary tissue has been reported in this condition.

Sarcoidosis

Etiology. Sarcoidosis represents a granulomatous disease of obscure cause. Although cutaneous manifestations of this disease were recognized as early as 1875, it was later demonstrated that sarcoidosis was a systemic disorder involving visceral tissues as well.

Although no specific cause has been identified, it has been suggested that this disease represents an infection or a hypersensitivity response to atypical mycobacteria. As many as 90% of patients in some studies showed significant titers of serum antibodies to these organisms. In some patients with sarcoidosis, a transmissible agent from human sarcoid tissue has been identified. Using molecular biologic techniques, mycobacteria DNA and RNA have been identified in sarcoidal tissues, raising the possibility of *Mycobacterium tuberculosis* or a related organism as a causative agent.

Susceptibility related to human leukocyte antigens (HLA) has been studied. Patients with some histocompatibility antigens (HLA-B7, HLA-B5, HLA-A9) may have a greater frequency of sarcoidosis than do others. It has also been found that most patients with sarcoidosis are anergic, demonstrating decreased levels of cutaneous sensitization to dinitrochlorobenzene, as well as to tuberculin, mumps virus, *Candida* antigen, and pertussis antigen.

Clinical Features. The protean manifestations of this disease are well known. Clinical courses range from spontaneous resolution to chronic progression. The disease may affect individuals at any age, although most are affected in the second and fourth decades. Females show a higher incidence than do males, and African-Americans are more frequently affected than whites.

Sarcoidosis is usually a self-limiting, benign disease with an insidious onset and protracted course. Patients may complain of lethargy, chronic fatigue, and anorexia, with specific signs and symptoms related to the organ involved.

Pulmonary manifestations are generally considered to be the most characteristic of this disease. They are typified by bilateral, hilar, and less commonly paratracheal lymphadenopathy. The disease may stabilize at this point, or it may advance to pulmonary fibrosis and a more ominous prognosis. The most serious complications of sarcoidosis are pulmonary hypertension, respiratory failure, and cor pulmonale.

The skin may be involved in approximately 25% of cases; most commonly, an erythema nodosum of acute onset and short duration is seen. Skin plaques characterized by nontender, dark purple, elevated areas on limbs, abdomen, and buttocks may appear. Another form of cutaneous pathology includes lesions known as *lupus pernio,* a term used to describe symmetric, infiltrative, violaceous plaques on the nose, cheeks, ears, forehead, and hands.

Ocular involvement may be seen but is variable in extent. Inflammation of the anterior uveal tract is the most common occurrence. This may be associated with parotid gland swelling and fever, so-called *uveoparotid fever* or *Heerfordt's syndrome.*

Hepatic involvement is quite common, with approximately 60% of patients showing granulomatous lesions on liver biopsy. However, clinical evidence of hepatic involvement appears in fewer than 50% of patients as demonstrated in abnormal liver function test results.

Osseous lesions are uncommonly noted, with a 5% occurrence rate in most studies. When present, punched-out lesions involving the distal phalanges with erosions of cancellous bone and an intact cortex are seen. Destruction of alveolar bone with tooth mobility may be evident within the maxilla and mandible.

Oral soft tissue lesions of sarcoidosis are nodular and generally indistinguishable from those seen in Crohn's disease. Parotid swelling may occur either unilaterally or bilaterally with about equal frequency (Fig. 8–17*A* and Table 8–2). This is often associated with lassitude, fever, gastrointestinal upset, joint pains, and night sweats, which may precede glandular involvement by several days to weeks. Other salivary glands may also be involved by the granulomatous inflammatory process, leading to xerostomia.

The upper aerodigestive tract may be involved, with lesions developing in the nasal mucosa, especially in the inferior turbinate and septal regions.

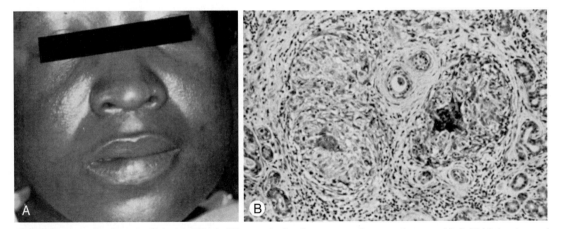

Figure 8–17. *A,* Sarcoidosis of the parotid. *B,* Micrograph showing noncaseating granulomas, epithelioid histiocytes, and giant cells.

Granulomas may also occur in the nasal sinuses, pharynx, epiglottis, and larynx.

Serum chemistry, radiographic studies, and biopsy are useful laboratory tests. Serum chemistry studies should include calcium (for evidence of hypercalcemia) and angiotensin-I converting enzyme, lysozyme, and adenosine deaminase levels (for evidence of macrophage activity within granulomas). Gallium scintiscanning and routine chest radiographs and intraoral films may be used to demonstrate bone involvement.

Histopathology. Consistent microscopic findings of sarcoidosis are noncaseating granulomas (Fig. 8–17B). The granulomas may be well demarcated and discrete or sometimes coalescent. Within the granulomas are macrophages and multinucleated giant cells, usually of the Langhans type. A diffuse lymphocytic infiltrate may be seen around the periphery of the granulomas. Absent is the caseation-type necrosis that is typical of tuberculosis.

Table 8–2. Conditions Associated with Chronic Salivary Gland Enlargement

---

Sjögren's syndrome
  Benign lymphoepithelial lesion
Neoplasms
  Epithelial: adenomas, carcinoma
  Lymphoma
Sarcoidosis
Infections
  Bacterial
  Actinomycosis
  Tuberculosis
Metabolic conditions
  Malnutrition, including anorexia and bulimia
  Diabetes mellitus
  Chronic alcoholism

Lip biopsy may occasionally provide evidence of sarcoid involvement of minor salivary glands in support of clinical impression of pulmonary disease.

Diagnosis. The Kveim test has traditionally been used to establish the diagnosis of sarcoidosis. An antigenic extract of spleen tissue is prepared from a patient with confirmed sarcoidosis and injected intradermally into the forearm of a patient with an undiagnosed case. In positive circumstances, a nodule develops at the injection site in 4 to 6 weeks. When this nodule is excised, it shows noncaseating granulomas. An 80 to 85% level of positivity is noted in patients with pulmonary involvement; a 2% chance of false-positive reaction occurs in individuals with other granulomatous diseases.

Use of a laboratory assay of the angiotensin-converting enzyme level has proved to provide reliable evidence in sarcoidosis. Elevation of this enzyme in conjunction with a positive chest radiograph has a high diagnostic reliability.

The histologic differential diagnosis includes tuberculosis, leprosy, cat-scratch disease, fungal infections (blastomycosis, coccidioidomycosis, and histoplasmosis) and parasitic diseases such as toxoplasmosis. Granulomas seen in association with beryllium and talc exposure must also be considered.

Treatment and Prognosis. Spontaneous resolution occurs in a significant number of patients. Corticosteroids are generally considered beneficial and remain the drugs of choice in treating symptomatic pulmonary sarcoidosis. Other agents may be used in addition to or instead of corticosteroids. Chloroquine has been found useful in the management of this disease, either alone or in combination with corticosteroids. Immunosuppressive drugs have been used with good results in individuals not responding to corticosteroid management. Immunomodulators such as levamisole may be useful in the management of arthritic symptoms caused by sarcoidosis.

In general, the prognosis for sarcoidosis is good, but patients must be monitored periodically with chest radiographs and serum angiotensin-I converting enzyme determinations. Clinical relapses are not usual in cases in which spontaneous resolution has occurred.

METABOLIC CONDITIONS

A group of disorders that may cause salivary gland enlargement is sometimes called *sialadenosis*. It usually affects the parotid glands bilaterally, typically in the absence of inflammatory symptoms. Conditions such as chronic alcoholism, dietary deficiency, obesity, diabetes mellitus, hypertension, and hyperlipidemia have been linked to this clinical salivary gland abnormality.

Alcoholic cirrhosis or chronic alcoholism and asymptomatic enlargement of the parotid glands occurs in 30 to 80% of patients. Salivary gland enlargement has been attributed to chronic protein deficiency. Comparable parotid gland enlargement in individuals with cirrhosis due to other causes does not apparently occur. Nutritional or protein deprivation may also lead to a similar salivary gland enlargement.

In diabetes mellitus, reduced flow rates have been reported in addition to bilateral parotid gland enlargement. The mechanism of acinar hypertrophy in this condition is unknown. Reduced flow rates from the parotid and other major salivary glands may lead to an increased risk of bacterial sialadenitis.

In cases of type I hyperlipoproteinemia, a sicca-like syndrome has been described. This is characterized primarily by parotid enlargement with mild oral or ocular sicca symptoms; it is generally attributed to the presence of fatty replacement of functional salivary gland parenchyma.

Another endocrine-related salivary gland enlargement may be noted in acromegaly. This may merely be a reflection of a generalized organomegaly encountered in this endocrine-mediated disturbance. Apparent parotid enlargement (acinar hypertrophy) and increased levels of parotid flow have also been noted in patients having chronic relapsing pancreatitis.

CONDITIONS ASSOCIATED WITH IMMUNE DEFECTS

Benign Lymphoepithelial Lesion

The term *benign lymphoepithelial lesion* (Mikulicz's disease), was coined in 1952 to characterize a unilateral or bilateral swelling of the parotid glands resulting from a benign infiltration of lymphoid cells. The lesion was originally believed to be inflammatory in origin. Later, neoplastic or pseudoneoplastic processes were believed to be responsible for this condition. The most recent evidence points to an immunologic abnormality. Benign lymphoepithelial lesion may be seen as a solitary salivary gland abnormality, or it may be one of the manifestations of Sjögren's syndrome and possibly HIV disease. Although the vast majority of lymphoepithelial lesions remain benign, malignant transformation of the lymphoid or the epithelial component has been described.

Etiology. The cause of the benign lymphoepithelial lesion is obscure. The most likely possibility involves genetic abnormalities or susceptibilities within the cell-mediated arm of the immune system. Postulated is either excessive T helper cell function or a depression of suppressor cell function, permitting T cell activation. An alternative theory relates to an antigenic challenge caused by viral alteration of glandular cell surface antigens. This in turn may result in stimulation of B cell antibody production that is directed to glandular tissue. This disorder may result from activation of both these events. The result is an immune-mediated process and a loss of salivary parenchymal tissue with subsequent alteration in function.

Clinical Features. Although the overall incidence of the benign lymphoepithelial lesion is low, it is most frequently noted in middle-aged women as a progressive, asymptomatic enlargement of the affected salivary glands. The process may initially be a unilateral one, but over time, it becomes bilateral. A frequent clinical marker is the appearance of superimposed bacterial infections secondary to reduction in flow rate. In this event, the gland involved becomes enlarged and firm. With repeated bouts of superimposed bacterial infections, the affected glands become nodular.

Histopathology. Microscopically, this process begins around intralobular ducts, producing a lymphocytic sialadenitis or parotitis. The result is dilatation of ducts and periductal lymphocytic sialadenitis (Fig. 8–18). Acinar atrophy, a conse-

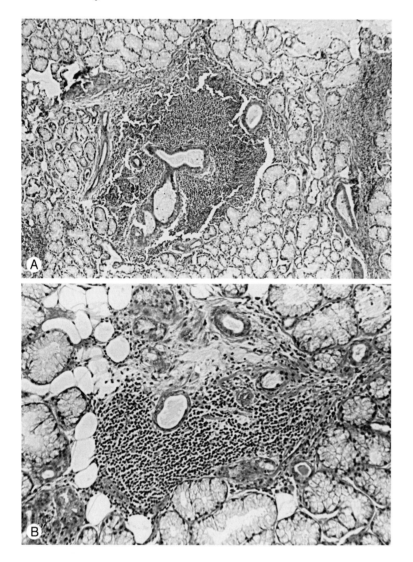

Figure 8–18. *A* and *B,* Early benign lymphoepithelial lesion showing periductal inflammation.

quence of ductal damage, is progressive and proportional to the degree of lymphocytic infiltration. As this takes place, squamous metaplasia occurs within the ductal segment, ultimately causing luminal obliteration and hyperplasia of duct lining cells. As a result of this process, so-called epimyoepithelial islands appear (Fig. 8–19). This is the histologic cornerstone for the diagnosis of benign lymphoepithelial lesion. A bright eosinophilic cuffing at the interface of the epimyoepithelial islands and the surrounding lymphocytic infiltrates may be striking at times. Late in this stage of the disease, increased interstitial fibrosis occurs, producing a chronic punctate or cavitary form of sialadenitis on sialographic examination. Rarely, amyloid deposits may be seen. The end result is complete loss of acinic tissues and secretory function.

Differential Diagnosis. Chronic bilateral en-largement of the salivary glands must be separated from sarcoidosis, lymphoma, gout, leukemia, diabetes mellitus, chronic alcohol abuse, and, rarely, hypertension. History and clinical examination are important in identifying the correct process. Serum chemistry studies may help separate sarcoidosis and gout from the other conditions. Peripheral blood counts help identify leukemia.

Treatment and Prognosis. Generally, treatment of patients with benign lymphoepithelial lesion is palliative. The management of a benign lymphoepithelial lesion has undergone some modification. This change is related to a better understanding of the natural history of this disease, specifically as it relates to its predisposition for neoplastic transformation. This predisposition has been emphasized by using laboratory techniques that investigate the presence of monoclonality of the lymphocytic infiltrate either by immunohisto-

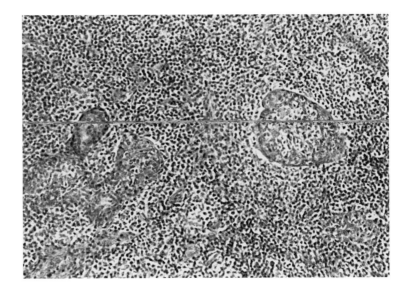

Figure 8–19. Advanced benign lymphoepithelial lesion showing residual epimyoepithelial islands surrounded by lymphocytes.

chemical or molecular or gene rearrangement studies. Although there are opposing views regarding the significance of monoclonality within a benign lymphoepithelial lesion, it is believed to be suggestive of low-grade B cell lymphoma of the mucosa-associated lymphoid tissue. These are low-grade lymphomas that are treated with irradiation when localized to salivary glands.

Sjögren's Syndrome

Sjögren's syndrome is the expression of an autoimmune process that principally results in rheumatoid arthritis, dry eyes (keratoconjunctivitis sicca), and dry mouth (xerostomia) owing to lymphocytic replacement of lacrimal and salivary glands. Microscopically, the glandular changes are identical to those of benign lymphoepithelial lesion. In some patients, this syndrome may present with vague symptoms related only to xerostomia and keratoconjunctivitis sicca; in others, the autoimmune process may take the form of severe multisystem illness. The lacrimal and salivary gland involvement is often one expression of a generalized exocrinopathy that is lymphocyte mediated.

Etiology. Although the specific cause of this syndrome is unknown, numerous immunologic alterations indicate a disease of great complexity. The generalized alteration relates to a polyclonal B cell hyperactivity that reflects a lack of regulation by T cell subpopulations. As with the benign lymphoepithelial lesion, the specific causes of this immunologic defect remain speculative.

This syndrome appears to be of autoimmune origin that may be limited to exocrine glands, or it may extend to include systemic connective tissue disorders. In instances of only exocrine involvement, this syndrome is known as *primary Sjögren's syndrome.* If, in addition to the xerostomia and keratoconjunctivitis sicca, there is an associated connective tissue disorder, regardless of the specific type, it is known as *secondary Sjögren's syndrome.*

Viruses, particularly retroviruses and Epstein-Barr virus, have been implicated in the etiology of Sjögren's syndrome. Evidence suggesting a role for retroviruses has come from the demonstration of antibodies against HIV-associated proteins in a subset of patients with Sjögren's syndrome and from the clinical similarity of HIV-associated salivary gland disease to Sjögren's syndrome. The significance of anti-HIV antibodies in some patients with Sjögren's syndrome has not been determined. It has been suggested that these antibodies may be stimulated by another retrovirus that is related to HIV or that they may represent cross-reacting autoantibodies.

Epstein-Barr virus has been demonstrated in salivary gland tissue of patients with Sjögren's syndrome. However, the virus has also been found in the salivary glands of normal individuals, thus weakening the contention that Epstein-Barr virus has a primary role in the cause of this condition. If Epstein-Barr virus is involved, its role is likely secondary in nature.

Clinical Features. Sjögren's syndrome occurs in all ethnic and racial groups. The peak age of onset is 50 years, and 90% of cases occur in women. Children and teenagers are rarely affected. Distinguishing between primary and secondary forms of the syndrome, especially those associated with rheumatoid arthritis, is usually not

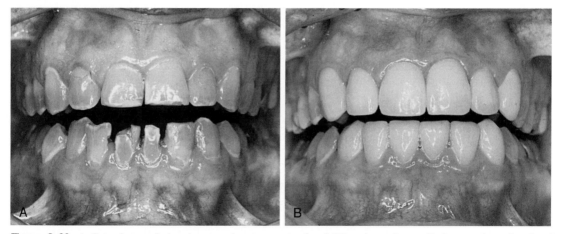

Figure 8–20. *A*, Extensive cervical caries secondary to xerostomia of Sjögren's syndrome. *B*, Same patient after dental restorations. (Courtesy of Dr. R. M. Courtney.)

difficult. This may be important because of an increased risk of lymphoreticular malignancy developing in the primary form—the relative risk is estimated to be approximately 44 times that of the general population. An interesting associated sign is a decrease in serum immunoglobulin levels accompanying or preceding the malignant change.

The chief oral complaint in Sjögren's syndrome is xerostomia, which may be the source of eating and speaking difficulties (see Table 8–1). These patients are also at greater risk for dental caries, periodontal disease, and oral candidiasis (Fig. 8–20). Parotid gland enlargement, which is often recurrent and symmetric, occurs in approximately 50% of patients (Fig. 8–21; see also Table 8–2). A significant percentage of these patients also

present with complaints of arthralgia, myalgia, and fatigue.

The salivary component of Sjögren's syndrome may be assessed by sialochemical studies, nuclear imaging of the glands, contrast sialography, flow rate analysis, and minor salivary gland biopsy. The most commonly used method currently is labial salivary gland biopsy.

Nuclear medicine techniques using a technetium pertechnetate isotope and subsequent scinti-scanning can yield important functional information relative to the uptake of the isotope by salivary gland tissue. Contrast sialography aids in detecting filling defects within the gland being examined. A punctate sialectasia is characteristic in individuals with Sjögren's syndrome (Fig. 8–

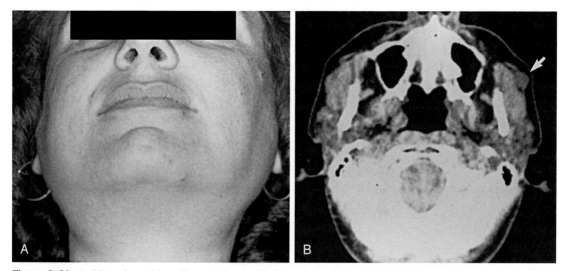

Figure 8–21. *A*, Bilateral parotid swelling associated with Sjögren's syndrome. *B*, Axial tomogram demonstrating symmetric bilateral parotid gland enlargement and unilateral periparotid lymph node enlargement *(arrow)* in a patient with Sjögren's syndrome.

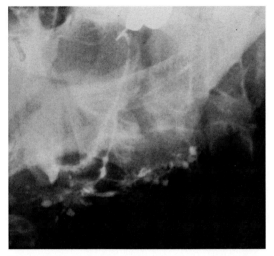

Figure 8–22. A parotid sialogram indicating severe globular and punctate sialectasia. The absence of functional acinic elements in addition to interstitial fibrosis prevents radiographic contrast medium from entering the intralobular portion of the gland. Duct wall damage presents as a globular outpouch formation in this patient with Sjögren's syndrome.

22). This latter finding reflects significant ductal and acinar damage, with only the interlobular ducts remaining in cases of moderate to advanced disease. Over time, with further parenchymal and ductal damage, focal areas of narrowing or stenosis of larger ducts takes place and may be seen on sialogram. Other forms of sialectasia may also be noted, including globular and cavitary types.

Other laboratory findings commonly found in primary and secondary Sjögren's syndrome include mild anemia, leukopenia, eosinophilia, elevated erythrocyte sedimentation rate, and diffuse elevation of serum immunoglobulin levels. Additionally, numerous autoantibodies may be found, including rheumatoid factor, antinuclear antibodies, and precipitating antinuclear antibodies such as anti–Sjögren's syndrome-A (SS-A) and anti–Sjögren's syndrome-B (SS-B). Antibodies SS-A and SS-B may be seen in association with both primary and secondary Sjögren's syndrome. Patients who have SS-B antibodies are more likely to develop extraglandular disease (secondary form of the syndrome).

In the secondary form, rheumatoid arthritis is the most common systemic autoimmune disease, although systemic lupus erythematosus is not infrequently encountered. Less commonly, diseases such as scleroderma, primary biliary cirrhosis, polymyositis, vasculitis, parotitis, and chronic active hepatitis may be associated with secondary Sjögren's syndrome (Table 8–3).

Immunogenetic typing studies have indicated statistically significant expressions of various his-

tocompatibility antigens in patients with primary and secondary forms of the syndrome. HLA-DR4 antigen is often identified in patients with secondary Sjögren's syndrome; those antigens found in those with the primary form are frequently HLA-B8, HLA-DR3 types.

Histopathology. In all the major salivary glands, the microscopic features of Sjögren's syndrome are well known and have been described under benign lymphoepithelial lesion. In individuals with Sjögren's syndrome, the benign lymphocytic infiltrate replaces major salivary gland parenchyma. Epimyoepithelial islands are present in approximately 40% of cases. Much less commonly, epimyoepithelial islands are seen in affected minor salivary glands.

The routine preparation of minor salivary gland tissue demonstrates a wide range in the degree of inflammatory cell infiltration and acinar replacement. The initial lesion is represented by a focal periductal aggregate of lymphocytes and fewer plasma cells. As inflammatory foci enlarge, a corresponding level of acinar degeneration is seen. With increasing lymphocytic infiltration, confluence of inflammatory foci occurs. Periductal and perivascular hyaline deposits may also be noted. Studies have shown a positive correlation in pattern and extent of infiltration between labial sali-

Table 8–3. Organ System Conditions in Sjögren's Syndrome

Skin
    Dryness and reduced sweat production
    Scleroderma
    Vasculitis and purpura
Salivary and lacrimal glands
    Enlargement
    Xerostomia
    Keratoconjunctivitis sicca
    Atrophy
Gastrointestinal tract
    Dental caries
    Oral candidiasis
    Hypochlorhydria
    Hepatosplenomegaly
    Biliary cirrhosis
Respiratory
    Rhinitis
    Pharyngitis
    Obstructive pulmonary disease
Cardiovascular system
    Raynaud's disease
    Lupus erythematosus
Hematopoietic system
    Anemia (megaloblastic, microcytic-hypochromic)
    Leukopenia
    Hypergammaglobulinemia
    Hypersedimentation
Musculoskeletal system
    Rheumatoid arthritis

vary glands and submandibular and parotid glands in patients with Sjögren's syndrome.

A grading system has been developed for assessing the salivary component (lymphocytic sialadenitis) of Sjögren's syndrome. A glandular area that contains 50 or more lymphocytes is designated as a *focus*. More than one focus in 4 mm² is regarded as being significant. Interpretation of labial gland biopsy specimens should be done with the knowledge that infiltrates may be seen both in normal glands and in glands that are inflamed for other reasons, including myasthenia gravis, bone marrow transplant, other connective tissue diseases, and obstructive phenomena.

Diagnosis. Diagnosis is dependent on laboratory data, clinical examination, and a detailed history. The classic triad of xerostomia, keratoconjunctivitis sicca, and rheumatoid disease remains valid. Labial salivary gland biopsy should be performed and must demonstrate one or more foci of lymphocytes per 4 mm² (i.e., a focus score of 1 or more).

An important consideration concerns the clinical manifestation of xerostomia. Although this is the main oral symptom and clinical sign in Sjögren's syndrome, other considerations of dry mouth must be evaluated. Additionally, major salivary gland enlargement is a feature of Sjögren's syndrome but may be episodic in nature, and in some patients it may not be present at all. The sialographic and salivary scintigraphic findings are generally not specific and should be incorporated into other clinical and laboratory studies, including minor salivary gland biopsy, as one considers the diagnosis of Sjögren's syndrome.

Treatment. Sjögren's syndrome and the complication of the sicca component are best managed symptomatically. Artificial saliva and artificial tears are available for this purpose. Preventive oral measures are extremely important relative to xerostomia. Scrupulous oral hygiene, dietary modification, topical fluoride therapy, and remineralizing solutions are important in maintaining oral and dental tissues. Use of sialagogues, such as pilocarpine, remains of limited value and may be contraindicated in some cases.

The prognosis of Sjögren's syndrome is complicated by an association with malignant transformation to lymphoma. This may occur in approximately 6 to 7% of cases; it is more common in those with only the sicca components of the syndrome. A predisposing factor in development of lymphoma appears to be related to prolonged immunologic and lymphoid hyperreactivity. Less frequently observed is the transformation of the epithelial component to undifferentiated carcinoma.

Generally, the course for Sjögren's syndrome is one of chronicity requiring long-term symptomatic management. Careful follow-up and management by a dentist, ophthalmologist, and rheumatologist, among others, are critical.

BENIGN NEOPLASMS

At approximately 5 months of development, a characteristic lobular architecture of salivary glands becomes established. As branching morphogenesis continues, terminal tubular elements differentiate toward acinar cell formation (Fig. 8–23). Coinciding with acinar granule formation is the early presence of flattened cellular elements, presumptive myoepithelial cells, which form between the acinar cells and surrounding basal lamina. These cells vary in configuration from strap-like to stellate. Early in their development, myoepithelial cells lack the characteristic myofilaments and are often optically clear. The origin of the myoepithelial cell is controversial; most investigators favor origin from terminal tubular cells.

Terminal tubular elements are ultimately responsible for the formation of striated intralobular ducts and intercalated ducts as well as acini and myoepithelial cells. Intralobular and interlobular ducts of the excretory system arise from the remaining progenitor stalk cells.

The microanatomy and the embryogenesis of the salivary glands are related to histogenesis of neoplasia as well as classification schemes of epithelial salivary gland tumors. A stem cell or reserve cell within the salivary duct system is believed by many to be the cell of origin of salivary gland neoplasms. Some believe that intercalated duct cells and acinar cells are capable of giving rise to these neoplasms. The role of the myoepithelial cell in the composition and growth of nu-

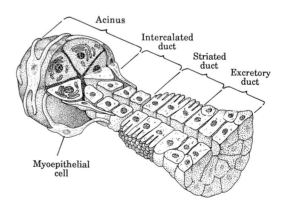

Figure 8–23. The basic mature salivary gland unit.

Table 8–4. Classification of Salivary Gland Adenomas

Benign mixed tumor (pleomorphic adenoma)
Monomorphic adenomas
    Basal cell adenoma
    Canalicular adenoma
    Myoepithelioma
    Sebaceous adenoma
    Oncocytoma
    Papillary cystadenoma lymphomatosum
Ductal papillomas
    Sialadenoma papilliferum
    Inverted ductal papilloma
    Intraductal papilloma

In modification of Seifert G, Brocheriou C, Cardesa A, Eveson JW. WHO International Classification of Tumors. Tentative histological classification of salivary gland tumors. Pathol Res Pract 186:555–581, 1990.

merous epithelial salivary tumors is thought to be considerable. Although it is not considered the primary cell of origin of salivary gland tumors, with the exception of the myoepithelioma, the myoepithelial cell has been shown to be an important participant in mixed tumor (pleomorphic adenoma), adenocystic carcinoma, salivary duct carcinoma, polymorphous low-grade adenocarcinoma, and epimyoepithelial carcinoma of intercalated duct origin.

The three major paired salivary glands—parotid, submandibular, and sublingual—plus the hundreds of small minor salivary glands located within the submucosa of the oral cavity and oropharynx are capable of giving rise to a wide range of neoplasms. The majority of salivary neoplasms are epithelial in origin and are considered to be of either ductal or acinar derivation. In addition to epithelial neoplasms, benign lesions may arise from salivary interstitial connective tissue elements, especially within the parotid gland. Rarely, the interstitial connective tissue components of major salivary glands can give rise to primary sarcomas, their behavior being identical to that of their extraglandular counterparts.

The overall incidence of minor salivary gland neoplasia is relatively low. The parotid gland, the most frequent site of salivary gland neoplasia, is more often involved with benign rather than with malignant neoplasms. On the other hand, submandibular gland and minor salivary gland neoplasms have a greater likelihood of being malignant. The overall figure relative to the incidence of malignancy in the parotid gland is 25%, in the submandibular gland 50%, and in minor salivary glands 60 to 75%. Although tumors of the sublingual glands are extremely uncommon, when they are present, they are usually malignant.

Benign Mixed Tumor (Pleomorphic Adenoma)

The benign mixed tumor, or pleomorphic adenoma, is the most common tumor of major and minor salivary glands (Tables 8–4 and 8–5). The parotid gland accounts for approximately 85% of these tumors, whereas the submandibular gland and the intraoral minor salivary glands account for 8% and 7%, respectively. Of those tumors arising within the oral cavity, the majority are noted in the palate.

The histogenesis of this lesion relates to a proliferation of cells with ductal and/or myoepithelial features. The myoepithelial-differentiated cell assumes an important role in determining the overall composition and appearance of mixed tumors. Most studies indicate a range of cell types in mixed tumors—those that are completely epithelial are on one end of a spectrum and those that are completely myoepithelial are on the other. Between these two extremes, less well-developed cells with features of both myoepithelial and ductal elements may be seen. It has been theorized that rather than simultaneous proliferation of neoplastic epithelial and myoepithelial cells, a single cell with the potential to differentiate toward either epithelial or myoepithelial cells may be responsible for these tumors.

Clinical Features. Mixed tumors occur at any age, favor women slightly more than men, and are most prevalent in the fourth to sixth decades of

Table 8–5. Benign Salivary Gland Tumors

TYPE	PAROTID	SUBMANDIBULAR	SUBLINGUAL	MINOR	TOTAL
Benign mixed tumor	3196	266	0	346	3808
Papillary cystadenoma lymphomatosum	431	6	0	0	437
Oncocytoma	45	2	0	0	47
Other monomorphic adenomas	131	5	1	48	185
Total	3803	279	1	394	4477

Compiled from Batsakis JG, et al. Head Neck Surg 1:260, 1979; Dardick I, et al. Hum Pathol 13:62, 1982; Eneroth CM. Cancer 27:1415, 1971; and Headington JT, et al. Cancer 39:2460, 1977.

life. They constitute approximately 50% of all intraoral minor salivary gland tumors. Generally, they are mobile except when they occur in the hard palate. They appear as firm, painless swellings and, in the vast majority of cases, do not cause ulceration of the overlying mucosa (Fig. 8–24). The palate is the most common intraoral site, followed by the upper lip and buccal mucosa. Intraoral mixed tumors, especially those noted within the palate, lack a well-defined capsule. Within the submandibular gland, mixed tumors present as discrete masses. It is clinically impossible to distinguish these from malignant salivary gland tumors during early stages of growth. They may also be difficult to distinguish from enlarged lymph nodes within the submandibular triangle.

When they arise within the parotid gland, mixed tumors are generally painless and slow growing. They are usually located below the ear and posterior to the mandible. Some tumors may be grooved by the posterior extent of the mandibular ramus, with long-standing lesions capable of producing pressure atrophy on this bone. When they are situated within the inferior pole or tail of the parotid, the tumors may present below the angle of the mandible and anterior to the sternocleidomastoid muscle.

Mixed tumors generally range from a few millimeters to several centimeters in diameter and are capable of reaching giant proportions in the major salivary glands, especially the parotid. The tumor is typically lobulated and enclosed within a connective tissue pseudocapsule that varies in thickness. In areas where the capsule is deficient, neoplastic tissue may lie in direct contact with adjacent salivary tissue.

Histopathology. Microscopically, mixed tumors demonstrate a wide spectrum of histologic features. The pleomorphic patterns within individual tumors are responsible for the synonym *pleomorphic adenoma.* Approximately one third of mixed tumors show an almost equal ratio of epithelial and mesenchymal elements (Fig. 8–25). The epithelial component may be arranged in numerous patterns, including those forming glands, tubules, ribbons, and solid sheets. (Fig. 8–26). An occasional finding is the presence of metaplastic epithelial change to squamous, sebaceous, or oncocytic elements. Adding to the histologic complexity are stromal admixtures of myxoid, chondroid, hyaline, and rarely adipose and osseous tissues (Fig. 8–27).

Myoepithelial cells also add to the complex patterns seen in benign mixed tumors. The myoepithelial component may be of two morphologic types—plasmacytoid cells (Fig. 8–28) and spindle cells. Plasmacytoid cells often tend to aggregate; grouped spindle cells tend to appear in parallel arrangements.

Examination of the limiting compressed fibrous connective tissue or pseudocapsule surrounding the tumor may demonstrate islands of tissue within it or extending through it. Such islands may appear as satellite nodules at a variable distance from the main tumor mass. Serial sectioning usually demonstrates that such satellites are, in fact, outgrowths or pseudopods continuous with the main tumor mass.

In studying whole organ sections of parotid gland mixed tumors, it was noted that no tumors possessed a smooth and complete surface capsule and that, on histopathologic analysis, areas of exposed capsule, capsular breaks, incompleteness of the capsule, and tumor ingrowth into the capsule

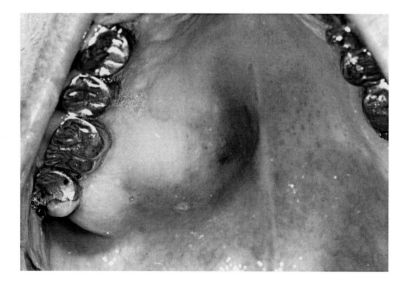

Figure 8–24. Mixed tumor of the hard palate.

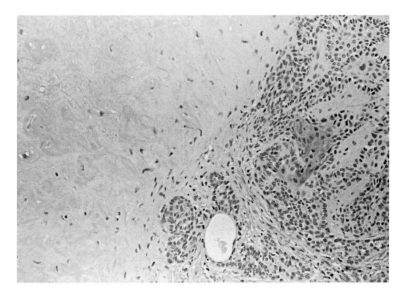

Figure 8–25. Mixed tumor showing a mesenchymal component (left) and an epithelial component (right).

were noted. As discussed later, this anatomic feature is the primary factor that guides treatment.

The histologic appearance of the mixed tumor in some cases resembles the monomorphic adenoma; in other cases, an adenoid cystic carcinoma type pattern may be seen. Features that suggest the possibility of malignant change include the presence of focal areas of necrosis, invasion, atypical mitoses, and extensive hyalinization.

Treatment and Prognosis. The treatment of choice for benign mixed tumor of minor or major salivary glands is surgical excision. Enucleation of parotid mixed tumors is not advisable because of risk of recurrence due to extension of tumor

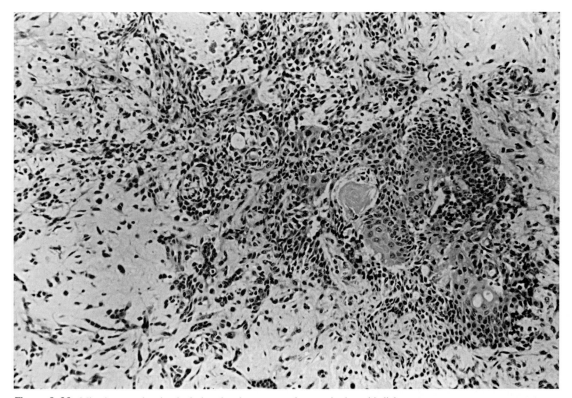

Figure 8–26. Mixed tumor showing both ductal and squamous elements in the epithelial component.

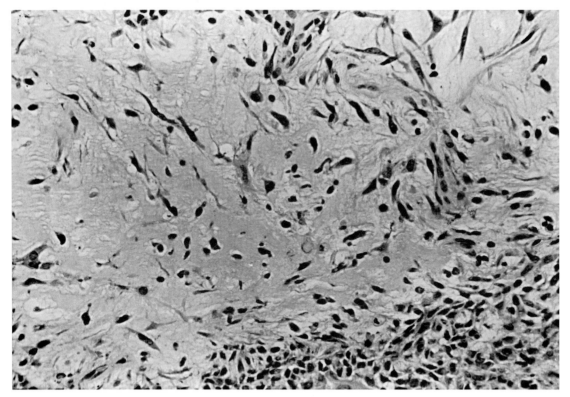

Figure 8–27. Myxoid area in a mixed tumor.

through capsular defects. Removal of mixed tumors arising within the parotid gland is complicated by the presence of the facial nerve. Any surgical approach, therefore, must include preservation of the uninvolved facial nerve. In most cases, superficial parotidectomy with preservation of the facial nerve is the most appropriate management for mixed tumors arising within the parotid.

Resection of the submandibular gland is the preferred treatment for benign mixed tumors in this location. Lesions of the palate or gingiva frequently involve periosteum or bone, making removal difficult. Other oral benign mixed tumors can be more easily removed; but such removal should include tissue beyond the pseudocapsule.

Inadequate initial removal of the mixed tumor

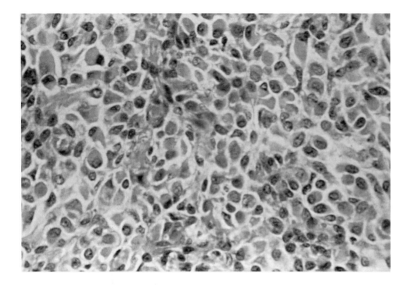

Figure 8–28. Plasmacytoid or oncocytoid cells in a mixed tumor.

in major glands may result in recurrence, often with multiple discrete tumor foci. These recurrent lesions may be widely distributed within the area of previous surgery and may occur in association with the surgical scar. The prime determinant of nonrecurrence is adequate surgical treatment at the initial phase. In most instances, the recurrent tumor maintains the original pathology; however, with each recurrence there is an increased possibility of malignant transformation. Also, approximately 25% of benign mixed tumors undergo malignant transformation *if lesions are untreated for an extended length of time.* The probability of such malignant change also increases if the area has previously been treated with surgery or radiotherapy.

Monomorphic Adenomas

Because monomorphic adenoma is composed of cells predominantly of one type and because of the absence of connective tissue changes, monomorphic adenoma has been separated from mixed tumors. Classification schemes may refer to overall histologic pattern or to histogenesis (Tables 8–4 and 8–6). Studies that used ultrastructural and immunohistochemical techniques have provided a different perspective on the histogenetic aspects of these lesions. Although some monomorphic adenomas are indeed composed of an isomorphic tumor cell population, others have a bimorphic pattern of differentiation in which there is minimal participation by myoepithelial-type cells.

BASAL CELL ADENOMAS

Basal cell adenomas constitute approximately 1 to 2% of all salivary gland adenomas. About 70%

Table 8–6. Histogenetic Classification of Monomorphic Adenoma

Terminal duct origin
  Basal cell adenomas
    Solid
    Trabecular-tubular
    Membranous (dermal analogue tumor)
  Canalicular adenoma
Terminal or striated duct origin
  Sebaceous adenoma
  Sebaceous lymphadenoma
Striated duct origin
  Oncocytoma
  Papillary cystadenoma lymphomatosum
Excretory duct origin
  Sialadenoma papilliferum/inverted ductal papilloma

are found within the parotid. In minor salivary glands, most occur in the upper lip, followed in frequency by the palate, buccal mucosa, and lower lip.

Clinical Features. Basal cell adenomas are generally slow growing and painless. The lesions tend to be clinically rather distinct on palpation, but they can be multifocal and multinodular. The age range of patients is between 35 and 80 years, with a mean of approximately 60 years. A distinct male predilection is noted.

The *membranous adenoma (dermal analogue tumor)* variant occurs in the parotid gland in more than 90% of cases, with no cases reported in the intraoral minor glands. These lesions vary from 1 to 5 cm in greatest dimension and generally present as an asymptomatic swelling. Several patients with this particular finding in the parotid gland have presented with synchronous or metachronous adnexal cutaneous tumors, including dermal cylindroma, trichoepithelioma, and eccrine spiradenoma.

Histopathology. Generally, the isomorphic pattern and absence of chondroid metaplasia and mucoid to myxoid stroma help to differentiate these lesions from the benign mixed tumor. In the *solid* variety, islands or sheets of basaloid cells frequently show peripheral palisading, with individual cells at the periphery appearing cuboidal to low columnar in profile (Fig. 8–29). Mitoses are inconspicuous. Nuclei are regular in shape and uniformly basophilic, and the amount of cytoplasm is generally minimal.

The *trabecular-tubular* form of basal cell adenoma presents with a distinctive morphology. Trabeculae or solid cords of epithelial cells alternate with ductal or tubular elements composed of two distinctive cell types (Fig. 8–30). The luminal surfaces of the small formed ducts are lined by cuboidal cells with a minimal amount of cytoplasm. A cuboidal basal cell layer separates the epithelial lining elements from the stroma. The trabeculae are often outlined by a prominent or thickened basement membrane.

The *membranous adenoma* differs from other subtypes in that it is generally multilobular, and it is encapsulated in approximately 50% of cases. The tumor grows in a nodular fashion, with individual nodes often separated by normal salivary gland tissue. Variable-sized islands of tumor tissue are embedded in and separated from each other by a thick hyaline and eosinophilic, periodic acid–Schiff (PAS)–positive membrane or investment. Similar, if not identical, eosinophilic hyaline material is also noted in droplet form within the intercellular areas of the tumor islands.

Treatment and Prognosis. Monomorphic ade-

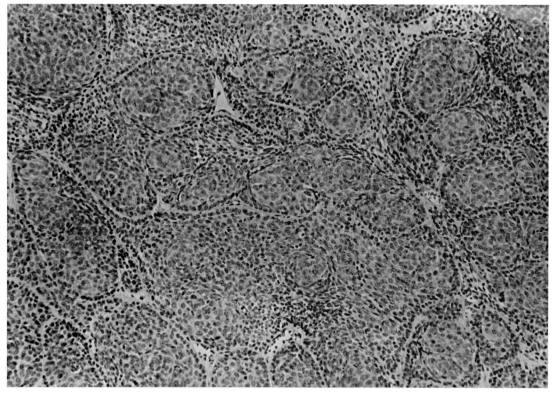

Figure 8–29. Solid variant of basal cell monomorphic adenoma.

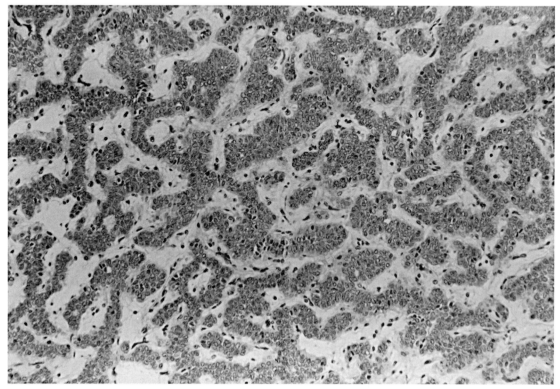

Figure 8–30. Trabecular-tubular variant of basal cell monomorphic adenoma.

nomas are benign and rarely recur. The membranous form of the basal cell adenoma, however, has a significant rate of recurrence because of its growth pattern and multifocal nature. Preferred management is conservative surgical excision including a rim or margin of normal uninvolved tissue.

CANALICULAR ADENOMA

The *canalicular adenoma,* a separate form of monomorphic adenoma, is distinguished from basal cell adenoma because it occurs almost exclusively within the oral cavity and has distinctive clinical and histologic features. Its biologic behavior is, however, similar.

Clinical Features. A narrow age range is noted in patients with canalicular adenomas. Most patients tend to be older than 50 years, and most patients are women. The upper lip is by far the most common site for the canalicular adenoma, with one series reporting 81% of lesions located in this region. The lesions tend to be freely movable and asymptomatic and range in size from a few millimeters to 2 to 3 cm.

The clinical differential diagnosis of this lesion includes mucus retention cyst and benign mixed tumor.

Histopathology. Characteristically, the canalicular adenoma shows bilayered strands of basaloid cells that branch and anastomose within a delicate and loose stroma that is highly vascular and contains few fibroblasts and little collagen (Fig. 8–31). Individual cells are characteristically columnar, with moderate to abundant amounts of eosinophilic cytoplasm. Canalicular adenoma oc-

casionally may not be totally encapsulated, and more than 20% of cases are also multifocal.

Treatment and Prognosis. The treatment of choice for canalicular adenoma is surgical excision with the inclusion of a cuff of clinically normal tissue. That more than 20% of lesions are multifocal may account for some recurrences.

MYOEPITHELIOMA

Benign salivary gland tumors composed entirely of myoepithelial cells are called *myoepitheliomas.* Although of epithelial origin, the phenotypic expression of the tumor cells is more closely related to smooth muscle. Reflective of this is the immunohistochemical staining of myoepithelioma cells with antibodies to actin, cytokeratin, and S-100 protein.

Most myoepitheliomas arise within the parotid gland and, less frequently, in the submandibular gland and intraoral minor salivary glands (Fig. 8–32). Clinically, myoepitheliomas present as circumscribed painless masses within the affected gland. An equal gender occurrence has been noted. A range of presentation from the third through ninth decades, with a median of 53 years, has been reported.

Microscopically, clusters of either plasmacytoid or spindle cells make up these lesions. Approximately 70% of cases contain spindle cells, and approximately 20% are composed of plasmacytoid cells (Fig. 8–33). In one study, 13% of myoepitheliomas were seen to contain both cell forms in approximately equal quantity. Growth patterns range from predominantly solid lesions with little background stroma to those with significant levels

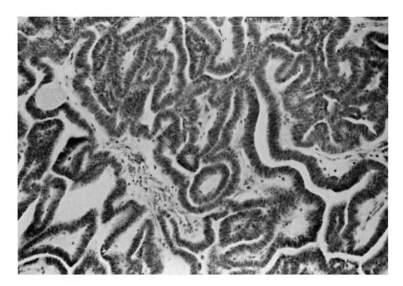

Figure 8–31. Canalicular adenoma.

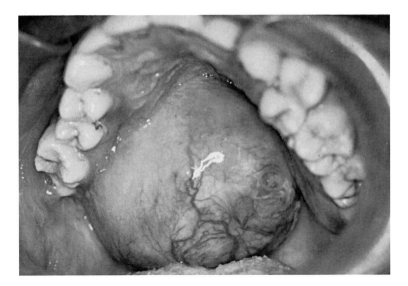

Figure 8–32. Myoepithelioma of the hard palate.

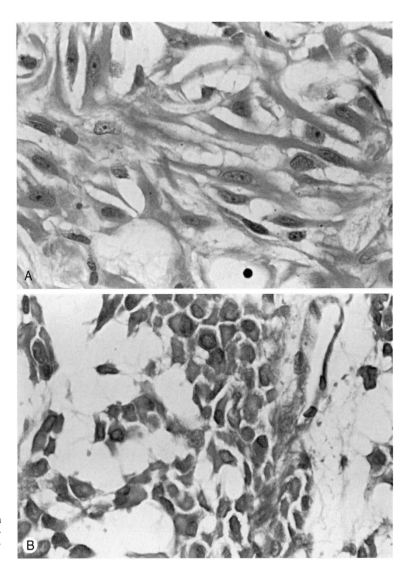

Figure 8–33. *A*, Myoepithelioma composed of spindle cells. *B*, Myoepithelioma composed of plasmacytoid cells.

of mucoid or myxoid elements interspersed between myoepithelial cells.

Ultrastructurally, a thin basal lamina is found between the tumor cells and the supportive stroma. Occasional hemidesmosomes and pinocytotic vesicles may be noted along the stromal aspect of the plasma membrane. Pools or dispersed forms of glycogen may be noted peripherally in the cytoplasm. Centrally, filamentous or fibrillar material within the spindle cells is arranged parallel to the long axis of the cells, producing an overall resemblance to smooth muscle cells. Within the plasmacytoid type of myoepithelial cell, filaments tend to be randomly scattered.

Treatment of this benign lesion is identical to that of the benign mixed tumor. Conservative excision of lesions arising in minor salivary glands is advised, including a thin rim of surrounding normal tissue. When lesions are noted within the parotid gland, superficial parotidectomy is indicated. Overall prognosis is excellent, and recurrences are not expected.

SEBACEOUS ADENOMA

The presence of sebaceous glands or evidence of sebaceous differentiation has been noted in submandibular and parotid salivary glands. This particular tissue, thought to originate in intralobular ducts, gives rise to the sebaceous adenoma and other sebaceous neoplasms designated as sebaceous lymphadenoma, sebaceous carcinoma, and sebaceous lymphadenocarcinoma. These are rare lesions composed predominantly of sebaceous gland–derived cells; they are well differentiated in the benign forms and moderately to poorly differentiated in the malignant forms. In sebaceous lymphadenoma, a benign lymphoid component is seen. The parotid gland is the site of chief involvement, although intraoral examples have been reported. These lesions range from a few millimeters to several centimeters in diameter. Parotidectomy is the treatment of choice when lesions arise in this gland. Surgical excision is used in cases of intraoral neoplasms.

ONCOCYTOMA

The oncocytoma or oxyphilic adenoma, a rare lesion arising within salivary gland tissue, is seen predominantly in the parotid gland. As the name implies, this lesion is composed of cellular elements termed *oncocytes,* which are large granular acidophilic cells. Such cells are normally found in salivary glands in the intralobular ducts, and they usually increase in number with age. Oncocytes are found in mucous glands of the aerodigestive tract as well as in minor and major salivary glands of the oral and perioral regions. The histogenetic origin of this lesion is believed to be from the salivary duct epithelium, in particular the striated duct.

Clinically, the oncocytoma tends to be a solid, round to ovoid encapsulated lesion usually less than 5 cm in diameter when it is noted within major salivary glands. These lesions are rarely seen intraorally. In some instances, bilateral occurrence may be noted.

Within individual glands (most often the parotid), a nonneoplastic and multicentric cellular change known as *oncocytosis* may be seen. This metaplasia of salivary duct and acinar cells is seen in the context of an otherwise normal gland. As oncocytic foci enlarge, confusion with oncocytoma may occur.

Microscopically, the oncocytoma cells are characterized as swollen or enlarged, with granular eosinophilic cytoplasm (Fig. 8–34). The outline of the cells is generally polyhedral, with a pyknotic hyperchromatic nucleus. Ultrastructural studies often provide an unequivocal diagnosis by finding abundant numbers of mitochondria within the cytoplasm of the tumor cells. Careful examination of the mitochondria shows them to be abnormal, with unusual or atypical outlines and large numbers of cristae.

Owing to the near-universal benign course and slow growth rate, treatment is generally conservative, with superficial parotidectomy as the treatment of choice for parotid lesions. In minor salivary glands, removal of the tumor with a margin of normal tissue is deemed to be adequate. Recurrence is rarely noted.

The malignant oncocytic tumor or so-called malignant oncocytoma is rare. The diagnosis is based on atypical nuclear changes in conjunction with overall oncocytic cellular features. Malignant change may arise *de novo* or may occur in preexisting benign oncocytomas.

PAPILLARY CYSTADENOMA LYMPHOMATOSUM (WARTHIN'S TUMOR)

The papillary cystadenoma lymphomatosum, also known as Warthin's tumor, accounts for approximately 7% of epithelial neoplasms of salivary glands, with the vast majority occurring within the parotid gland. Intraorally, this lesion is rare. The papillary cystadenoma lymphomatosum is thought to arise within lymph nodes as a result

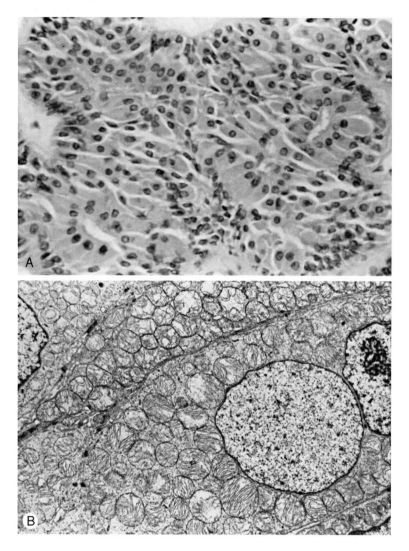

Figure 8–34. *A,* Oncocytoma. *B,* Ultrastructure of the same lesion showing tumor cells with abundant cytoplasmic mitochondria.

of entrapment of salivary gland elements early in development. This theory is supported by the occasional case of multicentricity as well as normal lymph node architecture surrounding many early or developing tumors. It is believed that some intraoral lesions may arise in an area of reactive lymphoid hyperplasia secondary to chronic inflammation.

When it occurs in the parotid, this tumor presents typically as a doughy to cystic mass in the inferior pole of the gland, adjacent and posterior to the angle of the mandible (Fig. 8–35). In this situation, the proximity of the submandibular gland may give the impression that the lesion has developed within this gland rather than within the parotid.

There is a distinct male predilection for Warthin's tumor, with an average male-to-female ratio of 5 to 1 noted in many older series. More re-

cently, however, case studies and larger series have reported more equal gender distribution, with only slight male predominance. The average age of onset is generally between the fifth and eighth decades of life. When bilaterality is noted (2 to 6% of cases), the growths may be multiple and synchronous or metachronous.

This lesion is also characterized on nuclear scan as being capable of technetium-99 uptake, and therefore it may appear as a so-called "hot" nodule. This tumor is encapsulated and has a smooth to lobulated surface and a round outline. Microscopically, numerous cystic spaces of irregular outline contain papillary projections lined by columnar eosinophilic cells (oncocytes) (Fig. 8–36). The lining cells are supported by reserve cells that are cuboidal and centrally nucleated. Squamous metaplasia of the lining cells may occasionally be seen. At the base of the cuboidal cell layer, a

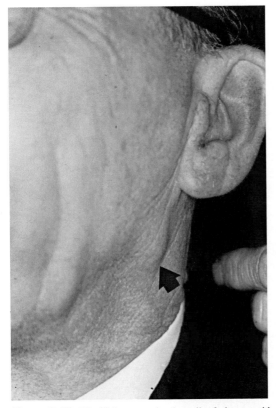

Figure 8–35. Warthin's tumor in the tail of the parotid gland *(arrow)*.

basement membrane separates the epithelium from an underlying lymphoid stroma. Germinal centers and sinusoidal spaces are typically seen.

The basis for the cytoplasmic granularity of the epithelial component relates to the presence of a large number of mitochondria within the cytoplasm. The lymphoid element is overwhelmingly composed of B lymphocytes.

Recurrences have been documented but are believed to represent second primary lesions or an expression of multiple lesions. Malignant transformation or carcinoma arising within this lesion is rarely encountered, but it may follow radiotherapy to the region. The type of malignancy arising in the majority of cases is squamous cell carcinoma, with fewer cases of adenocarcinoma and mucoepidermoid carcinoma reported.

Ductal Papillomas

Ductal papillomas consist of sialadenoma papilliferum, inverted ductal papilloma, and intraductal papilloma. These rare tumors are thought to arise within the interlobular and excretory duct portion of the salivary gland unit.

Sialadenoma papilliferum is an unusual benign salivary gland neoplasm first reported in 1969 as a distinct entity of minor and major salivary gland origin. The majority of cases reported subsequently have been found intraorally; the buccal mucosa and palate are the most common sites.

Sialadenoma papilliferum usually presents as a painless exophytic papillary lesion. Most cases have been reported in men between the fifth and eighth decades of life. In most reported cases, the clinical impression before removal is that of a simple papilloma, owing to its frequent keratotic appearance and papillary surface configuration.

This tumor appears to originate from the superficial portion of the salivary gland excretory duct. Papillary processes develop, forming convoluted clefts and spaces (Fig. 8–37). Each papillary projection is lined by a layer of epithelium approximately two to three cell layers thick and is supported by a core of fibrovascular connective tissue. The more superficial portions of the lesion demonstrate a squamous epithelial lining; deeper portions show more cuboidal to columnar cells, often oncocytic in appearance. As growth continues, the overlying mucous membrane becomes papillary to verrucous in nature, much like a squamous papilloma. This lesion generally resembles the syringocystadenoma papilliferum of the scalp, a lesion of eccrine sweat gland origin.

The behavior of this lesion is benign. Management is by conservative surgery; there is little chance for recurrence.

A related papillary lesion of salivary duct origin is the *inverted ductal papilloma*. This is a rare entity that presents as a nodular submucosal mass resembling a fibroma or lipoma. It is seen in adults and has an equal gender distribution.

Microscopically, the inverted ductal papilloma resembles the sialadenoma papilliferum (Fig. 8–38). Below an intact surface, a marked proliferation of ductal epithelium into the surrounding stromal tissue is noted. Crypts and cyst-like spaces lined by columnar cells with polarized nuclei are interspersed with goblet cells and transitional forms of cuboidal to squamous cells.

The third form of ductal papilloma is the *intraductal papilloma*. This rare lesion arises deeper from the surface, within the ductal system, often presenting as a salivary obstructive process. Histologically, a single or double layer of cuboidal to columnar epithelium covers several papillary fronds that project into a cystic space with no evidence of proliferation into the wall of the cyst. There is a striking histologic similarity of this lesion to intraductal papilloma of breast. Treatment for this lesion as well as the inverted ductal

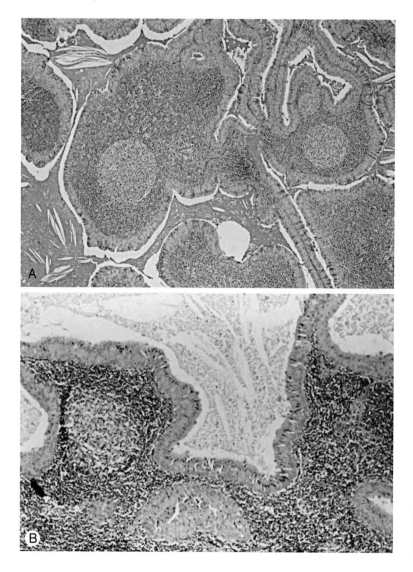

Figure 8–36. *A* and *B,* Warthin's tumor. Note the cystic spaces lined by columnar cells supported by lymphoid tissue.

papilloma is simple excision. There is little risk of recurrence.

MALIGNANT NEOPLASMS

The classification of malignant neoplasms is shown in Table 8–7.

Mucoepidermoid Carcinoma

The mucoepidermoid carcinoma has been a somewhat controversial lesion of salivary gland origin with respect to its biologic behavior and natural history. Evidence supports the opinion that all grades of mucoepidermoid lesions are carcinomas and have the potential to metastasize.

However, low-grade mucoepidermoid carcinomas typically pursue a locally invasive, relatively non-aggressive course. As the name implies, muco-epidermoid carcinomas are epithelial mucin-producing tumors. They are believed to arise from reserve cells in the interlobular and intralobular segments of the salivary duct system. The name of this tumor accurately reflects its biphasic structure of epidermoid and mucus-secreting cells. The neoplastic mucous cells contain neutral glycoproteins, acidic mucins, and sulfomucins; the epidermoid cells contain keratin intermediate filaments.

Clinical Features. The most common site of the mucoepidermoid carcinoma is the parotid gland, where 60 to 90% of such lesions are encountered. This lesion represents the most common malignant tumor of salivary gland and is also the most common salivary gland malignancy of

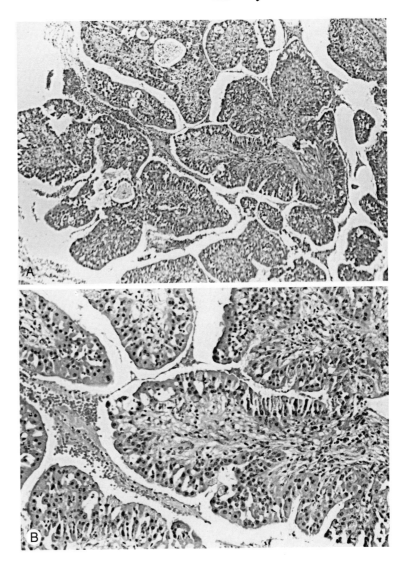

Figure 8–37. *A* and *B,* Sialadenoma papilliferum composed of epithelium-lined papillary projections.

childhood. Mucoepidermoid carcinomas account for approximately 34% of parotid malignancies, 20% of submandibular gland malignancies, and 29% of minor salivary gland malignancies (Table 8–8 and Figs. 8–39 and 8–40). This lesion may also arise centrally within the mandible (Fig. 8–41), presumably from embryonically entrapped salivary elements or from neoplastic transformation of mucous cells in odontogenic cysts.

The prevalence of mucoepidermoid carcinomas is noted to be highest in the third to fifth decades of life, and there is an equal gender representation. The mean duration between onset and diagnosis varies according to the histologic grade of the lesion—one study indicated a 6-year hiatus between onset and treatment. High-grade lesions demonstrate a 1.5-year interval before diagnosis.

The clinical manifestations of the mucoepidermoid carcinoma depend greatly on the grade of malignancy. Tumors of low-grade malignancy present with a prolonged period of painless enlargement. Within the oral cavity, the mucoepidermoid carcinoma often resembles an extravasation or retention-type mucocele that may at times be fluctuant as a result of cyst formation. Tumors of high-grade malignancy, on the other hand, grow rapidly and are often accompanied by pain and mucosal ulceration. Within the major salivary glands, high-grade tumors may present with evidence of facial nerve involvement or obstructive signs. In unusual circumstances in which mucoepidermoid carcinomas arise within the mandible or maxilla, they generally are detected as radiolucent lesions that are expansile and situated within the molar and premolar area. Radiographically, they must be separated from giant cell granuloma, odontogenic cysts, ameloblastoma, and other odontogenic tumors.

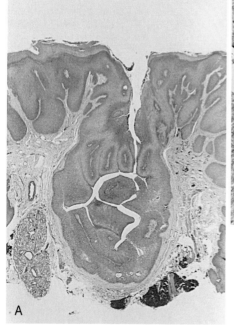

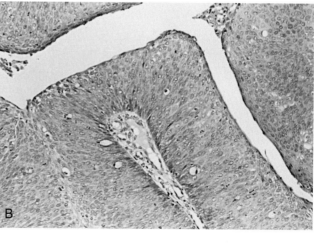

Figure 8–38. *A* and *B,* Inverted ductal papilloma.

Histopathology. Mucoepidermoid carcinomas are often well circumscribed, although the lesion typically demonstrates infiltration of adjacent tissue. Lesions are generally divided into high-grade and low-grade types. Intermediate-grade lesions have also been described and lie histologically and behaviorally between low- and high-grade lesions.

Most low-grade mucoepidermoid carcinomas are composed of mucus-secreting cells arranged around microcystic structures, often with an intermingling of intermediate or epidermoid cellular cells (Figs. 8–42 and 8–43). The mucin-containing cells are characterized by intracellular mucin, which may be demonstrated by PAS and mucicarmine positivity (Figs. 8–44 and 8–45). Coalescence of small cysts into large cystic spaces is typical of low-grade malignancy. These cysts may distend the surrounding supportive tissue and rupture, allowing escape of mucus into the surrounding tissues, with a concomitant reactive inflammatory response. At the margin of low-grade tumors, the pattern is often one of broad pushing fronts, a testament to the tumor's low-level invasiveness.

High-grade (and intermediate-grade) malignancies are characterized by neoplastic cell clusters

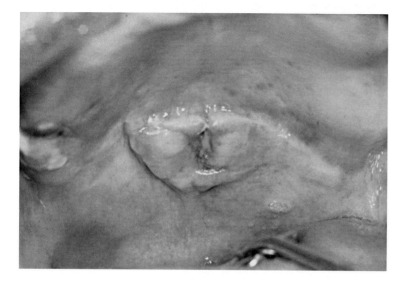

Figure 8–39. Mucoepidermoid carcinoma at the junction of the hard and soft palates.

Table 8–7. Classification of Malignant Neoplasms

CLASSIFICATION OF SALIVARY GLAND ADENOCARCINOMAS*

Mucoepidermoid carcinoma
Adenoid cystic carcinoma
Acinic cell carcinoma
Carcinoma ex-mixed tumor/malignant mixed tumor
Epimyoepithelial carcinoma
Polymorphous low-grade adenocarcinoma
Salivary duct carcinoma
Basal cell adenocarcinoma
Sebaceous adenocarcinoma
Oncocytic adenocarcinoma
Adenocarcinoma (*Not Otherwise Specified*)

CLASSIFICATION ACCORDING TO BIOLOGIC BEHAVIOR

Low grade
    Mucoepidermoid carcinoma (low grade)
    Acinic cell carcinoma
    Polymorphous low-grade adenocarcinoma
    Basal cell adenocarcinoma
Intermediate grade
    Mucoepidermoid carcinoma (intermediate grade)
    Epimyoepithelial carcinoma
    Sebaceous adenocarcinoma
High grade
    Mucoepidermoid carcinoma (high grade)
    Adenoid cystic carcinoma
    Carcinoma ex-mixed tumor/malignant mixed tumor
    Salivary duct carcinoma
    Squamous cell carcinoma
    Oncocytic adenocarcinoma

*In modification of Seifert G, Brocheriou C, Cardesa A, Eveson JW. WHO International Classification of Tumors. Tentative histological classification of salivary gland tumors. Pathol Res Pract 186:555–581, 1990.

that are more solid with fewer cystic spaces and mucous cells (Fig. 8–46). Larger numbers of epidermoid cells and intermediate cells are seen at the expense of more differentiated mucous cells.

Cellular pleomorphism, nuclear hyperchromatism, and mitotic figures may be noted within these tumors. In many high-grade mucoepidermoid carcinomas, much of the lesion may resemble squamous cell carcinoma, with only small numbers of mucous cells evident. In high-grade lesions, infiltration in the form of cords and strands of cells may be noted well beyond the obvious clinical focus of the tumor.

The pattern and proportion of mucous to epidermoid elements in metastatic foci may not resemble the primary lesion. Extremes of cellular type may be evident, with either mucous or epidermoid cells forming the predominant component.

Prognosis and Treatment. Prognostic significance may be ascribed to histologic grades of malignancy from low to high grade. Low-grade mucoepidermoid carcinomas characteristically follow a benign clinical course; however, in several instances low-grade lesions have metastasized widely. Clinical confirmation of the aggressiveness of high-grade carcinomas generally is evident within the first 5 years after the initial treatment, with local and distant metastases being evident in as many as 60% of cases. Incidences of metastases to cervical lymph nodes from mucoepidermoid carcinomas of the parotid gland (excluding low-grade lesions) have reached 44%. A 5-year survival of 95% or greater is associated with low-grade lesions. For high-grade lesions, however, survival rates are approximately 40%. In follow-up periods extended to 15 years, the cure rate for high-grade carcinomas drops to 25% or less.

Treatment of the primary malignancy is typically surgical. High-grade malignancies are usually managed with surgery plus postoperative radiotherapy to the primary site. Radical neck dissection is rarely performed in small lesions of

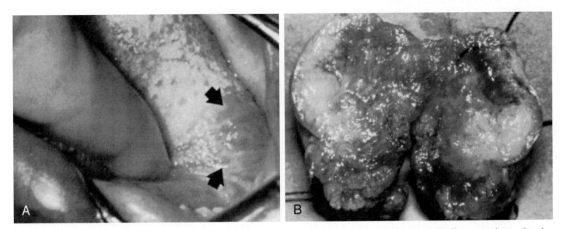

Figure 8–40. *A,* Mucoepidermoid carcinoma in the posterolateral aspect of the tongue *(arrows.)* *B,* Gross specimen showing infiltrative tumor as lighter-colored areas.

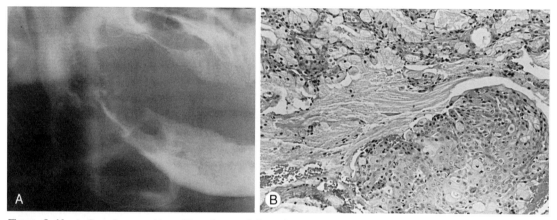

Figure 8–41. *A*, Central mucoepidermoid carcinoma of the molar-ramus area of the mandible. *B*, Biopsy specimen showing mucous and epidermoid cells in a low-grade tumor.

Table 8–8. Malignant Salivary Gland Tumors

TUMOR	PAROTID	SUBMANDIBULAR	SUBLINGUAL	MINOR	TOTAL
Mucoepidermoid carcinoma	593	73	8	253	927
Adenoid cystic carcinoma	180	148	7	388	723
Acinic cell carcinoma	241	8	8	25	282
Malignant mixed tumor	257	54	—	66	377
Adenocarcinoma	318	53	—	243	614
Squamous cell carcinoma	83	23	1	5	112
Other	60	17	—	38	115
Total	1732	376	24	1018	3150

Compiled from Chaudhry AP, et al. Cancer 58:72, 1986; Chen SY, et al. Cancer 42:678, 1978; Ellis GL, et al. Cancer 52:542, 1983; Evans HL, et al. Cancer 53:935, 1985; Luna MA, et al. Oral Surg Oral Med Oral Pathol 59:482, 1985; Perzin KH, et al. Cancer 42:265, 1978; Ranko RM, et al. Am J Surg 118:790, 1969; Spiro RH, et al. Am J Surg 130:452, 1975; and Spiro RH, et al. Cancer 39:388, 1977.

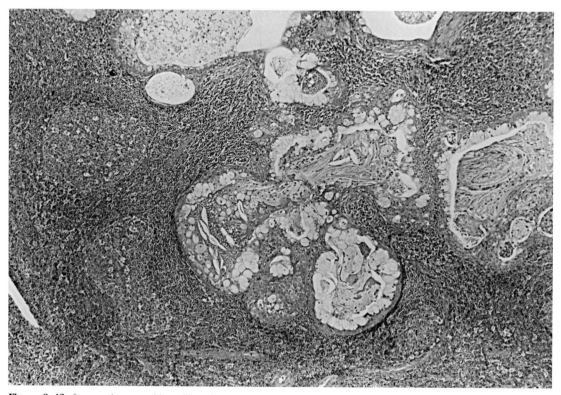

Figure 8–42. Low-grade mucoepidermoid carcinoma metastatic to a cervical lymph node.

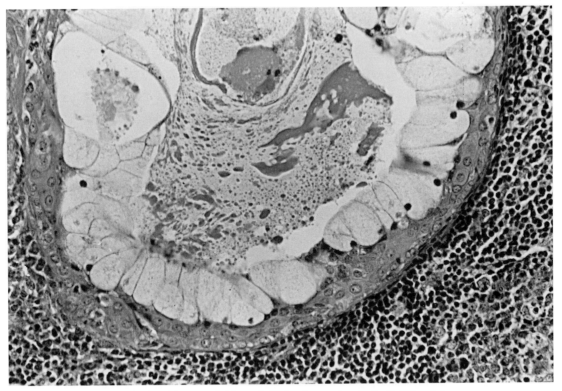

Figure 8–43. High magnification of the tumor in Figure 8–42 showing mucin goblet cell differentiation.

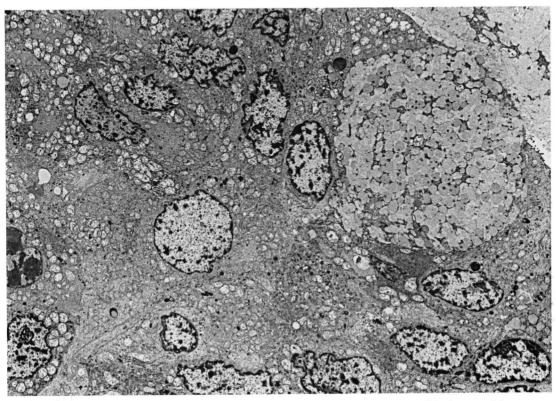

Figure 8–44. Electron micrograph of low-grade mucoepidermoid carcinoma. Note the mucous cell in the upper right.

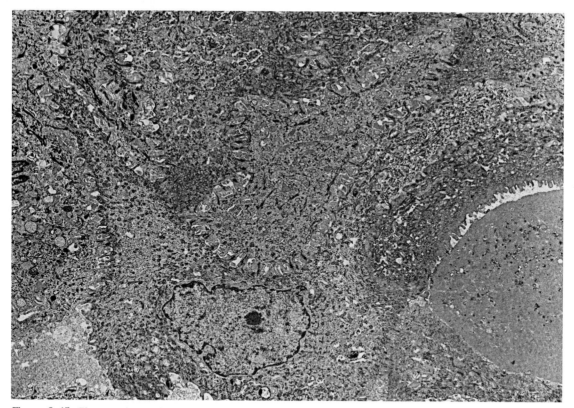

Figure 8–45. Electron micrograph of low-grade mucoepidermoid carcinoma. Tonofilaments can be seen in the cytoplasm of most cells, and desmosomes can be seen between cells.

low-grade malignancy; high-grade tumors usually require this form of management.

Central mucoepidermoid carcinomas are usually of low-grade behavior and histology. Most deaths were attributed to uncontrolled local recurrence, with occasional regional lymph node metastasis reported. This tumor, when arising in bone, has been associated with a 40% recurrence rate after simple curettage.

Adenoid Cystic Carcinoma

Adenoid cystic carcinoma (adenocystic carcinoma) has been portrayed as one of the most biologically deceptive and frustrating of all tumors in the head and neck region. This form of adeno-carcinoma is distinctive and merits separation from other forms of glandular neoplasia because of its microscopic appearance, behavioral characteristics, high rate of local recurrence, and systemic spread.

The origin of adenoid cystic carcinoma is thought to be from the intercalated duct reserve cell or terminal tubule complex. Differentiation is believed to be along the intercalated duct cell line.

Clinical Features. This lesion accounts for approximately 23% of all salivary gland carcinomas. Approximately 50 to 70% of all reported cases of adenoid cystic carcinoma occur in minor salivary glands of the head and neck. In the major salivary glands, the parotid gland is most often affected.

Most patients with adenoid cystic carcinoma are between the fifth and seventh decades of life. There is no gender predilection, although a slight female predominance is noted for lesions arising in the submandibular gland.

In the major salivary glands, the clinical appearance is usually that of a unilobular mass that is firm on palpation, occasionally with some pain or tenderness. These lesions generally are characterized by a slow growth rate; they have often been present for several years before the patient's seeking treatment. Facial nerve weakness or paralysis may occasionally be the initial presenting symptom, especially in late-stage lesions.

Bone invasion occurs frequently, initially without radiographic changes because of infiltration through marrow spaces. Distant spread to the lungs is more common than is metastasis to regional lymph nodes. Also of interest is the tendency for tumor invasion of perineural spaces,

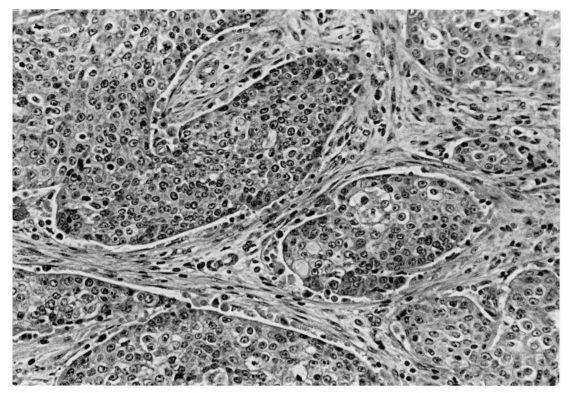

Figure 8–46. High-grade mucoepidermoid carcinoma.

with the neoplasm often found well beyond the site of clinical disease. A frequent feature of intraoral lesions, particularly those arising on the palate, is ulceration of the overlying mucosa, a point often used to help clinically distinguish this lesion from the more common benign mixed tumor (Fig. 8–47).

Histopathology. The standard light microscopic feature of adenoid cystic carcinoma is a cribriform of cylindromatous pattern (Figs. 8–48 and 8–49), a tubular-trabecular pattern, a solid basaloid pattern of growth, or a combination of these. Some controversy surrounds the prognosis relative to these histologic variants, but it is thought that the solid basaloid pattern is associated with a poorer overall outcome. Areas of central necrosis within solid clusters of cells may indicate a more aggressive form of disease. More important factors regarding prediction of behavior include size of the primary lesion, anatomic location, presence or absence of metastatic disease at time of diagnosis, and facial nerve involvement.

Individual cells composing the tumor are small and cuboidal, with disproportionately large isomorphic nuclei. Nuclear atypia is absent or minimal, and mitotic figures are usually not seen. Chromatin aggregation is dense, and nuclear contours are even.

The distinctive morphology of this neoplasm relates to formation of pseudocystic spaces that contain various acellular substances. This material consists chiefly of sulfated mucopolysaccharides that are ultrastructurally characterized by multilayered or replicated basal lamina material. Myoepithelial cells may represent a minor part of the cellular component of adenocystic carcinomas. Occasionally, both myoepithelial and ductal elements are arranged in a pattern that mimics normal ducts in which there is an inner row of small cuboidal cells surrounded by larger myoepithelial cells. An important distinctive microscopic feature is perineural and intraneural invasion (Fig. 8–50).

Treatment and Prognosis. Regardless of the site of the primary lesion, surgery is regarded as the treatment of choice for adenoid cystic carcinomas. When the parotid glands are involved, wide resection in the form of a superficial parotidectomy or superficial and deep lobectomy is recommended. In the parotid region, the debate is whether or not the facial nerve should be spared; most investigators recommend resection only if the tumor surrounds or invades this nerve.

Intraorally, wide excision, often with removal of underlying bone, is the treatment of choice. Radical surgical excision may be justified to obtain surgical margins that are free of tumor.

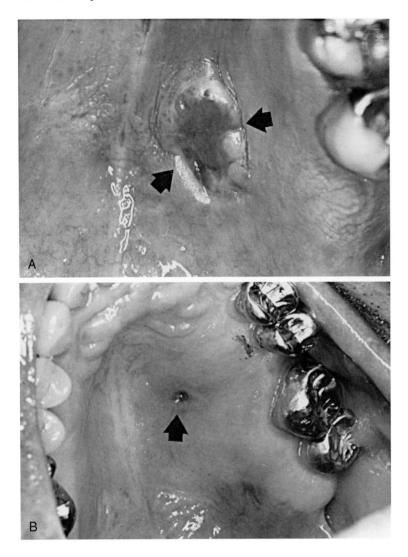

Figure 8–47. *A* and *B,* Adenoid cystic carcinomas of the hard palate *(arrows).*

Postsurgical radiation therapy has shown promising results and has a role in the management of recurrence. Chemotherapy is currently regarded as ineffective. Multiple-agent chemotherapy has, however, shown some promise in management of widely metastatic disease.

The prognosis for patients with adenoid cystic carcinoma must be judged not in terms of 5-year survival rates but rather in terms of 15- to 20-year survival rates. Survival rates at 5 years approximate 70%; at 15 years the rate is only 10%. Factors that negatively influence prognosis include the presence of tumor at the line of surgical excision, tumor size greater than 4 cm, and the presence of more than 30% of a solid pattern within the tumor. A long survival time has been positively correlated with a greater number of gland-like spaces per square millimeter within the tumor.

Acinic Cell Carcinoma

The acinic cell carcinoma is a distinctive neoplasm of salivary gland origin. The preponderance of cases are reported in major salivary glands, especially the parotid. The putative origin of the acinic cell carcinoma is from the intercalated duct reserve cell, although there is reason to believe that the acinic cell itself retains the potential for neoplastic transformation. It has been suggested that the acinic cell carcinoma may represent an integrated proliferation of intercalated and acinic precursors and, less commonly, myoepithelial cells. The neoplastic elements may be organized in a fashion simulating the acinar intercalated duct unit.

Clinical Features. The acinic cell carcinoma may be found in all age groups, including chil-

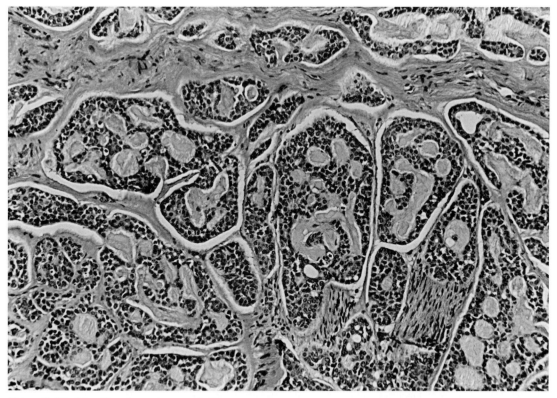

Figure 8–48. Adenoid cystic carcinoma, cribriform pattern.

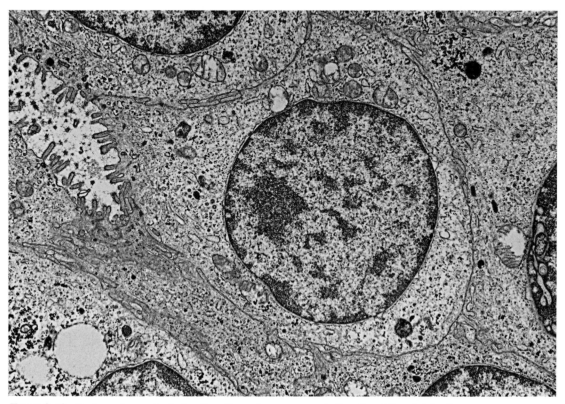

Figure 8–49. Electron micrograph of adenoid cystic carcinoma composed of small undifferentiated cells.

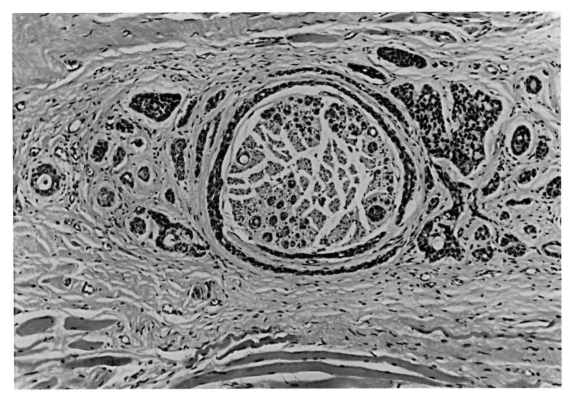

Figure 8–50. Adenoid cystic carcinoma showing perineural invasion.

dren, with the peak incidence noted within the fifth and sixth decades of life. There appears to be no gender predilection.

This lesion accounts for 14% of all parotid gland tumors and 9% of the total of salivary gland carcinomas of all sites. An unusual feature is its frequency of bilateral parotid gland involvement in approximately 3% of cases. Most cases develop within the superficial lobe and inferior pole of the parotid gland. Far fewer cases have been reported within the submandibular and intraoral minor salivary glands. Within the oral cavity, most cases occur in the palate and buccal mucosa.

Acinic cell carcinomas usually present as slow-growing lesions less than 3 cm in diameter. Although it is not indicative of prognosis, pain is a frequent presenting symptom. The interval between the initial appearance of the mass and treatment varies from 6 months to 5 years. In nearly half of all cases, the clinical impression is that of a benign lesion.

Histopathology. In at least one third of acinic cell carcinomas, a marked cystic growth pattern can be noted. Large lobules or nests of tumor cells with little intervening stroma are characteristic. The arrangement of neoplastic cells is quite variable, with several growth patterns evident. Generally, cells are arranged in solid masses with blunted or pushing margins. The solid pattern of growth is the most common (Fig. 8–51), followed closely by a trabecular pattern. Other variations include microcystic, papillary cystic, and follicular forms.

The predominant cell type is the well-differentiated acinar cell containing cytoplasmic granules varying from finely diffuse to large and coarse. Granules are PAS positive and identical to those found in normal acinic cells. Intercalated duct-type cells are seen in approximately one third of cases, and nonspecific and vacuolated cells are seen in nearly one fourth of cases. Many acinic cell carcinomas demonstrate occasional clear cell elements, and rare examples are found to be composed entirely of clear cells.

Ultrastructurally, acinic tumor cells reflect normal acinar elements with large amounts of rough endoplasmic reticulum, well-developed Golgi complexes, and secretory granule formation (Fig. 8–52). The granules demonstrate maturation as they approach the apical portion of the cytoplasm, where they ultimately fuse with the plasma membrane and lose their contents through exocytosis.

Treatment and Prognosis. Surgery is the preferred treatment. In general, acinic cell carcinomas seldom metastasize, yet they have a strong tendency to recur. Determinant survival rates of 89%

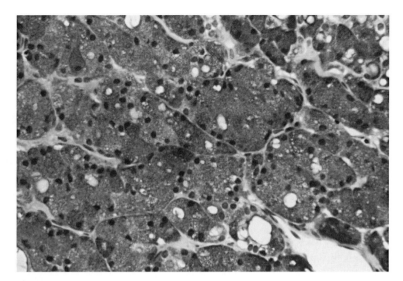

Figure 8–51. Acinic cell carcinoma. Tumor cell cytoplasm is granular and basophilic.

at 5 years and 56% at 20 years indicate their overall malignant nature. Metastases to regional lymph nodes occur in approximately 10% of cases, whereas distant metastases occur in approximately 15% of cases. It has been found that neither morphologic pattern nor cell composition is a predictable prognostic feature. Unfavorable prognostic features include pain or fixation to surrounding tissue, gross tumor invasion into adjacent tissue, and microscopic features of desmoplasia, cellular atypia, and increased mitotic activity.

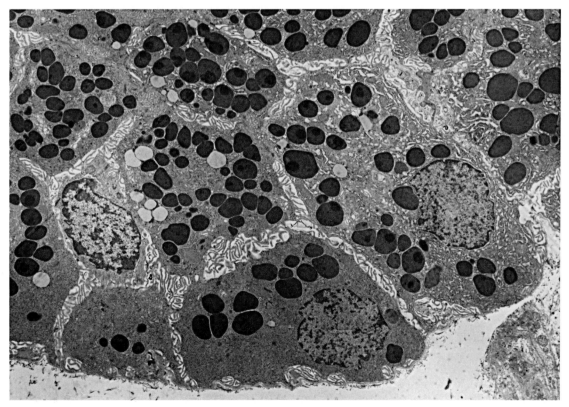

Figure 8–52. Electron micrograph of acinic cell carcinoma. Tumor cells contain dark secretory granules.

Carcinoma Ex-mixed Tumor/ Malignant Mixed Tumor

Carcinoma ex-mixed tumor represents an epithelial malignancy arising in a preexisting mixed tumor where such remnants may be identified. When metastatic disease occurs, only the malignant component metastasizes. This is more common than the so-called malignant mixed tumor.

Two types of *malignant mixed tumor* have been recognized. One type is a malignancy in which both the epithelial and the mesenchymal components are malignant; hence a carcinosarcoma designation could be used. In metastatic sites, both elements are present. The second type of malignant mixed tumor is characterized by a histologically benign mixed tumor that for some reason metastasizes while still retaining its bland, benign histologic appearance.

In summary, therefore, the malignant mixed tumor represents three separate entities that are histologically distinct. These include the carcinoma arising within a mixed tumor (carcinoma ex-mixed tumor), the carcinosarcoma or true malignant mixed tumor, and the metastasizing mixed tumor.

Clinical Features. The carcinoma ex-mixed tumor usually arises from an untreated benign mixed tumor known to be present for several years (Fig. 8–53) or from a benign mixed tumor that has had many recurrences over many years. Malignancy occurring within a previously benign tumor is heralded by rapid growth after an extremely long period of minimally perceptible increase.

Approximately 68% of carcinoma ex-mixed tumors and malignant mixed tumors are found in the parotid gland, and 18% are found in the minor intraoral salivary glands. The average age when malignancy becomes evident is 60 years, approximately 20 years beyond the age noted for benign mixed tumor. Suspicious signs of malignancy include fixation of the mass to surrounding tissues, ulceration, and regional lymphadenopathy.

Histopathology. The margins of carcinoma ex-mixed tumors and malignant mixed tumors are generally well defined, although infiltrative areas are likely to be present. Necrosis and hemorrhage with areas of dystrophic mineralization are frequently noted. Most areas of malignancy appear as adenoid cystic carcinoma, undifferentiated carcinoma, or a combination of both (Fig. 8–54).

When present, metastatic deposits histologically mimic the primary lesion. Chondroid patterns may be evident in metastatic deposits, also mimicking the primary tumor.

Treatment and Prognosis. Treatment is almost exclusively surgical, with radical neck dissection

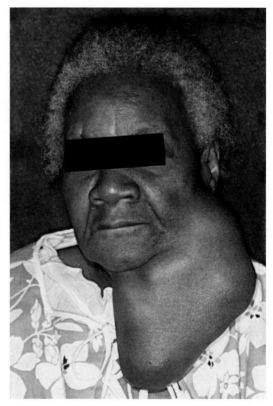

Figure 8–53. Carcinoma ex-mixed tumor occurring in a long-standing mixed tumor.

part of the initial treatment in patients with evidence of cervical lymph node involvement.

Local recurrence is a problem in nearly half of patients with primary parotid neoplasms and in nearly three fourths of patients with submandibular and minor salivary gland tumors. Approximately 10% of cases present with uncontrollable lymphatic disease, with nearly one third of these showing metastasis to distant sites, usually to lung and bone.

Determinant cure rates at 5, 10, and 15 years after treatment in one study were 40%, 24%, and 19%, respectively; in another study, 30% of those monitored for 10 years were free of disease.

Epimyoepithelial Carcinoma

Generally, salivary gland tumors composed of optically clear cells may be derived from intercalated duct cells, reserve cells, myoepithelial cells, mucous cells, sebaceous cells, and acinar cells. Cytoplasmic optical clarity is thought to result from minimal cellular differentiation and lack of organelles; from storage or accumulation of cytoplasmic elements such as glycogen, mucin, and

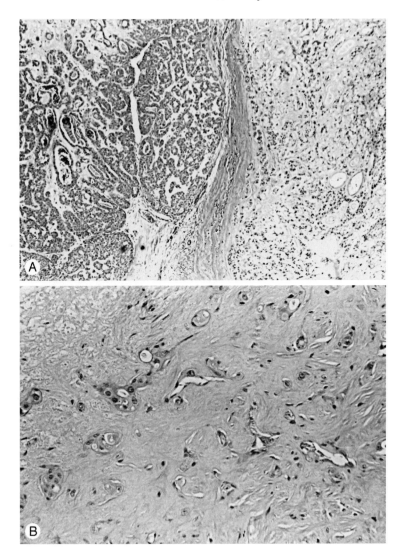

Figure 8–54. *A* and *B,* Carcinoma ex-mixed tumor. Neoplastic cells are hyperchromatic and pleomorphic.

lipid or clear secretory granules; or from fixation artifact. Clear cells may therefore be encountered in numerous salivary gland tumors, including mucoepidermoid carcinomas and sebaceous neoplasms, and in organelle-poor cells within benign mixed tumors, acinar cell carcinomas, and monomorphic adenomas. When these tumors are eliminated in a differential diagnosis of a clear cell tumor, most of the remainder probably belong in the epimyoepithelial carcinoma category, or possibly clear cell carcinoma.

Clear cell carcinoma (formerly, hyalinizing clear cell carcinoma) is a rare salivary gland tumor composed of a single cell type. Clear tumor cells form a trabecular or nested pattern and are PAS positive and mucin negative. Immunohistochemically, cells are keratin positive, but S-100 protein and muscle specific actin negative. A hyalinized stroma is often seen. This is a low grade malignancy and should be treated as such.

Clinical Features. The peak incidence of the epimyoepithelial carcinoma is within the seventh and eighth decades of life. There is a two-to-one female predilection. Approximately 5% occur within the intraoral minor salivary glands, whereas nearly 85% occur within the parotid gland, and the balance within the submandibular glands. Presentation is generally as a soft tissue mass and lack of symptoms with peripheral nerve involvement noted in approximately one fourth of cases.

Histopathology. A multinodular growth pattern characterizes epimyoepithelial carcinoma. Nodules of tumor are composed of two cell types, generally in a duct-like arrangement (Fig. 8–55). A row of cuboidal, darkly staining cells form

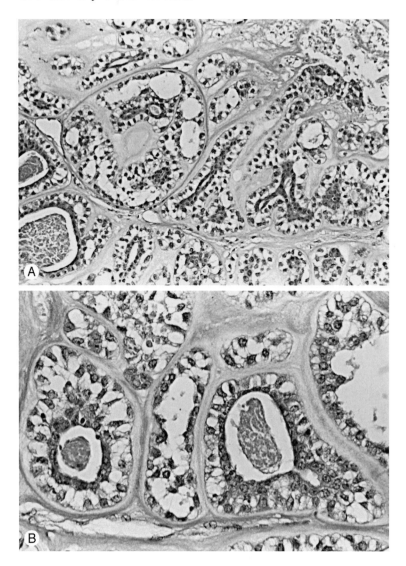

Figure 8–55. *A* and *B,* Epimyoepithelial carcinoma.

a lumen, often containing PAS-positive material. These ductal cells are surrounded by one or several layers of myoepithelial cells that are characterized by a columnar to ovoid outline with pale or clear cytoplasm. Large concentrations of cytoplasmic glycogen may be present in these cells. Immunohistochemical studies have shown the presence of actin and S-100 protein in the clear cell component, supporting their myoepithelial origin. Clusters or lobules of tumor epithelium are surrounded by a hyalinized, cell-poor matrix. Extensions of tumor beyond an incomplete capsule are frequently noted. Areas of necrosis may also be evident on occasion.

Ultrastructurally, both ductal and myoepithelial elements have been confirmed and substantiate the earlier conclusions about histogenesis and cellular origins of this lesion. Although such lesions usually appear in the parotid, they make up less than 1% of parotid gland neoplasms.

Treatment of epimyoepithelial carcinoma is essentially surgical. When it occurs in the parotid gland, superficial parotidectomy is the treatment of choice; neck dissection is reserved for patients demonstrating lymphadenopathy. Recurrences have most frequently been associated with lesions greater than 3 cm. The overall recurrence and metastasis rates, however, are low, with this lesion best regarded as a low-grade malignancy. Recurrences are common, but death as a direct result of widespread tumor is uncommon.

Polymorphous Low-Grade Adenocarcinoma

Polymorphous low-grade adenocarcinoma (lobular carcinoma, terminal duct carcinoma) has been recently segregated from other salivary tumors because of its distinctive clinical, histomorpho-

Table 8–9. Polymorphous Low-Grade Adenocarcinoma (1987)

LOCATION	NUMBER	PERCENT
Palate	39	62
Buccal mucosa	8	13
Upper lip	6	10
Retromolar	4	6
Base of tongue	2	3
Pterygomandibular raphe	2	3
Mandibular mucosa	1	1.5
Maxillary tuberosity	1	1.5

Compiled from Batsakis JG. Ann Otol Rhinol Laryngol 89:196, 1980; Eneroth CM. Cancer 27:1415, 1971; Eveson JW, et al. J Pathol 146:51, 1985; Freedman P, et al. Oral Surg Oral Med Oral Pathol 56:157, 1983; and Spiro RH. Head Neck Surg 8:177, 1986.

logic, and behavioral aspects. This tumor is generally considered to be a low-grade malignancy with a relatively indolent course and low risk of metastasis.

The origin of the polymorphous low-grade adenocarcinoma is believed to be the most proximal portion of the salivary duct. Both myoepithelial and ductal elements appear to participate in the growth of this tumor. In some areas, these lesions resemble other forms of salivary neoplasia that histogenetically arise from the intercalated duct reserve cell system.

Clinical Features. This neoplasm occurs in the fifth through eighth decades of life, with a mean age of 59 years. There is no gender predilection. The lesion occurs almost exclusively in minor salivary glands, with the palate being the most frequently reported site (Table 8–9). Polymorphous low-grade adenocarcinomas typically present as firm, elevated, nonulcerated, nodular swell-ings that are usually nontender. A wide range in size has been noted, but most are between 1 and 4 cm in diameter. The slow growth rate is evidenced by the long duration—many months to years—before diagnosis and treatment. Neurologic symptoms are usually not reported in association with this tumor.

Histopathology. Absence of encapsulation and a general lobular morphology characterize this group of low-grade adenocarcinomas. Infiltration into the surrounding salivary gland and connective tissue is evident at low-power examination (Fig. 8–56). In most areas, the tumor is composed of a homogeneous population of cells with prominent, bland nuclei and minimal cytoplasm. These cells are arranged in lobules as well as in solid nests (Fig. 8–57). Tubules lined by a single layer of cells are also typical of this tumor. Cribriform structures bearing a close resemblance to adenoid cystic carcinoma may also be seen. Tumor cells, often spindled, are also arranged in trabeculae and narrow cords. Striking patterns in which concentric arrangements of individual cells appear around blood vessels and nerves may be noted. The perineural pattern of growth is similar to that seen in the adenoid cystic carcinoma. In the latter, larger nerve trunks are generally involved; polymorphous low-grade adenocarcinoma seems to affect chiefly small nerve twigs. The epithelial and myoepithelial components of this lesion are scattered in a stroma that may be hyalinized. Necrosis and mitotic figures are usually absent.

Treatment and Prognosis. The indolent nature of this tumor mandates conservative surgical excision. Perineural invasion by this malignancy does not appear to affect prognosis. In the rare cases in

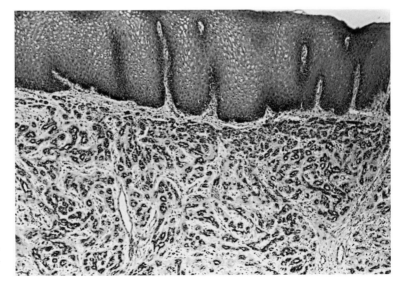

Figure 8–56. Polymorphous low-grade adenocarcinoma in oral mucous membrane.

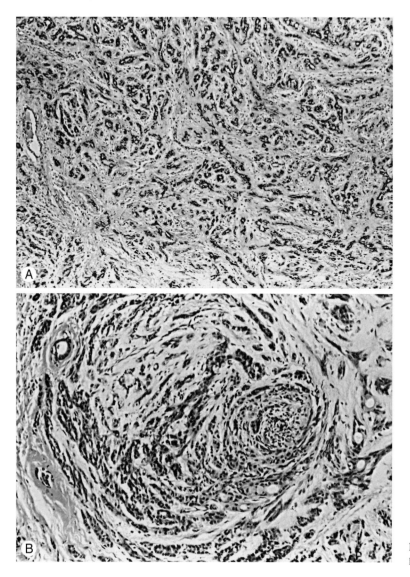

Figure 8–57. *A* and *B,* Polymorphous low-grade adenocarcinoma.

which cervical lymph node involvement is noted, appropriate surgical dissection is indicated.

The prognosis of this low-grade malignancy is generally good, although long-term follow-up should be part of patient management.

Salivary Duct Carcinoma

Salivary duct carcinoma is a high-grade malignancy of major salivary glands.

Clinical Features. The salivary duct carcinoma is characterized clinically by a distinctive predominance in the parotid gland (over 80% of cases); the submandibular gland accounts for the balance. Nearly 80% of cases have been recorded in males, and the overall peak incidence is in the seventh decade. The lesion arises as a firm, painless mass. It is generally brought to the clinician's attention within 1 year of onset.

Histopathology. A striking microscopic resemblance to ductal carcinomas originating in the breast is noted, with architectural features that include papillary cribriform and solid growth patterns along with a desmoplastic stroma and comedo necrosis (Fig. 8–58). Cellular features include an eosinophilic cytoplasm and occasional accumulations of intracytoplasmic mucin. Nuclear atypia is noted. In general, few mitoses are seen. Most tumors have infiltrative margins, with neural invasion evident in approximately 50% of cases (Fig. 8–59).

Surgical excision is indicated for this lesion, with concomitant neck dissection or postoperative

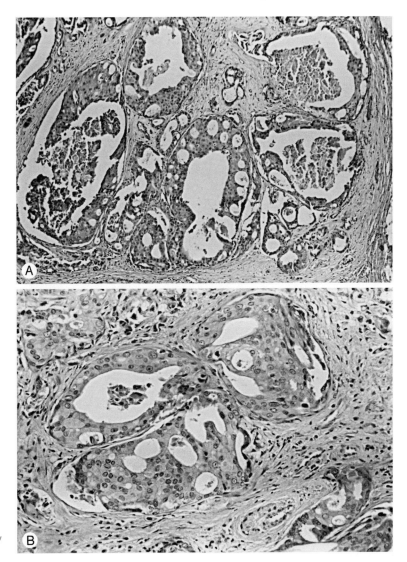

Figure 8–58. *A* and *B,* Salivary duct carcinoma.

irradiation or both. The role of chemotherapy is yet to be determined. In cases of advanced disease, combination therapy has not altered prognosis. Large series indicate that more than 50% of patients die of their disease within 5 months to 6 years after treatment. Pulmonary and osseous metastases are frequently noted.

Squamous Cell Carcinoma

Squamous cell carcinoma arising within the salivary glands is a rare event. The submandibular gland is most commonly involved, followed by the parotid. Obstructive sialadenitis (more common in the submandibular gland) has been thought to be a predisposing condition. Most patients tend to be in the seventh decade of life or beyond.

Squamous cell carcinomas of the parotid gland and submandibular glands are generally well to moderately well differentiated with no evidence of mucin production. Metastatic squamous cell carcinoma and high-grade mucoepidermoid carcinoma are usually alternative diagnoses.

Local recurrence and regional lymph node metastasis are common events, and distant metastasis is unusual. Surgery is the treatment of choice. As with most other salivary gland malignancies, ultimate survival relates more to the clinical stage than to histologic differentiation.

Basal Cell Adenocarcinoma

This rare tumor of major salivary glands is believed to be the malignant counterpart of the basal cell adenoma. It appears microscopically similar to the basal cell adenoma, except that it

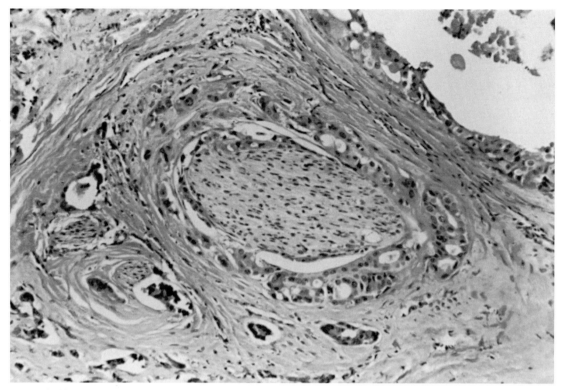

Figure 8–59. Salivary duct carcinoma showing perineural invasion.

exhibits an infiltrative growth pattern and has the ability to metastasize. These tumors are composed of nests, cords, and solid zones of basaloid cells. Two cytologic types of cells are frequently seen: small compact cells and larger polygonal cells. The former may frequently be seen surrounding the latter, often in a palisaded fashion. The feature that separates this tumor from the basal cell adenoma is the finding of small nests of neoplasm in adjacent normal structures. Infiltration of nerve is also seen. Local recurrence and distant metastasis seem to be distinct potentials for basal cell adenocarcinoma. Nonetheless, this tumor is generally regarded as a low-grade malignancy. With adequate surgical treatment, patients should have a favorable outcome.

Adenocarcinoma

By definition, any malignancy arising from salivary duct epithelium or within salivary glands of epithelial origin is an adenocarcinoma. This term, however, is less commonly used as a specific diagnostic entity, because most classification systems have broken down this complex group of neoplasms into discrete entities. The entities may be defined primarily by structure but also by be-

havior. After recognition of polymorphous low-grade adenocarcinoma, salivary duct carcinoma, and epimyoepithelial carcinoma, the small remaining group of salivary carcinomas with no specific designation may be categorized as adenocarcinomas.

The utility of the "not otherwise specified" adenocarcinoma heading relates to the undifferentiated carcinoma. Owing to a near-total lack of differentiation, placement in existing categories becomes impossible. High-grade malignancies, such as salivary duct carcinomas and mucoepidermoid carcinomas, may have similar features but also may have other microscopic elements that permit their diagnosis.

Microscopically, undifferentiated carcinomas vary from solid to trabecular, with cell types ranging from spindle to round and small. The small cell carcinoma, although suggesting a neuroectodermal origin, has yet to be shown to possess the appropriate neurosecretory granular component necessary for that diagnosis. Most authorities believe that the small cell carcinoma of salivary gland origin merely represents a variant of anaplastic carcinoma. Because undifferentiated adenocarcinomas are of a high-grade type, a correspondingly poor prognosis is noted, even with radical or combination therapy.

Bibliography

Reactive Lesions (Noninfectious)

Allard RHB, van der Kwast WAM, van der Waal I. Mucosal antral cysts: review of the literature and report of a radiographic survey. Oral Surg Oral Med Oral Pathol 51:2–9, 1981.

Brannon R, Fowler C, Hartman K. Necrotizing sialometaplasia: a clinico-pathologic study of sixty-nine cases and review of the literature. Oral Surg Oral Med Oral Pathol 72:317–325, 1991.

Buchner A, Merrel PW, Carpenter WM, Leider AS. Adenomatoid hyperplasia of minor salivary glands. Oral Surg Oral Med Oral Pathol 71:583–587, 1991.

Epstein J, Schubert M. Synergistic effect of sialogogues in management of xerostomia after radiation therapy. Oral Surg Oral Med Oral Pathol 64:179–182, 1987.

Eveson JW. Superficial mucoceles: pitfall in clinical and microscopic diagnosis. Oral Surg Oral Med Oral Pathol 66:318–322, 1988.

Gardner DG. Pseudocysts and retention cysts of the maxillary sinus. Oral Surg Oral Med Oral Pathol 58:561–567, 1984.

Jensen JL. Superficial mucoceles of the oral mucosa. Am J Dermatopathol 12:88–92, 1990.

McClatchey KD, Appelblatt NH, Zarbo RJ. Plunging ranula. Oral Surg Oral Med Oral Pathol 57:408–412, 1984.

Stephens LC, Schultheiss TE, Price RE, et al. Radiation apoptosis of serous acinar cells of salivary and lacrimal glands. Cancer 67:1539–1543, 1991.

Wolff A, Fox PC, Ship JA, et al. Oral mucosal status and major salivary gland function. Oral Surg Oral Med Oral Pathol 70:49–54, 1990.

Infectious Conditions

DeLuke DM, Sciubba JJ. Oral manifestations of sarcoidosis: report of a case masquerading as a neoplasm. Oral Surg Oral Med Oral Pathol 59:184–188, 1985.

Drosos AA, Constantopoulos SH, Psychos D, et al. The forgotten cause of sicca complex: sarcoidosis. J Rheumatol 16:1548–1557, 1989.

Galili D, Marmary Y. Spontaneous regeneration of parotid gland following juvenile recurrent parotitis. Oral Surg Oral Med Oral Pathol 60:605–607, 1985.

Gronhagen-Riska C, Fyhrquist F, von Willebrand E. Angiotensin I-converting enzyme: a marker of highly differentiated monocytic cells. Ann N Y Acad Sci 465:242–249, 1986.

Harvey J, Catoggio L, Gallagher PJ, Maddison PJ. Salivary gland biopsy in sarcoidosis. Sarcoidosis 6:47–50, 1989.

Marder M, Barr C, Mandel I. Cytomegalovirus presence and salivary composition in acquired immunodeficiency syndrome. Oral Surg Oral Med Oral Pathol 60:372–376, 1985.

Mitchell I, Turk J, Mitchell D. Detection of mycobacterial rRNA in sarcoidosis with liquid-phase hybridization. Lancet 339:1015–1017, 1992.

Saboor S, Johnson N, McFadden J. Detection of mycobacterial DNA in sarcoidosis and tuberculosis with polymerase chain reaction. Lancet 339:1012–1015, 1992.

Conditions Associated with Immune Defects

Alexander EL, Hirsch TJ, Arnett FC, et al. Ro (SSA) and La (SSB) antibodies in the clinical spectrum of Sjögren's syndrome. J Rheumatol 9:239–246, 1982.

Atkinson JC, Travis WD, Pillemer SR, et al. Major salivary function in primary Sjögren's syndrome and its relationship to clinical features. J Rheumatol 17:318–322, 1990.

Caselitz J, Osborn M, Wustrow J, et al. Immunohistochemical investigations on the epimyoepithelial islands in lymphoepithelial lesions. Lab Invest 55:427–432, 1986.

Daniels T. Clinical assessment and diagnosis of immunologically mediated salivary gland disease in Sjögren's syndrome. J Autoimmun 2:529–541, 1989.

Daniels TE, Fox PC. Salivary and oral components of Sjögren's syndrome. Rheum Dis Clin North Am 18:571–589, 1992.

Daniels TE, Whitcher JP. Association of patterns of labial salivary gland inflammation with keratoconjunctivitis sicca. Arthritis Rheum 37:869–877, 1994.

Falzon M, Isaacson PG. The natural history of benign lymphoepithelial lesion of the salivary gland in which there is a monoclonal population of B-cells. Am J Surg Pathol 15:59–65, 1991.

Fishleder A, Tubbs R, Hesse B, Levine H. Uniform detection of immunoglobulin-gene rearrangement in benign lymphoepithelial lesions. N Engl J Med 316:1118–1121, 1987.

Fox PC, van der Ven PF, Sonies BC, et al. Xerostomia evaluation of a symptom with increasing significance. J Am Dent Assoc 110:519–525, 1985.

Fox RI, Howell FV, Bone RC, et al. Primary Sjögren's syndrome: clinical and immunopathologic features. Semin Arthritis Rheum 14:77–105, 1984.

Fox RI, Luppi M, Kang HI, Pisa P. Reactivation of Epstein-Barr virus in Sjögren's syndrome. Springer Semin Immunopathol 13:217–231, 1991.

Fox RI, Robinson CA, Curd JG, et al. Sjögren's syndrome: proposed criteria for classification. Arthritis Rheum 29:577–585, 1986.

Garry RF, Fermin CD, Darrenn JH, et al. Detection of a human intracisternal A-type retroviral particle antigenically related to HIV. Science 250:1127–1129, 1990.

Hernandez Y, Daniels T. Oral Candidiasis in Sjögren's syndrome: prevalence, clinical correlations, and treatment. Oral Surg Oral Med Oral Pathol 68:324–329, 1989.

Jordan R, Diss TC, Lench NJ, et al. Immunoglobulin gene rearrangements in lymphoplasmacytic infiltrates of labial salivary glands in Sjögren's syndrome. Oral Surg Oral Med Oral Pathol 79:723–729, 1995.

Reichlin M. Significance of the Ro antigen system. J Clin Immunol 6:339–348, 1986.

Schiodt M. HIV-associated salivary gland disease: a review. Oral Surg Oral Med Oral Pathol 73:164–167, 1992.

Talal N. Immunologic and viral factors in Sjögren's syndrome. Clin Exp Rheumatol 8(Suppl 5): 23–26, 1990.

Talal N, Dauphinee MJ, Dang H, et al. Detection of serum antibodies to retroviral proteins in patients with primary Sjögren's syndrome (autoimmune exocrinopathy). Arthritis Rheum 33:774–781, 1990.

Benign Neoplasms

Batsakis JG, Luna MA, El-Naggar AK. Basaloid monomorphic adenomas. Ann Otol Rhinol Laryngol 100:687–690, 1991.

Chau MNY, Radden BG. Intraoral salivary gland neoplasms: a retrospective study of 98 cases. J Oral Pathol 15:339–342, 1986.

Daley TD. The canalicular adenoma: considerations on differential diagnosis and treatment. J Oral Maxillofac Surg 42:728–730, 1989.

Eveson JW, Cawson RA. Salivary gland tumors. A review of 2,410 cases with particular reference to histologic types, site, age, and sex distribution. J Pathol 146:51–58, 1985.

Noguchi S, Aihara T, Yoshino K, et al. Demonstration of monoclonal origin of human parotid gland pleomorphic adenoma. Cancer 77:431–435, 1996.

Spiro RH. Salivary neoplasms: overview of a 35-year experience with 2,807 patients. Head Neck Surg 8:177–184, 1986.

Malignant Neoplasms

Aberle AM, Abrams AM, Bowe R, et al. Lobular (polymorphous low-grade) carcinoma of minor salivary glands. Oral Surg Oral Med Oral Pathol 60:387–395, 1985.

Auclair PL, Goode RK, Ellis GL. Mucoepidermoid carcinoma of minor salivary glands. Cancer 69:2021–2030, 1992.

Batsakis JG, El-Naggar AK. Terminal duct adenocarcinomas of salivary tissues. Ann Otol Rhinol Laryngol 100:251–253, 1991.

Batsakis JG, Luna MA. Low grade and high grade adenocarcinomas of the salivary duct system. Ann Otol Rhinol Laryngol 98:162–163, 1989.

Batsakis JG, Pinkston GR, Luna MA, et al. Adenocarcinomas of the oral cavity: a clinicopathologic study of terminal duct carcinomas. J Laryngol Otol 97:825–835, 1983.

Brandwein MS, Jagirdar J, Patil J, et al. Salivary duct carcinoma (cribriform salivary carcinoma of excretory ducts). Cancer 65:2307–2314, 1990.

Brookstone MS, Huvos AS. Central salivary gland tumors of the maxilla and mandible: a clinicopathologic study of 11 cases with an analysis of the literature. J Oral Maxillofac Surg 50:229–236, 1992.

Callendar DL, Frankenthaler RA, Luna MA, et al. Salivary gland neoplasms in children. Arch Otolaryngol Head Neck Surg 118:472–476, 1992.

Chau MNY, Radden BG. Intraoral salivary gland neoplasms: a retrospective study of 98 cases. J Oral Pathol 15:399–342, 1986.

Chaudhry AP, Cutler LS, Liefer C, et al. Ultrastructural study of the histogenesis of salivary gland mucoepidermoid carcinoma. J Oral Pathol 18:400–409, 1989.

Chaudhry AP, Leifer C, Cutler LS, et al. Histogenesis of adenoid cystic carcinoma of the salivary glands. Light and electron microscopic study. Cancer 58:72–82, 1986.

Corio RL, Sciubba JJ, Brannon RB, et al. Epithelial-myoepithelial carcinoma of intercalated duct origin. Oral Surg Oral Med Oral Pathol 53:280–287, 1982.

Dardick I, George D, Jeans MTD, et al. Ultrastructural morphology and cellular differentiation in acinic cell carcinoma. Oral Surg Oral Med Oral Pathol 53:325–334, 1987.

Dardick I, Gliniecki MR, Heathcote J, Burford-Mason A. Comparative histogenesis and morphogenesis of mucoepidermoid carcinoma and pleomorphic adenoma. Virchows Arch [A] 417:405–417, 1990.

Ellis GL, Corio RL. Acinic cell adenocarcinoma. A clinicopathologic analysis of 294 cases. Cancer 52:542–549, 1983.

Evans HL, Batsakis JG. Polymorphous low-grade adenocarcinomas of minor salivary glands: a study of 14 cases of a distinctive neoplasm. Cancer 53:935–942, 1985.

Eveson JW, Cawson RA. Salivary gland tumors. A review of 2,410 cases with particular reference to histologic types, site, age, and sex discrimination. J Pathol 146:51–58, 1985.

Frierson HF, Mills SE, Garland TA. Terminal duct carcinoma of minor salivary glands. Am J Clin Pathol 84:8–14, 1985.

Greiner TC, Robinson RA, Maves MD. Adenoid cystic carcinoma. A clinicopathologic study with flow cytometric analysis. Am J Clin Pathol 92:711–720, 1989.

Hamper K, Lazar F, Dietel M, et al. Prognostic factors for adenoid cystic carcinoma of the head and neck. J Oral Pathol Med 19:101–107, 1990.

Hui KK, Batsakis JG, Luna MH, et al. Salivary duct adenocarcinoma: a high-grade malignancy. J Laryngol Otol 100:105–114, 1986.

Lewis JE, Olsen KD, Weiland LH. Acinic cell carcinoma. Clinicopathologic review. Cancer 67:172–179, 1991.

Luna MA, Batsakis JG, Ordonez NG, et al. Salivary gland adenocarcinomas. A clinicopathologic analysis of three distinctive types. Semin Diagn Pathol 4:117–135, 1987.

Luna MA, Ordonez NG, MacKay B, et al. Salivary epithelial-myoepithelial carcinoma of intercalated ducts: a clinical, electron microscopic, and immunocytochemical study. Oral Surg Oral Med Oral Pathol 59:482–490, 1985.

Milchgrub S, Gnepp DR, Vuitch F, et al. Hyalinizing clear cell carcinoma of salivary gland. Am J Surg Pathol 18:74–82, 1994.

Nascimento AG, Amaral ALP, Prado ALF, et al. Adenoid cystic carcinoma of salivary glands. A study of 61 cases with clinicopathologic correlation. Cancer 57:312–319, 1986.

Norberg LE, Burford-Mason AP, Dardick I. Cellular differentiation and morphologic heterogeneity in polymorphous low-grade adenocarcinoma. J Oral Pathol Med 20:373–379, 1991.

Ogawa Y, Hong S-S, Toyosawa S, et al. Expression of major histocompatibility complex class II antigens and interleukin-1 by epithelial cells of Warthin's tumor. Cancer 66:2111–2117, 1990.

Santucci M, Bondi R. New prognostic criterion in adenoid cystic carcinoma of salivary gland origin. Am J Clin Pathol 91:132–138, 1989.

Seifert G, Brocheriou C, Cardesa A, Eveson JW. WHO International Classification of Tumors. Tentative histological classification of salivary gland tumors. Pathol Res Pract 186:555–581, 1990.

Simpson RHW, Clarke TJ, Sarsfield PTL, Gluckman PGC. Epithelial-myoepithelial carcinoma of salivary glands. J Clin Pathol 44:419–423, 1991.

Simpson R, Sarsfield P, Clarke T, Babajews A. Clear cell carcinoma of minor salivary glands. Histopathology 17:433–438, 1990.

Spiro RH. Salivary neoplasms: overview of a 35-year experience with 2,807 patients. Head Neck Surg 8:177–184, 1986.

Stephen J, Batsakis JG, Luna MA, et al. True malignant mixed tumors (carcinosarcoma) of salivary glands. Oral Surg Oral Med Oral Pathol 61:597–602, 1986.

Szanto PA, Luna MA, Tortoledo ME, et al. Histologic grading of adenoid cystic carcinoma of the salivary glands. Cancer 54:1062–1069, 1984.

van der Waal JE, Snow GB, van der Waal I. Intraoral adenoid cystic carcinoma. The presence of perineural spread in relation to site, size, local extension and metastatic spread in 22 cases. Cancer 66:2031–2033, 1990.

Vincent SD, Hammond HL, Finkelstein MW. Clinical and therapeutic features of polymorphous low-grade adenocarcinoma. Oral Surg Oral Med Oral Pathol 77:41–47, 1994.

Waldron CA, Koh ML. Central mucoepidermoid carcinoma of the jaws: Report of four cases with analysis of the literature and discussion of the relationship to mucoepidermoid, sialodontogenic and glandular odontogenic cysts. J Oral Maxillofac Surg 48:871–877, 1990.

9

Lymphoid Lesions

REACTIVE LESIONS

In this section, three primary groupings—reactive, developmental, and neoplastic—are considered. Important in the discussion of lymphoid lesions involving the oral cavity and adjacent areas is that many lesions, especially those arising in lymph nodes, are capable of simulating malignancy.

Lymphoid Hyperplasia

It is sometimes difficult to distinguish reactive from neoplastic lymphoid proliferations, especially when occurring in unusual sites such as the peritonsillar area, palate, buccal mucosa, lymph nodes, and salivary glands. There is also is an increasing incidence of cystic benign lymphoepithelial lesions within the parotid and submandibular gland in patients with the acquired immunodeficiency syndrome (AIDS).

One of the normal sites of lymphoid tissue is the posterolateral portion of the tongue. The aggregations of lymphoid tissue within this area are part of the *foliate papillae* or lingual tonsil. They may be distinguished from other lymphoid tissues by deep crypts lined by stratified squamous epithelium. These papillae occasionally become inflamed or irritated, with associated enlargement and tenderness. In such instances, patients may become symptomatic. On examination, these areas are enlarged and somewhat lobular in outline, with an intact overlying mucosa and prominent superficial vessels. In instances in which such lesions

are removed for diagnostic purposes, the chief finding is reactive lymphoid hyperplasia. Within the enlarged germinal centers, mitoses and macrophages containing cellular debris may be seen. In addition to the foliate papillae, other zones where lymphoid tissue is found include the anterior floor of the mouth on either side of the lingual frenum, the anterior tonsillar pillar, and the posterior portion of the soft palate. Because lymphoid tissues are not always found in these areas, they are usually regarded as ectopic. The term *oral tonsil* also refers to this tissue.

Reactive lymphoid hyperplasia (oral tonsil) has male predominance and is noted within the second and third decades of life. In one study, a mean of 23 years was found. The lesions range from 1 to 15 mm in diameter and may persist for years.

The *buccal* or *facial lymph node* is often the site of a reactive hyperplastic process. This is characterized as a freely movable submucosal nodule usually adjacent to the second premolar and first molar teeth. The cause of the process is unknown, but it may be a reaction to irritation or localized trauma. Gingivitis or periapical pathology may occasionally stimulate or initiate enlargement of this particular lymph node.

Management should be directed toward elimination of the cause of the problem if it can be identified, followed by simple observation.

Follicular lymphoid hyperplasia may be seen in the palate. This reactive polyclonal proliferation of lymphocytes is often difficult to separate from *lymphoproliferative disease of the palate,* a condition that may signify lymphoma. Histologically, follicular lymphoid hyperplasia of the palate is characterized by irregularly sized, well-demarcated germinal centers with a crisply defined rim or mantle of small, mature lymphocytes (Fig. 9–1). Within the germinal centers, macrophages contain phagocytosed nuclear debris. Using immunohistochemical techniques, polyclonal light chains are expressed by the B lymphocytes. Additionally, the mantle zones are composed of both mature and immature B cells, while the extramantle zones contain both B and T lymphocytes, plasma cells, macrophages, and eosinophils. Indefinite follow-up is prudent because of possible confusion of lymphoid hyperplasia with lymphoproliferative disease/lymphoma.

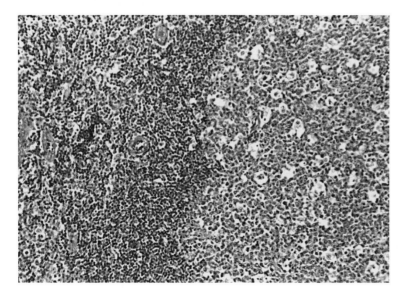

Figure 9–1. Lymphoid hyperplasia. Note the germinal center (left) with numerous light-staining macrophages.

Angiolymphoid Hyperplasia with Eosinophilia (ALHE)

This condition, also known as *epithelioid* or *histiocytoid hemangioma,* was first described in 1948 as a nodular subcutaneous benign disease in young men. Later, however, cases with the same clinical and histologic features were reported in the oral cavity. In addition to nodular aggregates of lymphocytes and eosinophils, regional lymphadenopathy and blood eosinophilia are noted. Similar findings were also noted under the headings of *Kimura's disease,* eosinophilic granuloma of soft tissue, and eosinophilic lymphofolliculosis. Because Kimura's disease was originally described as having a distinct male predilection without the associated regional lymphadenopathy, some clinicians believe that the two conditions represent different entities: Histologically, some differences have also been described, adding to the tendency to split ALHE into two separate but related entities.

Etiology. Because of vascular proliferation and an intensive inflammatory infiltrate, a reactive etiology has been suggested. Increased serum IgE levels and deposition of IgE within the lymphoid follicles further suggest a reactive immune cause. Also demonstrated has been the presence of anti–*Candida albicans* antibody within the lesions and improvement after hyposensitization to this allergen.

Clinical Features. ALHE is found predominantly in the head and neck area, accounting for approximately 85% of all cases. However, oral mucous membrane involvement is rare. The labial mucosa is the oral site most commonly affected. In Asians, there is a distinct male predominance.

There is a wide age range from 7 to 79 years and a mean age of 35 years. Lesions generally are solitary, with a mean size of 1.7 cm reported. Peripheral eosinophilia greater than 4% has been noted in 60% of the cases in which peripheral blood counts have been included. The clinical course is characterized by the presence of a painless, mobile, submucosal nodule that enlarges gradually. Multiple lesions have been reported in more than 40% of cases.

Histopathology. Lesions are circumscribed and usually are grossly separable from surrounding tissue. A nodular mass of hyperplastic lymphoid tissue with well-developed lymphoid follicles containing germinal centers may be seen. Proliferating capillaries with plump endothelial cells are found in a dense, patchy infiltrate of lymphocytes, with eosinophils and fewer numbers of macrophages noted. Toward the periphery, this infiltrate may extend into surrounding soft tissue. Arterial intimal proliferation and disruption of the internal elastic lamina may be seen. Early lesions or those in an active growth phase may be dominated by a vascular element; older or quiescent lesions may contain a larger percentage of inflammatory cells.

Differential Diagnosis. When it involves the labial mucosa, ALHE's characteristic nodule may be indistinguishable from a minor salivary gland neoplasm or a mucus retention cyst or mucocele. Other benign soft tissue neoplasms, such as lipoma and schwannoma, might be included in the differential diagnosis.

Because of the presence of eosinophils within tissue, microscopic differential diagnosis should include eosinophilic granuloma and traumatic (eosinophilic) granuloma.

Treatment. Excision is the treatment of choice. Intralesional steroid injections have also been used with variable results. Recurrences are occasionally noted. The presence of blood or peripheral eosinophilia has generally been reported with numerous or recurrent lesions.

DEVELOPMENTAL LESIONS

Lymphoepithelial Cyst

The lymphoepithelial cyst is an uncommon lesion of the mouth, major salivary glands, and neck. It is thought to arise from an entrapment of epithelium within lymph nodes or lymphoid tissue during development. Subsequent epithelial proliferation results in a clinically evident mass.

The oral lymphoepithelial cyst (see also the discussion on ectopic lymphoid tissue in Chapter 3) presents as an asymptomatic mucosal elevation that is well defined and yellowish-pink. The site most commonly affected is the floor of the mouth, where approximately 50% of cases are found. The ventral and posterolateral portions of the tongue constitute an additional 40% of the cases; the balance is shared among the soft palate, mucobuccal fold, and anterior faucial pillars. A wide age range is noted from adolescence to the seventh decade of life. The gender distribution is essentially equal. Except for the small central cystic space, these lesions are identical to ectopic lymphoid aggregates.

A marked increase in the incidence of lymphoepithelial cysts of the major salivary glands has been noticed recently, particularly in those testing positive for the human immunodeficiency virus (HIV). The mechanism of cyst formation is unclear.

Histopathology. The lymphoepithelial cyst is lined by stratified squamous epithelium that is often parakeratotic. There may be focal areas of pseudostratified columnar cells or mucous cells. The epithelial lining is surrounded by a discrete, well-circumscribed lymphoid component, often with germinal center formation and a sharply defined zone of mantle lymphocytes. Additionally, the cyst wall may contain variable proportions of lymphocytes, macrophages, plasma cells, and occasional multinucleated giant cells. Continuity of the cyst lining with the surface oral epithelium may occasionally be noted.

Differential Diagnosis. In the anterior floor of the mouth, a sialolith may be similar in appearance to a lymphoepithelial cyst. However, a history of pain and swelling would be expected with a salivary duct stone. Developmental anomalies such as teratoma or dermoid cyst, benign mesenchymal neoplasms, and salivary gland tumors might also be considered in a differential diagnosis for floor of mouth soft tissue mass. When involving the parotid gland, the lymphoepithelial cyst must be distinguished from salivary lymphoma, Warthin's tumor, and cystic neoplasms of salivary origin.

Treatment. Conservative excisional biopsy is generally used for definitive diagnosis as well as for treatment. Recurrence is not expected.

NEOPLASMS

Lymphoma

Lymphomas arising within the oral cavity account for fewer than 5% of oral malignancies. In the head and neck, lymphomas may be seen within regional lymph nodes and within extranodal lymphoid sites in areas known as the gut-associated or mucosa-associated lymphoid tissue (MALT), which extend from the oral cavity to the anal region. Within the oral cavity, lymphoid tissue is chiefly represented in Waldeyer's ring; elsewhere within the oral cavity it appears as unencapsulated lymphoid tissue within the base of the tongue and soft palate, as well as within the major and minor salivary glands where lymphoid tissue has been arranged in duct-associated aggregates. Of importance is that lymphoma can occur in either nodal or extranodal sites.

There are many histologic classifications of lymphomas. These neoplasms are derived from lymphocytes of B or T cell lineage; they may rarely be of macrophage origin. Some classifications are based on histologic features alone, whereas others include immunologic characteristics or correlation with probable biologic behavior. Lymphomas are separated into two groups: those of Hodgkin's type and those considered non-Hodgkin's lymphomas.

HODGKIN'S LYMPHOMA

Hodgkin's disease rarely involves the oral cavity, although there are cases in which this disease has appeared in the soft tissues as well as in the mandible and maxilla. On occasion, the oral manifestations may represent the primary site of involvement; in other cases, associated cervical lymphadenopathy or more widespread Hodgkin's disease may be noted concurrently.

Clinical Features. Generally, Hodgkin's disease occurs over a wide age spectrum, with clustering of patients between 15 to 35 years and beyond 55 years. There is a slight male predilec-

Table 9–1. Ann Arbor Staging System of Hodgkin's Disease (Modified)

Stage I:	Involvement of a single lymph node region. I_e—Involvement of single extralymphatic site.
Stage II:	Involvement of two or more lymph node regions on the same side of the diaphragm. II_e—Involvement of an extralymphatic site or organ and one or more lymph node regions on the same side of the diaphragm.
Stage III:	Regional involvement of lymph nodes on both sides of the diaphragm. III_e—Involvement of localized extralymphatic organ.
Stage IV:	Disseminated involvement of one or more extralymphatic organs or tissues with or without associated lymph node enlargement.

Table 9–2. Hodgkin's Disease (Lukes-Butler Histologic Classification [Rye Modification])

Lymphocyte predominance
Nodular sclerosis
Mixed cellularity
Lymphocyte depletion
Unclassified

tion. Clinically, Hodgkin's disease is characterized by painless enlargement of lymph nodes or extranodal lymphoid tissue. Within the oral cavity, tonsillar enlargement, usually unilateral, may be seen in the early phases. When extranodal sites are involved, submucosal swellings may be seen, sometimes with mucosal ulceration or erosion of underlying bone. Subsequent to microscopic diagnosis, clinical staging must be undertaken. This may consist of physical examination, radiographic imaging, lymphangiography, and laparotomy. After the staging procedure, a definitive treatment plan is established. Table 9–1 provides details of the Ann Arbor system of clinical staging.

Histopathology. Of greatest significance is the identification of the Reed-Sternberg cell, which must be present for the diagnosis of Hodgkin's disease to be established. This cell of lymphocytic origin is characterized by its large size and bilobed nucleus; each lobe contains a large amphophilic or eosinophilic nucleolus (Fig. 9–2). The nuclear chromatin pattern is vesicular and condensed at the periphery. Other Reed-Sternberg cells may be characterized by two nuclei with a prominent nucleolus or by multiple nuclei. Cells similar to Reed-Sternberg cells may be seen in certain viral diseases such as infectious mononucleosis and Burkitt's lymphoma, as well as in patients with treated lymphocytic lymphoma, chronic lymphocytic leukemia, and some benign immunoblastic proliferations.

The Lukes-Butler histologic classification of Hodgkin's disease that was modified by Rye recognizes four subtypes (Table 9–2): (1) lymphocyte predominance, (2) nodular sclerosis, (3) mixed cellularity, and (4) lymphocyte depletion. The lymphocyte-predominant type has the most favorable prognosis, and the lymphocyte-depletion type has the least favorable prognosis. In the lymphocyte-predominant form, a small mature lymphocyte is the most prevalent cell, but it is mixed with scattered macrophages (Fig. 9–3). Few Reed-Sternberg cells are seen in this form of the disease.

The most frequent form of Hodgkin's disease is the nodular-sclerosing type. It is characterized by bands of collagen that originate from the periphery and penetrate into the lymph node, subdividing it into islands of tumor that contain Reed-Sternberg cells (Fig. 9–4).

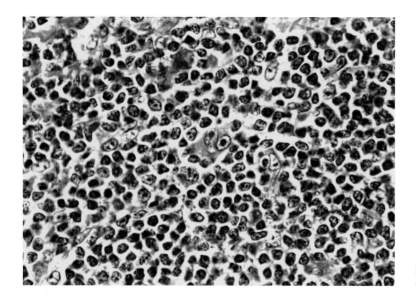

Figure 9–2. Reed-Sternberg cell (center) in Hodgkin's disease.

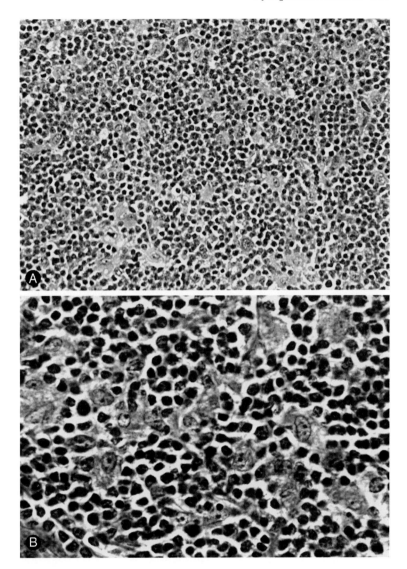

Figure 9–3. *A* and *B,* Hodgkin's disease, lymphocyte predominance.

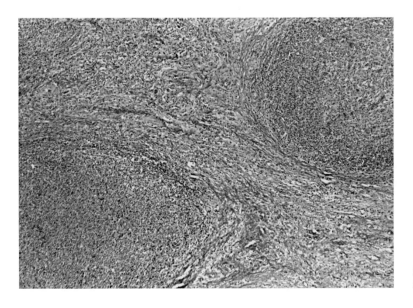

Figure 9–4. Hodgkin's disease, nodular sclerosing type.

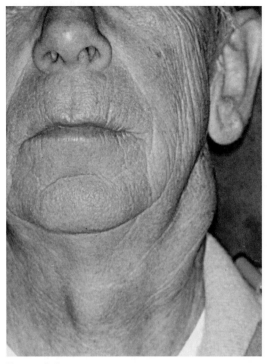

Figure 9–5. Lymphoma (non-Hodgkin's) of the cervical lymph nodes.

The mixed-cellularity type of Hodgkin's disease contains a combination of lymphocytes, eosinophils, neutrophils, plasma cells, macrophages, and many Reed-Sternberg cells. The mixed-cellularity type of Hodgkin's disease carries the third best prognosis, intermediate between the nodular-sclerosing type and the lymphocyte-depletion form.

In the lymphocyte-depletion form of Hodgkin's disease, the chief microscopic characteristic is abundant pleomorphic Reed-Sternberg cells and relatively few lymphocytes.

Differential Diagnosis. Cervical lymphadenopathy would suggest conditions ranging from inflammatory to neoplastic. Specified entities that can produce lymph node enlargement include chronic lymphadenitis, infectious diseases, and lymphoma. In young patients infectious mononucleosis should be considered. Nonlymphoid lateral neck lesions that could be included in a clinical differential include salivary gland tumors, cervical lymphoepithelial cyst, and carotid body tumor.

Treatment and Prognosis. The clinical staging and histologic classification of Hodgkin's disease (and non-Hodgkin's lymphoma) are critical in determining management and prognosis. The lymphocyte-predominant form of the disease carries with it the most favorable prognosis, and the lymphocyte-depletion form the worst prognosis. Stage I disease has the best prognosis; stage IV (disseminated disease) has the worst. Generally, clinical stage has a greater influence on overall prognosis than does histologic subtype.

Management of Hodgkin's disease consists of external radiation therapy and multiple-agent chemotherapy. What was once a fatal illness with poor survival statistics has become a curable disease. Most patients with Hodgkin's disease are cured because of treatment with intensive radiotherapy and/or chemotherapy.

NON-HODGKIN'S LYMPHOMA

Non-Hodgkin's lymphomas are relatively common neoplasms (53,600 new cases estimated for 1997), and often occur in extranodal head and

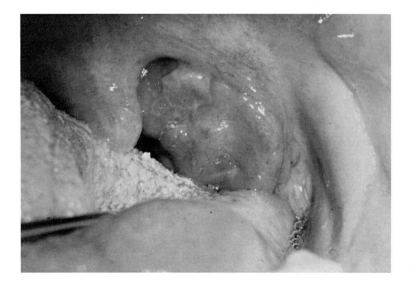

Figure 9–6. Lymphoma (non-Hodgkin's) of the left tonsil.

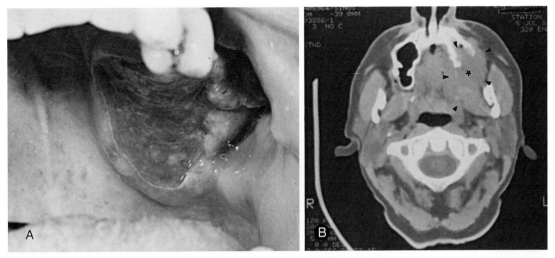

Figure 9–7. *A,* Lymphoma (non-Hodgkin's) of the sinus with oral presentation. *B,* Computed tomographic scan showing a large destructive mass (*). Lateral, medial, and posterior walls of the maxillary sinus have been destroyed by the tumor.

neck sites, especially in HIV-infected (AIDS) patients. Until recently, extranodal oral lymphomas, presenting either as primary or secondary oral disease, have been uncommon. With the emergence of HIV infection, oral HIV-associated lymphomas are now encountered with increased frequency and have been accompanied by a distinct shift to predominately high-grade tumors and a positive correlation with the presence of Epstein-Barr virus in the lesion.

Clinical Features. Middle-aged and elderly individuals are most commonly affected by non-Hodgkin's lymphoma, except for Burkitt's lymphoma, which can be encountered in children. Studies show that males have a slight preponderance over females. Nodal disease is characterized by gradual asymptomatic enlargement that may become static for a considerable period before diagnosis (Fig. 9–5). Without intervention, additional lymph nodes will become involved. The rate of enlargement will depend on the type of lymphoma. Oral non-Hodgkin's lymphomas may appear in mucosa-associated lymphoid tissue (Waldeyer's ring), or they may develop as infiltrates in nonlymphoid tissue. Oral lymphomas are characterized by an absence of symptoms and by tumescence, often with overlying ulceration (Figs. 9–6 and 9–7). After tonsil, palate is the most common oral site (Table 9–3). If bone is the primary site, alveolar bone loss and tooth mobility are often presenting signs. Swelling, pain, numbness of the lip, and pathologic fracture may also be associated with bone lesions. The condition originally reported as *lymphoproliferative disease of the hard palate* is now considered to represent a *bona fide* lymphoma (Fig. 9–8). Microscopically,

this condition may be difficult to separate from lymphoid hyperplasia (Fig. 9–9).

After the diagnosis of lymphoma is established, a staging procedure similar to that used in Hodgkin's lymphoma is performed. Stage I disease represents involvement of a single lymph node region or a single extralymphatic site. Stage II disease involves two or more lymph node chains; stage III involvement demonstrates positive disease on both sides of the diaphragm. Stage IV correlates with diffuse or disseminated involvement of one or more extralymphatic organs, other than spleen, spine, Waldeyer's ring, or appendix. The involvement of bone marrow or liver likewise indicates a stage IV disease.

Histopathology. For non-Hodgkin's lymphoma, numerous classification schemes have evolved. Those that are now most commonly used include the Kiel Classification, the National Institutes of Health International Working Formulation (Table 9–4), and the most recently proposed Revised European-American Classification of Lymphoid Neoplasms (REAL). The working formulation inte-

Table 9–3. Oral Soft Tissue Sites Affected by Non-Hodgkin's Lymphoma

Tonsil	55%
Palate	30%
Buccal mucosa	10%
Tongue	2%
Floor of mouth	2%
Retromolar region	2%

Compiled from Eisenbud L, et al. Oral Surg 56:151, 1983; and Fierstein JT, et al. Laryngoscope 88:582, 1978.

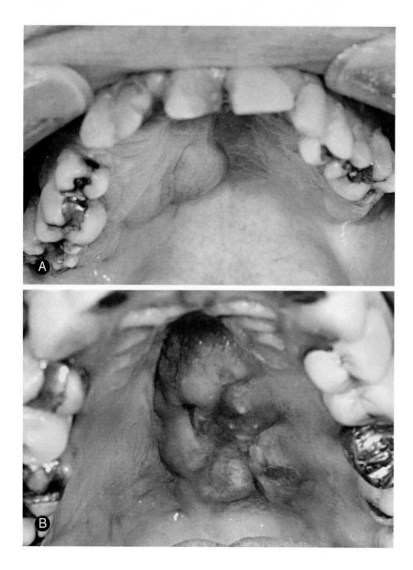

Figure 9–8. *A* and *B*, Lymphomas (non-Hodgkin's) of the hard palate.

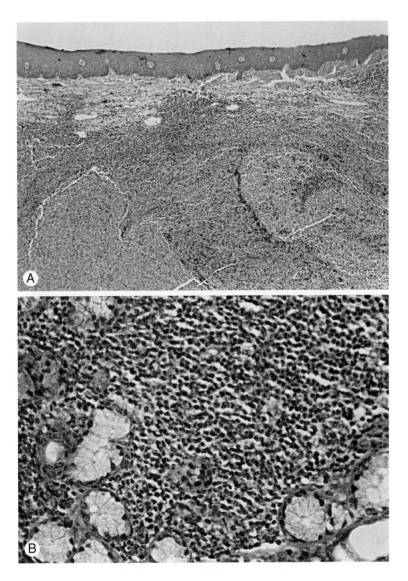

Figure 9–9. *A* and *B*, Nodular, small lymphocytic cell lymphoma of the hard palate (low grade).

Table 9–4. Working Formulation for Non-Hodgkin's Lymphoma

	Behavioral	Histologic
I	Low grade	Small lymphocytic
		Follicular, small cleaved cell
		Follicular, mixed: small cleaved and large cell
II	Intermediate grade	Follicular, large cell
		Diffuse, small cleaved cell
		Diffuse, mixed small and large cell
		Diffuse large cell
III	High grade	Large cell, immunoblastic
		Lymphoblastic
		Diffuse, small noncleaved cell

grates microscopic features along with expected clinical behavior. The REAL classification (like the Keil) is based on a combination of tumor cell morphology and immunologic findings. Features include division of lymphomas into B and T cell subtypes, inclusion of the low-grade MALT lymphomas, and inclusions of Hodgkin's disease.

In general, two basic morphologic groups of lymphoma are recognized, nodular (follicular) and diffuse forms; the former shows a more favorable prognosis (Figs. 9–10 and 9–11). Nodular lymphomas show malignant cells arranged in a pattern characterized by regular nodules distributed throughout a lymph node or extranodal site. In lymphomas showing a diffuse pattern, abnormal cells are distributed uniformly throughout the involved tissue. In either case, the normal architecture of the lymphoid tissue is destroyed. Cytology or predominant cell type within the lesion is of great significance.

Nodular Lymphomas. Nodular lymphomas may be divided into three subtypes: poorly differentiated lymphocytic, mixed lymphocytic-histiocytic, and histiocytic. Common to all subtypes are various numbers of atypical small lymphoid cells and large lymphoid cells (histiocytes). The small cells show scanty cytoplasm and an irregular cleaved or indented nucleus along with coarse, condensed chromatin. Because of the size and nuclear characteristics of the larger cells, they were originally considered histiocytes but have been shown to represent transformed B lymphocytes.

It is important to subdivide nodular lymphomas because of clinical and prognostic considerations. It has been shown that patients with nodular lymphoma, poorly differentiated lymphocytic type, usually present with generalized disease; yet, despite extensive disease, these patients have a relatively favorable prognosis. The least favorable prognosis is associated with the so-called histiocytic or large cell subtype. Despite the fact that these tumors are more often localized at the time of diagnosis, they are most prone to progress from a nodular to a diffuse pattern, which has a significantly poorer prognosis. Immunologic studies have shown through antigenic markers that nodular lymphomas are neoplasms of follicular B lymphocytes, with the majority composed of follicular center cells.

Diffuse Lymphomas. Most oral lymphomas exhibit a diffuse pattern and are of B cell lineage. In Japanese populations, a proportionally high incidence of T cell lymphomas has been reported. Diffuse lymphomas are a heterogeneous group of tumors, both morphologically and clinically. Various cell types participate in these neoplasms, and these allow subclassification into several

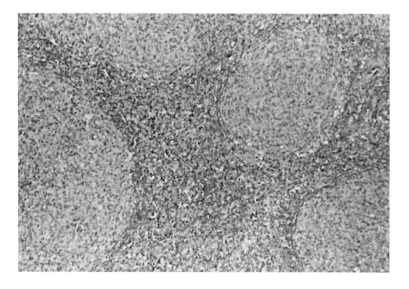

Figure 9–10. Follicular large cell lymphoma (intermediate grade).

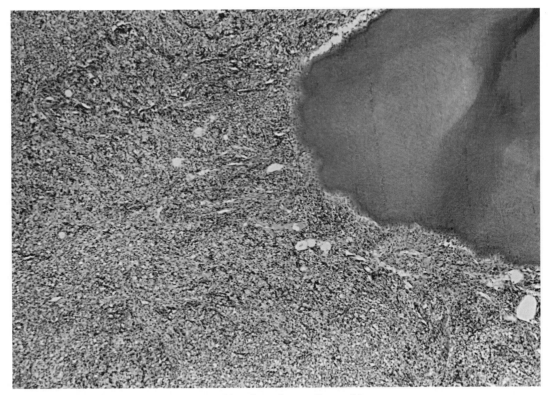

Figure 9–11. Diffuse, mixed small and large cell lymphoma (intermediate grade).

groups: lymphocytic (well and poorly differentiated types) (Fig. 9–12), histiocytic (large cell) (Fig. 9–13), mixed lymphocytic-histiocytic, lymphoblastic, and undifferentiated (includes Burkitt's lymphoma).

The histiocytic or diffuse large cell lymphoma is the most common type in the head and neck region. As a general rule, the incidence of large cell lymphomas increases with age and positive HIV status. The clinical course is usually aggressive, and the prognosis is poor, although this type frequently presents with disease limited to one side of the diaphragm. Histologically, the neoplastic cell is a large lymphocyte that exhibits considerable variation in nuclear shape and cellular size. Cells frequently contain two or more nuclei, often with a single large eosinophilic nucleolus. The nuclear chromatin tends to be vesicular, and mitotic figures are often numerous with a high proliferation rate. The presence of macrophages containing phagocytic cytoplasmic inclusions known as tingible bodies is characteristic.

Within the Working Formulation, architectural subsets have been reordered according to expected behavior (Table 9–4). Under the low-grade category, subtypes include a well-differentiated small lymphocyte type of lymphoma and a nodular or follicular lymphoma that contains a predominant small cleaved lymphocyte population. Also, a nodular or follicular architectural pattern composed of a mixture of small cleaved and large cells is included. Within the intermediate-grade category, follicular tumors composed predominantly of large cells is represented, as well as diffuse lesions composed of small cleaved cells. Also within the intermediate grade are two other subsets, both with diffuse architecture. These two forms include a mixture of large and small cells in one and a large cell population in the other. The high-grade category within the working formulation consists of three variants—an immunoblastic large cell type, a lymphoblastic type, and small, noncleaved type that encompasses both the Burkitt's and the non-Burkitt's equivalents.

Treatment and Prognosis. The treatment of non-Hodgkin's lymphoma depends on the outcome of the clinical staging procedure. Local radiation therapy is generally used for stage I disease. Some clinicians recommend no treatment for some low-grade tumors because of their very slow growth and poor response to therapy. Treatment of other stages of lymphoma may be with irradiation only or with a combination of irradiation and multiple-agent chemotherapy.

Cumulative relapse-free 5-year survival rates in stage I non-Hodgkin's lymphoma treated with

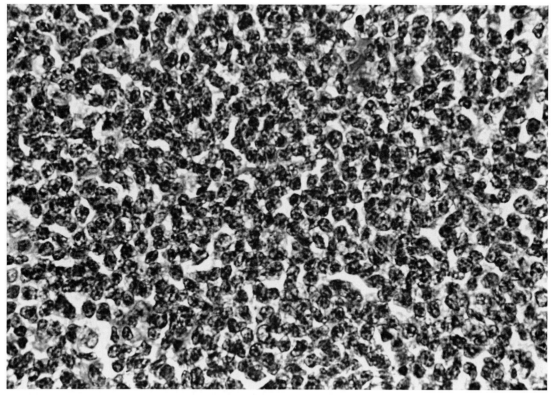

Figure 9–12. Small lymphocytic lymphoma (low grade).

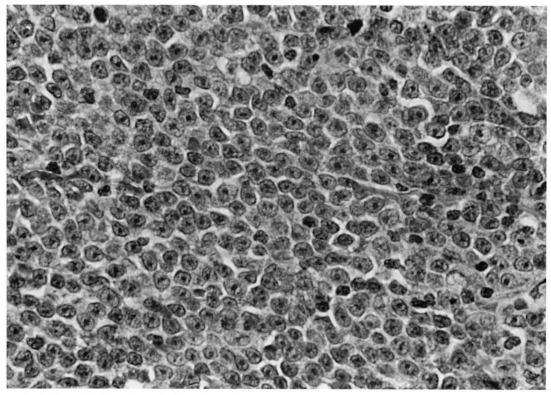

Figure 9–13. Diffuse large cell lymphoma (intermediate grade).

primary radiation have ranged from 50 to 90%. Patients with more advanced disease (stages II, III, and IV) have survival rates ranging between 30 and 60%. AIDS-associated lymphomas, which are usually high-grade lesions, are generally associated with a poor prognosis.

BURKITT'S LYMPHOMA

This form of non-Hodgkin's lymphoma is separated from the other forms because it occurs as a distinctive clinical-pathologic condition in children (Figs. 9–14 and 9–15). It was originally described in tropical Africa but is now known to occur elsewhere in the world. In the head and neck, this condition occurs in the mandible and maxilla and is therefore described in Chapter 14.

Myeloma/Plasmacytoma

Myeloma is a tumor composed of terminally differentiated B lymphocytes or plasma cells that generally present as multiple bone lesions (multiple myeloma, myelomatosis) (Fig. 9–16). The neoplastic population of plasma cells is termed *mono-*

clonal because the cells are from a single clone and produce homogeneous immunoglobulin composed of a single class of heavy and light chains (Fig. 9–17). Plasma cell tumors are subclassified into three types: solitary plasmacytoma of bone (Fig. 9–18), multiple myeloma, and extramedullary (soft tissue) plasmacytoma. The bone lesions are discussed in detail in Chapter 14.

Extramedullary plasmacytomas typically occur in the soft tissue of the upper respiratory tract and, rarely, the oral cavity. They present as lobulated masses in a broad age range that includes children and young adults. Generally, laboratory studies for extramedullary plasmacytoma yield negative results.

In multiple myeloma, chemotherapy, including use of alkylating agents and prednisone, is a mainstay of treatment, either alone or in combination with local radiation. For solitary plasmacytoma and extramedullary plasmacytoma, radiation or surgery is the standard mode of therapy. Progression of the solitary bone lesions to multiple myeloma is the rule, and progression of extramedullary lesions to multiple myeloma is the exception.

A complication not infrequently associated with multiple myeloma is *amyloidosis.* Similar but not identical amyloid protein deposits may be seen in several other unrelated conditions. The common

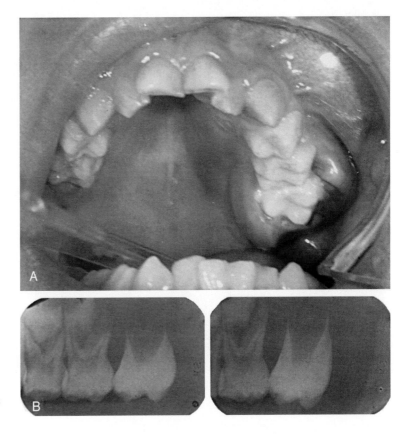

Figure 9–14. *A* and *B,* Burkitt's lymphoma.

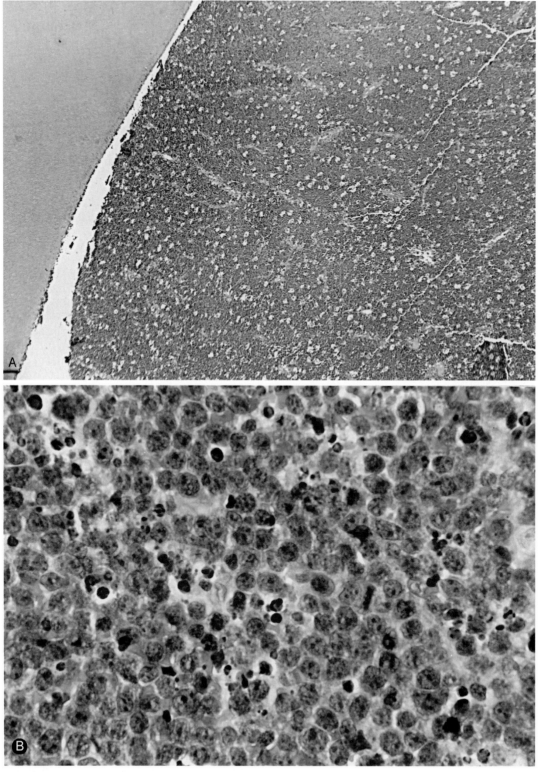

Figure 9–15. *A* and *B*, Burkitt's-type lymphoma (high-grade, diffuse, small noncleaved lymphoma).

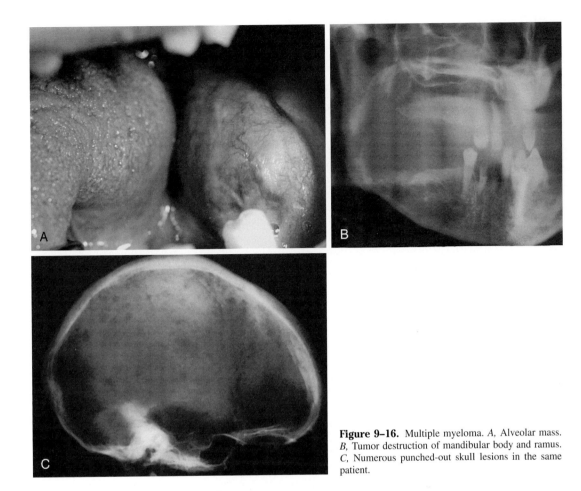

Figure 9–16. Multiple myeloma. *A,* Alveolar mass. *B,* Tumor destruction of mandibular body and ramus. *C,* Numerous punched-out skull lesions in the same patient.

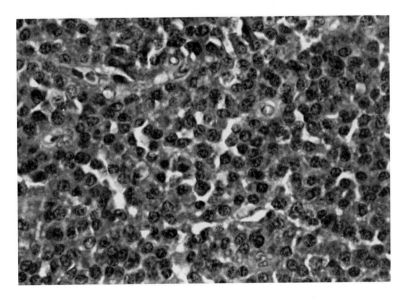

Figure 9–17. Multiple myeloma showing neoplastic plasma cells.

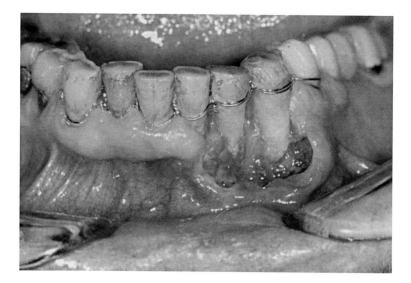

Figure 9–18. Plasmacytoma of mandibular alveolar bone.

denominator of the various forms of amyloidosis is organ dysfunction as deposits replace normal tissue.

Bibliography

Reactive Lesions

Bradley G, Main JHP, Birt BD, et al. Benign lymphoid hyperplasia of the palate. J Oral Pathol 16:18–26, 1987.

d'Agay MF, de Roquancourt A, Peuchamaur M, et al. Cystic benign lymphoepithelial lesion of the salivary glands in HIV-positive patients. Virchows Arch [A] 417:353–356, 1990.

Dannaker C, Piacquadio D, Willoughby CW, Goltz RW. Histiocytoid hemangioma: a disease spectrum. J Am Aàcad Dermatol 21:404–409, 1989.

Finfer MD, Gallo L, Perchick A, et al. Fine needle aspiration of cystic benign lymphoepithelial lesion of the parotid gland in patients at risk for the acquired immune deficiency syndrome. Acta Cytol 34:821–826, 1990.

Googe P, Harris N, Mihm M. Kimura's disease and angiolymphoid hyperplasia with eosinophilia: two distinct histopathological entities. J Cutan Pathol 14:263–271, 1987.

Napier SS, Newlands C. Benign lymphoid hyperplasia of the palate: report of two cases and immunohistochemical profile. J Oral Pathol Med 19:221–225, 1990.

Peters E, Altini M, Kola AH. Oral angiolymphoid hyperplasia with cosinophilia. Oral Surg Oral Med Oral Pathol 61:73–79, 1986.

Developmental Lesions

Elliott JN, Oertel YC. Lymphoepithelial cysts of the salivary glands. Histologic and cytologic features. Am J Clin Pathol 93:39–43, 1990.

Hong SS, Ogawa Y, Yagi T, et al. Benign lymphoepithelial lesion with large cysts. Oral Surg Oral Med Oral Pathol 19:266–270, 1990.

Neoplasms

Batsakis JG. Plasma cell tumors of the head and neck. Ann Otol Rhinol Laryngol 92:311–313, 1983.

Carbone A, Vaccher E, Barzan L, et al. Head and neck lymphomas associated with human immunodeficiency virus infection. Arch Otolaryngol Head Neck Surg 121:210–218, 1995.

Dardick I, Moher D, Cavell S, et al. An ultrastructural morphometric study of follicular center lymphocytes: III. The control of lymphocyte nuclear size in reactive hyperplasia and non-Hodgkin's lymphoma. Mod Pathol 3:176–185, 1990.

Economopoulos T, Asprou N, Stathakis N, et al. Primary extranodal non-Hodgkin's lymphoma in adults: clinicopathological and survival characteristics. Leukemia Lymphoma 21:131–136, 1996.

Fukuda Y, Ishida T, Fujimoto M, et al. Malignant lymphoma of the oral cavity: clinicopathologic analysis of 20 cases. J Oral Pathol 16:8–12, 1987.

Eisenbud L, Sciubba JJ, Mir R, et al. Oral presentations in non-Hodgkin's lymphoma: a review of 31 cases. Part I. Data analysis. Oral Surg 56:151–156, 1983.

Green JD, Neel HB, Witzig TE. Lymphoproliferative disorders of the head and neck. Am J Otolaryngol 12:26–32, 1991.

Green TL, Eversole LR. Oral lymphomas in HIV-infected patients: association with Epstein-Barr virus. Oral Surg Oral Med Oral Pathol 67:437–442, 1989.

Grogan TM, Miller TP, Fisher RI. A southwest oncology group perspective on the revised European-American Lymphoma Classification. Hematol/Oncol Clin North Am 11:819–842, 1997.

Hamilton-Dutoit SJ, Pallesen G, Franzmann MB, et al. AIDS-related lymphoma. Am J Pathol 138:149–163, 1991.

Handlers JP, Howell RE, Abrams AM, et al. Extranodal oral lymphoma. Part I. A morphologic and immunoperoxidase study of 34 cases. Oral Surg Oral Med Oral Pathol 61:362–367, 1986.

Ioachim HL, Dorsett B, Cronin W, et al. Acquired immunodeficiency syndrome-associated lymphomas: clinical, pathologic, immunologic, and viral characteristics of 111 cases. Hum Pathol 22:659–673, 1991.

Jaffe ES. An overview of the classification of non-Hodgkin's lymphomas. *In* Jaffe ES (ed). Surgical Pathology of the Lymph Nodes and Related Organs. Philadelphia, WB Saunders, 1985, pp 135–145.

Kaplan HS. Hodgkin's Disease, 2nd ed. Cambridge, Mass, Harvard University Press, 1980.

Lozada-Nur F, de Sanz S, Silverman S, et al. Intraoral non-Hodgkin's lymphoma in seven patients with acquired immunodeficiency syndrome. Oral Surg Oral Med Oral Pathol 82:173–178, 1996.

Parker SL, Tong T, Bolden S, Wingo PA. Cancer statistics, 1997. CA Cancer J Clin 47:5–27, 1997.

Portlock CS. Deferral of initial therapy for advanced indolent lymphomas. Cancer Treat Rep 66:417–419, 1982.

Raphael M, Gentilhomme O, Tuillez M, et al. Histopathologic features of high-grade non-Hodgkin's lymphomas in acquired immunodeficiency syndrome. Arch Pathol Lab Med 115:15–20, 1991.

Regezi JA, Zarbo RJ, Stewart JCB. Extranodal oral lymphomas: histologic subtypes and immunophenotypes (in routinely processed tissue). Oral Surg Oral Med Oral Pathol 72:702–708, 1991.

Rosenberg SA, Hoppe R, Glatstein RF, et al. National Cancer Institute sponsored study of non-Hodgkin's lymphomas: summary and description of a working formulation for clinical usage. Cancer 49:2112–2135, 1982.

Said JW, Shintaku IP, Teitelbaum A, et al. Distribution of T-cell phenotypic subsets and surface immunoglobulin-bearing lymphocytes in lymph nodes from male homosexuals with persistent generalized lymphoadenopathy. Hum Pathol 15:785–790, 1984.

Serraino D, Pezzotti P, Dorrucci M, et al. Cancer incidence in a cohort of human immunodeficiency virus seroconverters. Cancer 79:1004–1008, 1997.

Soderholm AL, Lindqvist C, Heikinheimo K, et al. Non-Hodgkin's lymphomas presenting through oral symptoms. Int J Oral Maxillofac Surg 19:131–134, 1990.

10

Cysts of the Oral Region

A cyst may be simply defined as an epithelium-lined pathologic space. Cysts of the maxilla, mandible, and perioral regions vary markedly in histogenesis, frequency, behavior, and treatment. Although most cysts in these regions are true cysts (they have an epithelial lining), some entities represent pseudocysts because they are not epithelium-lined.

ODONTOGENIC CYSTS

Periapical (Radicular) Cyst

Periapial (radicular or apical periodontal) cysts are by far the most common cysts of the jaws. These inflammatory cysts derive their epithelial linings from proliferation of small odontogenic epithelial residues (rests of Malassez) within the periodontal ligament.

Etiology and Pathogenesis. The periapical cyst develops from a preexisting *periapical granuloma* (Fig. 10–1), which represents a focus of chronically inflamed granulation tissue in bone at the apex of a nonvital tooth. The periapical granuloma is initiated and maintained by the degradation products of necrotic pulp tissue. Stimulation of the resident epithelial rests of Malassez occurs in response to the products of inflammation. Cystification occurs as the epithelium proliferates, to help separate the inflammatory stimulus (necrotic pulp) from surrounding bone.

Breakdown of cellular debris within the cyst lumen raises the protein concentration, producing an increase in osmotic pressure. The result is fluid transport across the epithelial lining to the lumen from the connective tissue side. Fluid ingress assists in outward growth of the cyst. With osteoclastic bone resorption, the cyst expands. Other bone-resorbing factors, such as prostaglandins, interleukins, and proteinases, from inflammatory cells and cells in the peripheral portion of the lesion permit additional cyst enlargement.

Clinical Features. Periapical cysts constitute approximately half to three fourths of all cysts in most large series. The age distribution peaks in the third through sixth decades. Of interest is the relative rarity of radicular cysts in the first decade even though caries and nonvital teeth are rather frequent in this age group. A majority of cases have been noted in males. Most cysts are located in the maxilla, especially the anterior region, followed by the maxillary posterior region, the mandibular posterior region, and finally the mandibular anterior region.

Most periapical cysts are asymptomatic and are often discovered incidentally during routine dental radiographic examination (Fig. 10–2). These cysts cause bone resorption but generally do not produce bone expansion. By definition, a nonvital pulp is necessary for the clinical diagnosis of a periapical cyst.

Radiographically, the periapical cyst cannot be differentiated from a periapical granuloma.

The radiolucency associated with a periapical cyst is generally round to ovoid, with a narrow, opaque margin that is contiguous with the lamina dura of the involved tooth. This radiopaque component may not be apparent if the cyst is rapidly

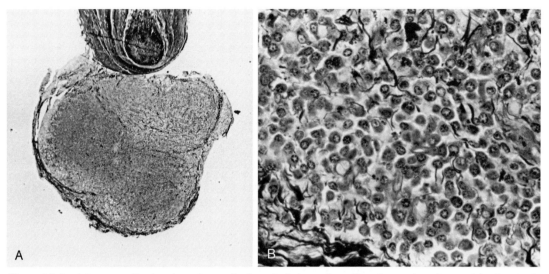

Figure 10–1. *A,* Low-magnification photomicrograph of a periapical granuloma. Note the root tip at the top of the photograph. *B,* High magnification shows inflammatory cells, mostly plasma cells.

enlarging. Cysts range from 5 mm or less to several centimeters in diameter, although the majority tend to be less than 1.5 cm. In long-standing cysts, root resorption of the offending tooth and occasionally adjacent teeth may be noted (Fig. 10–3).

Histopathology. The periapical cyst is lined by nonkeratinized stratified squamous epithelium of variable thickness (Figs. 10–4 and 10–5). Variable degrees of spongiosis (intercellular edema) may be seen. Transmigration of inflammatory cells through the epithelium is a common finding, with

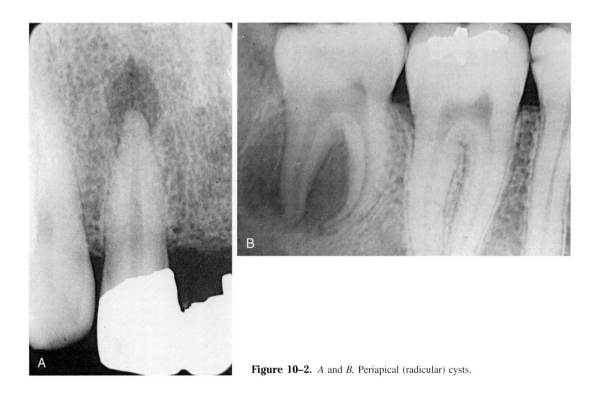

Figure 10–2. *A* and *B,* Periapical (radicular) cysts.

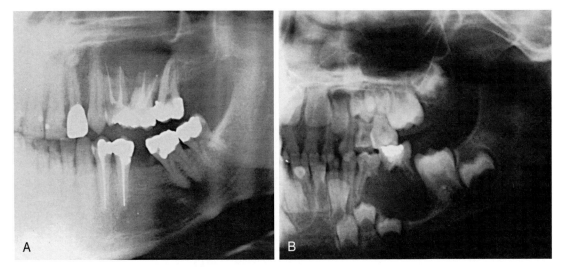

Figure 10–3. *A,* Radicular cyst of the maxilla. (Lesion did not resolve after endodontic therapy.) *B,* Periapical associated with a primary molar.

large numbers of polymorphonuclear leukocytes and fewer numbers of lymphocytes involved in this process. The underlying supportive connective tissue may be focally or diffusely infiltrated with a mixed inflammatory cell population. Toward the epithelium, polymorphonuclear leukocytes dominate; deeper within the connective tissue, lymphocytes are more common. Plasma cell infiltrates and associated refractile and spherical *Russell bodies* are found frequently and sometimes dominate the microscopic picture. Foci of dystrophic calcification, cholesterol clefts, and multinucleated giant cells may be seen subsequent to hemorrhage in the cyst wall (Fig. 10–6).

In a small percentage of periapical cysts (and dentigerous cysts), hyaline bodies, so-called *Rushton bodies,* may be found (Fig. 10–7). Such bodies within the epithelial lining are characterized by a hairpin or slightly curved shape, concentric lamination, and occasional basophilic mineralization. The origin of such bodies is believed to be related to previous hemorrhage.

Differential Diagnosis. Radiographically, the differential diagnosis of the radicular cyst must include the periapical granuloma. In areas of previously treated apical pathology, a surgical defect or periapical scar might also be considered. In the anterior mandible, a periapical radiolucency

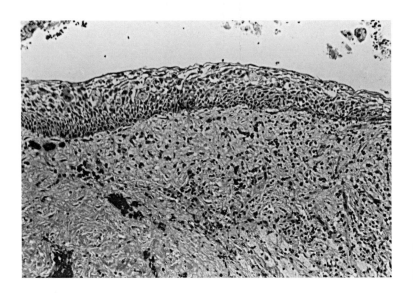

Figure 10–4. Periapical cyst lined with nonkeratinized stratified epithelium.

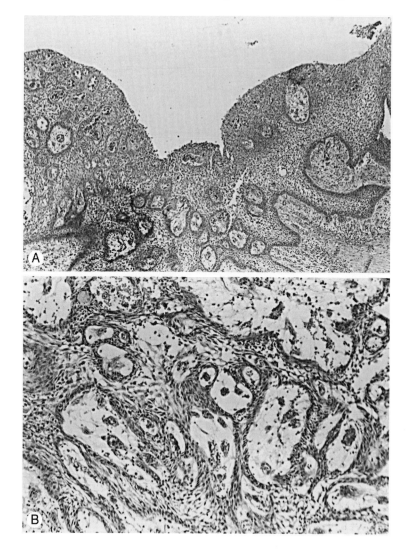

Figure 10–5. *A* and *B*, Hyperplastic epithelium lining a periapical cyst.

should be distinguished from the early phase of periapical cemental dysplasia. In the posterior quadrants, apical radiolucencies must be distinguished from the traumatic bone cyst. Occasionally, odontogenic tumors, giant cell lesions, metastatic disease, and primary osseous tumors may mimic a periapical cyst radiographically. In all the above considerations, teeth are vital.

Treatment and Prognosis. The periapical lesion (cyst/granuloma) may be successfully managed by extraction of the associated nonvital tooth and curettage of the epithelium in the apical zone. Alternatively, a root canal filling may be performed in association with an apicoectomy to permit direct curettage of the cystic lesion. The third and most frequently used option involves performing a root canal filling only, since most periapical lesions are granulomas and resolve after

removal of the inflammatory stimulus (necrotic pulp). Surgery (apicoectomy and curettage) is done only for lesions that are persistent, indicating the presence of a cyst or inadequate endodontics.

With incomplete removal of cystic epithelium, a *residual cyst* may develop from months to years after the initial treatment (Fig. 10–8). If either a residual cyst or the original periapical cyst remains untreated, continued growth can cause significant destruction and weakening of the mandible or maxilla. Complete bone repair is usually seen in adequately treated radicular and residual cysts.

Dentigerous Cyst

The dentigerous or follicular cyst is the second most common odontogenic cyst. By definition, a

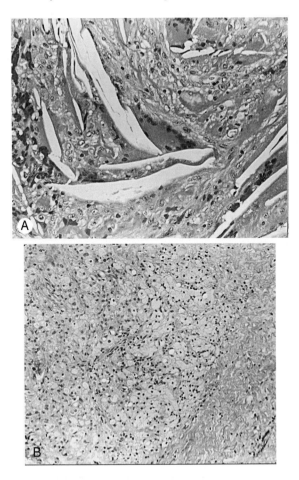

Figure 10–6. Cholesterol clefts and giant cells *(A)* and lipid-filled macrophages *(B)* in the wall of a periapical cyst.

dentigerous cyst is associated with the crown of an unerupted or developing tooth. The cyst enclosing the crown of the unerupted tooth is attached to the tooth cervix (enamel-cementum junction).

Etiology and Pathogenesis. The dentigerous cyst develops from proliferation of the enamel organ remnant or reduced enamel epithelium.

As with other cysts, expansion of the dentiger-

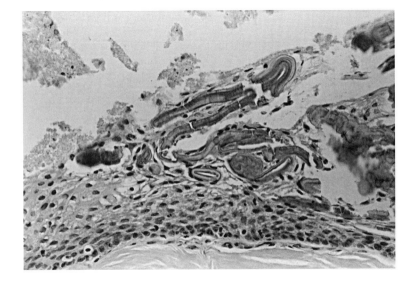

Figure 10–7. Hyaline bodies (Rushton bodies) in the lining of a periapical cyst.

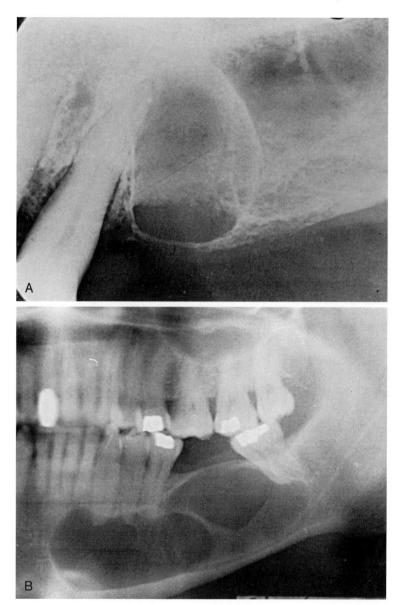

Figure 10–8. *A* and *B,* Residual cysts.

ous cyst is related to epithelial proliferation, release of bone-resorbing factors, and an increase in cyst fluid osmolality as a result of passage of inflammatory cells and desquamated epithelial cells into the cyst lumen.

Clinical Features. Dentigerous cysts are most commonly seen in association with third molars and maxillary canines, the most frequently impacted teeth (Fig. 10–9). The highest incidence of dentigerous cysts occurs during the second and third decades. There is a greater frequency in males, with a ratio of 1.6 to 1 reported.

Symptoms are generally absent, with late eruption a frequent indication of possible dentigerous

cyst formation. This particular cyst is capable of achieving significant size, occasionally with associated cortical bone expansion. Lesions may rarely achieve a size that predisposes to a pathologic fracture.

Radiographically, the dentigerous cyst presents as a well-defined, unilocular and occasionally multilocular radiolucency in association with the crown of an unerupted tooth (Fig. 10–10). The unerupted tooth is frequently displaced. In the mandible, the associated radiolucency may extend superiorly from the third molar site into the ramus or anteriorly and inferiorly along the body of the mandible. In maxillary dentigerous cysts involving

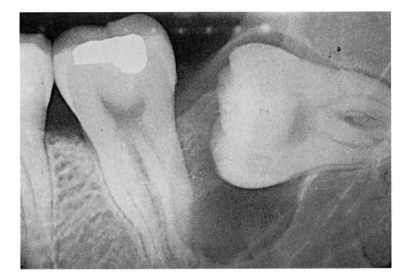

Figure 10–9. Dentigerous cyst.

the canine region, extension into the maxillary sinus or to the orbital floor may be noted.

Resorption of roots of adjacent erupted teeth may occasionally be seen.

A variant of the dentigerous cyst, the *paradental cyst* arises when there is partial eruption of the involved tooth. These cysts are usually found along the buccal root surface of mandibular third molars. Radiographically, they are well-circumscribed radiolucencies. These cysts are often associated with developmental enamel ridges or projections along the buccal bifurcation of the molar roots.

Histopathology. The supporting fibrous connective tissue wall of the cyst is lined by stratified squamous epithelium (Fig. 10–11). In an uninflamed dentigerous cyst, the epithelial lining is nonkeratinized and tends to be approximately four to six cell layers thick. On occasion, numerous cells, ciliated cells, and rarely sebaceous cells may be found in the lining epithilium. The epithelium-connective tissue junction is generally flat, al-

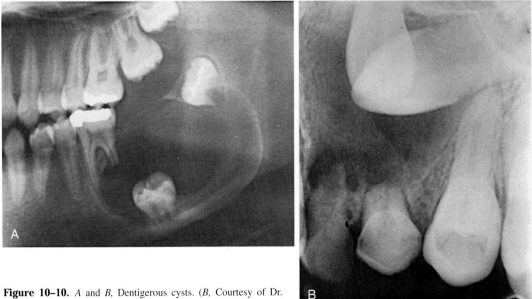

Figure 10–10. *A* and *B*, Dentigerous cysts. (*B*, Courtesy of Dr. W. G. Sprague.)

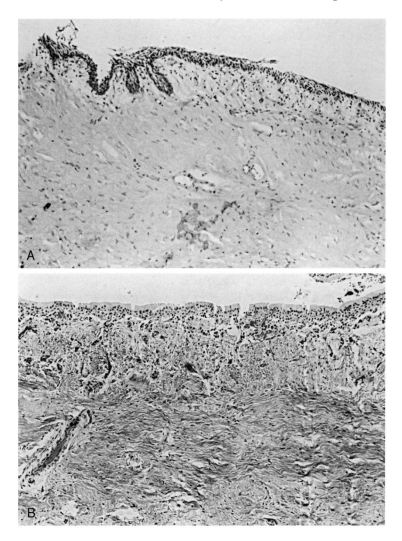

Figure 10–11. *A,* Stratified squamous epithelial lining of a dentigerous cyst. *B,* Reduced enamel epithelial lining of a follicular sac over the crown of an unerupted tooth.

though in cases in which there is secondary inflammation, epithelial hyperplasia may be noted (Fig. 10–12).

Differential Diagnosis. Differential diagnosis of pericoronal radiolucency should include: odontogenic keratocyst, ameloblastoma, and other odontogenic tumors. Ameloblastic transformation of a dentigerous cyst lining should also be part of the differential diagnosis. Adenomatoid odontogenic tumor would be a serious consideration with anterior pericoronal radiolucencies, and ameloblastic fibroma would be a possibility when occurring in the posterior jaws of young patients.

Treatment. Removal of the associated tooth and enucleation of the soft tissue component is definitive therapy in most instances. In cases in which cysts affect significant portions of the mandible, an acceptable early treatment approach involves exteriorization or marsupialization of the cyst to allow for decompression and subsequent shrinkage of the lesion, thereby reducing the extent of surgery to be done at a later date.

Potential complications of the untreated dentigerous cyst are of considerable significance. Transformation of the epithelial lining of the dentigerous cyst into an ameloblastoma is possible. Rarely, carcinomatous transformation of the lining epithelium may be noted. In cases in which mucous cells are present, potential is believed to exist for development of the rarely seen intraosseous mucoepidermoid carcinoma.

The specific complication of ameloblastoma arising in a dentigerous cyst is frequently a difficult histopathologic problem. Identification of early ameloblastomatous transformation has been associated with the following microscopic findings:

1. Nuclear hyperchromatism of the basal cell nuclei.

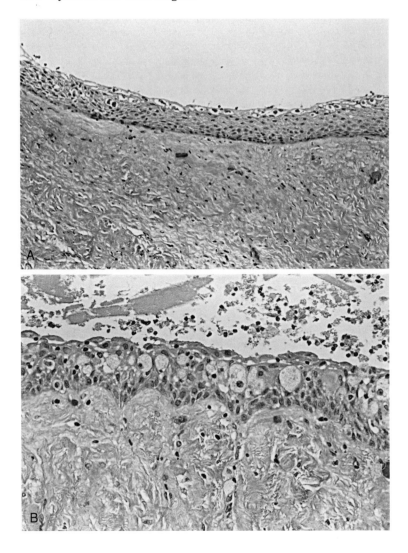

Figure 10–12. *A* and *B*. Epithelial linings of dentigerous cysts. Note mucous cells in *B*.

2. Palisading of the basal cells with nuclear polarization away from the basement membrane.

3. Cytoplasmic vacuole formation within the basal cells, generally between the nuclei and basement membrane.

4. Increased width of intercellular space within the epithelial layers (spongiosis).

ERUPTION CYST

The eruption cyst is essentially a type of dentigerous cyst that results from fluid accumulation within the follicular space of an erupting tooth (Fig. 10–13). The epithelium lining this space is simply reduced enamel epithelium. With trauma, blood may appear within the tissue space, forming a so-called *eruption hematoma.* No treatment is needed because the tooth erupts through the le-

sion. Subsequent to eruption, the cyst disappears spontaneously without complication.

Lateral Periodontal Cyst

The lateral periodontal cyst is defined as a nonkeratinized developmental cyst occurring adjacent or lateral to the root of a tooth. Discussion of the *gingival cyst of adulthood* appears with the discussion of lateral periodontal cyst because of the close histogenetic relationship between these lesions.

Etiology and Pathogenesis. The origin of this cyst is believed to be related to proliferation of rests of dental lamina. The lateral periodontal cyst has been pathogenetically linked to the gingival cyst: the latter is believed to arise from dental lamina remnants in soft tissue between the oral

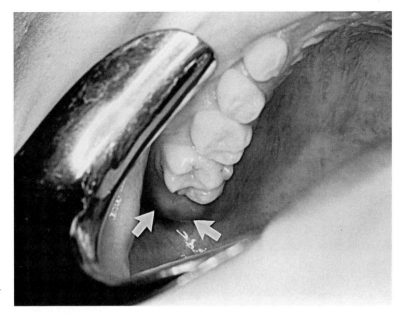

Figure 10–13. Eruption cyst over a molar *(arrows).*

epithelium and the periosteum, and the former from dental lamina remnants within bone and separate from the periodontal ligament. The relationship between the gingival and lateral periodontal cysts is further supported by their similar distribution where there is a corresponding higher concentration of dental lamina rests (rests of Malassez are more plentiful around the apices of teeth).

Clinical Features. The majority of lateral periodontal cysts and gingival cysts of the adult occur in the mandibular premolar and cuspid region and occasionally in the incisor area (Fig. 10–14). In the maxilla, lesions are noted primarily in the lateral incisor region. A distinct male predilection is noted for the lateral periodontal cyst, with a greater than 2 to 1 distribution. The adult gingival cyst shows a nearly equal gender predilection. The median age for both the lateral periodontal and the gingival cysts occurs between the fifth and sixth decades of life, with a range of 20 to 85 years for the lateral periodontal cyst and 40 to 75 years for the gingival cyst of the adult.

Clinically, the gingival cyst appears, as a small soft tissue swelling within or slightly inferior to the interdental papilla. It may assume a slightly bluish discoloration when it is relatively large. Most cysts are less than 1 cm in diameter (Fig. 10–15).

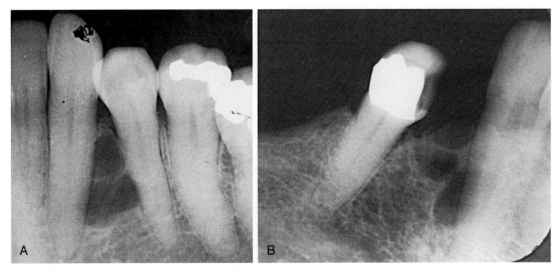

Figure 10–14. *A* and *B,* Lateral periodontal cysts. Note the multilocularity.

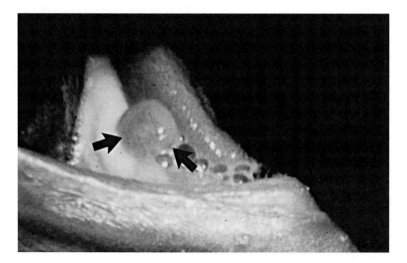

Figure 10–15. Gingival cyst in an edentulous adult *(arrows)*.

The lateral periodontal cyst presents as an asymptomatic, well-delineated, round or teardrop-shaped unilocular (and occasionally multilocular) radiolucency with an opaque margin along the lateral surface of a vital tooth root. Root divergence is rarely seen. The term *botryoid odontogenic cyst* is sometimes applicable when the lesion is multilocular.

Histopathology. Both the lateral periodontal cyst and the gingival cyst of the adult are lined by a thin, nonkeratinized epithelium (Fig. 10–16). Clusters of glycogen-rich clear epithelial cells may be noted in nodular thickenings of the cyst lining. Of interest is that the botryoid odontogenic cyst is similar in histologic appearance and location to the lateral periodontal cyst, supporting the belief that it represents a multilocular variant. A possible explanation of multilocularity is that several clusters of dental lamina remnants undergo cystic degeneration and subsequent fusion.

Differential Diagnosis. The lateral periodontal cyst must be distinguished from a cyst resulting from an inflammatory stimulus through a lateral root canal of a nonvital tooth (a lateral radicular cyst), an odontogenic keratocyst along the lateral root surface, and radiolucent odontogenic tumors. The differential diagnosis for the gingival cyst would include gingival mucocele, Fordyce's granules, parulis, and possibly a peripheral odontogenic tumor.

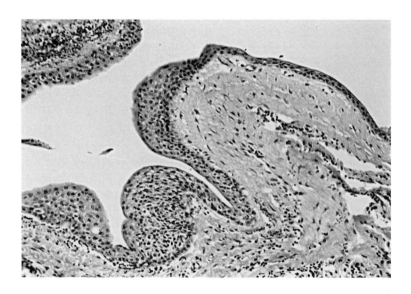

Figure 10–16. Epithelial lining of a lateral periodontal cyst. Note the occasional epithelial tufts in an otherwise thin lining.

Treatment and Prognosis. Local excision of both the gingival and the lateral periodontal cysts is generally curative. The multlocular variant *botryoid odontogenic cyst* seems to have some recurrence potential. Follow-up, therefore, is suggested for treated botryoid odontogenic cysts.

Glandular Odontogenic Cyst

The glandular odontogenic cyst, or the *sialo-odontogenic cyst,* described in 1987, shares some features with both the botryoid odontogenic cyst and a mucus-producing salivary gland tumor.

Clinical Features. A strong predilection is seen for the mandible (80%), especially the anterior mandible (Fig. 10–17). Maxillary lesions tend to be localized to the anterior segment. Jaw expansion is not uncommon, particularly in the mandible. The gender ratio is approximately 1 to 1. The mean age is 50 years, with a wide age range from the second through the ninth decades.

Radiographic Features. Most cases are radiographically multiloculated. In cases in which a unilocular radiolucency has been noted initially, recurrent lesions have tended to be multiloculated. Lesions reported have exhibited a wide variation in size, from some less than 1 cm to those involving most of the mandible bilaterally. Radiographic margins may be well defined and sclerotic. More aggressive lesions have shown an ill-defined peripheral border.

Histopathology. Histologically, this multilocular cyst is lined by nonkeratinized epithelium with focal aggregates or nodular thickenings within which the epithelial cells assume a swirled appearance similar to those seen in the lateral periodontal cyst and the botryoid odontogenic cyst (Fig. 10–18). The epithelial lining consists of cuboidal cells, often with cilia at the free surface. Mucous cells and clear cells are scattered or clustered along the cyst lining along with mucin pools. The overall histomorphology is reminiscent of a cystic low-grade mucoepidermoid carcinoma.

Treatment and Prognosis. This lesion should be considered locally aggressive, and therefore, surgical management should be dictated by the clinical and radiographic extent of the disease. Where adequate healthy bone remains beyond the extent of the cystic lesion, a peripheral curettage or marginal excision is appropriate. Long-term follow-up is essential given the local aggressiveness and recurrence-rate (approximately 25%) of this lesion.

Gingival Cyst of the Newborn

The gingival cyst of the newborn has also been designated as the dental lamina cyst of the newborn or Bohn's nodules. Such cysts appear typically as multiple nodules along the alveolar ridge in neonates. The consensus is that fragments of the dental lamina that remain within the alveolar ridge mucosa after tooth formation proliferate to form small, keratinized cysts. It is important to note that such proliferation is limited in overall

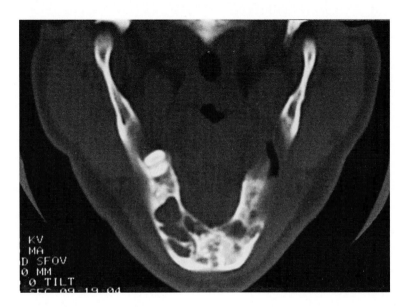

Figure 10–17. Computed tomography scan of a glandular odontogenic cyst. Note the multilocular lucency that crosses the midline of the mandible.

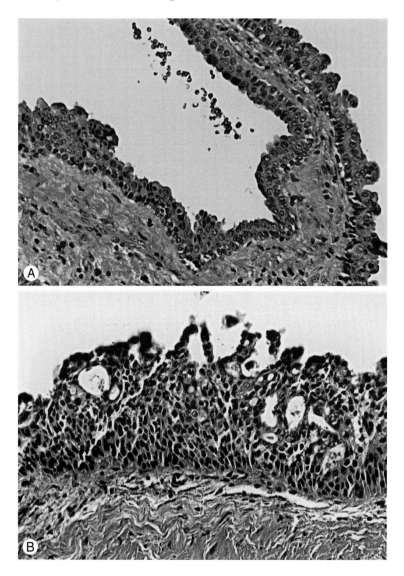

Figure 10–18. *A,* Glandular odontogenic cyst featuring apocrine-like cells, papillary surface, and nodular thickenings. *B,* Nodular areas contain mucous cells and mucous cysts.

extent and potential. In the vast majority of cases, these cysts degenerate and involute or rupture into the oral cavity.

Histologically, this cyst is lined by a thin epithelium, usually two to three cell layers thick (Fig. 10–19). Treatment is not necessary, because nearly all involute spontaneously or rupture before 3 months of age.

Similar epithelial inclusional cysts may occur along the midline of the palate (*palatine cysts of the newborn or Epstein's pearls*). These are of developmental origin but are derived from epithelium that is included in the fusion line between the palatal shelves and the nasal processes. These cysts also contain keratin and show a thin, attenuated epithelial lining. No treatment is necessary,

because they fuse with the overlying oral epithelium and resolve spontaneously.

Odontogenic Keratocyst

The odontogenic keratocyst has engendered a great deal of discussion in terms of its relationship to the *primordial cyst* that occurs in place of a tooth. It has been shown that primordial cysts are microscopically, odontogenic keratocysts. Confusion arose because other odontogenic cysts, including dentigerous, radicular, and residual cysts, occasionally contain keratinized cells. The odontogenic keratocyst, however, is regarded as a distinctive entity because of its characteristic histology,

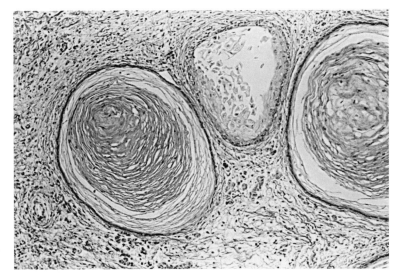

Figure 10–19. Gingival cysts of the newborn.

proliferation kinetics, and behavior. Therefore, although keratinization may be present in many other types of cysts, the specific histologic pattern of the odontogenic keratocyst separates it from all others.

Etiology and Pathogenesis. There is general agreement that the origin of the odontogenic keratocyst comes from dental lamina remnants in the mandible and maxilla. However, origin of this cyst from extension of basal cells of the overlying oral epithelium has also been suggested.

Clinical Features. Generally, odontogenic keratocysts have a benign, but aggressive behavior with a significant recurrence rate, and they may be an indicator of the *nevoid basal cell carcinoma syndrome.* This cyst seems to occur at any age and has a peak incidence within the second and third decades. Lesions found in children are often reflective of multiple odontogenic keratocysts as a component of the *nevoid basal cell carcinoma syndrome.* In the context of multiple odontogenic keratocysts, this particular syndrome must be ruled out (discussed later).

Odontogenic keratocysts are found in the mandible, in approximately a 2-to-1 ratio. In the mandible, the posterior portion of the body and the ramus region are most commonly affected, and in the maxilla the third molar area is most frequently affected.

Radiographically, the odontogenic keratocyst characteristically presents as a well-circumscribed radiolucency with smooth radiopaque margins (Fig. 10–20). Multilocularity is often present and tends to be seen more frequently in larger lesions.

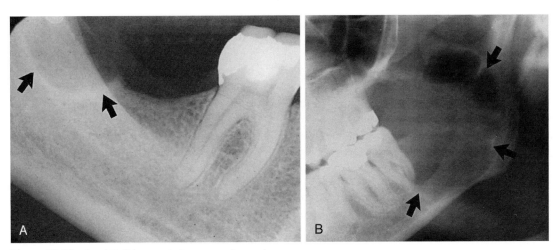

Figure 10–20. *A* and *B,* Odontogenic keratocysts *(arrows).*

Most lesions, however, are unilocular, with as many as 40% noted adjacent to the crown of an unerupted tooth (dentigerous cyst position). Approximately 30% of maxillary and 50% of mandibular lesions produce buccal expansion. Mandibular lingual enlargement is occasionally seen.

Histopathology. The epithelial lining is uniformly thin, generally ranging from 8 to 10 cell layers thick. The basal layer exhibits a characteristic palisaded pattern with polarized and intensely stained nuclei of uniform diameter. The luminal epithelial cells are parakeratinized and produce an uneven or corrugated profile. Focal zones of orthokeratin have been described. Additional histologic features that may occasionally be encountered include budding of the basal cells into the connective tissue wall and microcyst formation (Fig. 10–21). The fibrous connective tissue component of the cyst wall is often free of an inflammatory cell infiltrate and is relatively thin (Fig. 10–22). The epithelium-connective tissue interface is characteristically flattened, with no epithelial ridge formation.

An *orthokeratinized odontogenic cyst* has been described and is about one-twentieth as common as the odontogenic keratocyst (Fig. 10–23). Histologic distinction between the parakeratinized and orthokeratinized cysts is made because the latter is less aggressive, has a lower rate of recurrence, and is generally not syndrome-associated. In the orthokeratotic odontogenic cyst, a prominent granular layer is found immediately below a flat, noncorrugated surface. The basal cell layer is less

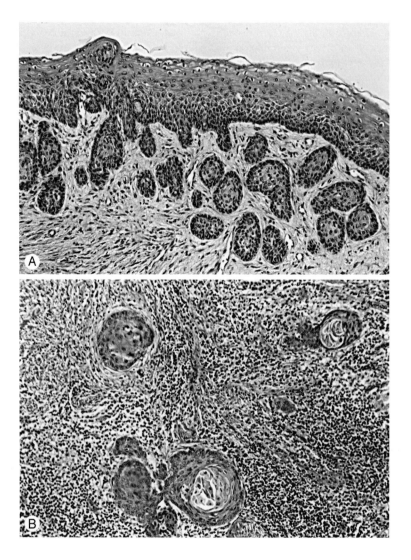

Figure 10–21. Odontogenic keratocyst histologic variations. *A,* Budding. *B,* Satellite cysts in the cyst wall.

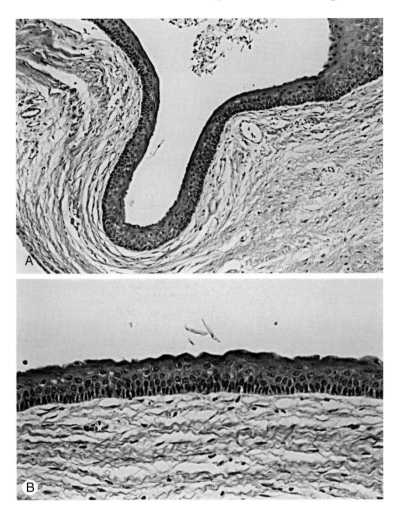

Figure 10–22. *A* and *B,* Parakeratotic epithelium typical of odontogenic keratocysts.

prominent, with a more flattened or squamoid appearance in comparison with the parakeratotic type.

Differential Diagnosis. When closely associated with teeth, several entities might be considered, such as dentigerous cyst, ameloblastoma, minimally calcified calcifying odontogenic cyst, adenomatoid odontogenic tumor, ameloblastic fibroma, and other rare odontogenic tumors. Lucent, nonodontogenic tumors, such as central giant cell granuloma, traumatic bone cyst, and aneurysmal bone cyst might be included in young patients.

Treatment and Prognosis. Surgical excision with peripheral osseous curettage or ostectomy is the preferred method of management. This more aggressive approach for a cystic lesion is justified because of the high recurrence rate associated with odontogenic keratocyst. The reason for high recurrence rates, ranging from 5 to 62%, remains unclear but may be related to one of several possibilities. The friable, thin connective tissue wall of

the cyst may lead to incomplete removal. Small dental lamina remnants or satellite cysts in the bone adjacent to the primary lesion may contribute to recurrence. Also, cystic proliferation of the overlying oral epithelial basal cell layer, if not excised during cyst removal, is thought by some to be significant. The actual biologic qualities of the cyst epithelium, such as mitotic index and production of bone-resorbing factors, may be associated with recurrences.

Follow-up examinations are important for patients with this lesion. Patients should be evaluated for completeness of excision, new keratocysts, and the nevoid basal cell carcinoma syndrome. Most recurrences become clinically evident within 5 years of treatment. Aside from recurrence potential, ameloblastic transformation is a rare complication.

Studies indicate that patients with multiple keratocysts have a significantly higher rate of recurrence than do those with single keratocysts: 35%

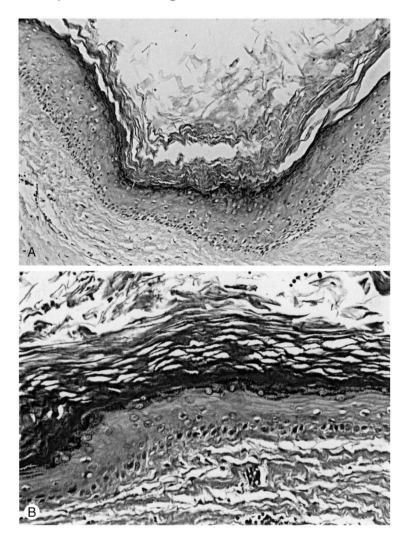

Figure 10–23. *A* and *B*, Orthokeratinized odontogenic cyst. Note the prominent granular layer.

and 10%, respectively. In such circumstances, it is necessary to rule out the presence of the nevoid basal cell carcinoma syndrome. Approximately 7% of patients with multiple odontogenic keratocysts are afflicted with this syndrome.

Briefly, the *nevoid basal cell carcinoma syndrome* includes multiple odontogenic keratocysts, bone defects, and multiple basal cell carcinomas. The syndrome is further characterized by cutaneous abnormalities including palmar and plantar keratotic pitting, multiple milia, and dermal calcinosis. Common bone defects include bifid ribs as well as vertebral and metacarpal abnormalities. Mild mandibular prognathism has been recorded in a small percentage of cases. Facial dysmorphogenesis including a broad nasal bridge with corresponding ocular hypertelorism and laterally displaced inner ocular canthi (dystopia canthorum) may be seen. Neurologic abnormalities including medulloblastoma, dysgenesis or agenesis of the

corpus callosum, calcification of the falx cerebri and, less frequently, of the falx cerebelli have also been documented.

Calcifying Odontogenic Cyst

The calcifying odontogenic cyst (COC) is a developmental odontogenic lesion that, because of occasionally reported aggressive behavior, has been viewed by some as having a behavior similar to a neoplasm, prompting the term *odontogenic ghost cell tumor.*

Etiology and Pathogenesis. The COC is believed to be derived from odontogenic epithelial remnants within the gingiva or within the mandible or maxilla. "Ghost cell keratinization," the characteristic microscopic feature of the COC, is also a defining feature of the cutaneous lesion known as *calcifying epithelioma of Malherbe* or *pilomatrixoma.* In the jaws, ghost cells may be seen in many odontogenic tumors, including odontomas, ameloblastomas, adenomatoid odontogenic tumors, ameloblastic fibro-odontomas, and ameloblastic fibromas.

Clinical Features. There is a wide age range for this cyst, with a peak incidence in the second decade. It usually appears in individuals younger than 40 years and has a decided predilection for females. More than 70% of COCs are seen in the maxilla. Approximately one fourth of these lesions present extraosseously as localized masses involving the gingiva. Those presenting in an extraosseous or peripheral location are usually noted in individuals older than 50 years and are found anterior to the first molar region.

Radiographically, COC may present as a unilocular or multilocular radiolucency with discrete, well-demarcated margins. Within the radiolucency may be scattered, irregularly sized calcifications (Fig. 10–24). Such opacities may produce a salt-and-pepper type of pattern, with an equal and diffuse distribution. In some cases, mineralization may develop to such an extent that the radiographic margins of the lesion are difficult to determine.

Histopathology. Most lesions present as well-delineated cystic proliferations with a fibrous connective tissue wall lined by odontogenic epithelium. Intraluminal epithelial proliferation occasionally obscures the cyst lumen, thereby producing the impression of a solid tumor (Fig. 10–25). The epithelial lining is of variable thickness. The basal epithelium may focally be quite prominent, with hyperchromatic nuclei and cuboidal to columnar pattern. Above the basal layer are more loosely arranged epithelial cells sometimes bearing similarity to the stellate reticulum of the enamel organ. The most prominent and unique microscopic feature is the presence of so-called ghost cell keratinization. The ghost cells are anucleate and retain the outline of the cell membrane. These cells undergo dystrophic mineralization characterized by fine basophilic granularity, which may eventually result in large sheets of calcified material. On occasion, ghost cells may become displaced in the connective tissue wall, eliciting a foreign-body giant cell response.

Differential Diagnosis. In the early stages of formation, the COC may have little or no mineralization and therefore may present as a radiolucency. Differential diagnosis would include dentigerous cyst, odontogenic keratocyst, and ameloblastoma. In later stages when a mixed radiolucent-radiopaque appearance is present, the differential would include adenomatoid odontogenic tumor, a partially mineralized odontoma, calcifying epithelial odontogenic tumor, and ameloblastic fibro-odontoma.

Treatment and Prognosis. Because of the unpredictable biologic behavior of this lesion, treatment is usually more aggressive than simple curettage. Patients should be monitored indefinitely, because recurrences are not uncommon. Management of the extraosseous or peripheral variant is conservative because recurrence is not characteristic.

NONODONTOGENIC CYSTS

Globulomaxillary Lesions

A "globulomaxillary cyst" was once considered a fissural cyst, located between the globular and maxillary processes. The old theory of origin related to epithelial entrapment within a line of embryologic closure with subsequent cystic change. Evidence now shows that this type of cyst is more likely derived from odontogenic epithelium located between the maxillary lateral incisor and the canine teeth. Globulomaxillary radiolucencies when reviewed microscopically include radicular cysts, periapical granulomas, lateral periodontal cysts, odontogenic keratocysts, central giant cell granulomas, calcifying odontogenic cysts, and odontogenic myxomas. The term *globulomaxillary* is used as a clinical term, with definitive diagnosis made from microscopic examination.

Radiologically, the globulomaxillary lesion appears as well-defined radiolucency, often producing divergence of the roots of the maxillary lateral incisor and canine teeth. Radicular cyst and peri-

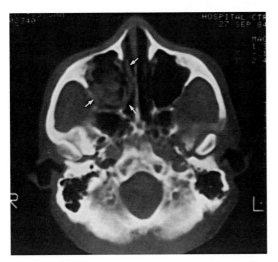

Figure 10–24. Computed tomography scan of a maxillary (right) calcifying odontogenic cyst *(arrows).*

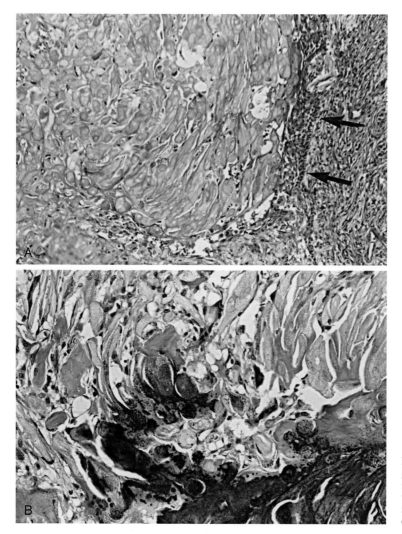

Figure 10–25. Calcifying odontogenic cyst. *A,* The epithelium *(arrows)* is thin, and the lumen (left) is filled with ghost cells. *B,* Ghost cell keratinization showing a focus of dystrophic calcification (bottom).

apical granuloma can be ruled out with pulp vitality testing.

Because of the array of potential diagnoses, the histology varies considerably from case to case. Specific histologic features of the differential diagnoses offered are found in the discussions of these entities.

Treatment and prognosis are determined by the definitive microscopic diagnosis.

Nasolabial Cyst

The nasolabial cyst is a soft tissue cyst of the upper lip. The occasionally used term *nasoalveolar cyst* would be inaccurate, because it does not involve alveolar bone.

The pathogenesis of the nasolabial cyst is unclear, although it was considered to arise from epithelial entrapment at the fusion site of the soft tissue components of the globular and maxillary processes. It was thought to represent the soft tissue counterpart of the globulomaxillary cyst. Because this is embryologically unsound, it is now believed to develop from remnants of the solid cord of cells that ultimately form the nasolacrimal duct.

The nasolabial cyst is a rare lesion with a peak incidence noted in the fourth and fifth decades. There is a distinct female predilection of nearly 4 to 1. The chief clinical sign is a soft tissue swelling that may present in the soft tissue over the canine region or the mucobuccal fold. Occasionally, the patients may complain of discomfort or some minor degree of nasal obstruction. If untreated, the cyst continues to grow at a slow rate and may ultimately distort the ala of the nose.

Radiographically, bone alteration may result from pressure resorption along the labial aspect of the anterior maxilla.

The epithelial lining of this cyst is characteristically a pseudostratified columnar type with numerous goblet cells (Fig. 10–26). Stratified squamous epithelium may be present in addition to cuboidal epithelium in some cases.

Differential Diagnosis. Salivary gland neoplasms and benign cutaneous adnexal tumors and cysts would be included in a differential diagnosis of the upper lip mass. This lesion should be surgically excised, and recurrence is unexpected.

Median Mandibular Cyst

The median mandibular cyst, like the globulomaxillary cyst, was once considered a fissural cyst.

Justification for a fissural origin was based on the no longer tenable theory of epithelial entrapment in the midline of the mandible during the "fusion" of each half of the mandibular arch. There is embryologic evidence of an isthmus of mesenchyme between the mandibular processes that is gradually eliminated as growth continues and, therefore, no fusion.

Cases diagnosed clinically as median mandibular cysts represent a microscopic spectrum similar to that seen with globulomaxillary lesions. Radicular cysts, lateral periodontal cysts, odontogenic keratocysts, and residual cysts have been noted in this area. Detection of mucous cells and ciliated epithelium in cysts found in the midline of the

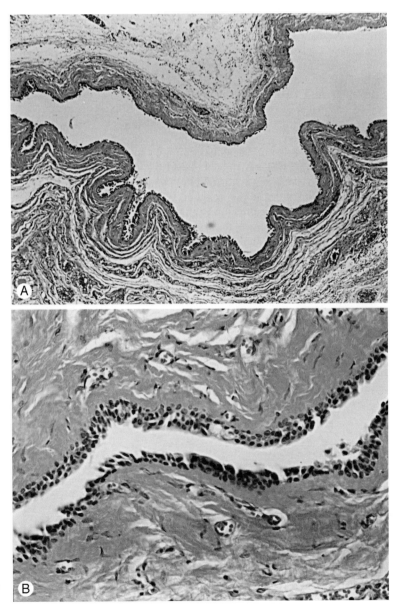

Figure 10–26. *A* and *B,* Nasolabial cysts.

mandible does not preclude an odontogenic origin, because both cell types can be found in other odontogenic cysts of the mandible and maxilla.

Nasopalatine Canal Cyst

The nasopalatine canal cyst, also known as *incisive canal cyst,* is located within the nasopalatine canal or within the palatal soft tissues at the point of the opening of the canal, where it is called *cyst of the palatine papilla.* The so-called *median palatine cyst* is believed to represent a more posterior presentation of a nasopalatine canal cyst rather than cystic degeneration of epithelial rests in the line of fusion of the palatine shelves. The rare *median alveolar cyst* is believed to be a true cyst of the alveolar process anterior to the incisive canal. This cyst in all probability represents an odontogenic cyst, possibly a primordial cyst of supernumerary (mesiodens) tooth bud origin.

Etiology and Pathogenesis. The development of the nasopalatine canal cyst comes from the proliferation of epithelial remnants of paired embryonic nasopalatine ducts within the incisive canal. The canal itself forms secondary to the fusion of the premaxilla with the right and left palatal processes. The anatomic exit of the canal is slightly posterior to the incisive papilla.

The stimulus for cyst formation from the epithelial remnants of the nasopalatine canals is uncertain, although bacterial infections and/or trauma are thought to have a role. Alternatively, it has been suggested that the mucous glands within the lining may cause cyst formation as a result of mucin secretion.

Clinical Features. A symmetric swelling in the anterior region of the palatal midline is characteristic of this lesion. The overall frequency of nasopalatine canal cysts in the general population ranges from 0.08 to 1.3%, as determined from analysis of specimen skulls. The majority of cases occur between the fourth and sixth decades of life. Males are more frequently affected than females—differences ranged as high as 3 to 1.

Most cases are asymptomatic, with the clinical sign of swelling usually calling attention to the lesion. Symptoms may follow secondary infection. Sinus formation and drainage is not uncommon and usually occurs at the most prominent portion of the palatine papilla.

Radiographically, the nasopalatine canal cyst is purely radiolucent, with sharply defined margins (Fig. 10–27). It may produce divergence of the roots of the maxillary incisor teeth and less commonly induce external root resorption. The anterior nasal spine is often centrally superimposed on the lucent defect, producing a heart shape. The radiolucency may occasionally be unilateral, with the midline forming the most medial aspect of the radiolucency.

Histopathology. The epithelial lining of this cyst ranges from stratified squamous to pseudostratified columnar when located near the nasal cavity (Fig. 10–28). In many instances, a mixture of two or more types of lining cells is seen. The connective tissue wall contains small arteries and nerves representing the nasopalatine neurovascular bundle.

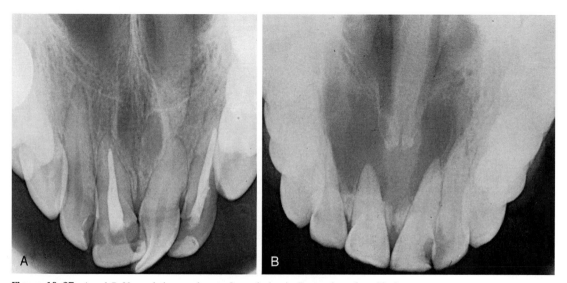

Figure 10–27. *A* and *B,* Nasopalatine canal cysts. Large lesion in *B* extends to the midpalate.

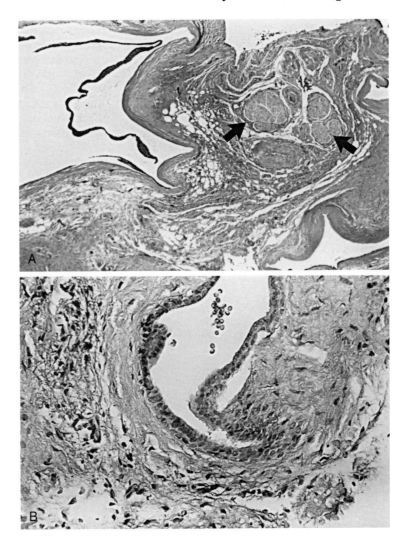

Figure 10–28. *A* and *B,* Nasopalatine canal cysts. Note the nerve bundles *(arrows)* and vascular channels in the cyst wall *(A).*

Differential Diagnosis. Periapical granuloma and cyst must be separated from the nasopalatine canal cyst. This can be done simply by determining tooth vitality. A normal but widened canal might also be considered. Additionally, primordial cysts resulting from degradation of a mesiodens or supernumerary tooth may potentially present in a similar fashion.

Treatment and Prognosis. This cyst requires surgical enucleation. In cases of large cysts, marsupialization may be considered before definitive enucleation. Recurrence rate is very low.

PSEUDOCYSTS

Aneurysmal Bone Cyst

The aneurysmal bone cyst is classified as a pseudocyst because it appears radiographically as a cyst-like lesion but microscopically exhibits no epithelial lining. It represents a benign lesion of bone that may arise in the mandible, maxilla, or other bones. The incidence in the cranial and maxillofacial area is approximately 5% of bone lesions; in all other sites this cyst represents 3% of all bone lesions. Within the craniofacial complex, approximately 40% of these lesions are located in the mandible, 25% in the maxilla.

Etiology and Pathogenesis. Although the pathogenesis of the aneurysmal bone cyst is obscure, it is generally regarded as a reactive process. An unrelated antecedent primary lesion of bone that is believed to initiate a vascular malformation frequently exists, resulting in a secondary lesion or aneurysmal bone cyst. Preexisting fibrous dysplasia, central giant cell granuloma, nonossifying fibroma, chondroblastoma, and other primary bone lesions have been described as antecedent lesions to aneurysmal bone cysts.

Clinical Features. The aneurysmal bone cyst typically affects persons younger than 30 years. The peak incidence occurs within the second decade of life. There is a slight female predilection.

When the mandible and maxilla are involved, the more posterior regions are affected, chiefly the molar areas. Pain is described in approximately half the cases, and a firm, nonpulsatile swelling is a frequent clinical sign. On auscultation, a bruit is not heard, and on firm palpation, crepitus may be noted.

Radiographic features include the presence of a destructive or osteolytic process with slightly irregular margins (Fig. 10–29). A multilocular pattern is noted in some instances, although it is usually unilocular. When the alveolar segment of the mandible and maxilla is involved, teeth may be displaced with or without concomitant external root resorption.

Histopathology. A fibrous connective tissue stroma contains variable numbers of multinucleated giant cells. Sinusoidal blood spaces are found (Fig. 10–30). That the sinusoidal spaces are not lined by endothelial cells has been confirmed by ultrastructural and immunohistochemical studies. Instead, fibroblasts and macrophages (histiocytes) line the sinusoids. The tissue between the vascular or sinusoidal elements often contains large numbers of multinucleated giant cells, fibroblasts, extravasated erythrocytes, and hemosiderin in a pattern reminiscent of central giant cell granuloma. Reactive new bone formation not unlike that seen in ossifying fibroma or fibrous dysplasia is also frequently noted.

Differential Diagnosis. Odontogenic keratocyst, central giant cell granuloma, and ameloblastic fibroma should be included in a differential diagnosis. Ameloblastoma and odontogenic myxoma could be included, although these lesions more typically appear in older patients.

Treatment and Prognosis. A relatively high recurrence rate has been associated with simple curettage. Excision or curettage with supplemental cryotherapy is the treatment of choice.

Traumatic (Simple) Bone Cyst

The traumatic bone cyst is an intrabony dead space that lacks an epithelial lining. The designation of pseudocyst relates to its cystic radiographic appearance and its gross surgical presentation. This lesion is quite uncommon in the mandible and maxilla, but it occurs relatively frequently in the humerus and other long bones.

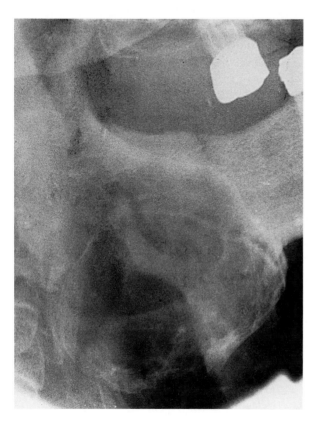

Figure 10–29. Aneurysmal bone cyst located in the angle of the mandible.

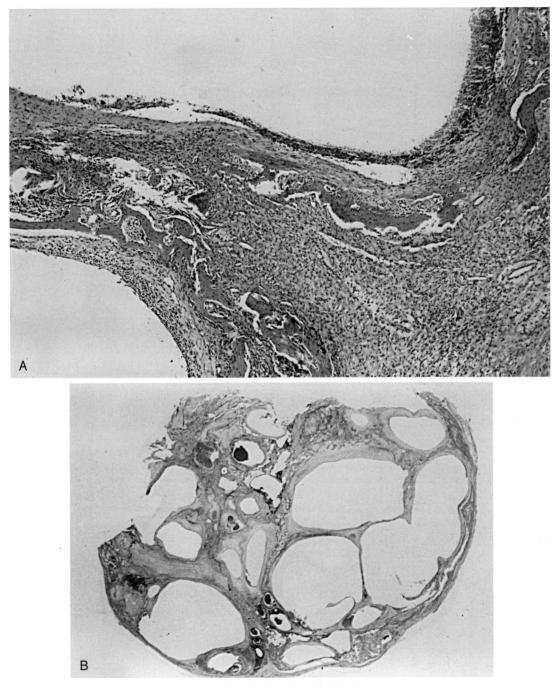

Figure 10–30. *A* and *B,* Aneurysmal bone cysts. Note the large sinusoidal blood spaces.

Pathogenesis. The pathogenesis of this lesion is not known, although most believe that it is associated with an antecedent traumatic event. Assuming this to be the case, it has been hypothesized that a traumatically induced hematoma forms within the intramedullary portion of bone. Rather than organizing, the clot breaks down, leaving an empty bony cavity. Alternative devel-opmental pathways include cystic degeneration of primary tumors of bone, such as central giant cell granuloma, disorders of calcium metabolism, and ischemic necrosis of bone marrow.

Clinical Features. Teenagers are most commonly affected, although traumatic bone cysts have been reported over a wide age range. An equal gender distribution has been noted.

By far the most frequent site of occurrence is the mandible. It may be seen in either anterior or posterior regions. Rare bilateral cases have been described. Swelling is occasionally seen, and pain is infrequently noted.

Radiographically, a well-delineated area of radiolucency with an irregular but defined edge is noted (Fig. 10–31). Minimal to prominent interradicular scalloping may be seen and occasionally slight root resorption.

Traumatic bone cysts have been frequently seen in association with florid osseous dysplasia. The relationship between these two entities is not understood.

Histopathology. Grossly, only minimal amounts of fibrous tissue from the bony wall are seen (Fig. 10–32). The lesion may occasionally contain blood or serosanguineous fluid. Microscopically delicate, well-vascularized, fibrous connective tissue without evidence of an epithelial component is identified.

Treatment and Prognosis. Once entry into the cavity is accomplished, the clinician need merely establish bleeding into the lesion before closure.

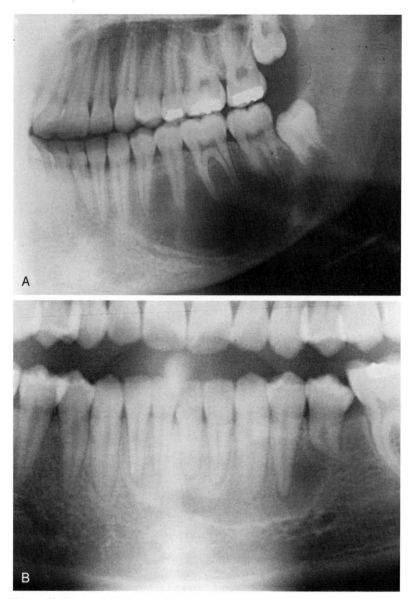

Figure 10–31. *A* and *B,* Traumatic bone cysts.

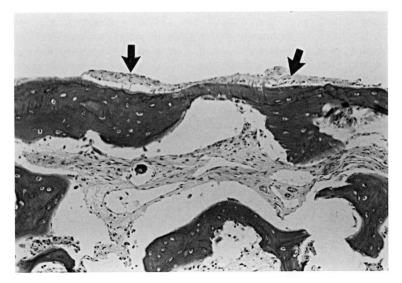

Figure 10–32. Wall of a traumatic bone cyst. Note the connective tissue lining the lesion *(arrows)*.

Organization of the bony clot results in complete bony repair without recurrence.

Static Bone Cyst

The static bone cyst is an anatomic indentation of the posterior lingual mandible that represents an entity that appears cystic on radiographic examination. This developmental depression of the mandible is believed to be secondary to entrapment of salivary gland or other soft tissue during the development of the mandible. These defects may occasionally be noted bilaterally and rarely, anterior to the first molar region of the mandible.

This lesion is entirely asymptomatic and is often observed incidentally in Panorex films. The location and appearance of the static bone cyst are distinctive and essentially are pathognomonic. When it is observed over time, there is no change in size, hence the term *static*.

The radiographic presentation is one of a sharply circumscribed oval radiolucency beneath the level of the inferior alveolar canal, with encroachment on the inferior border of the mandible (Fig. 10–33). Other depressions of the cortical surface of the mandible have been reported, albeit rarely, in association within the parotid gland along the lateral or facial aspect of the mandibular ramus.

The microscopic examination of material from these defects typically reveals normal submandibular salivary gland tissue or other resident soft tissue. Because the static bone cyst is diagnostic radiographically, biopsy is not necessary. Similarly, no treatment is required.

Focal Osteoporotic Bone Marrow Defect

The focal osteoporotic defect is an uncommon lesion that typically presents as a focal radiolu-

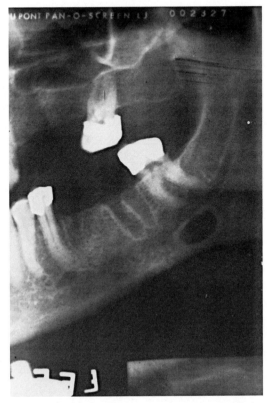

Figure 10–33. Static bone cyst in a characteristic location inferior to the mandibular canal.

cency in areas away from normal hematopoietic marrow (angle of the mandible and maxillary tuberosity). Approximately 70% occur in the posterior mandible; 70% occur in females.

The pathogenesis of the osteoporotic marrow defect is unknown, although three theories have been proposed. One theory states that abnormal healing following tooth extraction may be responsible. The fact that most lesions are noted within areas of previous extractions supports this theory of aberrant bone regeneration (Fig. 10–34). Another theory states that residual remnants of fetal marrow may persist into adulthood, thus presenting as a focal lucency. The third theory suggests that these defects are actually foci of marrow hyperplasia that are responsive in nature.

Microscopic findings in most cases are those of a cellular hematopoietic marrow with cell-to-fat ratios greater than 1 to 1. Within the cellular marrow, small lymphoid aggregates may be found as well as megakaryocytes.

The differential diagnosis includes osteomyelitis, traumatic bone cyst, and ameloblastoma. Owing to the radiographically nonspecific findings,

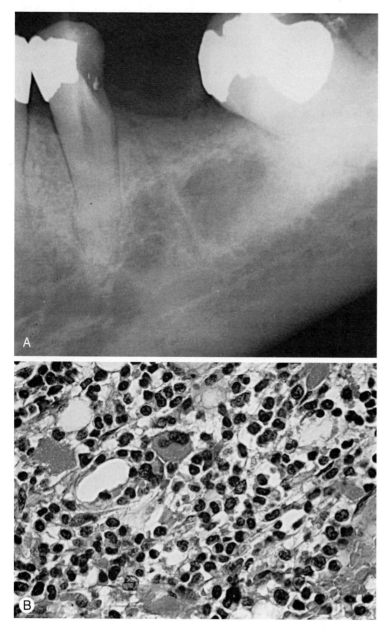

Figure 10–34. *A,* Focal osteoporotic bone marrow defect in an edentulous area of the mandible. *B,* Hematopoietic marrow from the defect.

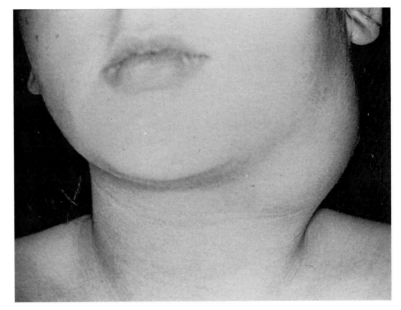

Figure 10–35. Branchial (lympho-epithelial) cyst.

diagnosis by incisional biopsy is desirable. Subsequent to this diagnosis, no further treatment is necessary.

SOFT TISSUE CYSTS OF THE NECK

Branchial Cyst/Cervical Lymphoepithelial Cyst

The branchial (cleft) cyst or cervical lymphoepithelial cyst is located in the lateral portion of the neck, usually anterior to the sternomastoid muscle (Fig. 10–35). It may also appear in the submandibular area, adjacent to the parotid gland, or around the sternomastoid muscle.

The traditional theory about the genesis of the branchial cyst relates to incomplete obliteration of the branchial clefts, arches, and pouches, with remnants of buried epithelial rests ultimately undergoing cystic change. The majority of such cysts arise from either the cervical sinus or the second branchial cleft or pouch.

An alternative, more current theory of origin proposes that epithelium is entrapped within cervical lymph nodes during embryogenesis. This epithelium, thought to be of salivary origin, would undergo cystic change at a later date.

The branchial cyst has an intraoral counterpart known as the *lymphoepithelial cyst.* The floor of the mouth is the most common site for these lesions, followed by the posterior lateral tongue

(Fig. 10–36). Rarely, lymphoepithelial cysts have also been reported in the parotid gland.

Clinical Features. These asymptomatic cysts usually become clinically apparent in late childhood or young adulthood as a result of enlargement. Drainage may occur through a small opening along the anterior margin of the sternomastoid muscle.

Histopathology. The branchial cyst is lined with stratified squamous epithelium, pseudostratified columnar epithelium, or both (Fig. 10–37). The epithelium is supported by connective tissue containing lymphoid aggregates usually with well-formed germinal centers.

Differential Diagnosis. Preoperative diagnoses may include cervical lymphadenitis, skin inclusion cyst, lymphangioma, and tumor of the tail of the parotid. Laterally displaced thyroglossal tract cyst and dermoid cyst might also be considered.

Treatment is surgical excision.

Dermoid Cyst

Dermoid cyst is a development that may occur in many areas of the body. When found in the oral cavity, they are usually in the anterior portion of the floor of the mouth in the midline. The overall incidence of this type of cyst in the head and neck is rather low, accounting for less than 2% of all dermoid cysts. The cause of the dermoid cyst in this area is believed to be developmental entrapment of multipotential cells or possibly implantation of epithelium.

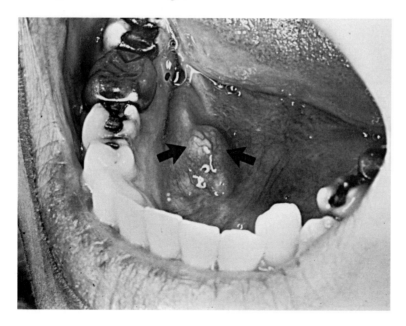

Figure 10–36. Oral lymphoepithelial cyst *(arrows).*

Clinical Features. Clinically, these cysts, when located above the mylohyoid muscle, displace the tongue superiorly and posteriorly, with resultant difficulties in function. When they are located below the mylohyoid muscle, a midline swelling of the neck occurs (Fig. 10–38). These cysts are painless and slow growing; there is no gender predilection. Lesions are generally less than 2 cm in diameter; however, extreme examples may range up to 8 to 12 cm. On palpation, the cysts are soft and doughy owing to keratin and sebum in the lumen.

Histopathology. Microscopically, the dermoid cyst is lined by stratified squamous epithelium supported by a fibrous connective tissue wall. Numerous secondary skin structures, including hair follicles, sebaceous glands, and sweat glands, (and occasionally teeth) may be found (Fig. 10–39).

Treatment. Treatment is surgical excision. Most lesions can be removed through the mouth with little risk of recurrence.

Thyroglossal Tract Cyst

The thyroglossal tract cyst is the most common developmental cyst of the neck, accounting for nearly three fourths of such lesions. The basis of this cystic pathology relates to thyroid gland development. The thyroid tissue becomes evident in the fourth week of gestation where derivatives of first and second branchial arches form the posterior portion of the tongue in the region of the foramen caecum. The thyroid anlage grows downward to its permanent location in the neck from the foramen caecum. Between the foramen caecum and the cervical location of the thyroid gland is the embryonic tract of the thyroid tissue. The developing gland passes through the base of the tongue and the hyoid bone to the midneck. By the tenth week of gestation, the tract or duct breaks up or involutes. Residual epithelial elements that do not completely atrophy may give rise to cysts in later life that may present in the posterior portion of the tongue *(lingual thyroid)* or in the neck itself.

Clinical Features. Approximately 30% of cases are found in patients older than 30 years, with a similar percentage in patients younger than 10 years. Most cysts occur in the midline, with 60% over the thyrohyoid membrane and only 2% within the tongue itself (Fig. 10–40). The overriding majority (70 to 80%) occur below the level of the hyoid bone. These cysts are generally asymptomatic; when they are attached to the hyoid bone and tongue, they may retract on swallowing or extension of the tongue. If they are infected, drainage through a sinus tract may occur. Rarely, malignant transformation has been described in these lesions.

Histopathology. Microscopic findings vary depending on the location of the cyst. Lesions occurring above the level of the hyoid bone demonstrate a lining chiefly of stratified squamous epithelium. A ciliated or columnar type epithelium usually is found in cysts occurring below the hyoid bone (Fig. 10–41). However, wide variation may be seen within a single cyst. Thyroid tissue

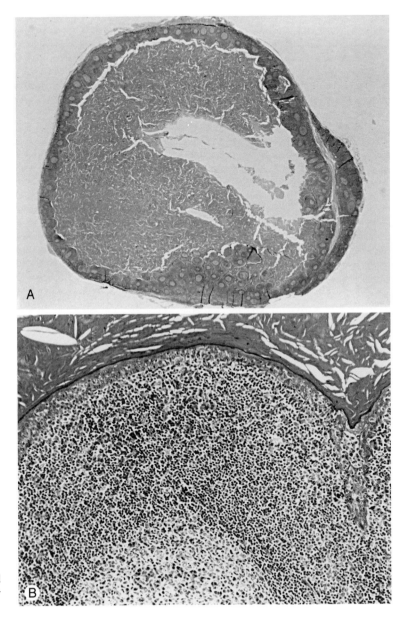

Figure 10–37. *A* and *B*. Branchial cysts. Note the lymphoid tissue subjacent to the thin epithelial lining.

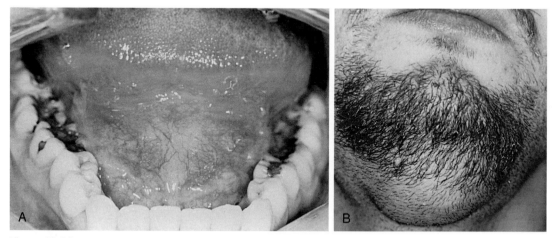

Figure 10–38. *A,* Dermoid cyst presenting in the midline of the floor of the mouth. *B,* Dermoid cyst presenting in the midline of the neck.

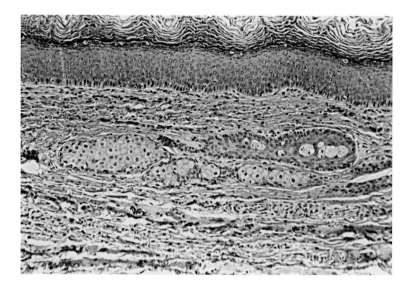

Figure 10–39. Dermoid cyst. Note the keratinized epithelium and sebaceous elements in the supporting connective tissue.

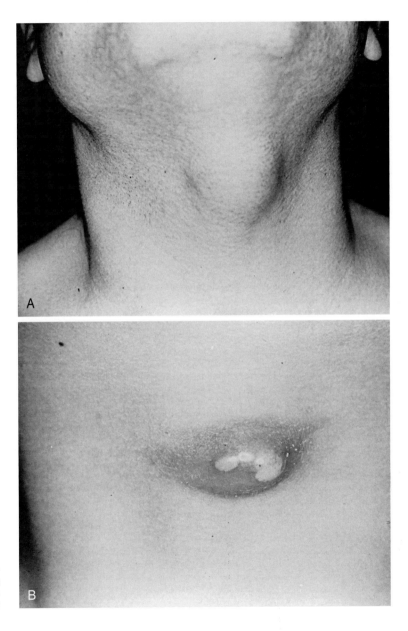

Figure 10–40. *A* and *B,* Thyroglossal tract cysts in the midline of the neck. Cyst in *B* is secondarily infected. (Courtesy of Dr. J. N. Attie.)

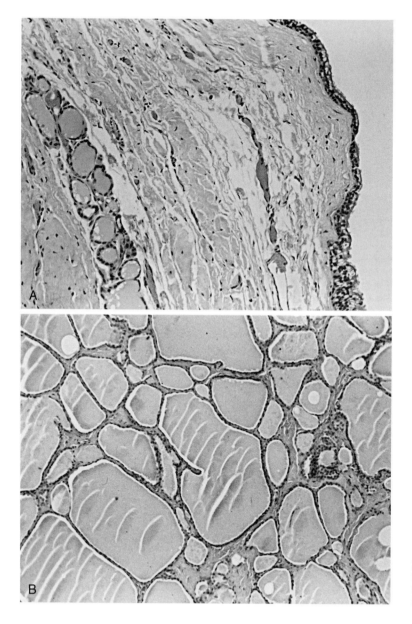

Figure 10–41. *A,* Thyroglossal tract cyst. Note the lumen (right) and thyroid acini (left). *B,* Thyroid tissue in a lingual thyroid.

may be seen within the connective tissue wall. Malignancy arising within the thyroglossal tract cyst may occur, usually in the form of papillary adenocarcinoma.

Differential Diagnosis. The differential diagnosis of the thyroglossal tract cyst should include dermoid cyst, thyroid neoplasm, branchial cyst, and sebaceous cyst.

Treatment. Treatment is surgical excision. Because the lesion may be rather tortuous in configuration, recurrence may be seen. It is often recommended that the central portion of the hyoid bone be removed in an effort to eliminate any residual thyroglossal tract epithelium from this site.

Bibliography

Odontogenic Cysts

Androulakis M, Johnson JT, Wagner RL. Thyroglossal duct and second branchial cleft anomalies in adults. Ear Nose Throat J 69:318–322, 1990.

Buchner A. The central (intraosseous) calcifying odontogenic cyst: an analysis of 215 cases. J Oral Maxillofac Surg 49:330–339, 1991.

Buchner A, Hansen LS. The histomorphologic spectrum of the gingival cyst in the adult. Oral Surg 48:532–539, 1979.

Crowley TE, Kaugars GE, Gunsolley JC. Odontogenic keratocysts: a clinical and histologic comparison of the parakeratin and orthokeratin variants. J Oral Maxillofac Surg 50:22–26, 1992.

Fantasia JE. Lateral periodontal cysts, botryoid odontogenic cysts and glandular odontogenic cysts. Oral Maxillofac Surg Clin North Am 3:127–136, 1991.

Forsell K, Forsell H, Kahnberg K-E. Recurrence of keratocysts—a long term follow up study. Int J Oral Maxillofac Surg 17:25–28, 1988.

Fowler CB, Brannon RB. The paradental cyst: a clinicopathologic study of six new cases and review of the literature. J Oral Maxillofac Surg 47:243–248, 1989.

Gardner DG, Kessler HP, Morency R, et al. The glandular odontogenic cyst and isolated periodontal defects. J Periodontol 53:145–151, 1982.

Gorlin RJ. Nevoid basal-cell carcinoma syndrome. Medicine 66:98–113, 1987.

Greer RO, Johnson M. Botryoid odontogenic cyst: clinicopathologic analysis of ten cases with three recurrences. J Oral Maxillofac Surg 46:574–579, 1988.

Kenealy JF, Torsiglieri AJ Jr, Tom LW. Branchial cleft anomalies: a five year retrospective review. Trans Pa Acad Ophthalmol Otolaryngol 42:1022–1025, 1990.

Main DM. Epithelial jaw cysts: ten years of the WHO classification. J Oral Pathol 14:1–7, 1985.

Main DM. Follicular cysts of mandibular third molar teeth: radiological evaluation of enlargement. Dentomaxillofac Radiol 18:156–159, 1989.

Meghi S, Harvey W, Harris M. Interleukin 1–like activity in cystic lesions of the jaw. Br J Oral Maxillofac Surg 27:1–11, 1989.

Padayachee A, van Wyk CW. Two cystic lesions with features of both the botryoid odontogenic cyst and the central mucoepidermoid tumor: sialo-odontogenic cyst? J Oral Pathol 16:499–504, 1987.

Partridge M, Towers JF. The primordial cyst (odontogenic keratocyst): its tumor-like characteristics and behavior. Br J Oral Maxillofac Surg 25:271–279, 1987.

Ramer M, Montazem A, Lane SL, Lummerman H. Glandular odontogenic cyst. Oral Surg Oral Med Oral Pathol 84:54–57, 1997.

Redman RS, Whitestone BW, Winne CE, et al. Botryoid odontogenic cyst report of a case with histologic evidence of multicentric origin. Int J Oral Maxillofac Surg 19:144–146, 1990.

Renard TH, Choucair RJ, Stevenson WD, et al. Carcinoma of the thyroglossal duct. Surg Gynecol Obstet 171:305–308, 1990.

Sadeghi EM, Weldon LL, Kwon PH, Sampson E. Mucoepidermoid odontogenic cyst. Int J Oral Maxillofac Surg 29:142–143, 1991.

Scharffeter K, Balz-Herrmann C, Lagrange W, et al. Proliferative kinetics—study of the growth of keratocysts. Morphofunctional explanation for recurrences. J Craniomaxillofac Surg 17:226–233, 1989.

Shamaskin RG, Svirsky JA, Kaugars GE. Intraosseous and extraosseous calcifying odontogenic cyst (Gorlin cyst). J Oral Maxillofac Surg 47:562–565, 1989.

Shear M. Cysts of the jaws: recent advances. J Pathol 14:43–59, 1985.

Spatafore CM, Griffin JA Jr, Keyes GG, et al. Periapical biopsy report: an analysis over a ten year period. J Endodon 16:239–241, 1990.

Stoelinga PJW. Studies on the dental lamina as related to its role in the etiology of cysts and tumors. J Oral Pathol 5:65–73, 1976.

Teronen O, Konttinen YT, Rifkin B, et al. Identification and characterization of gelatinase/type IV collagenases in jaw cysts. J Oral Pathol Med 24:78–84, 1995.

Trope M, Pettigrew J, Pewtras J, et al. Differentiation of radicular cyst and granulomas using computerized tomography. Endodon Dent Traumatol 5:69–72, 1989.

vanHeerden WFP, Raubenheimer EJ, Turner ML. Glandular odontogenic cyst. Head Neck 14:316–320, 1992.

Waldron CA, Koh ML. Central mucoepidermoid carcinoma of the jaws: report of four cases with analysis of the literature and discussion of the relationship to mucoepidermoid, sialo-odontogenic and glandular odontogenic cysts. J Oral Maxillofac Surg 48:871–877, 1990.

Wolf J, Hietanen J. The mandibular infected buccal cyst (paradental cyst): a radiographic and histologic study. Br J Oral Maxillofac Surg 28:322–325, 1990.

Woolgar JA, Rippin JW, Browne RM. A comparative histological study of odontogenic keratocysts in basal cell naevus syndrome and control patients. J Oral Pathol 16:75–80, 1987.

Wysocki GP, Brannon RB, Gardner DG, et al. Histogenesis of the lateral periodontal cyst and the gingival cyst of the adult. Oral Surg 50:327–334, 1980.

Yaskima M, Ogura M, Abiko Y. Studies on cholesterol accumulation in radicular cyst fluid—origin of heat-stable cholesterol-binding protein. Int J Biochem 22:165–169, 1990.

Nonodontogenic Cysts

Chamda RA, Shear M. Dimensions of incisive fossae on dry skulls and radiographs. J Oral Pathol 9:452–457, 1980.

DiFiore PM, Hartwell GR. Median mandibular lateral periodontal cysts. Oral Surg Oral Med Oral Pathol 63:545–550, 1987.

Gardner DG. An evaluation of reported cases of median mandibular cysts. Oral Surg Oral Med Oral Pathol 65:208–213, 1988.

Revel MP, Vanel D, Sigal R, et al. Aneurysmal bone cysts of the jaws: CT and MR findings. J Comput Assist Tomogr 16:84–86, 1992.

Tenca JI, Guinta JL, Norris LH. The median mandibular cyst and its endodontic significance. Oral Surg Oral Med Oral Pathol 60:316–321, 1985.

Wysocki GP. The differential diagnosis of globulomaxillary radiolucencies. Oral Surg 51:281–286, 1981.

Pseudocysts

Alles JU, Schulz A. Immunocytochemical markers (endothelial and histiocytic) and ultrastructure of primary aneurysmal bone cysts. Hum Pathol 17:39–45, 1986.

Barker GR. A radiolucency of the ascending ramus of the mandible associated with invested parotid salivary gland material and analogous with a Stafne bone cavity. Br J Oral Maxillofac Surg 26:81–84, 1988.

Correll RW, Jensen JL, Rhyne RR. Lingual cortical mandibular defects: a radiographic incidence study. Oral Surg Oral Med Oral Pathol 50:287–291, 1980.

Eisenbud LE, Attie JN, Garlick J, et al. Aneurysmal bone cyst of the mandible. Oral Surg Oral Med Oral Pathol 64:202–206, 1987.

Feinberg SE, Finkelstein MW, Page HL, et al. Recurrent "traumatic" bone cysts of the mandible. Oral Surg Oral Med Oral Pathol 57:418–422, 1984.

Gorab GN, Brahney C, Aria AA. Unusual presentation of a Stafne bone cyst. Oral Surg Oral Med Oral Pathol 61:213–220, 1986.

Kaugars GE, Cale AE. Traumatic bone cyst. Oral Surg Oral Med Oral Pathol 63:318–324, 1987.

Moule I. Unilateral multiple solitary bone cysts. J Oral Maxillofac Surg 46:320–323, 1988.

Struthers PJ, Shear M. Aneurysmal bone cyst of the jaws. I. Clinicopathologic features. Int J Oral Surg 13:85–91, 1984.

Struthers PJ, Shear M. Aneurysmal bone cyst of the jaws. II. Pathogenesis. Int J Oral Surg 13:92–100, 1984.

Soft Tissue Cysts of the Neck

Buchner A, Hansen LS. Lymphoepithelial cysts of the oral cavity. A clinicopathologic study of 38 cases. Oral Surg 50:441–449, 1980.

Fernandez JF, Ordonez NG, Schultz PN, et al. Thyroglossal duct carcinoma. Surgery 6:928–934, 1991.

Odontogenic Tumors

Odontogenic tumors are lesions derived from epithelial or mesenchymal elements, or both, that are part of the tooth-forming apparatus. They are therefore found exclusively in the mandible and maxilla (and gingiva on rare occasions) and must be considered in differential diagnoses of lesions involving these sites.

For the group, etiology and pathogenesis are totally obscure—no cause or stimulus has been elucidated. Clinically, odontogenic tumors are typically asymptomatic, but they may cause jaw expansion, movement of teeth, and bone loss. Knowledge of typical basic features such as age, location, and radiographic appearance of the various odontogenic tumors can be extremely valuable in developing a differential diagnosis (Table 11–1).

Like neoplasms elsewhere in the body, odontogenic tumors tend to mimic microscopically the cell or tissue of origin. Histologically, they may resemble soft tissues of the enamel organ or dental pulp, or they may contain hard tissue elements of enamel, dentin, or cementum or a mixture or composite of these.

Lesions in this group range from hamartomatous proliferations to malignant neoplasms with metastatic capabilities. An understanding of the biologic behavior of the various odontogenic tu- mors is of fundamental importance to the overall treatment of patients.

Several histologic classifications have been devised to help comprehend this complex group of lesions. Common to all schemes is the division of tumors into those that are composed of odontogenic epithelial elements, those that are composed of odontogenic mesenchyme, and those that are proliferations of both epithelial and mesenchymal tissues. A vast array of microscopic types of odontogenic lesions have been reported. However, many represent histologic variants of one of the major tumor groups. Because these variants are not biologically different, recognition as separate entities is cumbersome and unimportant. In the classification used in this chapter, histologic variants are discussed briefly under major entities.

EPITHELIAL TUMORS

Ameloblastoma

Historically, ameloblastoma has been known for many years, with reports dating back to the early nineteenth century. Its persistent local growth in the maxillofacial area and its ability to produce marked deformity before leading to serious debilitation probably account for its early recognition and numerous subsequent reports. Recurrence, especially after conservative treatment, has also contributed to the awareness of this lesion. Ever since the ameloblastoma was appreciated for its locally aggressive behavior, recurrence rate, and slight metastatic potential, controversy has centered around the most appropriate form of treatment. As clinical pathologic subtypes have been better defined, a rational basis has developed for treatment that provides an optimal cure rate with minimal patient morbidity.

This neoplasm originates within the mandible or maxilla from epithelium that is involved in the formation of teeth. Potential epithelial sources include enamel organ, odontogenic rests (rests of Malassez, rests of Serres), reduced enamel epithelium, and the epithelial lining of odontogenic cysts, especially the dentigerous cyst. The trigger or stimulus for neoplastic transformation of these

Table 11–1. Typical Clinical Features of Major Odontogenic Tumors

TUMOR	MEAN AGE	USUAL LOCATION	RADIOGRAPH
Ameloblastoma	40 years	Molar-ramus, mandible	Lucent, frequently multilocular
Calcifying epithelial odontogenic tumor	40 years	Molar-ramus, mandible	Lucent or with opaque foci
Adenomatoid odontogenic tumor	18 years	Anterior jaws	Lucent or with opaque foci
Myxoma	30 years	Any region	Lucent, often multilocular
Cementifying fibroma	40 years	Mandible	Lucent or with opaque foci
Cementoblastoma	25 years	Posterior mandible	Opaque
Periapical cemento-osseous dysplasia	40 years	Anterior mandible	Lucent to mixed to opaque
Odontoma	18 years	Any region	Opaque
Ameloblastic fibroma and fibro-odontoma	12 years	Molar-ramus, mandible	Lucent or with opaque focus

otherwise trivial epithelial structures is totally unknown.

Clinical Features. This is a lesion of adults, and it occurs predominantly in the fourth and fifth decades of life (Figs. 11–1 to 11–3). The age range is very broad, extending from childhood to late adulthood. Mean ages have been most commonly between 35 and 45 years. The rare lesions occurring in children are typically unicystic and appear clinically as odontogenic cysts. There appears to be no gender predilection for this tumor.

Ameloblastomas may occur anywhere in the mandible or maxilla, although the mandibular molar-ramus area is the most favored site (Fig. 11–4).

In the maxilla, the molar area is more commonly affected than are the premolar or anterior regions. Rarely, *extraosseous (peripheral) ameloblastomas* are found in the gingiva; a few have also been described in the buccal mucosa. These are seen in older adults, usually between 40 and 60 years of age. They may arise from overlying epithelium or rests of Serres and exhibit a benign, nonaggressive course. Peripheral lesions generally do not invade underlying bone, and they recur infrequently. Ameloblastomas are usually asymptomatic and are discovered either during routine radiographic examination or because of asymptomatic jaw expansion. Occasional tooth movement or malocclusion may be the initial presenting sign.

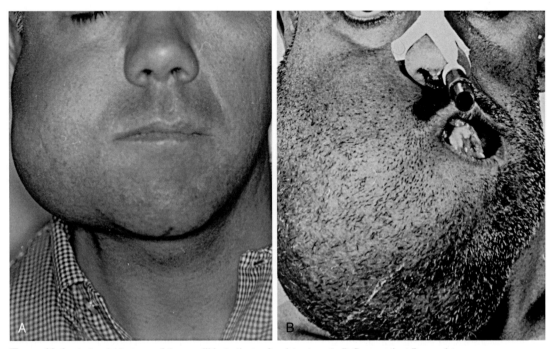

Figure 11–1. *A,* Ameloblastoma of the mandible (patient refused treatment). *B,* Same patient 7 years later.

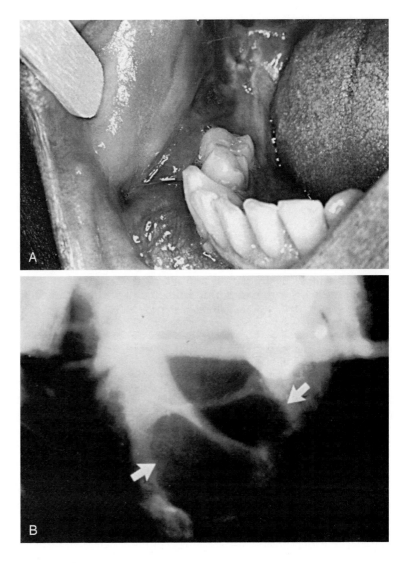

Figure 11–2. *A,* Intraoral view of the patient in Figure 11–1, showing movement of the teeth and filling of the vestibule. *B,* Lateral jaw radiograph showing multilocular radiolucency *(arrows).*

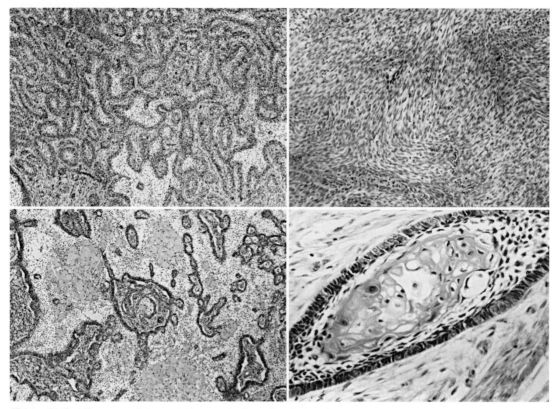

Figure 11–3. Microscopy of the ameloblastoma in the patient in Figure 11–1. *Upper left,* Follicular pattern. *Upper right,* Spindle pattern. *Lower left,* Granular cell change. *Lower right,* Keratinization of tumor island.

Radiographically, ameloblastomas appear as osteolytic processes (Fig. 11–5). These tumors, typically found in the tooth-bearing areas of the jaws, may exhibit a unilocular or multilocular appearance (Figs. 11–6 to 11–8). Because ameloblastomas are slow growing, the radiographic margins are usually well defined and sclerotic. In cases in which connective tissue desmoplasia occurs in conjunction with tumor proliferation, ill-defined radiographic margins are typically seen (this variety, known as *desmoplastic ameloblastoma,* also has a predilection for the anterior jaws). The generally slow tumor growth rate is also responsible for the movement of tooth roots. Root resorption may also appear in association with ameloblastoma growth.

Histopathology. Numerous histologic patterns have been described in ameloblastomas. Some may exhibit a single histologic subtype; others may display several histologic patterns within the same lesion. Common to nearly all subtypes is the polarization of cells around the proliferating nests in a pattern similar to ameloblasts of the enamel organ. Central to these cells are loosely arranged cells that mimic the stellate reticulum of the

enamel organ. Another typical feature is the budding of tumor cells from neoplastic foci in a pattern reminiscent of tooth development.

The microscopic subtype most commonly seen is the follicular type (Fig. 11–9). It is composed of islands of tumor cells that mimic the normal dental follicle. Central cystic degeneration of the follicular islands leads to a microcytic pattern (Fig. 11–10). The neoplastic cells occasionally develop into a network of epithelium, prompting the term *plexiform ameloblastoma.* When the central portions of the tumor islands become squamoid or elongated, the adjectives *acanthomatous* and *spindle* are sometimes used to modify the term *ameloblastoma.* Some tumors exhibit a pattern that is microscopically similar to basal cell carcinoma of the skin; these are *basal cell ameloblastomas.*

A subtype in which the central neoplastic cells exhibit prominent cytoplasmic granularity has been designated *granular cell ameloblastoma* (Fig. 11–11). Although one report suggested that this subtype of ameloblastoma may be more aggressive and may have a higher recurrence rate, this has not been substantiated. Optically clear

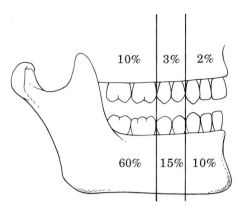

Figure 11–4. Approximate regional distribution of ameloblastomas.

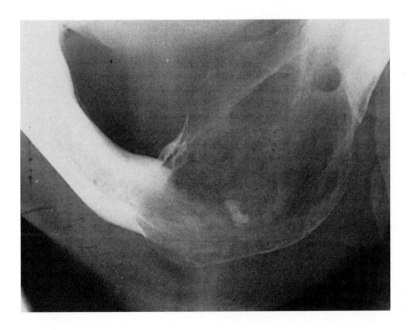

Figure 11–5. Ameloblastoma of the anterior mandible.

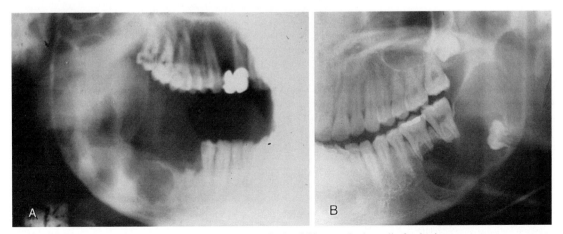

Figure 11–6. *A,* Ameloblastoma of the molar-ramus area. *B,* Ameloblastoma in the wall of a dentigerous cyst.

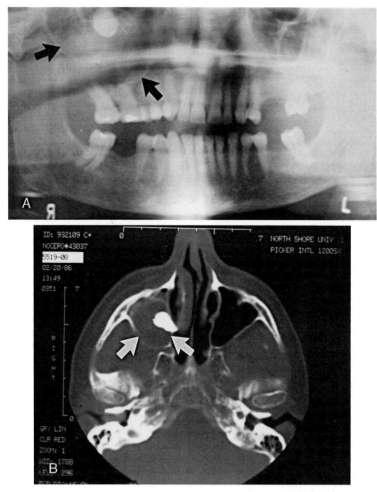

Figure 11–7. *A*, Maxillary ameloblastoma *(arrows)* associated with an impacted molar. *B*, Computed tomography scan of the lesion *(arrows)*.

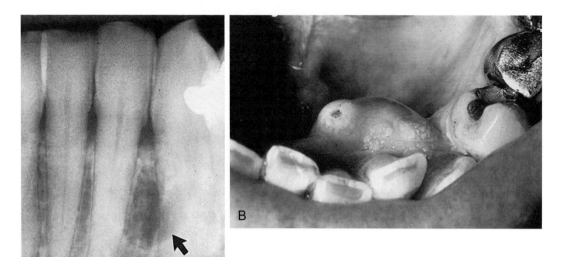

Figure 11–8. *A*, Ameloblastoma in a lateral root position *(arrow)*. *B*, Extension of the lesion into the lingual gingiva.

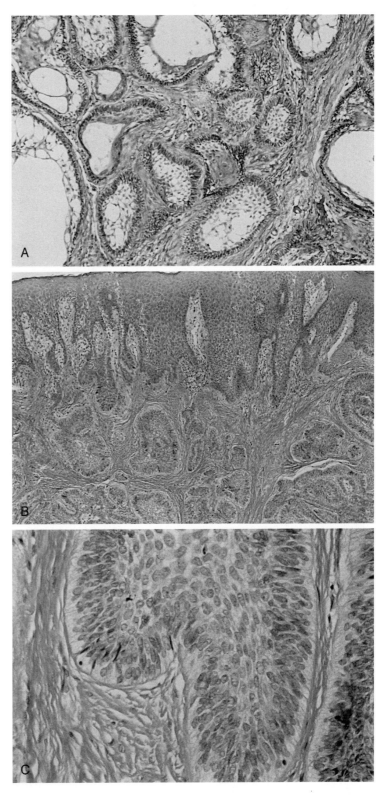

Figure 11–9. *A*, Ameloblastoma, follicular type. *B* and *C*, Peripheral (gingival) ameloblastoma.

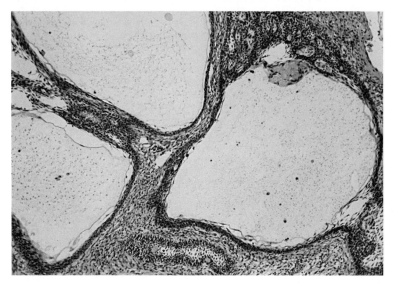

Figure 11–10. Ameloblastoma with microcystic change.

tumor cells and cells expressing ghost cell–type keratinization have also been seen in ameloblastomas (Fig. 11–12); the significance of this remains to be determined. Separation of ameloblastomas into the various microscopic groups described is essentially an academic exercise, because there appears to be no correlation between clinical behavior and these microscopic patterns.

Ameloblastomas have been subdivided into two biologic-microscopic subtypes—*solid* or *multilocular* and *cystic (unicystic).* There is significant justification for such subdivision, because treatment and prognosis differ. The solid or multicystic ameloblastoma, which may exhibit any or all of the microscopic patterns discussed, is more aggressive and requires more extensive treatment than its unicystic counterpart. It also has a relatively high recurrence rate (50 to 90%) if treated with curettage.

The cystic (unicystic) lesion, in contrast, is an ameloblastoma that has a major cystic space in which there may be intraluminal or mural growth. It may represent a cystic ameloblastoma that is unilocular, or it may represent an odontogenic cyst in which there has been ameloblastic transformation of the epithelial lining. A histologic variant

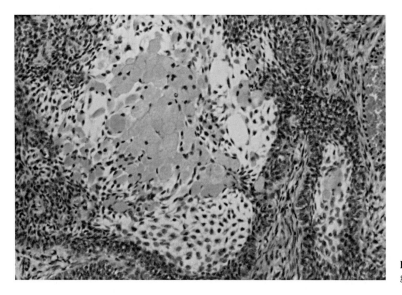

Figure 11–11. Ameloblastoma with granular cells.

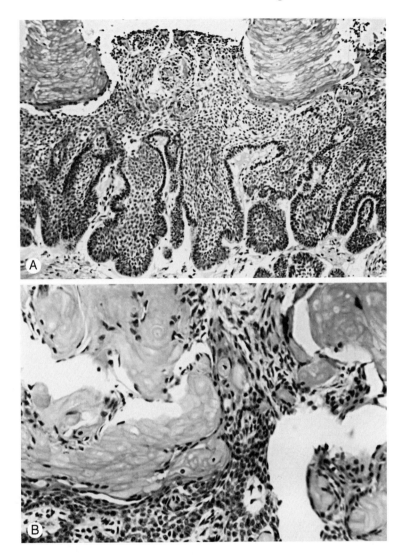

Figure 11–12. *A* and *B,* Ameloblastoma with ghost cell type of keratinization.

of this type is the *plexiform unicystic ameloblastoma,* in which the cyst wall exhibits a network of ameloblastic epithelium (Fig. 11–13). Unicystic ameloblastoma is seen in a younger age group (second to third decades) and typically in the mandibular molar area. It has a recurrence rate of less than 10% when curettage is the primary form of treatment. Diagnosis is often retrospective after enucleation for what appeared to be an odontogenic cyst. Follow-up is important because of persistent growth of residual tumor.

An additional subtype of ameloblastoma has been designated as *sinonasal ameloblastoma.* A mean age of 61 years and male dominance have been noted. Signs of nasal obstruction, epistaxis, and opacification are seen. The "totipotential" sinonasal lining cells are the putative site of origin. A plexiform microscopic pattern is most commonly seen.

Differential Diagnosis. When considering age, location, and radiographic features together, the clinical differential diagnosis can generally be limited to several entities in the three categories of jaw disease—odontogenic tumors, cysts, and benign nonodontogenic lesions. Among the odontogenic tumors, the calcifying epithelial odontogenic tumor (CEOT) (radiolucent variety) and odontogenic myxomas are prime considerations. The dentigerous cyst and the odontogenic keratocyst can also be included. In relatively young individuals, lesions that are radiographically similar to ameloblastoma include nonodontogenic lesions such as central giant cell granuloma, ossifying fibroma, central hemangioma, and possibly idiopathic histiocytosis.

Microscopically, some ameloblastomas, especially the plexiform unicystic and multicystic lesions, may be confused with odontogenic cysts in

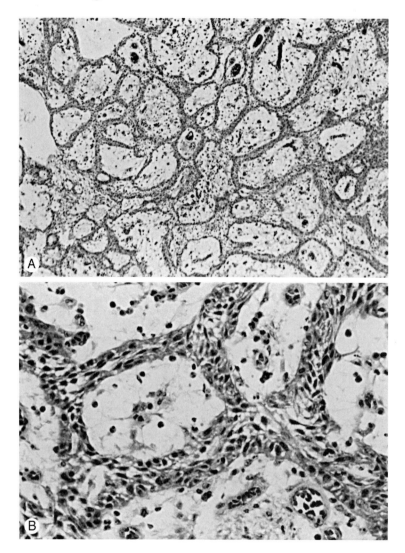

Figure 11–13. *A* and *B*, Plexiform unicystic ameloblastoma.

which there is hyperplasia of the lining. In the ameloblastoma, basal cell palisading is evident and inflammatory cells are usually scant. Maxillary ameloblastomas occasionally appear less differentiated, requiring separation from adenocarcinomas and squamous cell carcinomas of maxillary sinus origin (Fig. 11–14).

Treatment and Prognosis. No single standard type of therapy should be advocated for patients with ameloblastoma. Rather, each case should be judged on its own merits. Of prime consideration is whether the lesion is a solid-multicystic, unicystic, or extraosseous lesion. The solid-multicystic lesions require at least surgical excision, because recurrence follows curettage in 50 to 90% of cases. Block excision or resection should generally be reserved for larger lesions. Unicystic le-

sions, especially the smaller ones, require only enucleation and should not be overtreated. Peripheral ameloblastomas should also be treated in a similar conservative fashion.

Radiotherapy has been used to a very limited extent in the treatment of ameloblastomas, because it is generally believed that these tumors are radioresistant. Some evidence, however, shows that radiation levels of 45 Gy may produce significant therapeutic results. Until more is known about tumor responsiveness, radiation should be used in the exceptional case in which surgery may be unacceptably destructive, primarily maxillary lesions.

Malignant behavior by ameloblastomas is rarely encountered. These lesions occur in a younger age group (thirties) and appear in the mandible more frequently than in the maxilla. By definition, these

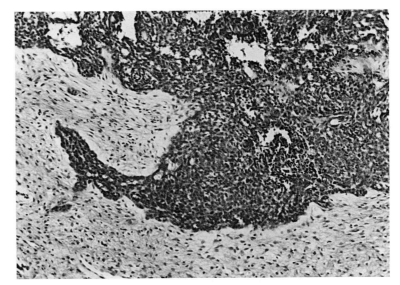

Figure 11–14. Atypical ameloblastoma of the maxilla.

are lesions that metastasize to local lymph nodes or distant organs (Fig. 11–15). Direct extension into contiguous areas does not qualify for a malignant classification. Malignant lesions have been divided into two subtypes: the *malignant ameloblastoma,* in which the primary and metastatic lesions are microscopically well differentiated with the characteristic histologic features of ameloblastoma; and *ameloblastic carcinoma,* in which the lesions (primary and metastatic) exhibit less microscopic differentiation, showing cytologic atypia and mitotic figures (Fig. 11–16). Malignant tumors are difficult to control locally and

infrequently metastasize. Metastases from malignant varieties of ameloblastoma appear usually in the lung, presumably owing to aspiration of tumor cells. Regional lymph nodes are the second most common metastatic site, followed by skull, liver, spleen, kidney, and skin.

Another epithelial odontogenic malignancy of the mandible and maxilla that is believed to arise from odontogenic rests has been designated as *primary intraosseous carcinoma.* This is regarded as a primary jaw carcinoma that does not have histologic features of ameloblastoma. It does not have its origin from a preexisting odontogenic

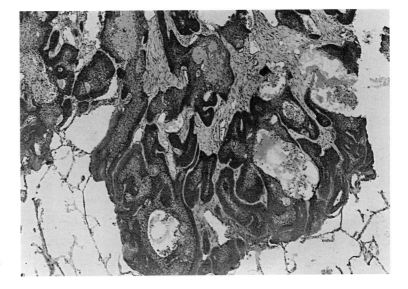

Figure 11–15. Metastatic ameloblastoma. Note the lung alveoli at the lower right and left.

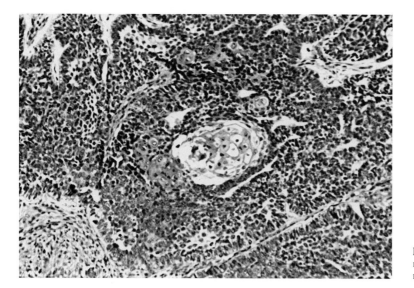

Figure 11–16. Ameloblastic carcinoma. Note the hypercellularity and nuclear hyperchromatism.

cyst. This rare adult lesion affects men more than women, and it is seen in the mandible more than the maxilla. Microscopically, about half these lesions exhibit keratin formation and about half show peripheral palisading of epithelial cell nests. This lesion must be differentiated microscopically from acanthomatous ameloblastoma and squamous odontogenic tumor. Prognosis is poor, with a 2-year survival rate reported at 40%.

A lesion known as *craniopharyngioma* is related to the ameloblastoma through similar origins. Both are ultimately derived from oral ectoderm—the ameloblastoma by way of dental lamina, and the craniopharyngioma by way of Rathke's pouch. The invagination of oral ectoderm (Rathke's pouch) is the initial embryonic expression of the development of part of the hypophysis. As the epithelium migrates to its final position in the base of the skull, epithelial rests may be left behind along the tract known as the *craniopharyngeal duct*. The rests, through some unknown mechanism, may proliferate to produce the rare neoplasm called *craniopharyngioma*. Biologically, this is a benign, slow-growing, infiltrative tumor similar to the ameloblastoma. Obviously, the location in the base of the skull makes it of greater significance relative to treatment and prognosis. Microscopically, the craniopharyngioma exhibits features of the ameloblastoma (Fig. 11–17). It also bears a striking resemblance to the calcifying odontogenic cyst through ghost cell keratinization and calcific deposits.

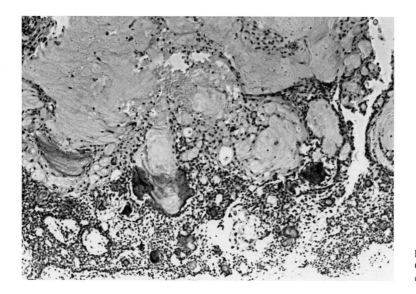

Figure 11–17. Craniopharyngioma. Ghost cell keratinization above and dark calcific deposits below.

Another lesion known as *adamantinoma of the tibia* was thought to be related to the ameloblastoma because of some histologic similarities. The adamantinoma (also an obsolete synonym for *ameloblastoma*) was also at one time thought to be endothelial, synovial, or mesenchymal in origin. However, based on the ultrastructural demonstration of desmosomes and tonofilaments and on the immunohistochemical demonstration of keratin (and negativity for factor VIII), an epithelial origin, most likely in basal epithelial cells or eccrine cells, appears most probable.

Squamous Odontogenic Tumor

Because this tumor involves the alveolar process, it is believed to be derived from neoplastic transformation of the rests of Malassez (Fig. 11–18). It occurs in the mandible and maxilla with equal frequency, favoring the anterior region of the maxilla and the posterior region of the mandible. Multiple lesions have been described in about 20% of affected patients, as have multicentric familial lesions.

The age range in which squamous odontogenic tumor has been described extends from the second through the seventh decades, with a mean of 40 years. There is no gender predilection. Patients usually experience no symptoms, although tenderness and tooth mobility have been reported. Radiographically, this lesion is typically a well-circumscribed, often semilunar lesion associated with the roots of teeth. Microscopically, it has some similarity to ameloblastoma, although the squamous odontogenic tumor lacks the columnar peripherally palisaded layer of epithelial cells. There

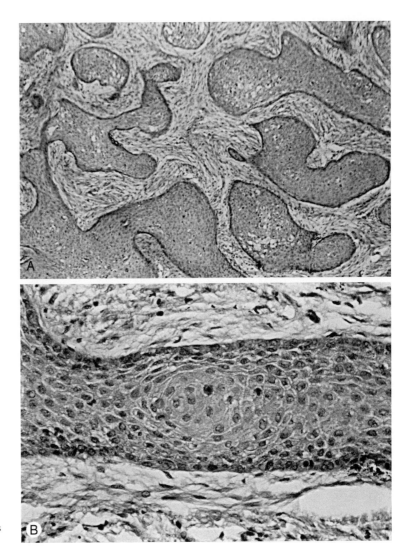

Figure 11–18. *A* and *B*, Squamous odontogenic tumor.

is also some similarity to proliferating odontogenic rests that are occasionally seen in periapical cysts.

This lesion has some invasive capacity and infrequently recurs after conservative therapy. Curettage or excision is the treatment of choice.

Calcifying Epithelial Odontogenic Tumor

This neoplasm, also known as *Pindborg tumor* after the oral pathologist who first described the entity, shares many features with the ameloblastoma. Microscopically, however, there is no resemblance to the ameloblastoma, and radiographically distinct differences will often be noted. The calcifying epithelial odontogenic tumor (CEOT) is

of odontogenic origin. The specific cell from which it is derived and the stimulus for growth are unknown, although the stratum intermedium of the enamel organ has been mentioned.

Clinical Features. The CEOT is seen in patients ranging in age from the second to the tenth decade, with a mean around 40 years. It has no gender predilection.

The mandible is affected twice as often as the maxilla. There is a predilection for the molar-ramus region, although any site may be affected. Peripheral lesions, usually in the anterior gingiva, have occasionally been identified.

Jaw expansion or incidental observation on routine radiographic survey is the usual way in which these lesions are discovered (Fig. 11–19). Radiographically, lesions are frequently associated with impacted teeth. The lesions may be unilocular or

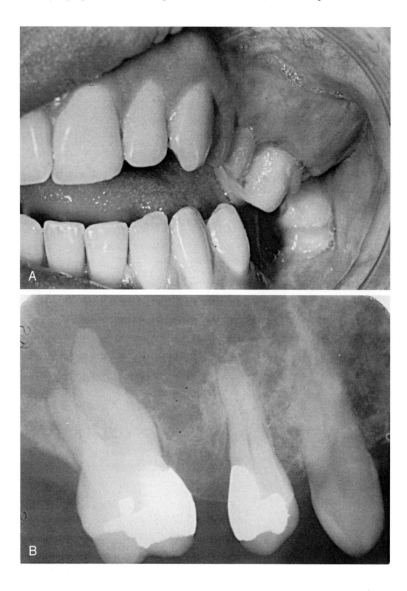

Figure 11–19. *A,* Calcifying epithelial odontogenic tumor of the maxilla. *B,* Radiograph showing a poorly defined lucency. (Courtesy of Dr. T. Pickens.)

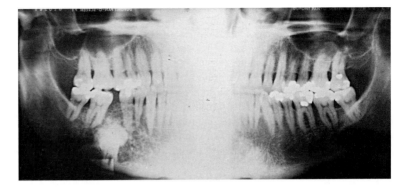

Figure 11–20. Mandibular calcifying epithelial odontogenic tumor showing a mixed lucent-opaque pattern.

multilocular. Small loculations in some lesions have prompted the use of the term *honeycomb* to describe this lucent pattern. The CEOT may be completely radiolucent, or it may contain opaque foci—a reflection of the calcified islands seen microscopically (Fig. 11–20). The lesions are usually well circumscribed radiographically, although sclerotic margins may not be evident.

Histopathology. A unique microscopic pattern typifies the CEOT. Sheets of large polygonal epithelial cells are usually seen (Fig. 11–21). Nuclei show considerable variation in size, shape, and

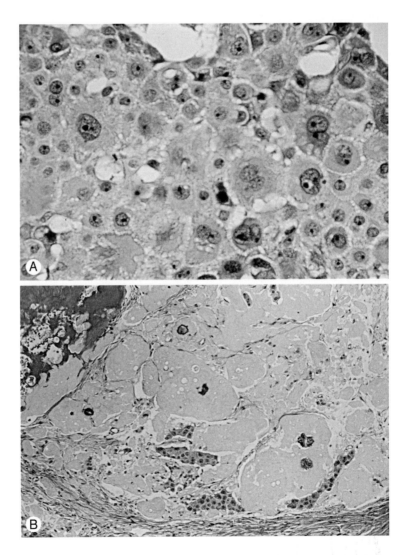

Figure 11–21. Calcifying epithelial odontogenic tumor. *A,* Bizarre epithelial cells. *B,* Amyloid component showing calcification (upper left).

number. Mitotic figures are rare. The cytoplasm is abundant and eosinophilic. Focal zones of optically clear cells can occasionally be seen in the microscopic clear cell variant.

Various amounts of an extracellular product that most investigators believe is amyloid are also typical of these tumors (Fig. 11–22). This homogeneous, pale-staining eosinophilic material stains positive for amyloid with Congo red stain in polarized light and with thioflavine T in ultraviolet light. Concentric calcific deposits (Liesegang rings) may be seen in the amyloid material. These rings, when sufficiently dense and large, are responsible for radiopacities.

Differential Diagnosis. When this lesion is radiolucent, it must be separated clinically from the dentigerous cyst, odontogenic keratocyst, ameloblastoma, and odontogenic myxoma. Some benign non-odontogenic jaw tumors might also be considered, but these would be less likely, based on age and location.

When a mixed radiolucent-radiopaque pattern is encountered, the calcified odontogenic cyst should be considered in a clinical differential diagnosis. Other less likely possibilities include adenomatoid odontogenic tumor (AOT), ameloblastic fibro-odontoma, ossifying fibroma, and osteoblastoma.

Treatment. This tumor has invasive potential but apparently not to the extent of the ameloblastoma. It is slow-growing and compromises the patient through direct extension. Metastases have

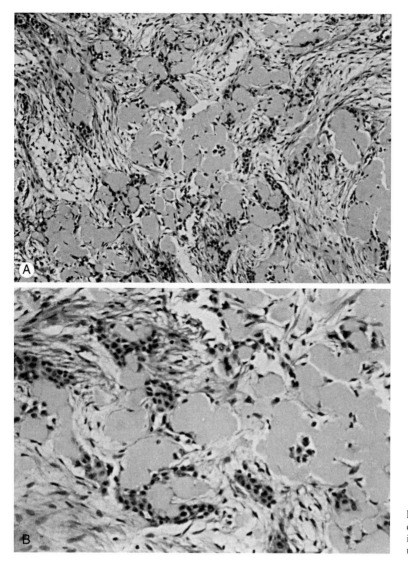

Figure 11–22. *A* and *B*, Calcifying epithelial odontogenic tumor showing strands of epithelium and globules of amyloid.

not been reported. Various forms of surgery, ranging from enucleation to resection, have been used
to treat CEOTs. The overall recurrence rate has
been less than 20%, indicating that aggressive
surgery is not indicated for the management of
most of these benign neoplasms.

Clear Cell Odontogenic Tumor (Carcinoma)

This is a rare neoplasm of the mandible and
maxilla. It has been found in women older than
60 years. It is a locally aggressive, poorly circumscribed neoplasm composed of sheets of optically
clear cells. Metastases to lung and regional lymph
nodes have been reported. Microscopic differential
diagnosis includes other jaw tumors that may have
a clear cell component, such as CEOT, central
mucoepidermoid carcinoma, metastatic acinic cell
carcinoma, metastatic renal cell carcinoma, and
ameloblastoma. Whether this neoplasm should be
regarded as a clear cell variant of the ameloblastoma or should be recognized as a distinct and
separate entity depends on further documentation
and follow-up of a larger number of cases.

Adenomatoid Odontogenic Tumor

Although the adenomatoid odontogenic tumor
(AOT) is of odontogenic origin, the presence of
unusual duct-like or gland-like structures has
given rise to numerous names that have been
modified by *adeno*. Until its distinctive characteristics were fully appreciated, the AOT was thought
to be a subtype of ameloblastoma and was known
by the name *adenoameloblastoma*. Clinically, microscopically, and behaviorally, it is clearly different from ameloblastoma. Some would classify this
lesion as a hamartoma rather than a neoplasm.

Clinical Features. The AOT is seen in a rather
narrow age range between 5 and 30 years, with
most cases appearing in the second decade. Females tend to be more commonly affected than
males. Most lesions appear in the anterior portion
of the jaws and more frequently in the anterior
maxilla, generally in association with the crowns
of impacted teeth (Fig. 11–23). From this position,
the tumor tissue typically proliferates into the lumen of a well-encapsulated cyst-like space.
Rarely, this lesion is seen in a peripheral gingival
location.

Radiographically, the AOT is a well-circum-

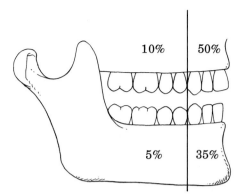

Figure 11–23. Approximate regional distribution of adenomatoid odontogenic tumor.

scribed unilocular lesion usually around the crown
of an impacted tooth (Fig. 11–24). The lesions are
typically radiolucent but may have small opaque
foci distributed throughout, reflecting the presence
of enameloid islands in the tumor tissue. When
they are located between anterior teeth, divergence
of roots may be seen (Fig. 11–25).

Histopathology. An epithelial proliferation is
composed of polyhedral to spindle cells. The pattern is often lobular but may appear as a reticulum
(Fig. 11–26). Rosettes or duct-like structures of
columnar epithelial cells give the lesion its characteristic microscopic feature (Fig. 11–27). Foci of
PAS-positive material are scattered throughout the
lesion. The number, size, and degree of calcification of these foci determine how the lesion presents radiographically.

Differential Diagnosis. Other lesions that
might be included in a differential diagnosis of
AOT are dentigerous cyst, because of frequent
association with impacted teeth, and lateral root
cyst, because of occasional location adjacent to
roots of anterior teeth. If opacities are evident, the
calcifying odontogenic cyst and the CEOT should
receive consideration.

Treatment. Conservative treatment (enucleation) is all that is required for this lesion. The
AOT is a totally benign encapsulated lesion that
only very rarely recurs.

MESENCHYMAL TUMORS

Odontogenic Myxoma

This odontogenic tumor is mesenchymal in nature and origin, mimicking microscopically the
dental pulp or follicular connective tissue. When
relatively large amounts of collagen are evident,
the term *fibromyxoma* may be used to designate

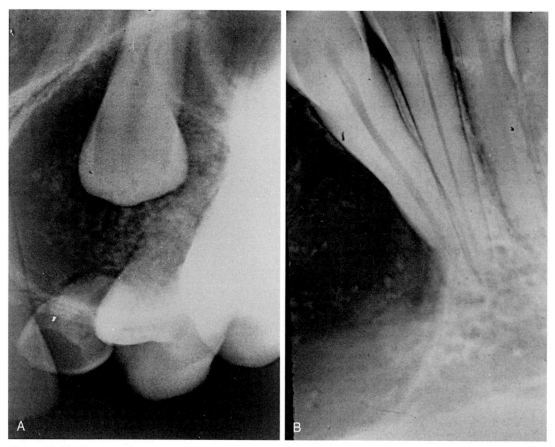

Figure 11-24. *A* and *B,* Adenomatoid odontogenic tumors. Note the opaque foci within the radiolucent lesions.

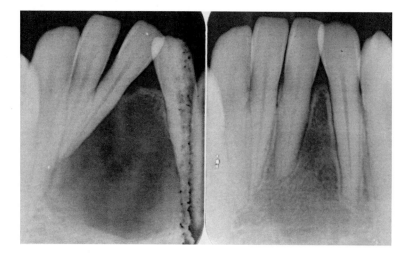

Figure 11-25. *Left,* Adenomatoid odontogenic tumor. *Right,* One year after enucleation.

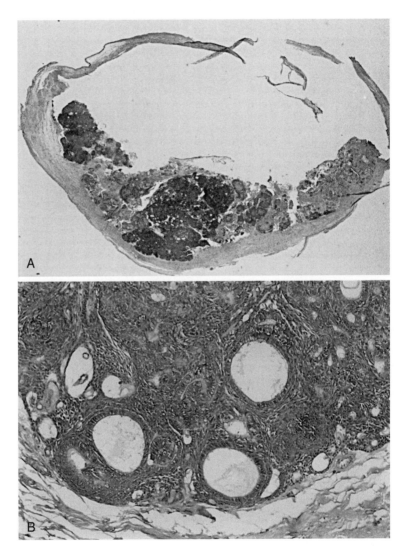

Figure 11–26. *A* and *B,* Adenomatoid odontogenic tumor proliferating into the lumen of the cystic space.

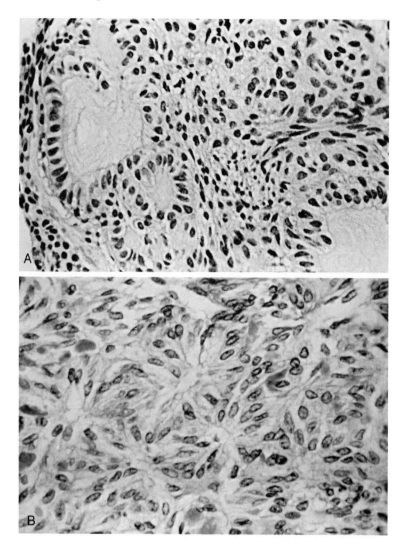

Figure 11–27. *A* and *B*, Two microscopic patterns of adenomatoid odontogenic tumor.

this entity. This is a benign neoplasm that may be infiltrative and aggressive and may recur.

Clinical Features. The age range in which this lesion appears extends from 10 to 50 years, with a mean of about 30. There is no gender predilection, and the lesions are seen anywhere in the mandible and maxilla, with about equal frequency (Fig. 11–28).

Radiographically, this lesion is always lucent, although the pattern may be quite variable. It may appear as a well-circumscribed or a diffuse lesion. It is often multilocular, frequently with a honeycomb pattern (Figs. 11–29 and 11–30). Cortical expansion (rather than perforation) and root displacement (rather than resorption) are the rule.

Histopathology. This tumor is composed of bland, relatively acellular myxomatous connective tissue (Fig. 11–31). Benign fibroblasts and myo-

fibroblasts with variable amounts of collagen are found in a mucopolysaccharide matrix. Bony islands, representing residual trabeculae, and capillaries are found scattered throughout the lesion. Odontogenic rests are very uncommon in these tumors. Their absence should not preclude the diagnosis.

Differential Diagnosis. Clinical differential diagnosis is essentially the same as that described for the ameloblastoma. Additionally, the central hemangioma is a serious consideration in honeycomb lesions. Important to consider microscopically when confronted with a myxomatous lesion from the central jaws are developing dental pulp and follicular connective tissue surrounding an impacted developing or mature tooth. This connective tissue may be a hyperplastic follicle and myxoid in character, closely mimicking the neo-

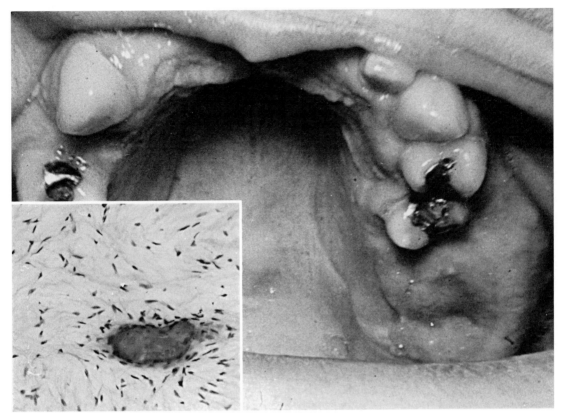

Figure 11–28. Myxoma of the left maxilla. *Inset,* Myxomatous tissue with a bony island.

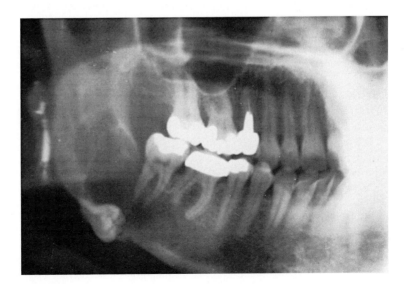

Figure 11–29. Radiograph showing a multilocular odontogenic myxoma of the body of the mandible.

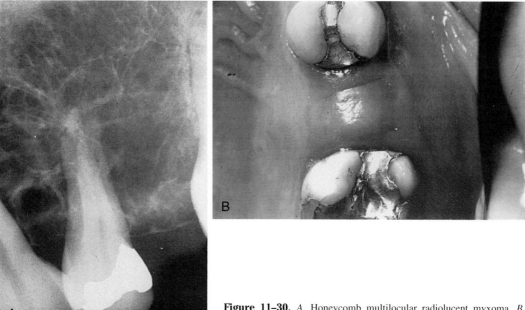

Figure 11–30. *A,* Honeycomb multilocular radiolucent myxoma. *B,* Oral expression of the lesion.

plasm (Fig. 11–32). History and radiographs are important aids in the definitive diagnosis of odontogenic myxomas.

Treatment. Surgical excision is the treatment of choice. Because of an often loose, gelatinous consistency, curettage may result in incomplete removal of viable neoplasm. The absence of encapsulation may also contribute to recurrence if the lesion is treated too conservatively. Although these lesions exhibit some aggressiveness and have a moderate recurrence rate, the prognosis is very good. Repeated surgical procedures do not appear to stimulate growth or cause metastasis.

Central Odontogenic Fibroma

This rare lesion is regarded as the central counterpart to the peripheral odontogenic fibroma. It has been seen in all age groups, and it is found in both the mandible and the maxilla. It results in a radiolucent lesion that is usually multilocular, often causing cortical expansion. Clinical differential diagnosis is similar to that described for ameloblastoma.

Microscopically, two patterns are generally ascribed to central odontogenic fibroma. In the simple type, the lesion is composed of a mass of mature fibrous tissue containing few epithelial rests. In the World Health Organization type, mature connective tissue contains abundant rests and

calcific deposits of what is regarded as dentin or cementum (Fig. 11–33). This microscopic differentiation may be academic, as there appears to be no difference in clinical behavior between the two subtypes. Microscopic differential would include *desmoplastic fibroma* (the bony counterpart of fibromatosis). This purely fibrous connective tissue lesion may be difficult to separate from central odontogenic fibroma because of overlapping microscopy. Clinical correlation should help, as desmoplastic fibroma would exhibit a more aggressive and recurrent behavior. Treatment of the odontogenic fibroma is enucleation or excision, and recurrence is very uncommon.

Cementifying Fibroma

Cementifying fibroma may be impossible to separate from ossifying fibroma and may in fact be just part of a spectrum of central fibrous lesions that contain calcified material. The only feature that has served to separate the two is the microscopic identification of cementum or bone in the lesion, a distinction that is unfortunately strictly subjective using current diagnostic tools. In any event, the separation appears to be essentially an academic exercise. The term *cemento-ossifying fibroma* may be used.

Clinical Features. The cementifying fibroma occurs chiefly in adults around the age of 40 years, but it has a fairly wide age range. There are

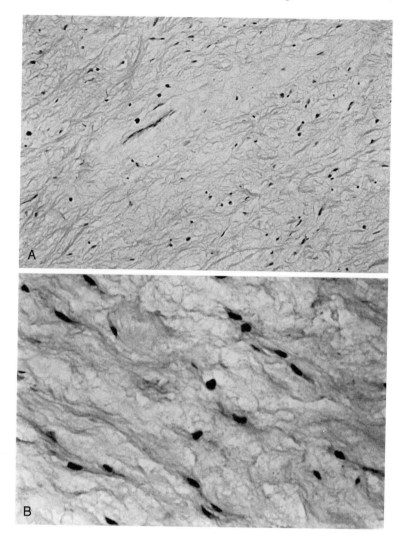

Figure 11–31. *A* and *B,* Odontogenic myxoma.

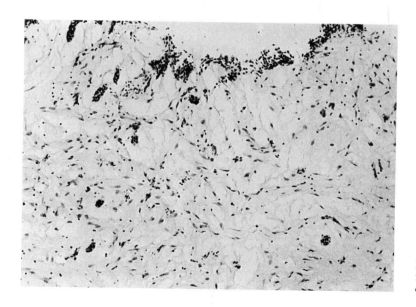

Figure 11–32. Myxomatous dental follicle. Note the remnants of the reduced enamel epithelium (top).

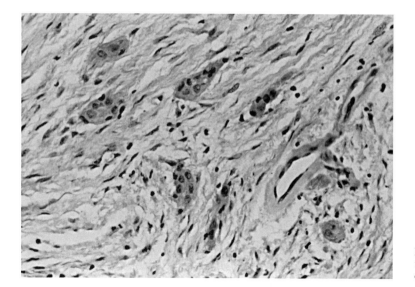

Figure 11–33. Central odontogenic fibroma. Note the fibrous stroma containing several odontogenic rests.

predilections for the mandible and for females. The lesion may cause tooth movement or cortical expansion. Radiographically, it may appear relatively radiolucent (Fig. 11–34), lucent with opaque foci, or diffusely opaque. The radiographic appearance is dependent on the size of the islands of cementum and the extent of calcification. The lesions are usually well circumscribed and are surrounded by a sclerotic margin.

Histopathology. A benign fibroblastic stroma typifies these lesions (Fig. 11–35). Cellularity may be high, but mitoses are rare. Cementum is usually identified as globules or oval islands of calcified material that are frequently surrounded by eosinophilic cementoid and cementoblasts. The cemental islands are evenly distributed throughout the lesion, but they may on occasion converge to form lobulated masses. Inflammatory cells are rarely seen.

Differential Diagnosis. Clinical differential diagnosis of cementifying fibroma should include cementoblastoma, ossifying fibroma, chronic osteomyelitis, and occasionally fibrous dysplasia. Conservative treatment is all that is required. Enucleation or excision should be curative. Recurrence is unexpected.

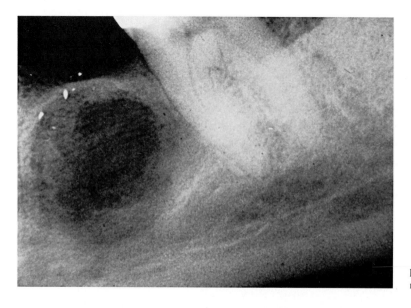

Figure 11–34. Cementifying fibroma in the body of the mandible.

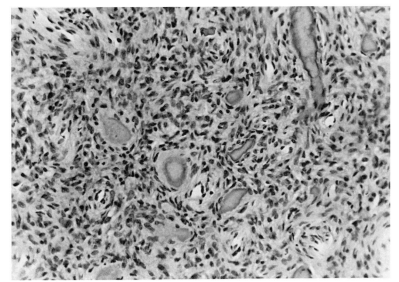

Figure 11–35. Cementifying fibroma composed of benign fibroblasts and islands of cementum.

Cementoblastoma

Clinical Features. The cementoblastoma, also known as *true cementoma,* is a rare benign neoplasm of cementoblast origin. It occurs predominantly in the second and third decades of life, typically before 25 years of age. There is no gender predilection. It is more often seen in the mandible than in the maxilla and more often in posterior than in anterior regions. It is intimately associated with the root of a tooth, and the tooth remains vital. The cementoblastoma may cause cortical expansion and, occasionally, low-grade intermittent pain.

Radiographically, this is an opaque lesion that replaces the root of the tooth (Fig. 11–36). It is usually surrounded by a radiolucent ring.

Histopathology. This lesion appears microscopically as a conglomeration of variably mineralized cementum-like material with numerous reversal lines. Intervening well-vascularized soft tissue contains cementoblasts, often numerous, large, and hyperchromatic. Cementoclasts are also evident.

Differential Diagnosis. The characteristic ra-

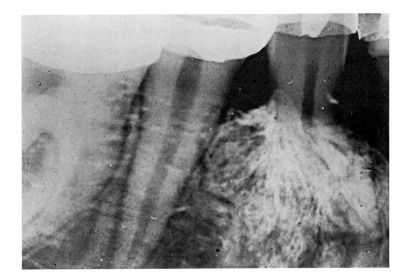

Figure 11–36. Cementoblastoma.

diographic appearance of this lesion is usually diagnostic. Other opaque lesions that share some features include odontoma, osteoblastoma, focal sclerosing osteomyelitis, and hypercementosis.

Treatment. Because of the intimate association of neoplasm with tooth root, this lesion cannot be removed without sacrificing the tooth. Bone relief is typically required to remove this well-circumscribed mass. Recurrence is not seen.

Periapical Cemento-Osseous Dysplasia

As the name implies, this lesion (formerly known as *cementoma*) represents a reactive or dysplastic process rather than a neoplastic one. This lesion appears to be an unusual response of periapical bone and cementum to some local factor.

Clinical Features. This is a relatively common phenomenon that occurs at the apex of vital teeth. Biopsy is unnecessary because the condition is usually diagnostic by clinical and radiographic features. Women, especially black women, are affected more than are men. Periapical cemento-osseous dysplasia appears in middle age (around 40 years) and rarely before the age of 20. The mandible, especially the anterior periapical region, is far more commonly affected than is the maxilla. More often, the apices of two or more teeth are affected.

This condition is typically discovered on routine radiographic examination, because patients are asymptomatic. This condition appears first as a periapical lucency that is continuous with the periodontal ligament space (Fig. 11–37). Although this initial pattern simulates radiographically a periapical granuloma or cyst, the teeth are always vital. As the condition progresses or matures, the lucent lesion develops into a mixed or mottled pattern owing to bone repair. The final stage appears as a solid opaque mass often surrounded by a thin, lucent ring. This process takes months to years to reach final stages of development and, obviously, may be discovered at any stage.

A less common condition described as *florid osseous dysplasia* (FOD) appears to be an exuberant form of periapical cemental dysplasia. FOD would represent the severe end of the spectrum of this unusual process. There is no apparent cause, and patients are asymptomatic except when the complication of osteomyelitis occurs. Females, especially black females, are predominantly affected, usually between 25 and 60 years of age. The condition is typically bilateral and may affect all four quadrants. A curious finding has been the concomitant appearance of traumatic (simple)

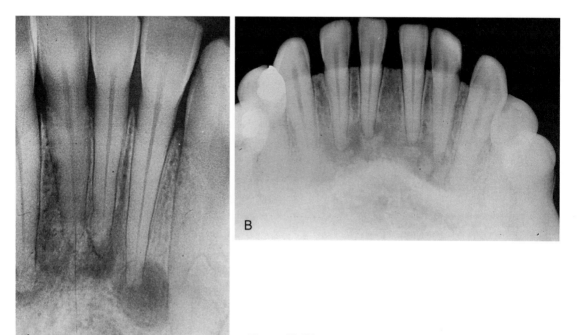

Figure 11–37. Periapical cemento-osseous dysplasia. *A,* Early lesions. *B,* More mature lesions.

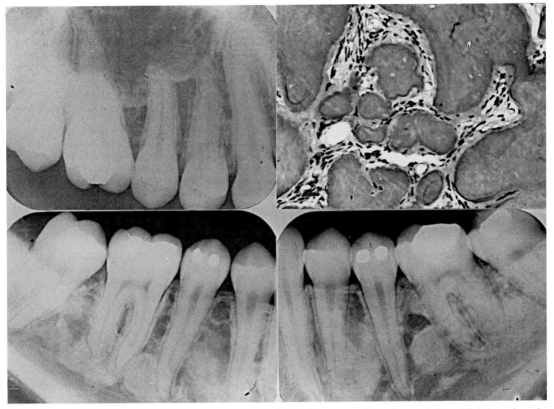

Figure 11–38. Florid osseous dysplasia. The maxilla is unaffected. Low-power photomicrograph *(top right)* shows irregular bony trabeculae in a benign fibrous matrix.

bone cysts in affected tissue. Radiographically, FOD appears as diffuse radiopaque masses throughout the jaw (Fig. 11–38). A ground-glass or cyst-like appearance may also be seen (Fig. 11–39).

Clinical differential diagnosis includes diffuse sclerosing osteomyelitis and Paget's disease. Paget's disease can be ruled out with biopsy and determination of serum alkaline phosphatase (normal in FOD). Chronic diffuse sclerosing osteomyelitis would be symptomatic. It may have a different radiographic appearance, and inflammatory cells would appear in biopsy tissue.

Microscopically, FOD consists of a benign fi-

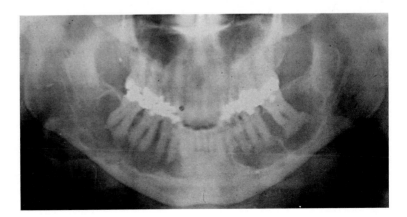

Figure 11–39. Florid osseous dysplasia. Note the lesions at the apex of the anterior teeth.

brous stroma containing irregular trabeculae of mature bone and cementum-like material. Because FOD is an asymptomatic, self-limited process, no treatment is required. In cases in which secondary infection occurs, antibiotics and sequestrectomy may be necessary.

Histopathology. Periapical cemento-osseous dysplasia is a mixture of benign fibrous tissue, bone, and cementum. The calcified tissue is arranged in trabeculae, spicules, or larger irregular masses. Reversal lines are eventually seen, and osteoblasts or cementoblasts, or both, line the islands of hard tissue. Chronic inflammatory cells may also be seen. Microscopically, periapical cemental dysplasia may appear very similar to chronic osteomyelitis and ossifying fibroma.

Differential Diagnosis. Age, gender, location, radiographic appearance, and tooth vitality considered together are diagnostic of this condition. When one or more of these factors are atypical, other diagnostic considerations include chronic osteomyelitis, ossifying fibroma, and periapical granuloma or cyst. In the opaque stage, odontoma, osteoblastoma, and focal sclerosing osteomyelitis are diagnostic possibilities.

Treatment. No treatment is required for this condition. Once the opaque stage is reached, the lesion stabilizes and causes no complications. Because teeth remain vital throughout the entire process, they should not be extracted, and endodontic procedures should not be done. Once clinical diagnosis is established, only observation is necessary.

MIXED (EPITHELIAL AND MESENCHYMAL) TUMORS

Odontoma

Odontomas are known as *mixed odontogenic tumors* because they are composed of tissue that is of both epithelial and mesenchymal origin. These tissues become fully differentiated, resulting in deposition of enamel by ameloblasts and dentin by odontoblasts. Although these cells and tissues appear normal, the architecture is defective. This abnormal organization of otherwise normal mature tissues has led to the opinion that odontomas should be regarded as hamartomas rather than neoplasms.

These calcified lesions take one of two general configurations. They may appear as numerous miniature or rudimentary teeth, in which case they are known as *compound odontomas,* or they may appear as amorphous conglomerations of hard tissue, in which case they are known as *complex odontomas.* As a group, they are the most common odontogenic tumors.

Clinical Features. Odontomas are lesions of children and young adults; most are discovered in the second decade of life. The range does, however, extend into later adulthood. The maxilla is affected slightly more often than the mandible. There is also a tendency for compound odontomas to occur in the anterior jaws and for complex odontomas to occur in the posterior jaws. There does not appear to be a significant gender predilec-

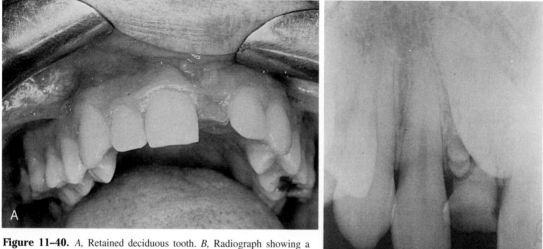

Figure 11–40. *A,* Retained deciduous tooth. *B,* Radiograph showing a retained tooth and a compound odontoma blocking an impacted central incisor.

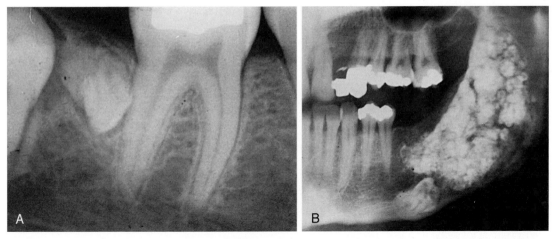

Figure 11–41. *A* and *B,* Complex odontomas. Note the impacted molar in *B* (bottom).

tion. Clinical signs that reflect the presence of an odontoma are a retained deciduous tooth (Fig. 11–40), an impacted tooth, and alveolar swelling. These lesions generally produce no symptoms.

Radiographically, the compound odontoma appears as several, and occasionally tens of, mature teeth in a single focus. This focus is typically in a tooth-bearing area, between roots or over the crown of an impacted tooth. Complex odontomas appear in the same regions but as amorphous opaque masses (Figs. 11–41 and 11–42). Lesions discovered during early stages of tumor development are primarily radiolucent, with focal areas of opacity representing early calcification of dentin and enamel.

Histopathology. Normal-appearing enamel, dentin, cementum, and pulp may be seen in these lesions (Fig. 11–43). Prominent enamel matrix and associated enamel organ are often seen before final maturation of hard tissues. So-called ghost cell keratinization is seen in epithelial cells of the enamel of some odontomas. This microscopic feature appears to have no significance other than to indicate the potential of these epithelial cells to keratinize.

Differential Diagnosis. Compound odontomas are diagnostic on radiographic examination. Complex odontomas usually present a typical radiographic appearance because of their solid opacification in relationship to teeth. However, differential diagnosis might include other opaque jaw lesions such as focal sclerosing osteomyelitis, osteoma, periapical cemental dysplasia, ossifying fibroma, and cementoblastoma.

Treatment. Odontomas have very limited growth potential, although an occasional complex lesion may cause considerable bone expansion.

Enucleation is curative, and recurrence is not a problem.

A rare variant known as *ameloblastic odontoma* has been described. This is essentially an ameloblastoma in which there is focal differentiation into an odontoma. Until more is known of the behavior of this rare lesion, it should be treated as an ameloblastoma.

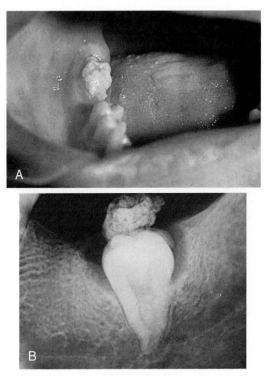

Figure 11–42. *A* and *B,* Erupted complex odontoma. (Courtesy of Dr. W. G. Sprague.)

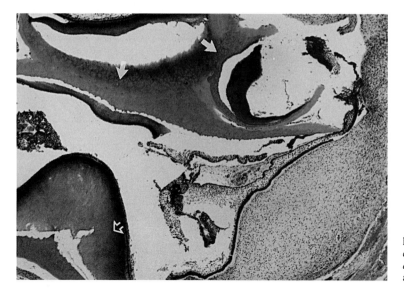

Figure 11–43. Complex odontoma composed of enamel matrix *(open arrow)* against dentin *(closed arrows)* and pulp tissue (lower right).

Ameloblastic Fibroma and Ameloblastic Fibro-Odontoma

These two lesions are considered together because they appear to be variations of the same process. Except for the presence of an odontoma, people affected with either of the two lesions share similar features of age, gender, and location. The biologic behaviors of these lesions are also similar. Both are mixed odontogenic tumors composed of neoplastic epithelium and mesenchyme with microscopically identical soft tissue compo-

nents. Both are regarded as benign neoplastic processes of odontogenic origin.

Clinical Features. These neoplasms occur predominantly in children and young adults. The mean age is about 12 years, and the upper age limit may be 40 years. The mandibular molar-ramus area is the favored location for these lesions, although any region may be affected. There is no gender predilection.

Radiographically, these lesions are well circumscribed and are usually surrounded by a sclerotic margin. They may be either unilocular or multilocular and may be associated with the crown of an impacted tooth (Fig. 11–44). An opaque focus

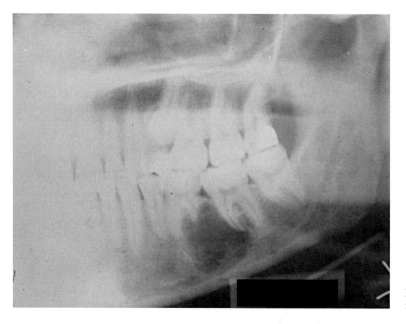

Figure 11–44. Ameloblastic fibroma of the mandible.

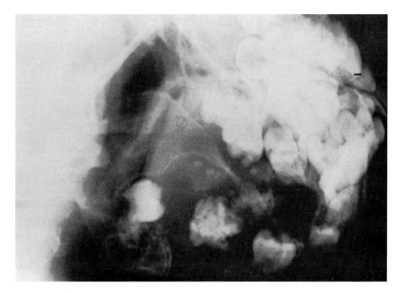

Figure 11–45. Lateral jaw radiograph from an 11-year-old boy, showing ameloblastic fibro-odontoma of the body and ramus of the mandible. (Courtesy of Dr. R. Hanna.)

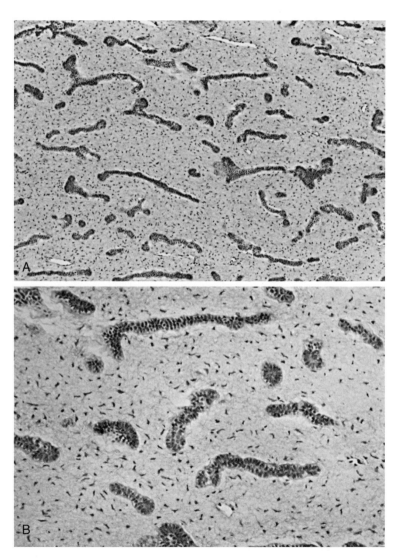

Figure 11–46. *A* and *B*, Myxomatous stroma of ameloblastic fibroma containing strands of odontogenic epithelium.

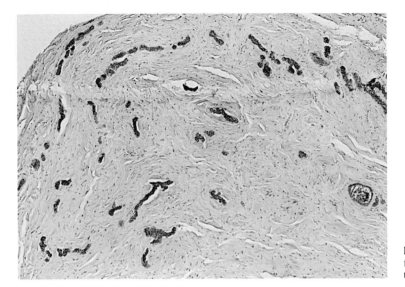

Figure 11–47. Fibrous sac (dental follicle) containing proliferative odontogenic rests.

appears within the ameloblastic fibro-odontoma owing to the presence of an odontoma (Fig. 11–45). This lesion therefore presents as a combined lucent-opaque lesion; the ameloblastic fibroma is completely lucent radiographically.

Histopathology. These lesions are lobulated in general configuration and are usually surrounded by a fibrous capsule. The tumor mass is composed predominantly of a primitive-appearing myxoid connective tissue (Fig. 11–46). The general absence of collagen gives this component a resemblance to dental pulp. Evenly distributed throughout the tumor mesenchyme are ribbons or strands of odontogenic epithelium that are typically two cells wide. The epithelial component has been compared microscopically with the dental lamina that proliferates from oral epithelium in the early stages of tooth development.

In the ameloblastic fibro-odontoma, cells in one or more foci continue the differentiation process and produce enamel and dentin. This may be in the form of a compound or complex odontoma, the presence of which does not alter the treatment or prognosis.

Differential Diagnosis. When ameloblastic fibroma (fibro-odontoma) presents with the age, location, and radiographic pattern typical for these lesions, diagnosis is usually apparent. When clinical features are outside the usual boundaries, a differential diagnosis for ameloblastic fibroma should include ameloblastoma, odontogenic myxoma, dentigerous cyst, odontogenic keratocyst,

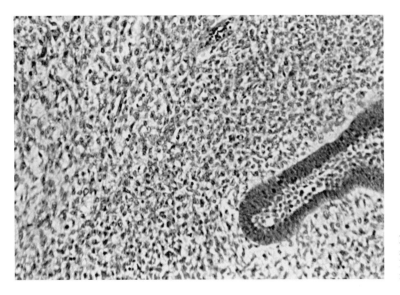

Figure 11–48. Ameloblastic fibrosarcoma. Fibrous stroma is hypercellular and hyperchromatic and contains numerous mitotic figures.

central giant cell granuloma, and histiocytosis. The differential diagnosis for ameloblastic fibroodontoma includes lesions with mixed radiographic patterns such as CEOT, calcifying odontogenic cyst, developing odontoma, and possibly AOT. Microscopically, this lesion must be differentiated from the more fibrous hyperplastic follicular sac, in which there is proliferation of odontogenic rests (Fig. 11–47).

Treatment. Because of tumor encapsulation and the general lack of invasive capacity, this lesion is treated with a conservative surgical procedure such as curettage or excision. Recurrences have been documented, but they are uncommon.

A rare malignant counterpart to these odontogenic tumors known as *ameloblastic fibrosarcoma* has been documented as arising in the jaws either *de novo* or from preexisting or recurrent ameloblastic fibroma. In this lesion, the mesenchymal component has the appearance of a fibrosarcoma and the epithelial component appears as it does in the benign lesion (Fig. 11–48). Clinically, the ameloblastic fibrosarcoma occurs at an age around 30 years and more often in the mandible than in the maxilla. Symptoms of pain and paresthesia may be present. This is a locally aggressive lesion that has metastatic potential. Resection is therefore the treatment of choice.

Bibliography

Ameloblastoma

Adekeye E, McCallum K. Recurrent ameloblastoma of the maxillofacial region. J Maxillofac Surg 14:153–157, 1986.

Atkinson C, Harwood A, Cummings B. Ameloblastoma of the jaw: a reappraisal of the role of megavoltage irradiation. Cancer 53:869–873, 1984.

Corio R, Goldblatt L, Edwards P, et al. Ameloblastic carcinoma: a clinicopathologic study and assessment of eight cases. Oral Surg Oral Med Oral Pathol 64:570–576, 1987.

Daley TD, Wysocki GP. Relative incidence of odontogenic tumors and oral and jaw cysts in a Canadian population. Oral Surg Oral Med Oral Pathol 77:276–228, 1994.

Eversole R, Leider A, Hansen L. Ameloblastomas with pronounced desmoplasia. J Oral Maxillofac Surg 43:735–740, 1984.

Gardner D. A pathologist's approach to the treatment of ameloblastoma. J Oral Maxillofac Surg 42:161–166, 1984.

Gardner D, Corio R. Plexiform unicystic ameloblastoma: a variant of ameloblastoma with a low recurrence rate after enucleation. Cancer 53:1730–1735, 1984.

Keszler A, Dominguez F. Ameloblastoma in childhood. J Oral Maxillofac Surg 44:609–613, 1986.

Leider A, Eversole L, Barkin M. Cystic ameloblastoma. Oral Surg Oral Med Oral Pathol 60:624–630, 1985.

Muller H, Slootweg P. The ameloblastoma, the controversial approach to therapy. J Maxillofac Surg 13:79–84, 1985.

Muller H, Slootweg P. Clear cell differentiation in an ameloblastoma. J Maxillofac Surg 14:158–160, 1986.

Philipsen H, Reichart P, Zhang K, et al. Adenomatoid odonto-genic tumor: biologic profile based on 499 cases. J Oral Pathol Med 20:149–158, 1991.

Ruskin J, Cohen D, Davis L. Primary intraosseous carcinoma: report of two cases. J Oral Maxillofac Surg 46:425–432, 1988.

Slootweg P, Muller H. Malignant ameloblastoma or ameloblastic carcinoma. Oral Surg 57:168–176, 1984.

Thompson IO, van Rensberg LJ, Phillips VM. Desmoplastic ameloblastoma: correlative histopathology, radiology, and CT-MR imaging. J Oral Pathol Med 25:405–410, 1996.

Ueno S, Nakamura S, Mushimoto K, et al. A clinicopathologic study of ameloblastoma. J Oral Maxillofac Surg 44:361–365, 1986.

Waldron C, El-Mofty S. A histopathologic study of 116 ameloblastomas with special reference to the desmoplastic variant. Oral Surg Oral Med Oral Pathol 63:441–451, 1987.

Waldron C, Small I, Silverman H. Clear cell ameloblastoma—an odontogenic carcinoma. J Oral Maxillofac Surg 43:707–717, 1985.

White R, Patterson J. Distant skin metastases in a long-term survivor of malignant ameloblastoma. J Cutan Pathol 13:383–389, 1986.

Woo S, Smith-Williams J, Sciubba J, et al. Peripheral ameloblastoma of the buccal mucosa: case report and review of the English literature. Oral Surg Oral Med Oral Pathol 63:78–84, 1987.

Other Epithelial Odontogenic Tumors

Ai-Ru L, Zhen L, Jian S. Calcifying epithelial odontogenic tumors. J Oral Pathol 11:399–406, 1982.

Bang G, Koppang H, Hansen L, et al. Clear cell odontogenic carcinoma: report of three cases with pulmonary and lymph node metastasis. J Oral Pathol Med 18:113–118, 1989.

Bernstein M, Buchino J. The histologic similarity between craniopharyngioma and odontogenic lesions: a reappraisal. Oral Surg Oral Med Oral Pathol 56:501–510, 1983.

Buchner A, Sciubba J. Peripheral epithelial odontogenic tumors: a review. Oral Surg Oral Med Oral Pathol 63:688–697, 1987.

Eisenstein W, Pitcock J. Adamantinoma of the tibia. Arch Pathol Lab Med 108:246–250, 1984.

Ellis G, Shmookler B. Aggressive (malignant?) epithelial odontogenic ghost cell tumor. Oral Surg Oral Med Oral Pathol 61:471–478, 1986.

Elzay R. Primary intraosseous carcinoma of the jaws. Oral Surg Oral Med Oral Pathol 54:299–303, 1982.

Eversole L, Belton C, Hansen L. Clear cell odontogenic tumor: histochemical and ultrastructural features. J Oral Pathol 14:603–614, 1985.

Goldblatt L, Brannon R, Ellis G. Squamous odontogenic tumor. Oral Surg Oral Med Oral Pathol 54:187–196, 1982.

Grodjesk J, Dolinsky H, Schneider L, et al. Odontogenic ghost cell carcinoma. Oral Surg Oral Med Oral Pathol 63:576–581, 1987.

Hansen L, Eversole L, Green T, et al. Clear cell odontogenic tumor—a new histologic variant with aggressive potential. Head Neck Surg 8:115–123, 1985.

Kristensen S, Andersen J, Jacobsen P. Squamous odontogenic tumor. J Laryngol Otol 99:919–924, 1985.

Leider A, Jonker A, Cook H. Multicentric familial squamous odontogenic tumor. Oral Surg Oral Med Oral Pathol 68:175–181, 1989.

Mills W, Davila M, Beuttenmuller E, et al. Squamous odontogenic tumor. Oral Surg Oral Med Oral Pathol 61:557–563, 1986.

Mori H, Yamamoto S, Hiramatsu K, et al. Adamantinoma of the tibia. Clin Orthop 190:299–310, 1984.

Norris L, Baghaei-Rad M, Maloney P. Bilateral maxillary

squamous odontogenic tumors and the malignant transformation of a mandibular radiolucent lesion. J Oral Maxillofac Surg 42:827–834, 1984.

Perez-Atayde A, Kozakewich H, Vawter G. Adamantinoma of the tibia. Cancer 55:1015–1023, 1985.

Mesenchymal and Mixed Odontogenic Tumors

Altini M, Thompson S, Lownie J, et al. Ameloblastic sarcoma of the mandible. J Oral Maxillofac Surg 43:789–794, 1985.

Dahl E, Wolfson S, Haugen J. Central odontogenic fibroma. J Oral Surg 39:120–124, 1981.

Dunlap C, Barker B. Central odontogenic fibroma of the WHO type. Oral Surg Oral Med Oral Pathol 57:390–394, 1984.

Handlers J, Abrams A, Melrose R, Danforth R. Central odontogenic fibroma. J Oral Maxillofac Surg 49:46–54, 1991.

Melrose R, Abrams A, Mills B. Florid osseous dysplasia. Oral Surg Oral Med Oral Pathol 41:62–82, 1976.

Regezi J, Kerr D, Courtney R. Odontogenic tumors: analysis of 706 cases. J Oral Surg 36:771–778, 1978.

Vincent S, Hammond H, Ellis G, et al. Central granular cell odontogenic fibroma. Oral Surg Oral Med Oral Pathol 63:715–721, 1987.

Zachariades N, Skordalaki A, Papanicolaou S, et al. Cementoblastoma: review of the literature and report of a case in a seven-year-old girl. Br J Oral Maxillofac Surg 23:456–461, 1985.

12

Benign Nonodontogenic Tumors

Jeffery C. B. Stewart

OSSIFYING FIBROMA
FIBROUS DYSPLASIA
DESMOPLASTIC FIBROMA
OSTEOBLASTOMA
OSTEOID OSTEOMA
CHONDROMA
OSTEOMA
CENTRAL GIANT CELL GRANULOMA
GIANT CELL TUMOR
HEMANGIOMA OF BONE
LANGERHANS CELL DISEASE
TORI AND EXOSTOSES
CORONOID HYPERPLASIA

OSSIFYING FIBROMA

Ossifying fibroma is a benign, slow-growing lesion of the jaws that is often clinically and microscopically similar, if not identical, to cementifying fibroma. This tumor is classified as one of the benign fibro-osseous lesions of the jaws and historically has been referred to as fibro-osteoma, osteofibroma, and benign fibro-osseous lesion of periodontal ligament origin.

Etiology and Pathogenesis. The ossifying fibroma is considered by many investigators to be a benign neoplasm that develops from undifferentiated cells of periodontal ligament origin. A neoplastic etiology is supported by examples of lesions that achieve a large size, exhibit aggressive behavior, and produce significant osseous destruction. Additionally, recurrences, though rare, have been described in some studies of ossifying fibroma. Chromosomal translocations have been identified in a few cases of ossifying fibroma. Others regard this lesion as an example of a localized dysplastic process in which bone metabolism is altered. The similarities between this lesion and the cementifying fibroma are numerous. Both tumors occur in similar age groups and locations and exhibit comparable clinical characteristics. The microscopic features are also indistinguish-

able in many instances. The distinction between these processes, most often based on the nature of the calcified product in the tumor, may in fact be academic, because their biologic behavior is identical. This has prompted many to use the term *cemento-ossifying fibroma* to describe this lesion.

Clinical Features. The ossifying fibroma is a slow-growing, expansile lesion that is usually asymptomatic when discovered. The lesions, with rare exceptions, arise in the tooth-bearing regions of the jaws, most often in the mandibular premolar-molar area. Some cases of ossifying fibroma have been reported in craniofacial bones other than the jaws. The slow growth of the tumor may ultimately produce expansion and thinning of the buccal and lingual cortical plates, although perforation and mucosal ulceration are rare. Ossifying fibromas are uncommon lesions that tend to occur during the third and fourth decades of life. A definite female predominance has been evident in several studies. These lesions occur most commonly in a solitary fashion, although rare instances of multiple synchronous lesions have been reported. The cases of multiple ossifying fibroma are most often sporadic, although rarely a familial tendency has been noted.

The most important radiographic feature of this lesion is the well-circumscribed, sharply defined border (Fig. 12–1). Ossifying fibromas otherwise present a variable appearance depending on the maturation or the amount of calcification present (Fig. 12–2). Early lesions may appear as unilocular or multilocular radiolucencies that bear considerable resemblance to odontogenic cysts. The initial radiolucent stage gradually progresses to a mixed radiolucent-radiopaque lesion as calcified material is deposited in the tumor. Mature lesions may consist of a dense, radiopaque mass surrounded by a well-defined, radiolucent rim. The roots of teeth may be displaced, and less commonly, the lesion may resorb tooth roots.

The well-circumscribed appearance of the ossifying fibroma is most evident at the time of sur-

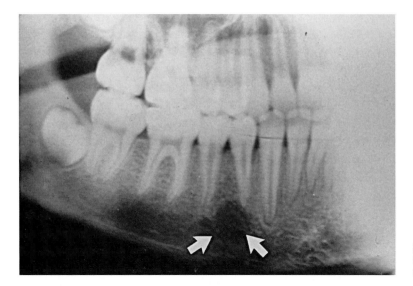

Figure 12–1. Ossifying fibroma in the premolar region of the mandible *(arrows).*

gery, when the lesion may easily be curetted or enucleated from the surrounding normal bone.

Histopathology. The tumor consists of a collagenous stroma that contains various numbers of uniform spindled or stellate cells (Fig. 12–3). Collagen fibers are often arranged haphazardly, although a whorled, storiform pattern may be evident. The stroma is well vascularized in many instances, although in some cases it is relatively fibrotic and avascular.

Calcific deposits are noted throughout the fibrous stroma (Fig. 12–4). The nature of the hard tissue is generally quite variable within a given tumor as well as between lesions. Irregular trabeculae of woven immature bone are most consis-

tently noted in these tumors, although lamellar bone is also present in a large percentage of cases. Osteoblasts may or may not be evident at the periphery of the bone deposits.

Additional patterns of calcified material include small, ovoid to globular, basophilic deposits and anastomosing trabeculae of cementum-like material. The observation of these deposits in many of these lesions has led some investigators to conclude that the ossifying fibroma and cementifying fibroma are similar if not identical lesions.

Most ossifying fibromas exhibit a mixture of the different types of calcified products, although a single morphologic type is evident in others.

Differential Diagnosis. Distinguishing between

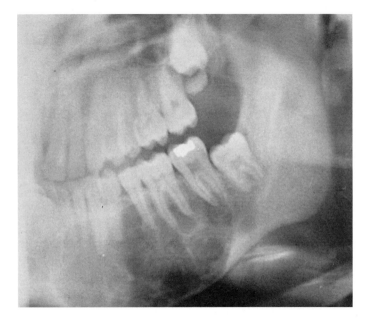

Figure 12–2. Ossifying fibroma of the mandible.

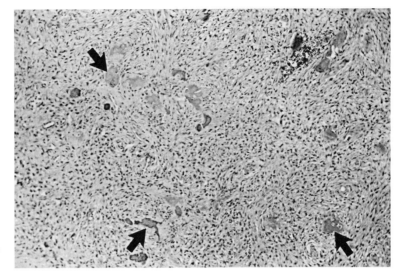

Figure 12–3. Ossifying fibroma composed of evenly distributed fibroblasts and several calcified foci of bone *(arrows).*

ossifying fibroma and fibrous dysplasia is the primary differential diagnostic challenge. Both processes may exhibit similar clinical, radiographic, and microscopic features. The most helpful feature distinguishing the two is the radiographic and clinically well-circumscribed appearance of ossifying fibroma and the ease with which it can be separated from normal bone. In most cases, the well-defined appearance of ossifying fibroma is evident radiographically. Historically, attempts at differentiating the two lesions were based only on histologic criteria. Fibrous dysplasia was reported to contain only woven bone, without evidence of osteoblastic rimming of bone. The presence of mature lamellar bone was believed to be characteristic of ossifying fibroma. Most authorities now acknowledge that these criteria are unreliable, be-

cause both types of bone may be found in either lesion.

Osteoblastoma and osteoid osteoma are evident in a slightly younger age group and are often characterized by pain. Additionally, osseous trabeculae in these lesions are rimmed by abundant plump osteoblasts. A central nidus is also evident in these lesions. Cementoblastoma may arise with a similar clinical and radiographic presentation; however, this lesion is fused to the root of the involved tooth.

It may occasionally be necessary to distinguish ossifying fibroma from focal sclerosing osteomyelitis. In general, a source of inflammation is evident, possibly accompanied by pain, tenderness, swelling, or lymphadenopathy.

Treatment and Prognosis. Treatment of ossi-

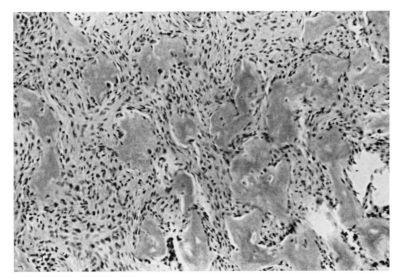

Figure 12–4. Ossifying fibroma composed of benign fibroblasts and irregular islands of new bone.

fying fibroma is most often accomplished by surgical removal using curettage or enucleation. As stated, the lesion can be separated easily from the surrounding normal bone. Recurrence is described only rarely after removal. The use of liquid nitrogen cryotherapy for the treatment of ossifying fibroma has also been reported. Long-term follow-up is advocated with conservative excision of lesions that might recur after curettage. A variant of ossifying fibroma, the *juvenile ossifying fibroma,* has been described in children and young adults. This lesion most commonly involves the paranasal sinuses and periorbital bones, resulting in exophthalmos, proptosis, sinusitis, and nasal symptoms. This rare lesion behaves in a more aggressive fashion than does the ossifying fibroma, and it may require more extensive therapy when encountered. Some investigators have attempted to clarify the microscopic features of juvenile ossifying fibroma. The presence of irregularly mineralized, cellular, osteoid strands lined by plump osteoblasts has been described as being characteristic of this lesion. The true relationship between these lesions awaits further elucidation.

FIBROUS DYSPLASIA

Fibrous dysplasia is a condition in which normal medullary bone is gradually replaced by an abnormal fibrous connective tissue proliferation. The mesenchymal tissue contains various amounts of osteoid and osseous material that presumably arises through metaplasia. The resultant fibro-osseous tissue is poorly formed and structurally inadequate.

Subsequent to the original description of this process, confusion about the criteria necessary for the diagnosis of fibrous dysplasia arose. As a result, many entities that appear to be distinct from fibrous dysplasia were included under this designation. Attempts to describe and define fibrous dysplasia more precisely continue.

Etiology and Pathogenesis. The precise cause of this condition remains unknown, although various theories have been proposed. Many authorities accept the premise that fibrous dysplasia represents a nonneoplastic, hamartomatous growth resulting from deranged mesenchymal cell activity or a defect in the control of bone cell activity. Several investigations have described the presence of an activating mutation in the gene that codes for the Gs alpha membrane–associated protein in patients with fibrous dysplasia. This alteration may result in altered proliferation and differentiation of osteoblastic cells in these patients. It has also been proposed that this lesion results from an arrest in

the maturation of mesenchymal tissue at the woven bone stage. Another hypothesis suggests that fibrous dysplasia is an abnormal reaction of bone to a localized traumatic episode. Alternatively, focal bone expression of a complicated endocrine disturbance has been suggested as a possible cause. The description of the presence of estrogen receptors in osteogenic cells of a patient with fibrous dysplasia suggests that this process may reflect a defect in the regulation of these receptors and consequently cellular activity. A hereditary basis for development of fibrous dysplasia has not been found.

Clinical Features. This disease most commonly presents as an asymptomatic, slow enlargement of the involved bone. Fibrous dysplasia may involve one bone or several bones concomitantly. *Monostotic fibrous dysplasia* is the designation used to describe the process as it occurs in one bone; *polyostotic fibrous dysplasia* applies to cases in which more than one bone exhibits evidence of the disorder. Polyostotic fibrous dysplasia is relatively uncommon; however, many patients have lesions of the skull, facial bones, or jaws as a component of the condition. *McCune-Albright syndrome* is a designation that has been applied to patients with polyostotic fibrous dysplasia, cutaneous melanotic pigmentations (café au lait macules), and endocrine abnormalities. The most commonly reported endocrine disorder consists of precocious sexual development in females. Acromegaly, hyperthyroidism, hyperparathyroidism, and hyperprolactinemia have also been described. *Jaffe-Lichtenstein syndrome* is characterized by multiple bone lesions of fibrous dysplasia and skin pigmentations.

Monostotic fibrous dysplasia is much more common than the polyostotic form, accounting for as many as 80% of the cases. Jaw involvement is common in this form of the disease. Other bones frequently affected are the ribs and femur. Fibrous dysplasia occurs within the maxilla more often than within the mandible. Maxillary lesions may extend to involve the maxillary sinus, zygoma, sphenoid bone, and floor of the orbit. This form of the disease, with involvement of several adjacent bones, has been referred to as *craniofacial fibrous dysplasia.* The most common site of occurrence with mandibular involvement is in the body portion.

The slowly progressive enlargement of the affected jaw is usually painless and typically presents as a unilateral swelling (Fig. 12–5). As the lesion grows, facial asymmetry becomes evident and may be the initial presenting complaint. The fusiform swelling of the affected jaw most commonly results from buccal cortical plate expan-

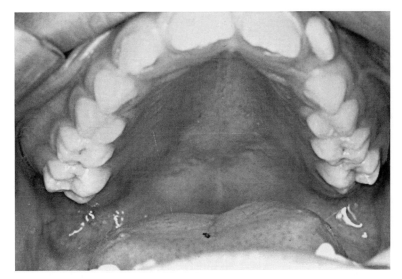

Figure 12–5. Monostotic fibrous dysplasia causing expansion of the right maxilla.

sion, and it rarely affects the lingual or palatal aspect. Displacement of teeth with resultant malocclusion and interference with normal eruption patterns may occur, although mobility of erupted teeth is not a feature of fibrous dysplasia.

This condition characteristically has its onset during the first or second decade of life. Rarely, the lesion is not evident until later in life, although this finding may only reflect the insidious, asymptomatic nature of fibrous dysplasia.

In a few instances, lesions of fibrous dysplasia may pursue a more aggressive clinical course, resulting in rapid growth, pain, nasal obstruction, and exophthalmos.

Monostotic fibrous dysplasia generally exhibits an equal gender distribution, and the polyostotic form tends to occur more commonly in females.

Fibrous dysplasia has a variable radiographic appearance that ranges from a radiolucent lesion to a densely radiopaque mass (Fig. 12–6). The classic presentation has been described as radiopaque, with numerous bony trabeculae imparting a ground-glass appearance. This characteristic feature, which becomes most identifiable on intraoral radiographs, is, however, not pathognomonic. Lesions of fibrous dysplasia may also present as unilocular or multilocular radiolucencies. A third pattern is one in which a mottled radiolucent and radiopaque appearance, similar to that noted in Paget's disease, predominates. Additional radiographic features that have been described include a fingerprint bone pattern and superior displacement of the mandibular canal in mandibular lesions.

An important distinguishing feature of fibrous dysplasia is the poorly defined radiographic and clinical margins of the lesion. The process appears to blend into the surrounding normal bone without evidence of a circumscribed border. Additionally, these lesions are frequently elliptical as opposed to spherical. Laboratory values, specifically serum calcium, phosphorus, and alkaline phosphatase, are within normal ranges for the patient's age group.

Histopathology. The histologic findings in fibrous dysplasia consist of a cellular, fibrous connective tissue proliferation that contains foci of irregularly shaped trabeculae of immature bone. A relatively constant ratio of fibrous tissue to bone throughout a given lesion has been described as characteristic. The collagen fibers may completely lack orientation or, alternatively, may be arranged in a storiform pattern of interlacing collagen bundles. The fibroblasts exhibit uniform spindle- to star-shaped nuclei. The bony trabeculae assume

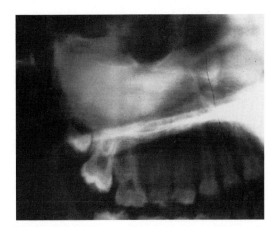

Figure 12–6. Diffuse maxillary opaque mass of fibrous dysplasia.

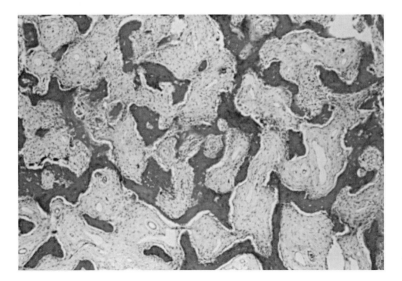

Figure 12–7. Irregular trabeculae of fibrous dysplasia.

bizarre, irregular shapes, likened to Chinese characters (Fig. 12–7). These trabeculae do not display any apparent functional orientation. The bone is predominantly woven bone that appears to arise directly from the collagenous stroma without prominent osteoblastic activity (Fig. 12–8). In a mature fibrous dysplasia lesion, lamellar bone may be found. Aneurysmal bone cysts have been noted in association with fibrous dysplasia in some reports. It should be noted that the microscopic features of fibrous dysplasia share many characteristics with those of ossifying fibroma.

Differential Diagnosis. The primary differential diagnosis for fibrous dysplasia of the jaws is ossifying fibroma. As previously noted, clinical, radiographic, and microscopic features must be considered together in order to distinguish these processes most accurately. The well-circumscribed appearance of ossifying fibroma in comparison with the ill-defined borders of fibrous dysplasia often serves as the differentiating factor. Additional features that aid in distinguishing these processes are listed in Table 12–1.

Paget's disease shares some features with fibrous dysplasia, but it occurs in a much older age group and typically exhibits a bilateral distribution. Alkaline phosphatase levels are characteristically increased in Paget's disease. Chronic osteomyelitis may mimic the mottled radiographic appearance of fibrous dysplasia. Inflammation is generally present and is accompanied by variable symptoms, including tenderness, pain, or purulent

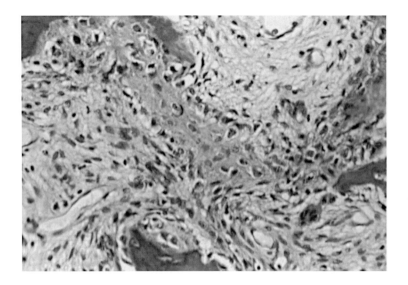

Figure 12–8. Fibrous dysplasia consisting of benign fibrous matrix and "metaplastic" bone.

Table 12–1. Differentiating Features of Ossifying Fibroma and Fibrous Dysplasia

FEATURE	OSSIFYING FIBROMA	FIBROUS DYSPLASIA
Age	Third and fourth decades	First and second decades
Gender predilection	Females	Equal (monostotic)
Location	Body of mandible favored	Maxilla favored slightly
Radiography	Well-defined margins	Poorly defined margins
Lesion shape	Roughly nodular or spherical jaw expansion	Fusiform or elliptical jaw expansion

drainage. The slowly progressive, asymptomatic nature of fibrous dysplasia usually allows differentiation from malignant tumors of bone.

Treatment and Prognosis. After a variable period of growth, fibrous dysplasia frequently stabilizes or slows considerably after the onset of puberty. Small lesions may therefore require no treatment other than biopsy confirmation and periodic follow-up. Large lesions that have caused cosmetic or functional deformity may be treated through a process of osseous recontouring. This procedure is generally reserved for the period of time after stabilization of the disease process. *En bloc* resections for complete removal are impractical and unnecessary because the lesions are relatively large and are generally regarded as nonneoplastic.

Malignant transformation is a rare complication of fibrous dysplasia (fewer than 1% of cases) that has been described usually in patients with the polyostotic type. Rapid enlargement of a lesion or onset of pain should suggest this possibility. Cystic degeneration within fibrous dysplasia may also cause increased swelling, however. Many of these patients were treated with radiation therapy, suggesting a role for radiation in the transformation process, although malignant change has been documented in the absence of radiation treatment.

DESMOPLASTIC FIBROMA

Desmoplastic fibroma is a benign, locally aggressive lesion of bone that shares many features with soft tissue desmoid tumor and fibromatosis. The tumor is rare and primarily affects the long bones and pelvis, although involvement of the jaws has been reported.

Etiology and Pathogenesis. The cause of desmoplastic fibroma is unknown. The lesion usually exhibits locally aggressive clinical behavior suggesting a neoplastic process. The potential role of genetic, endocrine, and traumatic factors in the pathogenesis of the lesion has led to speculation that it might represent an exuberant reactive proliferation.

Clinical Features. Most cases of desmoplastic fibroma of the jaws have occurred in patients under the age of 30 years, with a mean age of 14 years. No gender predilection has been noted. The mandible, usually the body-ramus region, is affected more frequently than the maxilla. Slowly progressive, asymptomatic swelling of the jaw is the usual presentation.

Radiographically, desmoplastic fibroma is typically a unilocular or multilocular radiolucency. The radiographic margins may be either well demarcated or poorly defined. Cortical perforation and root resorption may be seen.

Histopathology. The lesion consists of interlacing bundles and whorled aggregates of densely collagenous tissue that contains uniform spindled and elongated fibroblasts. Some areas may exhibit hypercellularity with plumper fibroblast nuclei. However, cytologic atypia and mitotic figures are not found. Bone is not produced by lesional tissue.

Differential Diagnosis. The radiographic features of a unilocular or multilocular radiolucency would prompt differential diagnostic consideration of odontogenic cysts and tumors as well as nonodontogenic lesions that typically occur in this age group. The presence of aggressive features, such as cortical perforation, or local symptoms might suggest the possibility of a malignancy. In some cases, histopathologic distinction between desmoplastic fibroma and well-differentiated fibrosarcoma may be difficult. The latter would exhibit increased mitotic rate, nuclear pleomorphism, and larger, densely aggregated fibroblasts. Some similarities are noted histologically with central odontogenic fibroma. The latter, however, may contain odontogenic rests and is typically nonaggressive clinically.

Treatment. Surgical resection of the lesion is generally reported as the treatment of choice. Curettage has been associated with a significant recurrence rate.

OSTEOBLASTOMA

Osteoblastoma is an uncommon primary lesion of bone that occasionally arises in the maxilla or the mandible. The term *giant osteoid osteoma* has been used at times to describe this lesion, because it is believed to represent a larger version of the osteoid osteoma. Osteoblastoma is a benign process that may exhibit a seemingly rapid onset and cause pain. These clinical features, as well as histologic findings, may on occasion cause confusion between this lesion and malignant tumors of bone.

Etiology and Pathogenesis. Although the cause of the osteoblastoma is unknown, most authorities consider this to be a true neoplasm of bone. The finding of a chromosomal translocation has been reported in one case of osteoblastoma. Reports of regression of lesions after biopsy or incomplete treatment have led some investigators to postulate that osteoblastoma represents an unusual reactive process within bone.

Clinical Features. Osteoblastoma arises most frequently in the vertebrae and the long bones of the body. These lesions involve the jaws and other craniofacial bones less commonly, but the mandible is the most frequent head and neck site. The posterior tooth-bearing regions of the maxilla or mandible are the usual sites of involvement. The midline areas of the jaws, coronoid processes, and condyle are rarely affected. Lesions have been reported as arising in either medullary or periosteal sites.

Most cases occur during the second decade of life, with 90% of osteoblastomas presenting before age 30. Males seem to be affected more commonly than females, by a ratio of approximately 2 to 1.

Osteoblastomas present with various signs and symptoms. Pain, often quite severe, is the most consistent symptom. Localized swelling may occur alone or along with the pain. The bony cortices may be expanded and tender to palpation, although mucosal ulceration is absent. Mobility of adjacent teeth has been noted. Unlike the pain occurring with those lesions that have been reported as osteoid osteoma, the pain associated with osteoblastoma is not often relieved by aspirin or nonsteroidal anti-inflammatory drugs. The classic nocturnal pain of osteoid osteoma is also uncommon with these lesions. Duration of signs or symptoms of osteoblastoma ranges from weeks to years.

The radiographic features are variable, consisting of combinations of radiolucent and radiopaque patterns (Fig. 12–9). The designation of osteoblastoma may be used for lesions greater than 2 cm in diameter, in contrast to smaller lesions, which are often referred to as *osteoid osteomas.* The well-circumscribed nature of the process is evident radiographically. A thin radiolucency may be noted, surrounding a variably calcified, central tumor mass. Sclerosis of perilesional bone, a constant feature of the smaller osteoid osteoma, is usually absent in osteoblastoma. A sun-ray pattern of new bone production, similar to that described in various malignant bone tumors, may be evident in these lesions.

Histopathology. The histologic appearance of osteoblastoma, like its radiographic appearance, is quite variable. Irregular trabeculae of osteoid and immature bone are present within a stroma containing a prominent vascular network (Fig. 12–10). The bony trabeculae exhibit various degrees of calcification. Remodeling of the osseous tissue may be evident in the form of basophilic reversal lines. Several layers of plump, hyperchromatic osteoblasts typically line the bony trabeculae. Pleomorphism and abnormal mitotic activity are

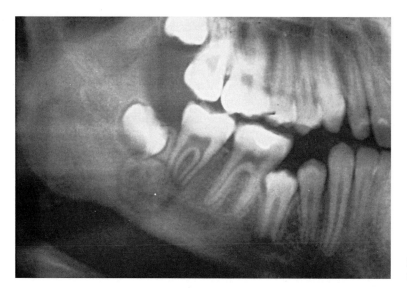

Figure 12–9. Osteoblastoma of the mandible.

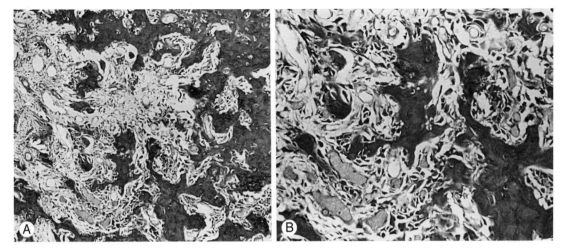

Figure 12–10. *A* and *B,* Osteoblastoma composed of irregular bony trabeculae surrounded by abundant hyperchromatic osteoblasts.

not features of these active osteoblasts, however. Stromal cells are generally small and slender, although osteoblast-like cells may be noted in these areas. An additional characteristic of osteoblastoma is the presence of numerous multinucleated giant cells scattered throughout the stroma.

Differential Diagnosis. Osteoblastoma must be differentiated from a number of bone-producing lesions, including cementoblastoma, ossifying fibroma, fibrous dysplasia, and osteosarcoma.

Osteoid osteoma bears considerable clinical, radiographic, and histologic similarity to osteoblastoma. Many experts, in fact, regard the two lesions as identical. Classically, the distinction rests primarily in the size of the lesion: osteoid osteoma, less than 2 cm, and osteoblastoma, larger than 2 cm. Nocturnal pain, frequently relieved by aspirin, is more commonly noted in osteoid osteoma. A sclerotic peripheral bone reaction is a significant feature of osteoid osteoma. Cementoblastoma can be differentiated from osteoblastoma because the former lesion arises from the surface of a tooth root and is fused to it. This intimate connection between lesion and tooth is unexpected in osteoblastoma.

Multilayered, plump osteoblasts lining bony trabeculae serve to distinguish osteoblastoma from ossifying fibroma. Most ossifying fibromas also contain small spherical, calcific structures. The clinical and radiographic features of these lesions may be similar, although pain is not a usual symptom of ossifying fibroma. Fibrous dysplasia has a poorly defined margin in contrast to the well-circumscribed appearance of osteoblastoma. Prominent osteoblastic activity is not a significant microscopic feature of fibrous dysplasia.

The relatively rapid onset and pain associated with some osteoblastomas necessitate differentiation from osteosarcoma. Radiographic and histologic similarities may also exist between given lesions. The hyperchromatic, large osteoblasts noted in osteoblastoma must be distinguished from the malignant tumor cells of osteosarcoma. Cytologic atypia, abnormal mitotic figures, and delicate osteoid adjacent to tumor cells are features of osteosarcoma.

Treatment and Prognosis. Surgical excision of osteoblastoma is the preferred method of treatment. A conservative approach, curettage or local excision, is curative in virtually all cases. Recurrence after adequate surgical intervention is uncommon. In rare instances, these tumors have been associated with a tendency to invade tissues locally and to recur subsequently. Some authorities have suggested the term *aggressive osteoblastoma* for such lesions, but others regard this as unnecessary subclassification. Rare examples of malignant transformation of osteoblastoma have also been reported.

OSTEOID OSTEOMA

This benign lesion of bone shares many features with osteoblastoma, as previously discussed. Distinction between these lesions has been described on the basis of size, site of occurrence, and radiographic appearance. These lesions, as they present in the jaws, are best regarded as closely related variants of the same process.

Etiology and Pathogenesis. Osteoid osteoma is idiopathic. This lesion is generally regarded as a true neoplasm, although the limited growth potential suggests an unusual reactive disorder.

Clinical Features. Osteoid osteoma is an uncommon bone lesion that, like osteoblastoma, occurs predominantly in individuals in the second and third decades of life. A definite male preponderance is also apparent. The tumor arises most commonly in the femur and tibia, with jaw lesions being rare. Any area of the mandible or maxilla may be involved, however.

Pain is the major symptom associated with osteoid osteoma. This symptom may be related to the effect of prostaglandins, because tissue extracts from both osteoid osteoma and osteoblastoma have been shown to contain increased concentrations of prostaglandin E_2. The pain may be described initially as intermittent, dull, and vague. It is frequently worse during the night and is often relieved with aspirin. Increasing severity of pain with time has been noted. Lesions located near the cortex may produce a localized tender swelling.

The classic radiographic appearance is that of a small ovoid radiolucency surrounded by a rim of sclerotic bone. The nidus of the tumor may exhibit various degrees of calcification, often presenting with a densely opaque center. Osteoid osteoma has a limited growth potential, not exceeding 2 cm in diameter.

Histopathology. Distinction between the histologic features of osteoid osteoma and osteoblastoma is essentially impossible. A richly vascular stroma invests trabeculae of osteoid and immature bone. The bone is rimmed by layers of active, plump osteoblasts. Some studies have suggested that osteoid osteoma contains fewer osteoblasts, reduced vascularity, and broader osseous trabeculae than does osteoblastoma. These differences have been difficult to appreciate in the experience of most pathologists. Electron microscopic studies have shown identical morphologic features in proliferating osteoblastic cells in both lesions.

Differential Diagnosis. The differential diagnosis for osteoid osteoma is similar to that for osteoblastoma. Lesions may occasionally resemble focal osteomyelitis on a radiographic basis. The absence of both inflammatory cells and fibrosis in the biopsy specimen of osteoid osteoma serves to distinguish the two processes.

Treatment and Prognosis. This benign process is treated by conservative surgical excision. Cure is expected after removal, because recurrence is rare. Spontaneous regression after no treatment or incomplete treatment has been reported. Surgical intervention, nonetheless, is the treatment of choice.

CHONDROMA

Chondromas are benign tumors composed of mature cartilage. The cause of these lesions is unknown. Chondromas have been reported in the jaws; however, these lesions are rare in this location, especially in comparison with their occurrence in other skeletal sites.

Clinical Features. The chondroma commonly presents as a painless, slowly progressive swelling. The gradual expansion of the lesion rarely results in mucosal ulceration. Most lesions of the craniofacial complex arise in the nasal septum and ethmoid sinuses. Chondromas of the maxilla are most frequently found in the anterior region, where cartilaginous remnants of development are located. Mandibular chondromas have been noted in the body and symphysis areas as well as the coronoid process and the condyle. Chondromas occur with equal incidence in both genders, with the majority of tumors appearing before 50 years of age.

The radiographic appearance of the chondroma is variable, the lesion most often presenting as an irregular radiolucent area. Foci of calcification may be evident within the radiolucent lesion. Resorption of the roots of adjacent teeth has been noted.

Histopathology. The lesion consists of well-defined lobules of mature hyaline cartilage. The cartilage may exhibit areas in which calcification has occurred. The chondrocytes are small cells that contain single, regular nuclei. Degeneration and necrosis may be present focally. The degree of cellularity varies considerably from one area to another within the chondroma.

Differential Diagnosis. The principal diagnostic dilemma rests in distinguishing the chondroma from a well-differentiated chondrosarcoma. Clinical and radiographic features often provide little useful information to distinguish these lesions. Considerable overlap may occur between these lesions histologically as well. Well-differentiated chondrosarcomas may be underdiagnosed as chondromas if the lesions are examined insufficiently.

Treatment and Prognosis. Surgical excision is the appropriate therapy for the chondroma. The difficulty in distinguishing histologically between this lesion and a well-differentiated chondrosarcoma suggests that wide, although not radical, surgical excision may be justified in some instances.

Prognosis for the chondroma is good after therapy, and recurrence is unusual. Recurrence should be cause for reconsidering the original diagnosis for the possibility of low-grade malignancy.

OSTEOMA

Osteomas are benign tumors that consist primarily of mature, compact, or cancellous bone.

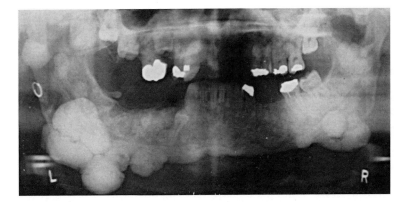

Figure 12–11. Multiple osteomas in Gardner syndrome. Note the impacted teeth.

Osteomas that arise on the surface of bone are referred to as *periosteal osteomas,* whereas those that develop centrally within bone are *endosteal osteomas.* Because these lesions are often small and asymptomatic, the true incidence involving the jaws is difficult to determine. Osteomas are generally thought to be relatively uncommon in this region, however.

Etiology and Pathogenesis. The cause of these lesions is unknown. Various causative factors that have been proposed include trauma, response to infection, and developmental abnormalities. None of these has been definitively shown to be the cause of all osteomas.

Clinical Features. Osteomas are most commonly identified during the second to fifth decades of life, although they may be found at any age. These tumors are reported to occur in males twice as frequently as in females, although a marked female predominance was noted in one study of osteomas of the jaws. These lesions most often occur in solitary fashion, except when associated with Gardner syndrome.

Gardner syndrome, inherited as an autosomal dominant disorder, is characterized by intestinal polyposis, multiple osteomas, fibromas of the skin, epidermal and trichilemmal cysts, impacted permanent and supernumerary teeth, and odontomas. The specific gene is present in a small region on the long arm of chromosome 5 (5q21). The majority of patients with Gardner syndrome do not exhibit the complete spectrum of clinical disease expression. The presence of numerous osteomas of the jaws and facial bones should lead one to investigate the possibility of this syndrome (Fig. 12–11). Osteomas may be found in the jaws, especially the mandibular angle, as well as in facial and long bones. The intestinal polyps associated with Gardner syndrome are commonly located in the colon and rectum. Significantly, the polyps, found microscopically to be adenomas, exhibit a very high rate of malignant transformation to invasive colorectal carcinoma.

Periosteal osteomas present clinically as asymptomatic, slow-growing, bony, hard masses. Asymmetry may be noted when lesions enlarge to sufficient proportion. Endosteal osteomas occurring within medullary bone may be discovered during routine radiographic examination as dense, well-circumscribed radiopacities, because extensive growth must take place before cortical expansion is evident. Osteomas may arise in the maxilla or mandible, as well as in facial and skull bones and within paranasal sinuses. Symptoms occasionally accompany these tumors. Headaches, recurrent sinusitis, and ophthalmologic complaints have been noted, dependent on lesion location.

Radiographically, both periosteal and endosteal osteomas appear as well-circumscribed, sclerotic, radiopaque masses.

Histopathology. Two distinct histologic variants of osteoma have been described. One form is composed of relatively dense, compact bone with sparse marrow tissue (Fig. 12–12). The other form consists of lamellar trabeculae of cancellous bone with abundant fibrofatty marrow spaces. Osteoblastic activity is usually prominent.

Differential Diagnosis. Osteomas should be distinguished from exostoses of the jaws. Exostoses are bony excrescences on the buccal aspect of alveolar bone. These lesions are of reactive or developmental origin and are not thought to be true neoplasms. Osteoblastomas and osteoid osteomas, which might also be considered in a differential diagnosis, are more frequently painful and may exhibit a more rapid rate of growth than osteomas. Osteomas may also be confused radiographically with odontomas or focal sclerosing osteomyelitis.

Treatment and Prognosis. The treatment of osteomas is surgical excision. Lesions should also be excised for the purpose of establishing the

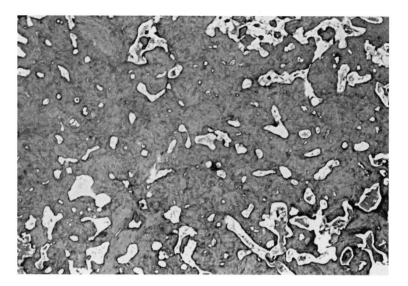

Figure 12–12. Dense mature bone in an osteoma from a patient with Gardner syndrome.

diagnosis. In some instances, periodic observation of small, asymptomatic osteomas is appropriate treatment. Osteomas do not recur following surgical removal.

CENTRAL GIANT CELL GRANULOMA

The central giant cell granuloma is a benign process that occurs almost exclusively within the jawbones. The tumor typically presents as a solitary radiolucent lesion of the mandible or maxilla.

Etiology and Pathogenesis. The true nature of the central giant cell granuloma remains unknown, despite considerable discussion and controversy in the literature. It has been proposed that the process represents a reparative response to intrabony hemorrhage and inflammation. Although the clinical progression of these lesions is inconsistent with repair, many investigators regard these lesions as reactive. A previous traumatic or inflammatory episode is not elicited in most cases, however. Other authorities view the central giant cell granuloma as a lesion related to the giant cell tumor of long bones, a lesion considered to be a true neoplasm. A third theory is that this lesion may represent a developmental anomaly closely related to the aneurysmal bone cyst. Experimental evidence suggests that the multinucleated giant cells may be derived variously from stromal mononuclear cells, myofibroblast-like cells, or immigrating osteoclasts. Proponents of osteoclast origin believe these lesions may involve an interaction between osteoblasts and the giant cells as part of a reactive response. The mononuclear cell component of these lesions has been shown to consist of a heterogeneous population of cells, most of which exhibit a fibroblastic or myofibroblastic phenotype.

Clinical Features. Central giant cell granuloma is an uncommon lesion and occurs less frequently than does peripheral giant cell granuloma. This process is found predominantly in children and young adults, with 64 to 75% of cases presenting before 30 years of age. Females are affected more frequently than males, with a ratio of 2 to 1.

The central giant cell granuloma is present almost exclusively in the maxilla and mandible, although isolated cases in facial bones and small bones of the hands and feet have been reported. Lesions occur more frequently in the mandible than in the maxilla. These lesions tend to involve the jaws anterior to the molar teeth, with occasional extension across the midline. Rarely, lesions involve the posterior jaws, including the mandibular ramus and condyle.

The central giant cell granuloma typically produces a painless expansion or swelling of the affected jaw. Cortical plates are thinned; however, perforation with extension into soft tissues is uncommon. The radiographic features of the central giant cell granuloma consist of a multilocular or, less frequently, unilocular radiolucency of bone (Fig. 12–13). The margins of the lesion are relatively well demarcated, often presenting a scalloped border. In some instances, central giant cell granulomas pursue a more aggressive clinical and radiographic course. These "aggressive" central giant cell granulomas may cause pain and may exhibit rapid growth, root resorption, perforation of cortical bone, and a tendency to recur after conservative surgical treatment.

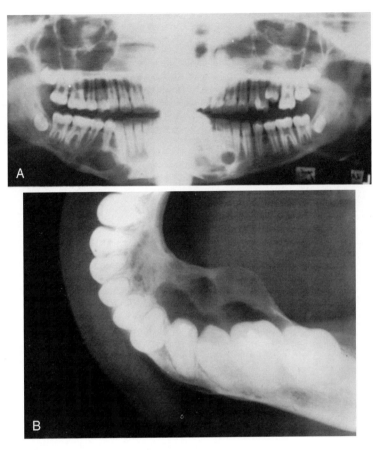

Figure 12–13. *A* and *B,* Central giant cell granuloma of the anterior mandible.

Histopathology. The lesion is composed of a proliferation of spindled fibroblasts in a stroma containing various amounts of collagen (Fig. 12–14). Numerous small vascular channels are evident throughout the lesion. Hemosiderin-laden macrophages are frequently noted, as well as extravasated erythrocytes. Multinucleated giant cells are present throughout the connective tissue stroma. The giant cells may be evenly dispersed; however, they are frequently aggregated around vascular channels. It has been proposed that aggressive central giant cell granulomas exhibit more dense populations of mononuclear and multinucleated giant cells with less fibrovascular tissue. Inflammatory cells are not prominent and, when they are seen, most likely are secondary in nature. Foci of osteoid may be present, scattered throughout the stroma.

Differential Diagnosis. The typical radiographic features of a solitary multilocular radiolucency indicate that ameloblastoma, odontogenic myxoma, odontogenic keratocyst, and aneurysmal bone cyst must be differentiated from this lesion. Cystic processes of the jaws should also be considered in a differential diagnosis, because some central giant cell granulomas may be unilocular.

The microscopic appearance of central giant cell granuloma is virtually identical to the giant cell lesion associated with hyperparathyroidism. These processes must be differentiated on the basis of biochemical tests. Increased serum calcium and alkaline phosphatase and decreased serum phosphorus values are indicative of primary hyperparathyroidism; normal serum chemistries are expected with central giant cell granuloma.

The giant cell tumor of bone may present with similar clinical and microscopic features, although many investigators believe careful examination allows differentiation. The giant cell tumor of bone is regarded as rare in the jaws in comparison with the central giant cell granuloma.

Treatment and Prognosis. Surgical management of these lesions with aggressive curettage is generally regarded as the treatment of choice. Curettage of the tumor mass followed by removal of the peripheral bony margins results in a good prognosis and a low recurrence rate. In some instances, presurgical endodontic therapy of involved teeth or their extraction may be necessary. A somewhat higher rate of recurrence has been reported in those lesions arising in children and young teens.

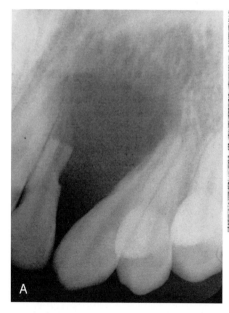

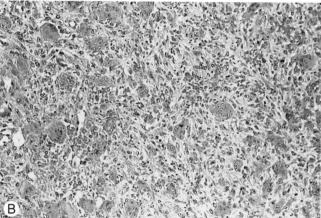

Figure 12–14. *A,* Central giant cell granuloma of the maxilla. *B,* Microscopy shows a benign fibroblastic matrix and numerous multinucleated giant cells.

Lesions with aggressive clinical features also exhibit a tendency to recur, frequently necessitating more extensive surgical approaches including resection. Intralesional injections of corticosteroids have been proposed as a nonsurgical method for management of these lesions, but the rationale of this therapy is questionable. The use of exogenous calcitonin may have some merit in the treatment of aggressive lesions. Preliminary data suggest that lesions may stabilize or regress after several months of therapy.

GIANT CELL TUMOR

Giant cell tumors are true neoplasms that arise most frequently in the long bones, especially in the area of the knee joint. These tumors exhibit a wide spectrum of biologic behavior from benign to malignant. The relationship between this lesion and the central giant cell granuloma is controversial. Some investigators regard the giant cell tumor as a distinct entity from the central giant cell granuloma, acknowledging the very rare occurrence of the giant cell tumor within the jaws. Other experts believe that these lesions represent two points in the spectrum of a single pathologic process.

Etiology and Pathogenesis. These neoplasms are thought to arise from undifferentiated mesenchymal cells exhibiting some characteristics of macrophages. These neoplastic proliferations are generally regarded as distinct from the central giant cell granuloma, which appears to be reactive. Some researchers, however, have considered the giant cell tumor of bone to be representative of the biologically more aggressive variant of the central giant cell granuloma.

Clinical Features. Giant cell tumors, although rare, have been reported to involve the jaws. Other sites of involvement in the head and neck include the sphenoid, ethmoid, and temporal bones. The giant cell tumor has been reported most frequently in the third and fourth decades of life.

These lesions may exhibit a wide range of biologic behavior and thus may present diverse clinical features. Benign variants may exhibit slow growth and bone expansion virtually identical to those of a giant cell granuloma. Aggressive or malignant variants may produce rapid growth, pain, or paresthesia. Radiographically, the giant cell tumor produces a radiolucent lesion similar in appearance to the central giant cell granuloma. Giant cell tumors have been noted in association with preexisting Paget's disease in both the jaws and the long bones.

Histopathology. Giant cell tumor is characterized by the presence of numerous multinucleated giant cells. The giant cells are dispersed evenly among mononuclear stromal cells. Nuclear morphology of both types of cells is virtually identical. Stromal cellularity is usually prominent, with minimal collagen production. Several studies have suggested that the giant cells in giant cell tumors are larger and contain more nuclei than the corresponding cells of central giant cell granuloma. Significant variation is noted in these findings, however, such that any given lesion may present diagnostic difficulty. Giant cell tumors may contain inflammatory cells and areas of necrosis while exhibiting a relative absence of hemorrhage and hemosiderin deposition. Osteoid formation is also noted less frequently than in giant cell granulomas.

Differential Diagnosis. Microscopically, the giant cell tumor must be differentiated from other conditions that contain multinucleated giant cells, including central giant cell granuloma, hyperparathyroidism, aneurysmal bone cyst, and cherubism.

Treatment and Prognosis. Surgical excision is the treatment of choice for the giant cell tumor. These lesions exhibit a greater tendency to recur after treatment than does the giant cell granuloma. Although too few cases have been reported in the jaws to predict recurrence rates, it is noteworthy that 30% of lesions in long bones recur after curettage. Finally, one case of a true malignant giant cell tumor has been reported in the jaws.

HEMANGIOMA OF BONE

Hemangiomas of bone are uncommon intraosseous lesions consisting of a proliferation of blood vessels. The central hemangioma occurs most frequently in vertebrae and in the skull. The mandible and the maxilla are the next most common sites of occurrence.

Etiology and Pathogenesis. The cause of central hemangiomas is unknown. Some lesions may represent true neoplasms; others are more probably developmental or traumatic in origin.

Clinical Features. More than half the central hemangiomas of the jaws occur in the mandible, with its posterior region being the most frequent site. The lesion occurs approximately twice as frequently in females as in males. The peak age of incidence is the second decade of life.

A firm, slow-growing, asymmetric expansion of the mandible or maxilla is the most common patient complaint. Spontaneous gingival bleeding around teeth in the area of the hemangioma may also be noted. Paresthesia or pain is occasionally evident, as well as mobility of involved teeth. Teeth may exhibit a pumping action such that, when depressed in an apical direction, the teeth rapidly resume their original position. Bruits or pulsation of large hemangiomas or arteriovenous malformations may be detected with careful auscultation or palpation of the thinned cortical plates. Significantly, hemangiomas may be present without any signs or symptoms.

Hemangiomas of the mandible and maxilla present a wide variety of radiographic appearances (Fig. 12–15). More than half occur as multilocular radiolucencies that have a characteristic soap-bubble appearance. A second form of these lesions consists of a rounded, radiolucent lesion in which bony trabeculae radiate from the center of the lesion, producing angular loculations. Less commonly, hemangiomas appear as cyst-like radiolucencies. The lesions may produce resorption of the roots of teeth in the area.

Histopathology. Hemangiomas of bone are composed of a proliferation of blood vessels. Most intrabony hemangiomas are of the cavernous type (Fig. 12–16). Dilated, thin-walled vascular spaces are lined by benign endothelial cells. Fibrous connective tissue stroma supports the blood-filled vascular spaces. Numerous small, capillary-sized vascular channels may be the prominent histologic feature. These lesions have been referred to as *capillary hemangiomas.* A mixture of both histo-

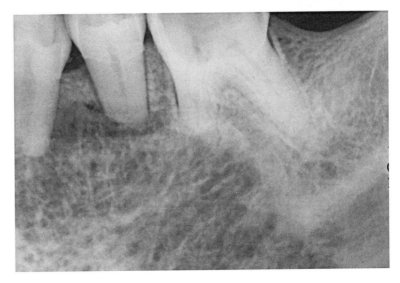

Figure 12–15. Hemangioma of the mandible, causing tooth resorption. (Courtesy of Dr. E. Ellis.)

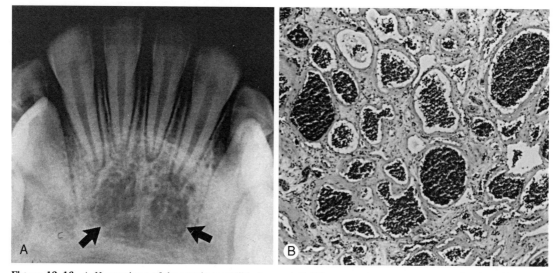

Figure 12–16. *A,* Hemangioma of the anterior mandible *(arrows). B,* Microscopy shows numerous vascular channels.

logic subtypes is frequently evident. The microscopic appearance of hemangiomas is academic because biologic behavior of the lesions is independent of this factor.

Differential Diagnosis. The differential diagnosis of the multilocular hemangioma of bone includes ameloblastoma, odontogenic myxoma, odontogenic keratocyst, central giant cell granuloma, and aneurysmal bone cyst. A unilocular lesion may be easily confused with other cystic processes that occur within jaws. Angiography often provides useful information in establishing the diagnosis of hemangioma.

Treatment and Prognosis. The most significant feature of hemangiomas of bone is that these lesions may prove life threatening if improperly managed. Extraction of teeth in an area involved by a central vascular lesion may result in potentially fatal bleeding. It is imperative to perform needle aspiration of any central lesion that potentially may be of vascular origin before performing a biopsy.

Methods used in the treatment of hemangioma of bone include surgery, radiation therapy, sclerosing agents, cryotherapy, and presurgical embolization techniques. The vascular supply of a given lesion, as well as its size and location, must be evaluated before the selection of a given treatment method.

LANGERHANS CELL DISEASE

Langerhans cell disease, also formerly known as *histiocytosis X* and *idiopathic histiocytosis,* is a disorder characterized by a proliferation of cells exhibiting phenotypic characteristics of Langerhans cells. The clinical manifestations of this process range from solitary or multiple bone lesions to disseminated visceral, skin, and bone lesions.

Historically, the term *histiocytosis X* was used to encompass three disorders: eosinophilic granuloma, Hand-Schüller-Christian syndrome, and Letterer-Siwe disease. These entities were grouped together owing to their similar microscopic appearance, despite the diverse manner of clinical disease expression. *Eosinophilic granuloma* has referred to solitary or multiple bone lesions only. *Hand-Schüller-Christian syndrome* has represented a specific clinical triad of lytic bone lesions, exophthalmos, and diabetes insipidus. Many affected persons also exhibited lymphadenopathy, dermatitis, splenomegaly, or hepatomegaly. *Letterer-Siwe disease* has been characterized by a rapidly progressive, usually fatal clinical course. Widespread organ, bone, and skin involvement by the proliferative process in infants has been the common presentation.

Most authorities do not currently consider this histiocytosis classification scheme as truly representative of this disease process. Letterer-Siwe disease, more recently referred to as the *acute disseminated form* of idiopathic histiocytosis, most likely represents a malignant neoplastic process. A minority of patients actually present with the classic triad of Hand-Schüller-Christian syndrome. This *chronic disseminated form* of the disorder is only one of various presentations in which lymph node, visceral, and bone involvement may occur. Less severe *chronic localized forms* of idiopathic histiocytosis appear to be represented by cases in which only multifocal or unifocal bone lesions are noted. Categorization of Langerhans cell disease has also been termed either *restricted* or *extensive,* based on clinical extent and site of disease involvement.

Etiology and Pathogenesis. The etiology and pathogenesis of Langerhans cell disease remain obscure. Investigations have, however, elucidated the cell of origin of this process. Ultrastructural and immunohistochemical similarities exist between the proliferative cell of this disorder and the Langerhans cell that normally resides in epidermis and mucosa. The dendritic (Langerhans) cells function in the processing and presentation of antigens to effector immune cells (T lymphocytes).

The acute form of this disease and some cases of the chronic forms are thought possibly to represent a neoplastic transformation. Abnormalities of DNA content in the proliferative cells have been demonstrated in only a few cases of Langerhans cell disease, however. More recent investigations in a limited number of patients have demonstrated a clonal proliferation of Langerhans cells, supporting the concept of a neoplastic process. It has also been suggested that the disease may result from exuberant reaction to an unknown antigenic challenge. Evidence regarding the possible role of viruses is conflicting, specifically human herpesvirus 6, in the etiology and pathogenesis of this disease. Evidence is emerging that some patients with Langerhans cell disease may exhibit defects in certain aspects of the cell-mediated arm of the immune system. A deficiency of suppressor T lymphocytes as well as low levels of serum thymic factor suggest the presence of a thymus abnormality in this disease. These immunologic defects may affect normal regulatory mechanisms, with resultant Langerhans cell proliferation.

Clinical Features. Langerhans cell disease is generally regarded as a condition of children and young adults that exhibits extreme clinical heterogeneity. An increased male predominance has been noted by some investigators. The monostotic and polyostotic forms of the disorder may affect virtually any bone of the body. The skull, mandible, ribs, vertebrae, and long bones are frequently involved. Oral changes may be the initial presentation in all forms of this disorder. Skin, mucosal, or bone involvement in the head and neck region was noted in more than 80% of children in one study. Tenderness, pain, and swelling are frequent patient complaints. Loosening of teeth in the area of the affected alveolar bone is a common occurrence. The gingival tissues are frequently inflamed, hyperplastic, and ulcerated. Oral mucosal lesions in the form of submucosal nodules, ulcers, and leukoplakia have also been described.

The jaws may exhibit solitary or multiple radiolucent lesions (Fig. 12–17). The lesions frequently affect the alveolar bone, causing the teeth to appear as if they are floating in space (Fig. 12–18). Bone lesions with a sharply circumscribed, punched-out appearance may also occur in the central aspects of the mandible or maxilla. These lesions are occasionally located exclusively in a periapical site, where they may be associated with periapical inflammatory lesions. Jaw lesions may be accompanied by bone involvement elsewhere in the skeleton. Radiographic skeletal surveys are useful for detecting widespread involvement. Cervical lymphadenopathy, mastoiditis, and otitis media are head and neck manifestations frequently present with multifocal involvement.

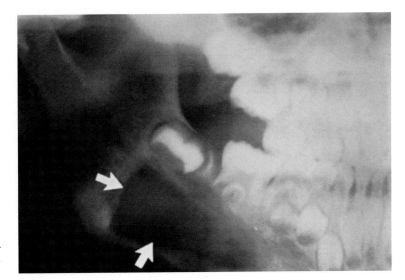

Figure 12–17. Langerhans cell disease of the mandible *(arrows).* (Courtesy of Dr. J. Hayward.)

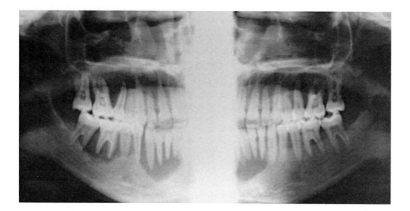

Figure 12–18. Langerhans cell disease of the mandible causing floating-teeth appearance.

Histopathology. The disorder is characterized by the proliferation of large cells with abundant cytoplasm, indistinct cell borders, and oval to reniform nuclei. These cells are most often arranged in sheets and may be admixed with various numbers of eosinophils and other inflammatory cells (Fig. 12–19). A second population of mononuclear phagocytes is frequently evident. These cells exhibit foamy, vacuolated cytoplasm in some cases. Multinucleated giant cells and foci of necrosis may be noted.

Electron microscopic study of the proliferative cells is significant because of the presence of rod-shaped cytoplasmic structures (Figs. 12–20 and 12–21). These Birbeck granules, normally present in Langerhans cells, are lamellated and exhibit central, periodic striations.

Immunohistochemical studies of tumor cells also support an origin from Langerhans cells. Phenotypic expression of CD1a antigens, S-100 protein, and HLA-DR antigens is shared by both normal cells and tumor cells. Identification of these and other specific antigenic markers along with the ultrastructural granules can provide useful diagnostic information.

Differential Diagnosis. Classic presentation of Langerhans cell disease in the jaws often results in loosening or premature exfoliation of teeth and precocious eruption of permanent teeth. Under these conditions, differential diagnosis must in-

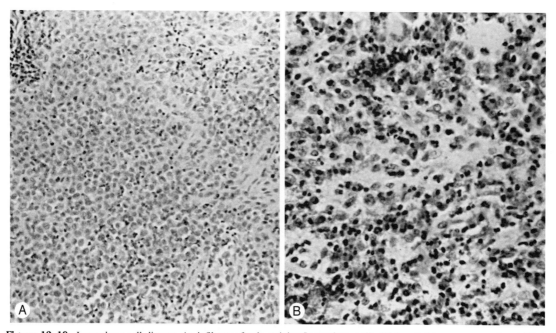

Figure 12–19. Langerhans cell disease. An infiltrate of pale-staining Langerhans cells *(A)* is noted in one zone and an infiltrate of Langerhans cells and eosinophils in another *(B)*.

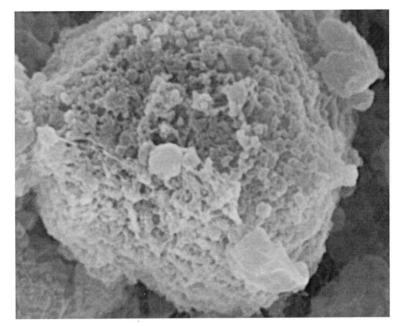

Figure 12–20. Scanning electron micrograph of Langerhans cell of Langerhans cell disease. Note the highly irregular cell surface.

clude juvenile or diabetic periodontitis, hypophosphatasia, leukemia, cyclic neutropenia, agranulocytosis, and primary or metastatic malignant neoplasms. Lesions located in a periapical site may be confused with inflammatory periapical lesions of pulpal origin. The presence of vital pulp in the involved tooth excludes the possibility of periapical granuloma or cyst.

Solitary radiolucent lesions in the central aspects of the jaws should be differentiated from odontogenic tumors and cysts. Numerous well-circumscribed radiolucencies may suggest multi-

ple myeloma, although this occurs in a much older age group. Histologic examination of tissue removed for biopsy generally serves to distinguish this disorder from the other entities listed. Disseminated disease also produces the signs and symptoms mentioned previously.

Treatment and Prognosis. The acute disseminated form commonly occurs during the first years of life and pursues a rapidly progressive course. The primary method of treatment involves use of several chemotherapeutic agents. The disease may be fatal despite intensive treatment. Pa-

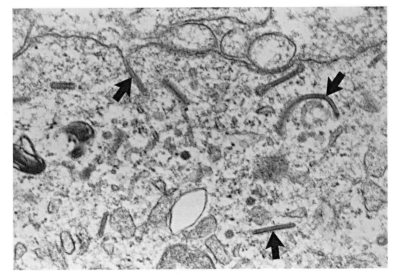

Figure 12–21. Transmission electron micrograph of Langerhans cell of Langerhans cell disease. Note the intracytoplasmic Langerhans cell granules *(arrows)*. Surface membrane (top) shows infoldings where granules presumably originate.

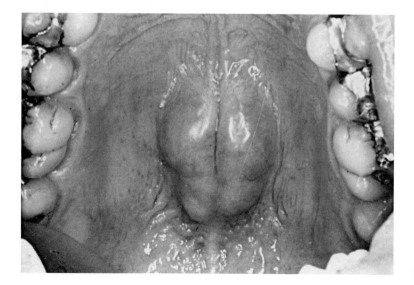

Figure 12–22. Torus palatinus.

tients with a poor prognosis have been treated with some success with allogeneic bone marrow transplantation.

Disseminated visceral and bone involvement in somewhat older children often behaves in a more chronic fashion. Individual lesions may be effectively managed with surgical curettage or low-dose radiation therapy. Cytotoxic agents such as vincristine sulfate, cyclophosphamide, and methotrexate often with systemic corticosteroids may be used for widespread or visceral involvement. The prognosis in this form of the disease is more optimistic, with half the patients surviving for 10 to 15 years.

The localized form of Langerhans cell disease occurs in older children, adolescents, and young adults. These lesions may be treated successfully with vigorous surgical curettage. Intralesional corticosteroid injections have also been used. Low-dose radiotherapy is used for lesions that are inaccessible to surgical treatment. Spontaneous regression of restricted disease has been reported. Therefore, treatment in some cases may be unnecessary. Involved teeth are generally sacrificed at the time of surgical therapy owing to the absence of bony support. The prognosis for this form of the disorder is good. These patients must be evaluated for additional bone or visceral involvement, which is usually manifested within the first 6 months after detection of the original lesion. Long-term follow-up is necessary to rule out the possibility of recurrent disease.

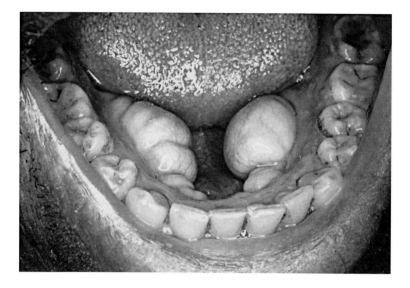

Figure 12–23. Torus mandibularis.

TORI AND EXOSTOSES

Tori and exostoses are nodular protuberances of mature bone; their precise designation depends on anatomic location. These lesions are of little clinical significance. They are nonneoplastic and rarely are a source of discomfort. The mucosa surfacing these lesions occasionally may be traumatically ulcerated, producing a slow-healing, painful wound or, less commonly, osteomyelitis. Surgical removal for the purpose of prosthetic rehabilitation may be necessary.

Etiology and Pathogenesis. The precise cause of these lesions remains obscure, although evidence has been presented to suggest that the torus may be an inherited condition. A simple dominant pattern of inheritance has been identified for palatal tori in a study of Venezuelan and Japanese populations. One investigator has indicated that both genetic and environmental factors determine the development of mandibular tori. The palatal torus is relatively prevalent in certain populations such as Asians, Native Americans, and Eskimos. The incidence in the general population of the United States is between 20 and 25%.

Mandibular tori are seen more commonly in certain groups such as blacks and some Asian populations. The overall incidence in the United States is estimated to be between 6 and 12%. The presence of mandibular tori was studied in patients with migraine headaches and temporomandibular disorders. A positive association suggested a possible role of parafunctional habits in the etiology of this condition.

The cause of exostoses is unknown. It has been suggested that the bony growths represent a reaction to increased or abnormal occlusal stresses of the teeth in the involved areas.

Clinical Features

Torus Palatinus. The palatal torus is a sessile, nodular mass of bone that presents along the midline of the hard palate (Fig. 12–22). This lesion occurs in females twice as often as it does in males in some populations. The palatal torus usually appears during the second or third decade of life, although it may be noted at any age. The bony mass exhibits slow growth and is generally asymptomatic. These lesions are frequently present in a symmetric fashion along the midline of the hard palate. Tori have been noted to form various configurations such as nodular, spindled, lobular, or flat. Large tori may be evident on radiographs as diffuse radiopaque lesions.

Torus Mandibularis. Mandibular tori are bony exophytic growths that present along the lingual aspect of the mandible superior to the mylohyoid ridge (Fig. 12–23). These tori are almost always bilateral, occurring in the premolar region. Infrequently, a torus may be noted on one side only. These lesions are asymptomatic, exhibiting slow growth during the second and third decades of life.

Mandibular tori may arise as solitary nodules or as multiple nodular masses that appear to coalesce. A significant gender predilection is not evident.

Exostoses. Exostoses are multiple (or single) bony excrescences that occur less commonly than do tori (Figs. 12–24 and 12–25). They are asymptomatic bony nodules that are present along the

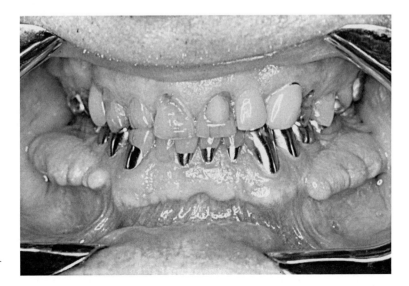

Figure 12–24. Mandibular exostoses.

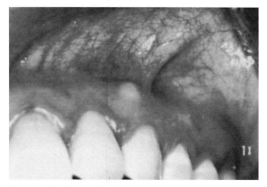

Figure 12–25. Maxillary exostosis.

buccal aspect of alveolar bone. Lesions are noted most frequently in the posterior portions of both the maxilla and the mandible. Exostoses have been reported as rare occurrences following skin graft vestibuloplasty gingival grafts, as well as beneath the pontic of a fixed bridge.

Histopathology. These lesions are composed of hyperplastic bone consisting of mature cortical and trabecular bone. The outer surface exhibits a smooth, rounded contour.

Treatment and Prognosis. Treatment of tori and exostoses is unnecessary, unless required for prosthetic considerations or in cases of frequent trauma to the overlying mucosa. Recurrence after surgical excision is only rarely seen.

CORONOID HYPERPLASIA

Hyperplasia of the coronoid processes of the mandible is an uncommon condition that is frequently associated with limitation of mandibular motion.

Etiology and Pathogenesis. The cause of this process remains unknown. A history of trauma is present in many instances; however, the precise relationship between the traumatic episode and the onset of coronoid enlargement has been difficult to establish. The coronoid enlargement appears to represent a hyperplastic process, although it has been suggested that the lesion may be neoplastic. Unilateral coronoid hyperplasia may be the result of a solitary osteochondroma; bilateral coronoid hyperplasia is apparently the result of a different process. The majority of cases have been reported in males, leading some investigators to suggest an X-linked inherited etiology. Subsequent cases have been reported in females, a finding that seems to preclude this possibility. Increased activity of the temporalis muscle with unbalanced condylar support has also been postulated as an etiologic factor.

Clinical Features. Hyperplasia of the coronoid processes is frequently bilateral, although unilateral enlargement has been noted. Bilateral coronoid hyperplasia typically results in limitation of mandibular movement, which is progressive over time.

The disorder is usually painless and, with a few exceptions, is not associated with facial swelling or asymmetry. Coronoid hyperplasia has been reported most frequently in young male patients. The age of onset is typically around puberty, although presentation for evaluation may be delayed for many years. Some cases have been noted, especially in females, before puberty and during adult life.

Enlarged and elongated coronoid processes are evident radiographically, although the general shape of the processes is usually normal. Unilateral coronoid hyperplasia often results in misshapen or mushroom-shaped coronoid processes on radiographs. Temporomandibular joint radiographs are unremarkable.

Histopathology. The enlarged coronoid processes consist of mature, hyperplastic bone. The bone may be partially covered by cartilaginous and fibrous connective tissue.

Differential Diagnosis. Bilateral coronoid hyperplasia rarely presents diagnostic difficulties. However, cases of unilateral coronoid hyperplasia must be differentiated from osseous and chondroid neoplasms.

Treatment and Prognosis. Treatment consists of surgical excision of the hyperplastic coronoid processes. Postoperative physiotherapy is also advocated. Long-term functional improvement has been variably successful as measured by an increase in mouth opening after surgical intervention. Recurrence has been rarely reported.

Bibliography

Auclair PL, Cuenin P, Kratochvil FJ, et al. A clinical and histomorphologic comparison of the central giant cell granuloma and the giant cell tumor. Oral Surg Oral Med Oral Pathol 66:197–208, 1988.

Barbujani G, Rolo M, Barrai I, Pinto-Cisternas J. Torus palatinus: a segregation analysis. Hum Hered 36:317–325, 1986.

Barnes L. Surgical Pathology of the Head and Neck. New York, Marcel Dekker, 1985, Chap 17.

Bridge JA. Cytogenetics and experimental models. Curr Opin Oncol 8:284–288, 1996.

Bunel K, Sindet-Pedersen S. Central hemangioma of the mandible. Oral Surg Oral Med Oral Pathol 75:565–570, 1993.

Candelere GA, Glorieux FH, Prud'homme J, St Arnaud R. Increased expression of the C-fos proto-oncogene in bone from patients with fibrous dysplasia. N Eng J Med 332:1546–1551, 1995.

Carl W, Sullivan MA. Dental abnormalities and bone lesions associated with familial adenomatous polyposis: report of cases. J Am Dent Assoc 119:137–139, 1989.

Chuong R, Kaban LB, Kozakewich H, Perez-Atayde A. Central giant cell lesions of the jaws: a clinicopathologic study. J Oral Maxillofac Surg 44:708–713, 1986.

Cleveland DB, Goldberg KM, Greenspan JS, et al. Langerhans cell histiocytosis: report of three cases with unusual oral soft tissue involvement. Oral Surg Oral Med Oral Pathol Oral Radiol Endod 82:541–548, 1996.

Clifford T, Lamey PJ, Fartash L. Mandibular tori, migraine and temporomandibular disorders. Br Dent J 180:382–384, 1996.

Consolini R, Cini P, Cei B, Bottone E. Thymic dysfunction in histiocytosis X. Am J Pediatr Hematol Oncol 9:146–148, 1987.

DiNardo LJ, Wetmore RF. Head and neck manifestations of histiocytosis-X in children. Laryngoscope 99:721–724, 1989.

Egeler RM, D'Angio GJ. Langerhans cell histiocytosis. J Pediatr 127:1–11, 1995.

Eggen S. Torus mandibularis: an estimation of the degree of genetic determination. Acta Odontol Scand 47:409–415, 1989.

Eisenbud L, Stern M, Rothberg M, Sachs SA. Central giant cell granuloma of the jaws: experiences in the management of 37 cases. J Oral Maxillofac Surg 46:376–384, 1988.

Engel JD, Supancic JS, Davis LF. Arteriovenous malformation of the mandible: life-threatening complications during tooth extraction. J Am Dent Assoc 126:237–242, 1995.

Eversole LR, Leider AS, Nelson K. Ossifying fibroma: a clinicopathologic study of 64 cases. Oral Surg Oral Med Oral Pathol 60:505–511, 1985.

Flanagan AM, Nui B, Tinkler SM, et al. The multinucleate cells in giant cell granulomas of the jaw are osteoclasts. Cancer 62:1139–1145, 1988.

Greer RO, Berman DN. Osteoblastoma of the jaws. Current concepts and differential diagnosis. J Oral Maxillofac Surg 36:304, 1978.

Harris M. Central giant cell granulomas of the jaws regress with calcitonin therapy. Br J Oral Maxillofac Surg 31:89–94, 1993.

Haug RH, Hauer C, DeCamillo AJ, Arenta M. Benign osteoblastoma of the mandible: report of a case. J Oral Maxillofac Surg 48:743–748, 1990.

Hegtvedt AK, Terry BC, Burkes EJ, Patty SR. Skin graft vestibuloplasty exostosis. A report of two cases. Oral Surg Oral Med Oral Pathol 69:149–152, 1990.

Hopkins KM, Huttula CS, Kahn MA, Albright JE. Desmoplastic fibroma of the mandible: review and report of two cases. J Oral Maxillofac Surg 54:1249–1254, 1996.

Huvos AG. Bone Tumors: Diagnosis, Treatment, and Prognosis. Philadelphia, WB Saunders, 1979.

Kaplan FS, Fallon MD, Boden SD, et al. Estrogen receptors in bone in a patient with polyostotic fibrous dysplasia (McCune-Albright syndrome). N Engl J Med 319:421–425, 1988.

Kaplan I, Calderon S, Buchner A. Peripheral osteoma of the mandible: a study of 10 new cases and analysis of the literature. J Oral Maxillofac Surg 52:467–470, 1994.

Kreutz RW, Sanders B. Bilateral coronoid hyperplasia resulting in severe limitation of mandibular movement. Report of a case. Oral Surg Oral Med Oral Pathol 60:482–484, 1985.

Krutchkoff DJ, Jones CR. Multifocal eosinophilic granuloma: a clinical pathologic conference. J Oral Pathol 13:472–488, 1984.

Lucas DR, Unni KK, McLeod RA, et al. Osteoblastoma: clinicopathologic study of 306 cases. Hum Pathol 25:117–134, 1994.

Marie PJ, dePollak C, Chanson P, Lomri A. Increased proliferation of osteoblastic cells expressing the activating Gs alpha mutation in monostotic and polyostotic fibrous dysplasia. Am J Pathology 150:1059–1069, 1997.

Marra LM. Bilateral coronoid hyperplasia, a developmental defect. Oral Surg Oral Med Oral Pathol 55:10–13, 1983.

Mascarello JT, Krous HF, Carpenter PM. Unbalanced translocation resulting in the loss of the chromosome 17 short arm in an osteoblastoma. Cancer Genet Cytogenet 69:65–67, 1993.

McLoughlin PM, Hopper C, Bowley NB. Hyperplasia of the mandibular coronoid process: an analysis of 31 cases and a review of the literature. J Oral Maxillofac Surg 53:250–255, 1995.

Misaki M, Shima T, Ikoma J, et al. Acromegaly and hyperthyroidism associated with McCune-Albright syndrome. Horm Res 30:26–27, 1988.

Nesbit ME, O'Leary M, Dehner LP, Ramsay NKC. The immune system and the histiocytosis syndromes. Am J Pediatr Hematol Oncol 3:141–149, 1981.

Ohkubo T, Hernandez JC, Ooya K, Krutchkoff DJ. "Aggressive" osteoblastoma of the maxilla. Oral Surg Oral Med Oral Pathol 68:69–73, 1989.

O'Malley M, Pogrel MA, Stewart JCB, et al. Central giant cell granulomas of the jaws: phenotype and proliferation-associated markers. J Oral Pathol Med 26:159–163, 1997.

Petrikowski CG, Pharoah MJ, Lee L, Grace MG. Radiographic differentiation of osteogenic sarcoma, osteomyelitis, and fibrous dysplasia of the jaws. Oral Surg Oral Med Oral Pathol Oral Rad Endod 80:744–750, 1995.

Pogrel MA. The management of lesions of the jaws with liquid nitrogen cryotherapy. J California Dental Assoc 23:54–57, 1995.

Rabkin MS, Wittwer CT, Kjeldsberg CR, Piepkorn MW. Flow-cytometric DNA content of histiocytosis X (Langerhans cell histiocytosis). Am J Pathol 131:283–289, 1988.

Riminucci M, Fisher LW, Shenker A, et al. Fibrous dysplasia of bone in the McCune-Albright syndrome. Am J Pathol 151:1587–1600, 1997.

Sciubba JJ, Younai F. Ossifying fibroma of the mandible and maxilla: review of 18 cases. J Oral Pathol Med 18:315–321, 1989.

Seah YH. Torus palatinus and torus mandibularis: a review of the literature. Aust Dent J 40:318–321, 1995.

Shapeero LG, Vanel D, Ackerman LV, et al. Aggressive fibrous dysplasia of the maxillary sinus. Skeletal Radiol 22:563–568, 1993.

Shatz A, Calderon S, Mintz S. Benign osteoblastoma of the mandible. Oral Surg Oral Med Oral Pathol 61:189–191, 1986.

Slootweg PJ, Muller H. Differential diagnosis of fibroosseous lesions. A histological investigation of 30 cases. J Craniomaxillofac Surg 18:210–214, 1990.

Slootweg PJ, Panders AK, Koopmans R, Nikkels PGJ. Juvenile ossifying fibroma. An analysis of 33 cases with emphasis on histopathological aspects. J Oral Pathol Med 23:385–388, 1994.

Smith RA, Hansen LS, Resnick D, Chan W. Comparison of osteoblastoma in gnathic and extragnathic sites. Oral Surg Oral Med Oral Pathol 54:285–298, 1982.

Stewart JCB, Regezi JA, Lloyd RV, McClatchey KD. Immunohistochemical study of idiopathic histiocytosis of the mandible and maxilla. Oral Surg Oral Med Oral Pathol 61:48–53, 1986.

Stoll M, Freund M, Schmid H, et al. Allogeneic bone marrow transplantation for Langerhans cell histiocytosis. Cancer 66:284–288, 1990.

Takeuchi T, Takenoshita Y, Kubo K, Iida M. Natural course of jaw lesions in patients with familial adenomatosis coli (Gardner's syndrome). Int J Oral Maxillofac Surg 22:226–230, 1993.

Terry BC, Jacoway JR. Management of central giant cell lesions: an alternative to surgical therapy. Oral Maxillofac Surg Clin North Am 6:579–600, 1994.

Ueno H, Ariji E, Tanaka T, et al. Imaging features of maxillary osteoblastoma and its malignant transformation. Skeletal Radiol 23:509–512, 1994.

Waldron CA. Fibro-osseous lesions of the jaws. J Oral Maxillofac Surg 43:249–262, 1985.

Waldron CA. Fibro-osseous lesions of the jaws. J Oral Maxillofac Surg 51:828–835, 1993.

Whitaker SB, Waldron CA. Central giant cell lesions of the jaws: a clinical, radiologic, and histopathologic study. Oral Surg Oral Med Oral Pathol 75:199–208, 1993.

Willman CL, Busque L, Griffith BB, et al. Langerhans'-cell histiocytosis (Histiocytosis X)—a clonal proliferative disease. N Engl J Med 331:154–160, 1994.

Wold LE, Pritchard DJ, Bergert J, Wilson DM. Prostaglandin synthesis by osteoid osteoma and osteoblastoma. Mod Pathol 1:129–131, 1988.

Worth HM, Stoneman DW. Radiology of vascular abnormalities in and about the jaws. Dent Radiogr Photogr 52:1–23, 1979.

Yih WY, Ma GS, Merrill RG, Sperry DW. Central hemangioma of the jaws. J Oral Maxillofac Surg 47:1154–1160, 1989.

Yih WY, Pederson GT, Bartley MH. Multiple ossifying fibromas: relationship to other osseous lesions of the jaws. Oral Surg Oral Med Oral Pathol 68:754–758, 1989.

13

Inflammatory Jaw Lesions

PULPITIS
PERIAPICAL ABSCESS
ACUTE OSTEOMYELITIS
CHRONIC OSTEOMYELITIS (OSTEITIS)
Garré's Osteomyelitis
Diffuse Sclerosing Osteomyelitis
Focal Sclerosing Osteomyelitis
    (Osteitis)

Osteomyelitis, by definition, is inflammation, not necessarily infection (microorganisms), of bone and bone marrow. The term *osteitis* may be substituted for *osteomyelitis* to indicate inflammation of bone. This term may, in fact, be more desirable, as osteomyelitis sometimes conjures up the picture of suppurative infection when that is usually not the intent. In the mandible and maxilla, most cases are related to a microbiologic (usually bacterial) infection that reaches the bone through nonvital teeth, periodontal lesions, or traumatic injuries. This, coupled with the patient's resistance factors, determines the clinical presentation, extent of the inflammatory process, and speed with which the infection develops. The recognized subtypes of osteomyelitis are closely related and essentially represent differences in etiologic agent and host response. The primary justification for separation of osteomyelitis into the various subtypes lies in the differences in treatment and prognosis for each. It is also important to be aware of clinical and radiographic presentations in making differential diagnoses of bone lesions.

PULPITIS

All the principles of inflammation that apply to any other body organ apply to lesions of the dental pulp. In addition, dental pulp has some unique features that make it unusually fragile and sensitive. First, it is encased by hard tissue (dentin/enamel) that does not allow for the usual swelling associated with the exudate of the acute inflammatory process. Second, there is no collateral circulation to maintain vitality when the primary blood supply is compromised. Third, biopsy and direct application of medications are impossible

without causing necrosis of the entire organ. Fourth, pain is the only sign that can be used to determine the severity of pulpal inflammation.

Because of referred pain, localizing the problem to the correct tooth can often be a considerable diagnostic challenge. Also of significance is the difficulty in relating clinical status of a tooth to histopathology. Unfortunately, no reliable symptoms or tests consistently correlate the two. The level of pulpal inflammation is determined through a combination of clinical criteria. Results of electric, heat, cold, and percussion tests must be added to patient history, clinical examination, and operator experience to arrive at the most appropriate diagnosis for the correct tooth. Generally, the more intense the pain and the longer the duration of symptoms, the greater the damage to the pulp. Severe symptoms usually indicate irreversible damage.

Etiology. In the dental pulp, inflammation is the response to injury, just as it is in any other organ. Additionally, the pulp response includes stimulation of odontoblasts to deposit reparative dentin at the site to help protect the pulp. If the injury is severe, the result is, instead, necrosis of these cells.

Caries is the most frequent form of injury that causes pulpitis. The degree of damage depends on the rapidity and extent of hard tissue destruction. Entry of bacteria into the pulpal tissue through a carious lesion is not necessary for pulpitis to occur, but this appears to be an important factor in the intensification of the inflammatory response. Pulpal microbiology adjacent to carious dentin demonstrates a diverse flora, including gram-positive anaerobes and *Bacteroides* species with low numbers of lactobacilli. Operative dental procedures in cavity and crown preparation may also trigger an inflammatory response in the dental pulp. The heat, friction, chemicals, and filling materials associated with restoration of teeth all are potential irritants. It is well known that less damage is done when a water spray is used during tooth preparation than when no water is used. It is also well established that an insulating base can provide significant protection of the pulp from irritating chemicals used with nonmetallic restorative materials and from heat transferred through large metallic fillings.

381

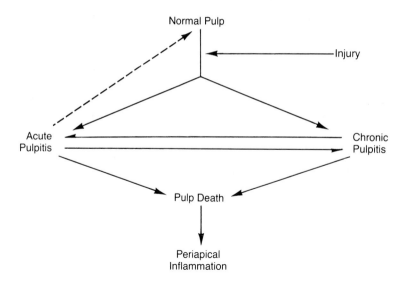

Figure 13–1. Pulpitis pathways.

Other types of injury that may trigger pulpitis are trauma, especially when it is severe enough to cause root or crown fracture, and periodontal disease that has extended to an apical or lateral root foramen.

Clinical and Histopathologic Features. Several detailed classifications of pulpitis that are based on histopathologic changes have been proposed. Because of the difficulty in correlating clinical features with microscopy, these schemes have proved to be of little practical value. Instead, most practitioners prefer a simple classification that is helpful in the clinical setting relative to treatment and prognosis (Fig. 13–1).

Focal Reversible Pulpitis. This acute, mild inflammatory pulpal reaction typically follows carious destruction of a tooth or placement of a large metallic filling. It causes teeth to be hypersensitive to thermal and electric stimuli (Table 13–1). The pain is mild to moderate and is typically intermittent. As the name implies, the changes are focal (subjacent to the injurious agent) and reversible if the cause is removed. Microscopically, the predominant feature is dilatation and engorgement of blood vessels (hyperemia). Exudation of plasma proteins also occurs, but this is difficult to appreciate in microscopic sections.

Acute Pulpitis. This inflammatory response may occur as a progression of focal reversible pulpitis, or it may represent an acute exacerbation of an already established chronic pulpitis. Pulpal damage may range in severity from simple acute inflammation marked by vessel dilatation, exudation, and neutrophil chemotaxis to focal liquefac-

Table 13–1. Features of Pulpitis and Periapical Disease

	PAIN	THERMAL/ ELECTRIC	RADIO- GRAPHS	MICROSCOPY	TREATMENT
Focal reversible pulpitis	Mild	Normal response	No PA change	Hyperemia	Remove irritant
Acute pulpitis	Constant, severe	Hyper to none	No PA change	PMNs, necrosis, exudation	RCT/extract
Chronic pulpitis	Mild, intermittent	Reduced response	No PA change	Lymphocytes, fibrosis	Remove irritant, obstruction, RCT/extract
Hyperplastic pulpitis	None	No response	No PA change	Granulation tissue	Extract/heroic RCT
Periapical abscess	Severe, pain on percussion	No response, necrotic pulp	Usually no PA change	Liquefaction of PA tissue, pus	RCT/extract
Periapical granuloma	None to slight	No response, necrotic pulp	Lucency	Granulation tissue, inflammatory cells	RCT/extract
Periapical cyst	None to slight	No response, necrotic pulp	Lucency	Epithelium-lined connective tissue	Cystectomy, RCT/extract

PA = periapical; RCT = root canal therapy; PMNs = polymorphonuclear neutrophils.

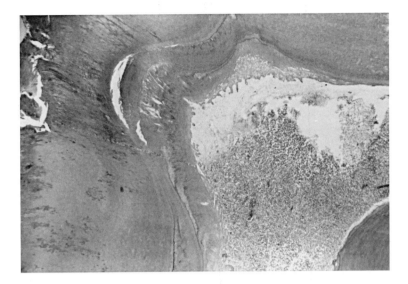

Figure 13–2. Abscess of the coronal pulp showing liquefaction and acute inflammatory cell infiltrate. Note the carious lesion and reparative dentin (left).

tion necrosis (pulp abscess) (Fig. 13–2) to total pulpal suppurative necrosis. Constant, severe tooth-associated pain is the usual presenting complaint. Pain is intensified with the application of heat or cold, although in cases in which liquefaction of the pulp has occurred, cold may, in fact, alleviate the symptoms. If there is an opening from the pulp to the oral environment, symptoms may be lessened because of the escape of the exudate that causes pressure on and chemical irritation of the pulpal and periapical nerve tissues.

In the early phases of acute pulpitis, the tooth may be hyperreactive to electric stimulation, but as pulp damage increases, sensitivity is reduced until there is no response. Because the exudate is confined primarily to the pulp rather than the periapical tissues, percussion tests generally elicit a response little different from normal.

Chronic Pulpitis. Chronic pulpitis is an inflammatory reaction that results from long-term, low-grade injury or occasionally from quiescence of an acute process. Symptoms, characteristically mild and often intermittent, appear over an extended period. A dull ache may be the presenting complaint, or the patient may have no symptoms at all. As the pulp deteriorates, responses to thermal and electric stimulation are reduced. Microscopically, lymphocytes, plasma cells, and fibrosis appear in the chronically inflamed pulp. Unless there is an acute exacerbation of the chronic process, neutrophils are not evident.

Chronic Hyperplastic Pulpitis. This special form of chronic pulpitis occurs in molar teeth (both primary and secondary) of children and young adults (Fig. 13–3). The involved teeth exhibit large carious lesions that open into the coro-

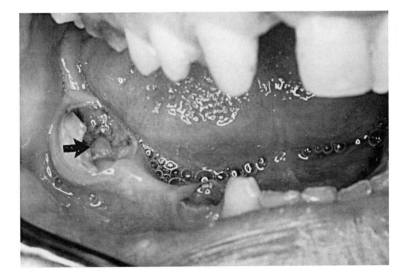

Figure 13–3. Hyperplastic pulpitis of a first permanent molar *(arrow).*

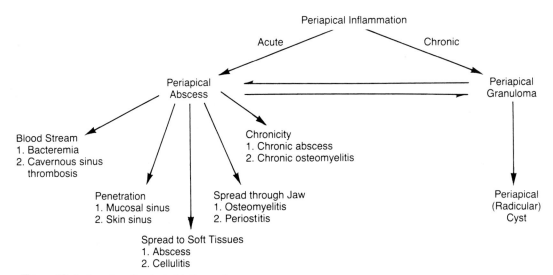

Figure 13–4. Sequelae of periapical inflammation.

nal pulp chamber. Rather than undergoing necrosis, the pulp tissue reacts in a hyperplastic manner, producing a red mass of reparative granulation tissue that extrudes through the pulp exposure. This type of reaction is believed to be related to the open root foramen, through which a relatively rich blood supply flows.

Symptoms seldom occur because there is no exudate under pressure, and there is generally no nerve tissue proliferating with the granulation tissue. Although the pulp tissue is viable, the process is not reversible and necessitates endodontic therapy or tooth extraction. The well-vascularized granulation tissue mass frequently becomes epithelialized, presumably by autotransplantation of epithelial cells from nearby mucosal surfaces.

Treatment and Prognosis. If the cause is identified and eliminated, focal reversible pulpitis should recede, returning the pulp to a normal state. If the inflammation progresses into an acute pulpitis with neutrophil infiltrates and tissue necrosis, recovery is unlikely regardless of attempts to remove the cause. Endodontic therapy or tooth extraction is the only treatment available at this stage.

With chronic pulpitis, pulpal death is the characteristic end result. Removal of the cause may slow the process or occasionally save the vitality of the pulp. Endodontic therapy or extraction is typically required. Chronic hyperplastic pulpitis is essentially an irreversible end stage that is treated with pulp extirpation and an endodontic filling or extraction.

PERIAPICAL ABSCESS

Etiology. Numerous sequelae may follow untreated pulp necrosis, all of which are dependent on the virulence of the microorganisms involved and the integrity of the patient's overall defense mechanisms (Fig. 13–4). From its origin in the pulp, the inflammatory process extends into the periapical tissues, where it may present as a granuloma or cyst, if chronic, or an abscess, if acute. Acute exacerbation of a chronic lesion may also be seen. The necrotic pulpal tissue debris, inflammatory cells, and bacteria, particularly anaerobes, all serve to stimulate and sustain the periapical inflammatory process.

Clinical Features. Patients with periapical abscesses typically have severe pain in the area of the nonvital tooth because of pressure and the effects of chemical mediators on nerve tissue (Table 13–1). The exudate and neutrophilic infiltrate of an abscess cause pressure on the surrounding tissue, frequently resulting in slight extrusion of the tooth from its socket. Pus associated with a lesion, if not focally constrained, seeks the path of least resistance and spreads into contiguous structures. The affected area of the jaw may be tender to palpation, and the patient may be hypersensitive to tooth percussion. The involved tooth is unresponsive to electric and thermal tests owing to pulp necrosis.

Because of the rapidity with which this lesion develops, there is generally insufficient time for significant amounts of bone resorption to occur. Therefore, radiographic changes are slight, usually limited to mild radiographic thickening of apical periodontal membrane space. However, if the lesion develops as an acute exacerbation of a chronic periapical granuloma, a radiolucent lesion is evident.

Histopathology. Microscopically, this lesion appears as a zone of liquefaction composed of proteinaceous exudate, necrotic tissue, and viable and dead neutrophils (pus). Adjacent tissue containing dilated vessels and a neutrophilic infiltrate surrounds the area of liquefaction necrosis.

The *periapical granuloma* represents the result of chronic inflammation at the apex of a nonvital tooth. It is composed of granulation tissue and scar infiltrated by variable numbers of chronic inflammatory cells (lymphocytes, plasma cells, macrophages) (Fig. 13–5). This lesion is to be distinguished from granulomatous inflammation, which is a distinctive type of chronic inflammation that is characteristic of certain diseases (e.g., tuberculosis, sarcoid, histoplasmosis) and features a predominance of macrophages (histiocytes) and often multinucleated giant cells. An acute flare of a periapical granuloma would show an abundant neutrophilic infiltrate in addition to granulation tissue and chronic inflammatory cells.

Treatment and Prognosis. Treatment of an acute periapical abscess requires observance of the standard principles of management of acute inflammation. Drainage should be established, either through an opening in the tooth itself or through the soft tissue surrounding the jaw if cellulitis has developed. Antibiotics directed against the offending organism are also required. Management must be thoughtful and skilled, because the consequences of delayed or inappropriate treatment can be significant and occasionally life threatening.

Spread of an abscess may be through one of several avenues. It may progress through the buccal cortical bone and gingival soft tissue, establishing a natural drain or sinus tract (Fig. 13–6). The same type of situation may occur in the palate or skin; this depends on the original location of the abscess and the path of least resistance (Fig.

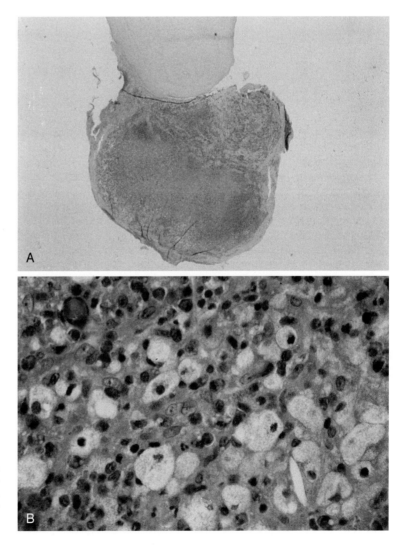

Figure 13–5. *A,* Periapical granuloma attached to a root tip. *B,* High magnification of the infiltrate, illustrating the chronic inflammatory cell infiltrate of lymphocytes, plasma cells, and macrophages (pale cytoplasm).

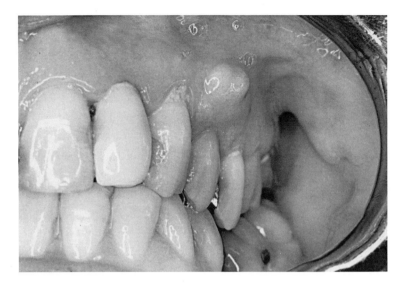

Figure 13–6. Parulis representing pus from the apex of a nonvital bicuspid.

13–7). If a drain is not established, the purulent exudate can cause an abscess (Fig. 13–8) or *cellulitis* (Fig. 13–9) in the soft tissues of the face, oral cavity, or neck. Cellulitis is an acute inflammatory process that is diffusely spread throughout the tissue rather than localized as with an abscess. This variant is the result of infection by virulent organisms that produce enzymes that allow rapid spread through tissue. Cellulitis of the submandibular space has been given the name *Ludwig's angina.*

A dangerous situation occurs when the acute infection involves major blood vessels. This may allow bacteria to enter the bloodstream, resulting in bacteremia. Also, retrograde spread of the infection through facial emissary veins to the cavernous sinus may set up the necessary conditions for thrombus formation. *Cavernous sinus thrombosis* is an emergency situation that is often fatal.

ACUTE OSTEOMYELITIS

Etiology. Acute inflammation of the bone and bone marrow of the mandible and maxilla results most frequently from extension of a periapical abscess. The second most common cause of acute osteomyelitis is physical injury, as occurs with fracture or surgery. Osteomyelitis may also result from bacteremia.

Most cases of acute osteomyelitis are infectious. Almost any organism may be part of the etiologic picture, although staphylococci and streptococci are the most frequently identified.

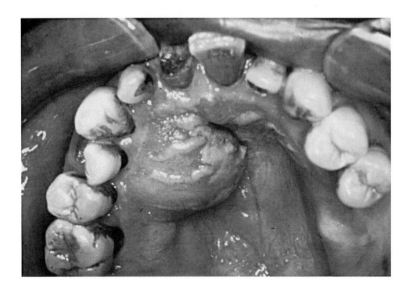

Figure 13–7. Palatal abscess originating from the apex of a nonvital bicuspid.

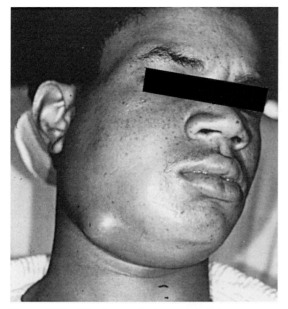

Figure 13–8. Skin abscess of odontogenic origin.

Clinical Features. Pain is the primary feature of this inflammatory process. Pyrexia, painful lymphadenopathy, leukocytosis, and other signs and symptoms of acute infection are also frequently present. Paresthesia of the lower lip occasionally occurs with mandibular involvement. In the development of a clinical differential diagnosis, the presence of this symptom should also suggest malignant mandibular neoplasms.

Unless the inflammatory process has been present for more than 1 week, radiographic evidence of acute osteomyelitis is usually not present. With time, diffuse radiolucent changes begin to appear.

Histopathology. A purulent exudate occupies the marrow spaces in acute osteomyelitis. Bony trabeculae show reduced osteoblastic activity and increased osteoclastic resorption. If an area of bone necrosis occurs (sequestrum), osteocytes are lost and the marrow undergoes liquefaction.

Treatment. Acute osteomyelitis is usually treated with antibiotics and drainage. Ideally, the causative agent is identified, and an appropriate antibiotic is selected through sensitivity testing in the laboratory. Surgery may also be part of the treatment, and it ranges from simple sequestrectomy to excision with autologous bone replacement. Each case should be judged individually because of variations in disease severity, organisms involved, and a patient's overall health.

CHRONIC OSTEOMYELITIS (OSTEITIS)

Etiology. Chronic osteomyelitis may be one of the sequelae of acute osteomyelitis (either untreated or inadequately treated), or it may represent a long-term, low-grade inflammatory reaction that never went through a significant or clinically noticeable acute phase. In either event, acute and chronic osteomyelitis have many similar etiologic factors. Most cases are infectious, and as in most infections, the clinical presentation and course are directly dependent on the virulence of the microorganism involved and the patient's resistance. Ana-

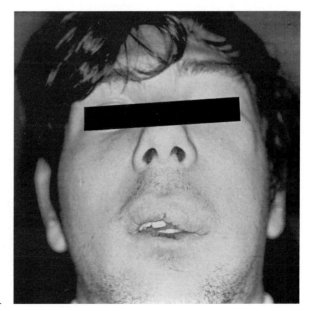

Figure 13–9. Cellulitis of odontogenic origin.

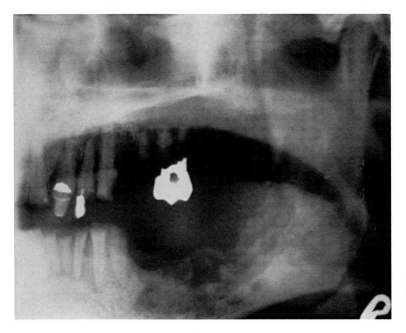

Figure 13–10. Chronic osteomyelitis in the mandible of a patient irradiated for oral cancer. Note the cervical caries.

tomic location, immunologic status, nutritional status, patient age, and the presence of preexisting systemic factors such as Paget's disease, osteopetrosis, and sickle cell disease are other factors affecting presentation and course.

Bone irradiated as part of head and neck cancer treatment is particularly susceptible to infection. Because of reduced vascularity and osteocyte destruction, osteoradionecrosis occurs in approximately 20% of patients who have undergone local irradiation (Fig. 13–10). Secondary infection generally follows. Typical precipitating or triggering events include periapical inflammation resulting from nonvital teeth, extractions (Fig. 13–11), periodontal disease, and fractures communicating with skin or mucosa.

Identification of a specific infectious agent involved in chronic osteomyelitis is usually difficult both microscopically and microbiologically. Sample error is significant either because of small, difficult-to-reach bacterial foci or because of contamination of the lesion by resident flora. Previously taken antibiotics also reduce the chances of culturing the causative organism. Although an etiologic agent is often not confirmed, most investigators believe that bacteria (e.g., staphylococci,

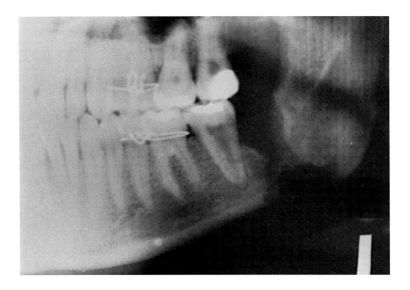

Figure 13–11. Chronic osteomyelitis at the site of a third molar extraction.

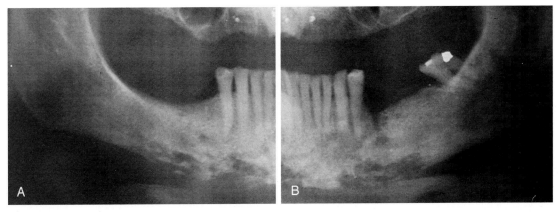

Figure 13–12. *A* and *B,* Chronic osteomyelitis.

streptococci, bacteroides, actinomyces) are responsible for the vast majority of chronic osteomyelitis cases.

Clinical Features. The mandible, especially the molar area, is much more frequently affected than is the maxilla. Pain is usually present but varies in intensity, and it is not necessarily related to the extent of the disease. Duration of symptoms is generally proportional to disease extension. Swelling of the jaw is a commonly encountered sign; loose teeth and sinus tracts are less frequently seen. Anesthesia is very uncommon.

Radiographically, chronic osteomyelitis appears primarily as a radiolucent lesion that may show focal zones of opacification. The lucent pattern is often described as moth-eaten because of its mottled radiographic appearance (Fig. 13–12). Lesions may be very extensive, and margins are often indistinct.

Histopathology. The inflammatory reaction in chronic osteomyelitis can vary from very mild to intense. In mild cases, microscopic diagnosis can be difficult because of similarities to fibro-osseous lesions such as ossifying fibroma and fibrous dysplasia (Fig. 13–13). Few chronic inflammatory cells (lymphocytes and plasma cells) are seen in a fibrous marrow (Fig. 13–14). Both osteoblastic and osteoclastic activity may be seen, along with irregular bony trabeculae—unlikely features of fibro-osseous lesions. In advanced chronic osteomyelitis, necrotic bone (sequestrum) may be present, as evidenced by both necrotic marrow and osteocytes (Fig. 13–15). Reversal lines reflect the waves of deposition and resorption of bone. Inflammatory cells are more numerous and osteoclastic activity more prominent than in mild cases.

Treatment. The basic treatment of chronic osteomyelitis centers around the selection of appropriate antibiotics and the proper timing of surgical intervention. Culture and sensitivity testing should

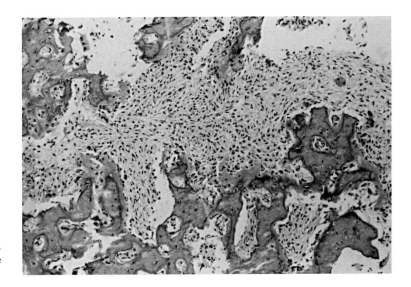

Figure 13–13. Chronic osteomyelitis showing irregular trabeculae and fibrous marrow.

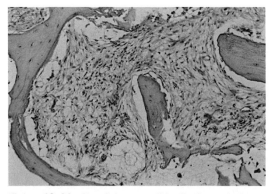

Figure 13–14. Chronic osteomyelitis showing typical scant chronic inflammatory cell infiltrate.

be carried out. Combinations of antibiotics may, on occasion, be more successful than single agents. Duration of antibiotic administration may also be relatively extended.

When a sequestrum occurs, surgery appears to hasten the healing process. Excision of other non-vital bone, sinus tracts, and scar has also been advocated. In cases in which pathologic fracture is a significant potential, immobilization is required.

In recalcitrant cases of chronic osteomyelitis and osteoradionecrosis, the use of *hyperbaric oxygen* has provided significant benefit for patients. In difficult cases, hyperbaric oxygen used in conjunction with antibiotics or surgery appears to be generally better than any of these methods used alone. The rationale for using hyperbaric oxygen is related to its stimulation of vascular proliferation, collagen synthesis, and osteogenesis. Contraindications include presence of viral infections,

optic neuritis, known residual or recurrent malignancies, and some lung diseases. The regimen typically used for this treatment adjunct involves placing a patient in a closed chamber with 100% oxygen at 2 atmospheres of pressure for 2 hours per day for several weeks. The elevated tissue oxygen levels achieved with this technique reach a limited maximum level by the end of therapy, but the effects appear to be long lasting.

Garré's Osteomyelitis

Etiology. Garré's osteomyelitis, or chronic osteomyelitis with proliferative periostitis, is essentially a subtype of chronic osteomyelitis that has a prominent periosteal inflammatory reaction as an additional component. It most often results from a periapical abscess of a mandibular molar. It has also followed infection associated with tooth extraction or partially erupted molars.

Clinical Features. This variety of osteomyelitis is uncommonly encountered. It has been described in the tibia, and in the head and neck, it is seen in the mandible. It typically involves the posterior mandible and is usually unilateral. Patients characteristically present with an asymptomatic bony hard swelling with normal-appearing overlying skin and mucosa (Fig. 13–16). On occasion, slight tenderness may be noted. This presentation necessitates the differentiation of this process from benign mandibular neoplasms. Radiographs and biopsy provide a definitive diagnosis.

Radiographically, the lesion appears centrally as a mottled, predominantly lucent lesion in a pattern consistent with chronic osteomyelitis (Fig. 13–17).

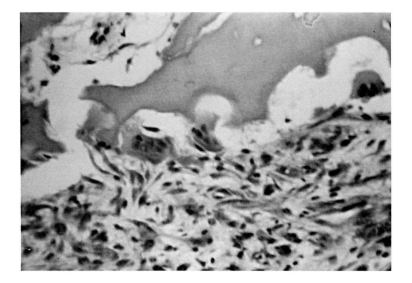

Figure 13–15. Sequestrum showing osteoclastic resorption.

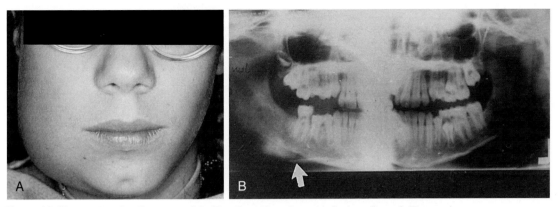

Figure 13–16. *A* and *B,* Garré's osteomyelitis. Note the periosteal reaction in the radiograph *(B, arrow).*

The feature that provides the distinctive difference is the periosteal reaction. This, best viewed on an occlusal radiograph, appears as an expanded cortex, often with concentric or parallel opaque layers (Fig. 13–18). Trabeculae perpendicular to the onion-skin layers may also be apparent.

Histopathology. Reactive new bone typifies the subperiosteal cortical response. Perpendicular orientation of new trabeculae to redundant cortical bone is best seen under low magnification (Fig. 13–19). Osteoblastic activity dominates in this area, and both osteoblastic and osteoclastic activity are seen centrally. Marrow spaces contain fibrous tissue with scattered lymphocytes and plasma cells. Inflammatory cells are often surprisingly scant, making microscopic differentiation from fibro-osseous lesions a diagnostic challenge.

Treatment. Identification and removal of the offending agent is of primary importance in Garré's osteomyelitis. Removal of the involved tooth is usually required. Antibiotics are generally in-

cluded early in this treatment also. The mandible then undergoes gradual remodeling without additional surgical intervention.

Diffuse Sclerosing Osteomyelitis

Etiology. Diffuse sclerosing osteomyelitis represents an inflammatory reaction in the mandible or maxilla, believed to be in response to a microorganism of low virulence. Bacteria are generally suspected as causative agents, although they are seldom specifically identified. Based on histologic changes, it has been suggested that hypersensitivity may be a plausible explanation of the cause. Important in the etiology and progression of diffuse sclerosing osteomyelitis is chronic periodontal disease, which appears to provide a portal of entry for bacteria. Carious nonvital teeth are less frequently implicated.

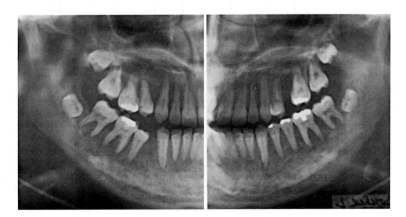

Figure 13–17. Garré's osteomyelitis. Note the mottled mandibular bone and expansion of the periosteum along the inferior border.

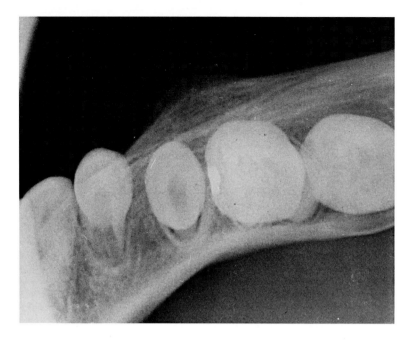

Figure 13–18. Garré's osteomyelitis showing the typical periosteal reaction.

Clinical Features. This condition may affect any age, sex, or race, but it tends to occur most frequently in middle-aged African-American women. The disease is typified by a protracted chronic course with acute exacerbations of pain, swelling, and occasional drainage.

Radiographically, this process is diffuse, typically affecting a large part of the jaw (Fig. 13–20). The lesion is ill defined. Early lucent zones may appear in association with sclerotic masses. In advanced stages, sclerosis dominates the radiographic picture. Periosteal thickening may also be seen. Scintigraphy may be particularly useful in evaluating the extent of this condition.

Histopathology. The microscopic changes of this condition are inflammatory. Fibrous replacement of marrow is noted. A chronic inflammatory cell infiltrate and occasionally a neutrophilic infiltrate are also seen. Bony trabeculae exhibit irregular size and shape and may be lined by numerous osteoblasts. Focal osteoclastic activity is also present. The characteristic sclerotic masses are composed of dense bone (Fig. 13–21), often exhibiting numerous reversal lines.

Differential Diagnosis. Chronic sclerosing osteomyelitis shares many clinical, radiographic, and histologic features with florid osseous dysplasia. The two should be separated, because the former is an infectious process and the latter a bony dysplastic process. Treatment and prognosis therefore are dissimilar. Florid osseous dysplasia appears to be an extensive form of periapical ce-

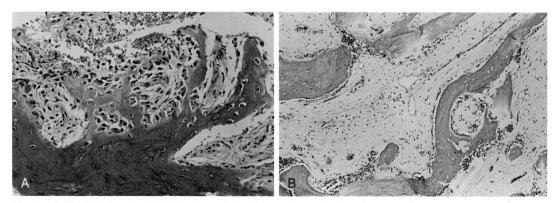

Figure 13–19. Garré's osteomyelitis showing a periosteal reaction *(A)* and fibrotic, mildly inflamed marrow *(B)*.

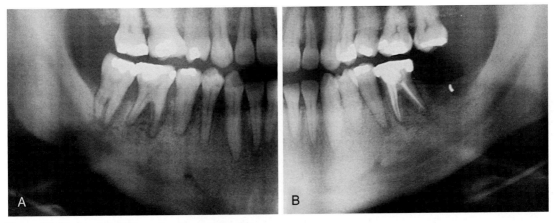

Figure 13-20. *A* and *B,* Diffuse sclerosing osteomyelitis.

mental dysplasia and, unlike diffuse sclerosing osteomyelitis, may exhibit anterior periapical lesions and traumatic or simple bone cysts. Further, florid osseous dysplasia is usually asymptomatic and lacks an inflammatory cell infiltrate.

Treatment. The management of diffuse sclerosing osteomyelitis is problematic because of the relative avascular nature of the affected tissue and because of the large size of the lesion. Even with treatment, the course is protracted.

If an etiologic factor such as periodontal disease or a carious tooth can be identified, it should be eliminated. Antibiotics are the mainstay of treatment and are especially helpful during painful exacerbations. Surgical removal of the diseased area is usually an inappropriate procedure because of the extent of the disease. Decortication of the

affected area has resulted in improvement in some cases. Low-dose corticosteroids have also been used with some success. Hyperbaric oxygen therapy may prove to be a valuable adjunct.

Focal Sclerosing Osteomyelitis (Osteitis)

Etiology. This is a relatively common phenomenon that is believed to represent a focal bony reaction to a low-grade inflammatory stimulus. It is usually seen at the apex of a tooth with long-standing pulpitis. This lesion may occasionally be adjacent to a sound unrestored tooth, suggesting that other etiologic factors such as malocclusion may be operative.

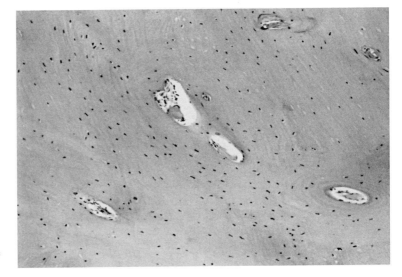

Figure 13-21. Dense sclerotic bone of diffuse sclerosing osteomyelitis.

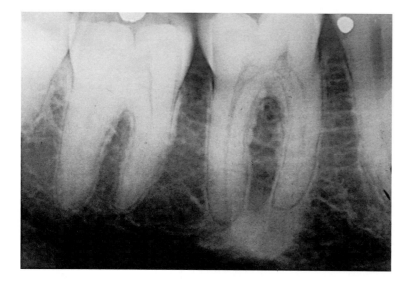

Figure 13–22. Focal sclerosing osteomyelitis, sometimes called *focal periapical osteopetrosis* when associated with normal teeth.

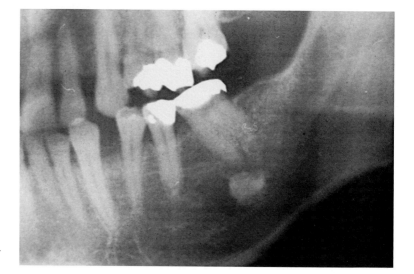

Figure 13–23. Focal sclerosing osteomyelitis.

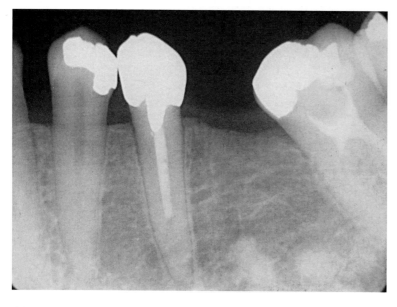

Figure 13–24. Focal sclerosing osteomyelitis.

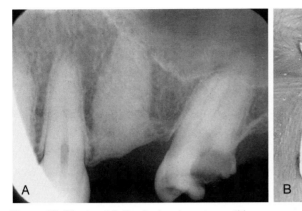

Figure 13–25. *A and B,* Focal sclerosing osteomyelitis.

Synonyms for focal sclerosing osteomyelitis include *bony scar, condensing osteitis,* and *sclerotic bone.* The term *focal periapical osteopetrosis* has also been used to describe the lesions associated with normal caries-free teeth (Fig. 13–22).

Clinical Features. Focal sclerosing osteomyelitis may be found at any age but is typically discovered in young adults. Patients are usually asymptomatic, and most lesions are discovered on routine radiographic examination. A majority are found at the apices of mandibular first molars, with a minority associated with mandibular second molars and premolars (Fig. 13–23). When teeth are extracted, these lesions remain behind indefinitely (Fig. 13–24).

Radiographically, one of several patterns may be seen. The lesion may be uniformly opaque; it may have a peripheral lucency with an opaque center; it may have an opaque periphery with a lucent center; or it may be composed of confluent or lobulated opaque masses.

Histopathology. Microscopically, these lesions are masses of dense sclerotic bone (Fig. 13–25). Connective tissue is scant, as are inflammatory cells.

Differential Diagnosis. Differential diagnosis should include periapical cemental dysplasia, osteoma, complex odontoma, cementoblastoma, osteoblastoma, and hypercementosis. In most cases, however, diagnosis can be made with confidence on the basis of historical and radiographic features.

Treatment. Because it is believed to represent a physiologic bone reaction to a known stimulus, the lesion need not be removed. Biopsy might be contemplated to rule out more significant lesions that received serious consideration in the differential diagnosis. The inflamed pulp that stimulated the focal sclerosing osteomyelitis should be treated. The decision about whether the tooth should be restored, treated endodontically, or extracted should be based on findings in a case-by-case basis.

Bibliography

Brook I, Frazier E, Gher M. Aerobic and anaerobic microbiology of periapical abscess. Oral Microbiol Immunol 6:123–125, 1991.

Cecic P, Hartwell G, Bellizzi R. Cold as a diagnostic aid in cases of irreversible pulpitis. Oral Surg Oral Med Oral Pathol 56:647–650, 1983.

Daramola J. Massive osteomyelitis of the mandible complicating sickle cell disease: report of a case. J Oral Surg 39:144–146, 1981.

Daramola J, Ajagbe H. Chronic osteomyelitis of the mandible in adults: a clinical study of 34 cases. Br J Oral Surg 20:58–62, 1982.

Eisenbud L, Miller J, Roberts I. Garré's proliferative periostitis occurring simultaneously in four quadrants of the jaws. Oral Surg 51:172–178, 1981.

Epstein J, van der Meij E, McKenzie M, et al. Postradiation osteonecrosis of the mandible. Oral Surg Oral Med Oral Pathol 83:657–662, 1997.

Eversole L, Stone C, Strub D. Focal sclerosing osteomyelitis/focal periapical osteopetrosis: radiographic patterns. Oral Surg 58:456–460, 1984.

Fattore L, Strauss R. Hyperbaric oxygen in the treatment of osteoradionecrosis: a review of its use and efficacy. Oral Surg Oral Med Oral Pathol 63:280–286, 1987.

Guernsey L, Clark J. Hyperbaric oxygen therapy with subtotal extirpation surgery in the management of osteonecrosis of the mandible. Int J Oral Surg 10(Suppl 1):168–177, 1981.

Hahn C, Falkler W, Minah G. Microbiological studies of carious dentin from human teeth with irreversible pulpitis. Arch Oral Biol 36:147–153, 1991.

Hyman J, Cohen M. The predictive value of endodontic diagnostic tests. Oral Surg 58:343–346, 1984.

Jacobsson S, Dahlen G, Moller A. Bacteriologic and serologic investigation in diffuse sclerosing osteomyelitis (DSO) of the mandible. Oral Surg 54:506–512, 1982.

Jacobsson S, Hollender L. Treatment and prognosis of diffuse sclerosing osteomyelitis (DSO) of the mandible. Oral Surg 49:7–14, 1980.

Kerley T, Mader J, Hulet W, et al. The effect of adjunctive hyperbaric oxygen on bone regeneration in mandibular osteomyelitis: report of a case. J Oral Surg 39:619–623, 1981.

Kim S. Neurovascular interactions in the dental pulp in health and inflammation. J Endod 16:48–53, 1990.

Lichty G, Langlais R, Aufdemorte T. Garré's osteomyelitis: literature review and case report. Oral Surg 50:310–313, 1980.

Marx RE, Carlson ER, Smith BR, Toraya N. Isolation of actinomyces species and *Eikenella corrodens* from patients with chronic diffuse sclerosing osteomyelitis. J Oral Maxillofac Surg 52:26–33, 1994.

Marx R, Johnson R. Studies in the radiobiology of osteoradionecrosis and their clinical significance. Oral Surg Oral Med Oral Pathol 64:379–390, 1987.

Marx R, Johnson R, Kline S. Prevention of osteoradionecrosis: a randomized prospective clinical trial of hyperbaric oxygen versus penicillin. J Am Dent Assoc 111:49–54, 1985.

Morton M. Osteoradionecrosis: a study of the incidence in the northwest of England. Br J Oral Maxillofac Surg 24:323–331, 1986.

Morton M, Simpson W. The management of osteoradionecrosis of the jaws. Br J Oral Maxillofac Surg 24:332–341, 1986.

Smith B, Eveson J. Paget's disease of bone with particular reference to dentistry. J Oral Pathol 10:233–247, 1981.

Steiner M, Gould A, Means W. Osteomyelitis of the mandible associated with osteopetrosis. J Oral Maxillofac Surg 41:395–405, 1983.

Triplett R, Branham G. Treatment of experimental mandibular osteomyelitis with hyperbaric oxygen and antibiotics. Int J Oral Surg 10(Suppl 1):178–182, 1981.

Wannfors K, Hammarstrom L. Infectious foci in chronic osteomyelitis of the jaws. Int J Oral Surg 14:493–503, 1985.

14

Malignant Nonodontogenic Neoplasms of the Jaws

Richard J. Zarbo

OSTEOSARCOMA
Juxtacortical (Surface) Osteosarcomas
  Parosteal Osteosarcoma
  Periosteal Osteosarcoma
CHONDROSARCOMA
Mesenchymal Chondrosarcoma
EWING'S SARCOMA
BURKITT'S LYMPHOMA
PLASMA CELL NEOPLASMS
Multiple Myeloma
Solitary Plasmacytoma of Bone
METASTATIC CARCINOMA

Malignant nonodontogenic neoplasms of the jaws, both primary and metastatic, are rare compared with tumors arising in the surrounding soft tissues. Despite the infrequent occurrence of these entities, a diagnosis of malignant jaw tumor has serious prognostic implications, often signaling a treatment plan requiring major therapeutic intervention. Tumors to be considered in this chapter are those arising from the hard tissues (osteosarcoma and chondrosarcoma) and those involving the marrow cavity of the mandible and maxilla (Ewing's sarcoma, Burkitt's lymphoma, plasma cell myeloma, and metastatic carcinoma).

OSTEOSARCOMA

Osteosarcomas account for approximately 20% of all sarcomas and, after plasma cell myeloma, are the most common primary bone tumors. Approximately 5% of osteosarcomas occur in the jaws, with an incidence of approximately 1 case in 1.5 million persons per year. Osteosarcomas arise in several clinical settings, including preexisting bone abnormalities such as *Paget's disease, fibrous dysplasia, giant cell tumor, multiple osteochondromas, bone infarct, chronic osteomyelitis,* and *osteogenesis imperfecta.* Some osteosarcomas have also been preceded by radiation therapy to

the affected bone for unrelated or antecedent disease. The vast majority of osteosarcomas involve the tubular long bones, especially those adjacent to the knee. Osteosarcomas can also be classified by site of origin into (1) the conventional type, arising within the medullary cavity; (2) juxtacortical tumors, arising from the periosteal surface; and (3) extraskeletal osteosarcomas, arising in soft tissue.

Clinical Features. Conventional osteosarcomas involving the mandible and maxilla display a predilection for males (62%). Although the peak incidence of osteosarcomas of the skeleton occurs in the second decade, those arising in the jaws present 1 to 2 decades later, with a mean age of 34 years. There is a nearly equal involvement of the maxilla (51%) and the mandible (49%). The majority (60%) of mandibular osteosarcomas arise in the body of the mandible; the remaining sites of predilection include the symphysis, angle of the mandible, ascending ramus, and temporomandibular joint. In the maxilla, there is a nearly equal incidence of tumors involving the alveolar ridge and maxillary antrum, with few affecting the palate.

Osteosarcomas involving the jaws present most commonly with swelling and localized pain. In some cases, there may be loosening and displacement of teeth as well as paresthesia due to involvement of the inferior alveolar nerve. Maxillary tumors display similar clinical symptoms but may cause paresthesia of the infraorbital nerve, epistaxis, nasal obstruction, or eye problems. Skin and mucosal ulceration are usually not a feature of osteosarcoma of the jaws. The average duration of symptoms is 3 to 4 months before diagnosis.

The radiographic appearance of conventional intramedullary osteosarcoma can be quite variable, reflecting the degree of calcification (Fig. 14–1). There appears to be little relationship between the radiographic pattern and the histologic subtype of osteosarcoma. Early osteosarcomas may be characterized by localized widening of the periodontal

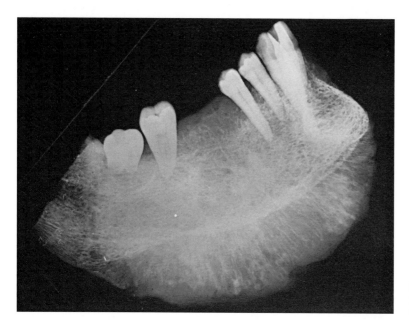

Figure 14–1. Osteosarcoma of the mandible showing radiating spicules of tumor bone in a sunburst pattern.

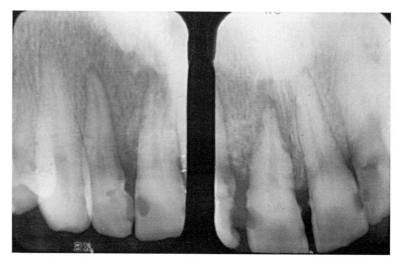

Figure 14–2. Osteosarcoma of the maxilla involving the alveolus of the central and lateral incisors.

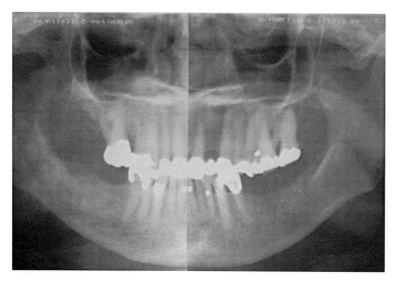

Figure 14–3. Osteosarcoma of the body and ramus of the mandible (left) exhibiting a mottled radiographic pattern.

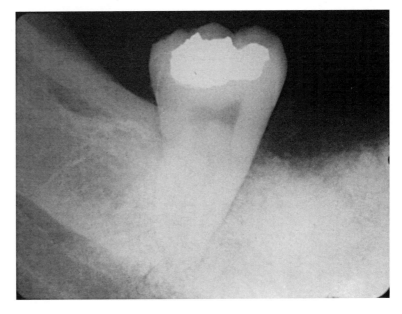

Figure 14–4. Osteosarcoma in an edentulous molar area showing extensive calcified tumor bone.

ligament space of one or two teeth (Fig. 14–2). The widened space results from tumor invasion of the periodontal ligament and resorption of the surrounding alveolar bone. Advanced tumors can be visualized as moth-eaten radiolucencies (Fig. 14–3) or irregular, poorly marginated radiopacities (Fig. 14–4). The majority of these neoplasms have mixed radiographic features. The typical sun-ray or sunburst radiopaque appearance due to periosteal reaction may be seen in jaw lesions but is not diagnostic of osteosarcoma.

Histopathology. Histologically, all osteosarcomas have in common a sarcomatous stroma directly producing tumor osteoid. Variable histologic

patterns dominate and have been designated osteoblastic (Fig. 14–5), chondroblastic (Fig. 14–6), and fibroblastic (Fig. 14–7). An additional variant has been designated telangiectatic—it displays multiple aneurysmal blood-filled spaces lined by malignant cells. This variant rarely occurs in the head and neck region.

Another rare variant with metastatic capability that may be encountered in the jaws histologically resembles osteoblastoma. This osteoblastoma-like osteosarcoma is characterized by permeative rather than circumscribed growth and lack of zonal maturation at the periphery.

Low-grade intra-osseous osteosarcoma is a re-

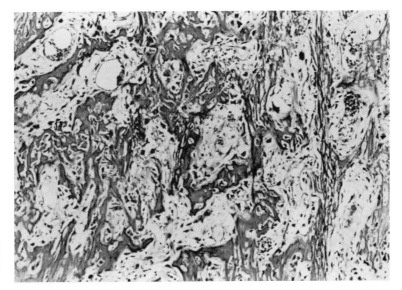

Figure 14–5. Osteoblastic variant of osteosarcoma characterized by an irregular network of calcifying osteoid trabeculae.

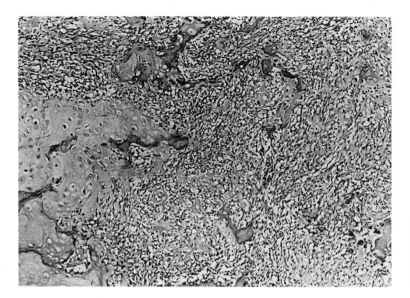

Figure 14–6. Chondroblastic variant of osteosarcoma dominated by neoplastic cartilage but containing diagnostic zones of malignant osteoid production by spindle cell stroma.

cently described variant that may involve the jaws of young patients in their twenties. Histologically, it resembles fibrous dysplasia because of the minimally atypical spindle cell proliferation with occasional mitotic figures and bone spicules. Unlike fibrous dysplasia, the radiographic appearance is that of an invasive intramedullary growth with poor margination and cortical destruction. However, some fibrous dysplasia-like osteosarcomas may exhibit a benign radiographic appearance. Unlike fibrous dysplasia, the proliferation permeates bone marrow, may extend through the periosteum, and may invade soft tissues. Recurrent tumor may histologically appear as a conventional high-grade osteosarcoma in 15% of patients. Recommended treatment is wide excision to avoid local recurrence.

All these histologic variants reflect the multipotentiality of the neoplastic mesenchymal cell in producing osteoid, cartilage, and fibrous tissue. Such histologic subclassification, however, bears no prognostic significance. Although osteoblastic histologic variants predominate in the skeleton, chondroblastic osteosarcomas are the most frequent histologic type (48%) occurring in the jaws. Most osteosarcomas of the mandible tend to be lytic (43%); those in the maxilla are osteoblastic (50%).

Overall, jaw osteosarcomas tend to be better differentiated than those of the skeleton. This dif-

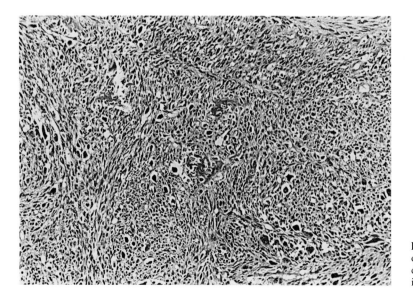

Figure 14–7. Fibroblastic variant of osteosarcoma with a malignant dense spindle cell stroma producing islands of osteoid.

ference appears to correspond to the poorer prognosis associated with osteosarcomas arising outside the jaws.

Differential Diagnosis. The uniform widening of the periodontal ligament space of involved teeth appears to be characteristic for early osteosarcoma. However, this focal radiographic defect may also have been seen with other malignancies surrounding teeth. Uniform widening of periodontal ligament spaces surrounding all teeth is seen in scleroderma. Moth-eaten radiolucencies are common to other malignancies, chronic osteomyelitis, and several benign neoplasms. A sclerotic radiographic appearance may be seen with some metastatic carcinomas and in Pindborg tumor, which is also often associated with an impacted tooth.

The histologic diagnosis hinges on finding the malignant osteoid production. Many jaw osteosarcomas are predominantly chondroblastic, however, and may be misdiagnosed as chondrosarcoma. Osteosarcomas with a predominant fibroblastic component may be misdiagnosed as fibrosarcoma or malignant fibrous histiocytoma of bone. Failure to recognize pathologic features of malignancy in the telangiectatic osteosarcoma has resulted in a misdiagnosis of aneurysmal bone cyst or giant cell tumor.

Treatment and Prognosis. Overall, 5-year survival rates of 25 to 40% are reported for jaw osteosarcomas in various series. Patients with mandibular tumors generally fare better than patients with maxillary tumors. Osteosarcomas are best treated by radical mandibulectomy or maxillectomy, with radiotherapy and chemotherapy for recurrences, soft tissue extension, or metastatic disease. As with most malignant jaw tumors, initial radical surgery results in a superior survival rate of 80% compared with 27% survival for local surgery. Treatment of mandibular osteosarcomas by presurgical insertion of radium needles has resulted in a 76% 5-year survival. Osteosarcomas of the jaws frequently recur (40 to 70%), with a metastatic rate of 25 to 50%. Osteosarcomas rarely metastasize to regional lymph nodes. The most common sites of metastases are lung and brain. Once the disease has become metastatic, the mean survival is 6 months. Nearly 80% of patients dying of the disease do so within the first 2 years. Local recurrences and isolated metastatic deposits are treated by surgical excision and chemotherapy.

Juxtacortical (Surface) Osteosarcomas

In contrast to the central intramedullary osteosarcomas, juxtacortical osteosarcomas arise at the periphery of bone at the periosteal surface, and they display distinct clinical, histologic, and radiographic features as well as a different biologic behavior. Juxtacortical osteosarcomas are uncommon neoplasms that compose approximately 5% of all osteosarcomas of the skeleton; they are rarely seen in the jaws. Most juxtacortical osteosarcomas arising in the jaws are the biologically low-grade parosteal subtype or rarely the periosteal subtype. Also recognized, but not commonly in the jaws, are a high-grade type of surface osteosarcoma and ''dedifferentiated'' parosteal osteosarcoma with an increased risk of local recurrence and metastasis.

PAROSTEAL OSTEOSARCOMA

Parosteal osteosarcoma occurs over a wide age range, with a peak incidence at 39 years. When the long bones are affected, there is a female predominance (3:2), but when the jaws are affected, males predominate. This variant of juxtacortical osteosarcoma most commonly involves the distal femoral metaphysis. The tumor presents as a slow-growing swelling or palpable mass, often accompanied by a dull aching sensation. Radiographically, the tumor is frequently radiodense and attached to the external surface of bone by a broad sessile base (Fig. 14–8). It is often more radiodense at the base than at the periphery. The broad pedicle is not continuous radiographically with the underlying marrow cavity. A radiolucent clear space, corresponding to the periosteum, can often be identified between the tumor and the normal bone cortex.

Histologically, parosteal osteosarcomas are well differentiated and characterized by a spindle cell stroma with minimal atypia and rare mitotic figures separating irregular trabeculae of woven bone having foci of osteoid and cartilage (Fig. 14–9). The periphery is less ossified than the base; it may have a lobulated cartilaginous cap or may be irregular because of linear extensions into soft tissue. Medullary involvement is unusual at initial presentation, but approximately 20% of tumors, especially recurrent ones, exhibit invasion of the underlying bone. This does not seem to affect prognosis adversely. The bland histologic appearance of parosteal osteosarcoma raises the possibility of osteoma, osteochondroma, heterotopic ossification, and myositis ossificans.

PERIOSTEAL OSTEOSARCOMA

Periosteal osteosarcoma occurs much less often than does parosteal osteosarcoma. It has a 2-to-1

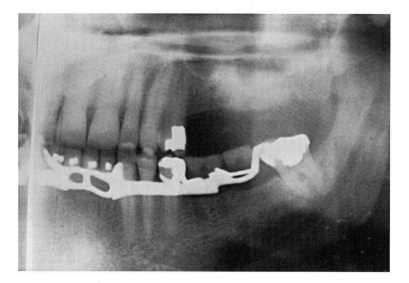

Figure 14–8. Parosteal osteosarcoma of the posterior maxillary alveolus. (Courtesy of Dr. K. Volz.)

male predominance and a peak age of occurrence of 20 years. These tumors commonly involve the upper tibial metaphysis. They are rarely seen in the jaws.

The radiographic appearance of periosteal osteosarcoma is distinct from that of parosteal osteosarcoma. The cortex of involved bone is radiographically intact and sometimes thickened, with no tumor involvement of the underlying marrow cavity (Fig. 14–10). The tumor is most often radiolucent, corresponding to its predominantly cartilaginous component, and has a more poorly defined periphery. On occasion, a periosteal reaction in the form of a Codman triangle may be noted, as well as variably sized perpendicular calcified

spicules of bone radiating from the cortex. Overall, the periosteal osteosarcoma tumor matrix is not as radiographically dense or homogeneous as that of the parosteal osteosarcoma.

Histologically, periosteal osteosarcoma is composed of lobules of poorly differentiated malignant cartilage; it often shows central ossification. The malignant cartilage and osteoid appear to radiate from an intact cortex (Fig. 14–11). The osteoid present in this variant is fine and lace-like, and it is found in the chondroid islands among intervening malignant spindle cells (Fig. 14–12). These histologic features can be identical to those of intramedullary osteosarcomas; therefore, radiographic correlation is necessary to make this diagnosis.

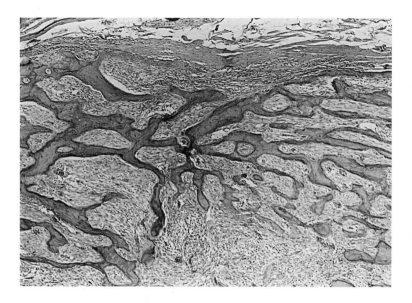

Figure 14–9. Parosteal osteosarcoma has radiating spicules of woven bone in a fibrocellular stroma that displays minimal cytologic atypia.

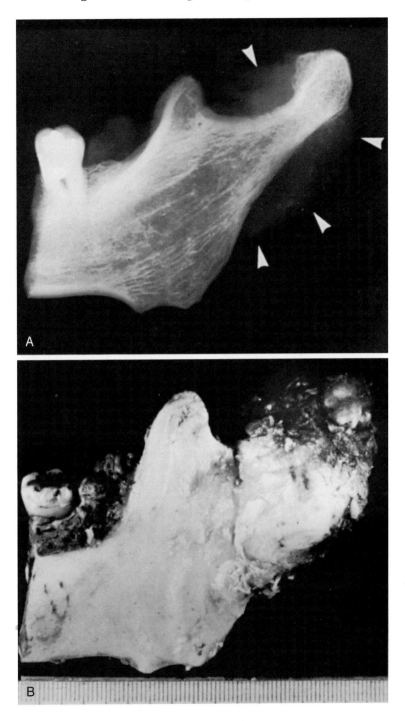

Figure 14–10. *A*, Radiograph of mandibulectomy specimen of periosteal osteosarcoma showing a lucent tumor mass overlying an intact cortex and medulla. *B*, Resected mandibular periosteal osteosarcoma showing white tumor involving the ramus but sparing the coronoid and condylar processes.

The malignant cytologic features also distinguish this variant of juxtacortical osteosarcoma from the parosteal type. In periosteal osteosarcoma, there is typically minimal tumor infiltration into cortical bone without medullary involvement. This feature helps differentiate this lesion from a chondroblastic intramedullary osteosarcoma that has permeated the cortex and formed a soft tissue mass.

The juxtacortical osteosarcoma must be completely removed by either *en bloc* resection or radical excision. A significant local recurrence rate can be expected if the underlying cortical bone is not removed with these lesions. The overall 5-year survival rate for juxtacortical osteosarcomas of the skeleton is 80%. In one series of juxtacortical osteosarcomas, pulmonary metastases devel-

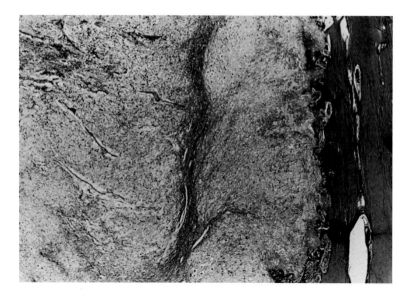

Figure 14–11. Periosteal osteosarcoma is a predominantly cartilaginous neoplasm overlying cortical bone without involvement of the marrow cavity. A poorly differentiated spindle cell component (upper left) is farthest from the cortex (right).

oped in 13% of patients with parosteal osteosarcomas and in 22% of patients with periosteal osteosarcomas. Overall, the survival rate for juxtacortical osteosarcomas is superior to that of conventional intramedullary osteosarcomas. However, it is not known if juxtacortical osteosarcomas of the jaws are substantially different in biologic behavior from those occurring in long bones. Meaningful conclusions comparing the treatment and prognosis of parosteal and periosteal osteosarcomas in the jaws cannot be made because of the few cases reported and the various methods of treatment used (curettage, local excision, and radical resection).

CHONDROSARCOMA

Chondrosarcomas arising in the mandible and maxilla are extremely rare and have accounted for approximately 1% of chondrosarcomas of the entire body. The appearance of benign chondrogenic tumors in the jaws is rare. The histologic distinction between a benign chondroma and a low-grade chondrosarcoma is not well defined, and clinical experience dictates that well-differentiated chondrogenic neoplasms in the jaws be considered potentially malignant and be handled accordingly.

Clinical Features. Chondrosarcomas more fre-

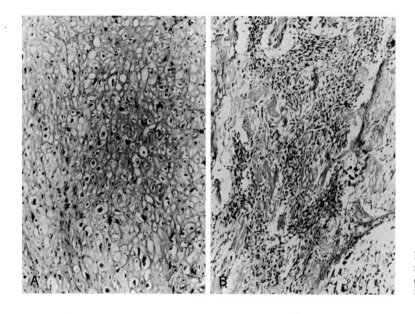

Figure 14–12. Cartilage component *(A)* and fine osteoid component *(B)* produced by spindle cell stroma in periosteal osteosarcoma.

quently involve the maxillofacial area (60%) than the mandible (40%). Lesions arising in the maxilla usually involve the anterior region (lateral incisor–canine region) and the palate. Mandibular chondrosarcomas occur most frequently in the premolar and molar regions, symphysis, coronoid process, and occasionally the condylar process (Fig. 14–13). There is no distinct gender predilection. Chondrosarcomas predominate in adulthood and old age. Although the mean age of occurrence of jaw chondrosarcomas is 60 years, almost half the cases have arisen in the third and fourth decades of life.

The most common signs are a painless swelling and expansion of the affected bones, resulting in loosening of teeth or ill-fitting dentures. Pain, visual disturbances, nasal signs, and headache may result from extension of chondrosarcomas from the jaw bones to contiguous structures.

The radiographic appearance of chondrosarcoma varies from moth-eaten radiolucencies that are solitary or multilocular to diffusely opaque lesions. Many chondrosarcomas contain mottled densities corresponding to areas of calcification

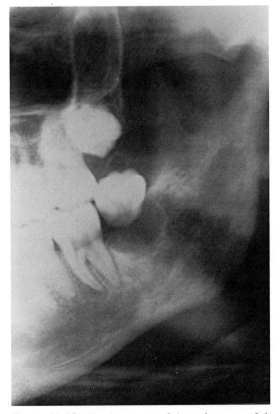

Figure 14–13. Chondrosarcoma of the molar-ramus of the mandible. Note extrusion of the third molar by tumor and a uniformly widened periodontal membrane space around the roots of the second molar.

and ossification. Localized widening of the periodontal ligament space may also be seen in chondrosarcoma. Computed tomographic visualization of cartilaginous neoplasms appears to be superior in defining the peripheral extent of the tumor compared with panoramic or flat-plate radiographs. A multilocular radiographic appearance may suggest a differential diagnosis of ameloblastoma, central giant cell granuloma, odontogenic myxoma, aneurysmal bone cyst, and keratocyst, whereas other patterns may suggest metastatic carcinoma, osteogenic sarcoma, and calcifying epithelial odontogenic tumor.

Histopathology. The histologic appearance of chondrosarcomas is variable. Most of these tumors arising in the jaws are well differentiated. The prognostic significance of the pathologic grading of chondrosarcomas is well established. The incidence of metastatic disease has been shown to be 0%, 10%, and 71% for chondrosarcomas of grade I, grade II, and grade III, respectively. Grade I chondrosarcomas often have a lobular architecture; they range from proliferations resembling benign cartilage to those with increased numbers of chondrocytes in a chondroid to myxomatous stroma (Fig. 14–14). Grade II tumors often have a myxoid stroma with enlarged chondrocyte nuclei displaying occasional mitotic figures (Fig. 14–15). Increased cellularity is frequently noted at the periphery of the cartilaginous lobules. Grade III chondrosarcomas are markedly cellular, often with a spindle cell proliferation. Mitotic figures may be numerous.

Differential Diagnosis. The histologic differential diagnosis of chondrosarcoma arising in the jaws may include benign enchondroma, which is rare in the jaws and should be considered only if the lesion is a small incidental finding. The histology more commonly evokes the possibility of the chondroblastic variant of osteosarcoma, which accounts for nearly 50% of the osteosarcomas in the jaws. This entity is recognized when adequate tissue sampling reveals foci of malignant osteoid formation. In addition, chondroid areas of pleomorphic adenoma arising in overlying soft tissues may mimic cartilaginous tumors of bone. Synovial chondromatosis involving the temporomandibular joint may also simulate chondrosarcoma.

Treatment and Prognosis. Because chondrosarcomas are considered to be radioresistant neoplasms, wide local or radical surgical excision is the treatment of choice. Therefore, the location of the primary lesion and the adequacy of surgical resection (tumor-free margins) are of prime prognostic significance for chondrosarcomas of the jaws. In addition, the pathologic grade of chondrosarcoma is indicative of its innate biologic behav-

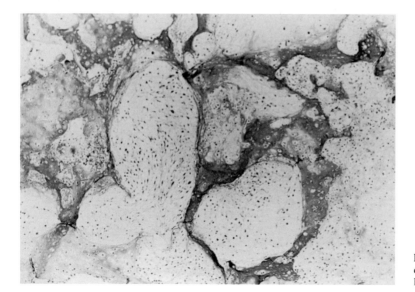

Figure 14–14. Low-grade chondrosarcoma showing lobulated proliferation of neoplastic cartilage.

ior and propensity for metastasis. The most common cause of death due to chondrosarcomas of the jaws is uncontrolled local recurrence and extension into adjacent vital structures. Metastasis, more common with high-grade chondrosarcomas, is generally to lungs or bone. The usual clinical course of chondrosarcomas is long, with recurrences not uncommonly occurring 5 years or even 10 to 20 years after therapy. The 5-year survival for chondrosarcomas of the jaws and craniofacial bones appears to be poorer than that for chondrosarcomas in other body sites. In addition, the 17% 5-year survival for patients with chondrosarcomas of the mandible is extremely poor—even worse than that of osteosarcomas involving the jaws.

Mesenchymal Chondrosarcoma

Mesenchymal chondrosarcoma is a very rare form of chondrosarcoma that is both histologically distinct and clinically unique compared with the chondrosarcomas arising in bone.

As many as one third of the mesenchymal chondrosarcomas arise in soft tissue. Those that arise in bone show a predilection for the maxilla, mandible, and ribs. In one series of 15 mesenchymal chondrosarcomas of bone, one third occurred in the jaws. Most tumors arise between the ages of 10 and 30 years, with a nearly equal gender distribution. This presentation is distinctly differ-

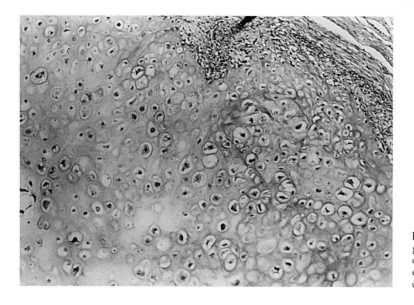

Figure 14–15. High-power micrograph of grade II chondrosarcoma displaying enlarged atypical chondrocyte nuclei and occasional binucleate forms.

ent from other forms of chondrosarcoma that occur with a mean age of 60 years.

Similar to the other malignant neoplasms discussed, pain and, at times, swelling are the usual presenting symptoms. The radiologic appearance is of a lytic lesion that may be ill defined or sharply defined. Most contain stippled or large areas of calcification.

The characteristic histologic appearance of mesenchymal chondrosarcoma is that of anaplastic small cell sarcoma containing zones of readily identifiable and often well-formed malignant cartilage. The undifferentiated small cell proliferation resembles Ewing's sarcoma and often displays a hemangiopericytoma-like growth pattern. It has been suggested that the small cell undifferentiated proliferation represents precartilaginous mesenchyme.

Appropriate sampling of these tumors demonstrates a bimorphic proliferation of undifferentiated small cells alternating with areas of cartilage. The latter finding distinguishes mesenchymal chondrosarcoma from similar-appearing Ewing's sarcoma, hemangiopericytoma, or even synovial sarcoma.

Mesenchymal chondrosarcoma is a highly malignant neoplasm that requires radical or wide surgical excision. Like other chondrosarcomas, it is relatively radioresistant, but the Ewing's sarcoma-like component may respond to radiation or chemotherapy. This is a highly lethal sarcoma, as evidenced by the fact that 80% of the patients in one series died of the disease. In addition to local recurrence, mesenchymal chondrosarcomas show a significant rate of distant metastases, often to lung and bones. Detection of metastatic disease in survivors may be delayed until 12 to 22 years after treatment of the primary tumor.

EWING'S SARCOMA

Ewing's sarcoma is a highly lethal round cell sarcoma that was first described by James Ewing in 1921. The cause is unknown, the cell of origin uncertain, and even the multipotentiality of antigenic expression controversial. Ewing's sarcoma is related to the peripheral primitive neuroectodermal tumor (PNET), sharing a common karyotype translocation t(11;12) (11;22) (q24;q12) in approximately 90% of these tumors. Ewing's sarcoma accounts for approximately 6% of all malignant bone tumors. Approximately 4% of Ewing's sarcomas have arisen in the bones of the head and neck, with 1% occurring in the jaws. Most involve the bones of the lower extremity or pelvis. When the jaws are involved, the predilection is for the ramus of the mandible, with few cases reported in the maxilla. Because Ewing's sarcoma has a propensity to metastasize to other bones, the possibility that jawbone involvement represents metastatic disease from another skeletal site should always be considered.

Clinical Features. Ninety percent of Ewing's sarcomas occur between the ages of 5 and 30 years, and more than 60% affect males. The mean age of occurrence for primary tumors involving the bones of the head and neck is 10.9 years. Pain and swelling are the most common presenting symptoms. Involvement of the mandible or maxilla may result in facial deformity, destruction of alveolar bone with loosening of teeth, and mucosal ulcers (Fig. 14–16). Radiographic findings in the jaws are nonspecific and may simulate an infectious process as well as a malignant process. The most characteristic appearance is that of a moth-eaten destructive radiolucency of the medulla and

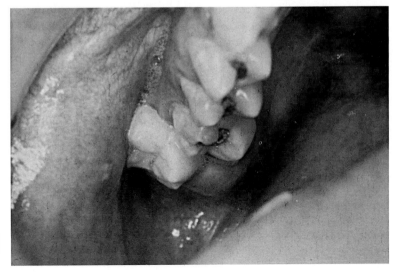

Figure 14–16. Ewing's sarcoma of the maxilla causing displacement of the second molar.

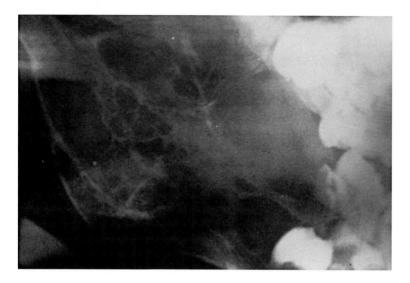

Figure 14-17. Lateral jaw radiograph of Ewing's sarcoma of the ramus of the mandible in a 4-year-old boy. Condyle in upper left and posterior teeth in lower right.

erosion of the cortex with expansion (Fig. 14–17). A variable periosteal onionskin reaction may also be seen. A significant number of patients additionally have a soft tissue mass.

Histopathology. With an adequate tissue bi-opsy, Ewing's sarcoma is recognized microscopically as a proliferation of uniform, closely packed cells that may be compartmentalized by fibrous bands (Fig. 14–18). The round to oval nuclei have finely dispersed chromatin and inconspicuous

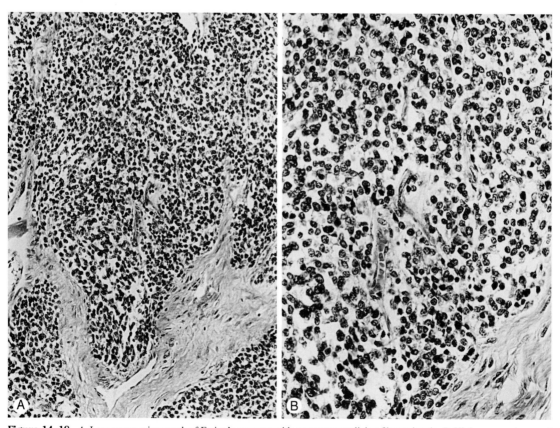

Figure 14-18. *A,* Low-power micrograph of Ewing's sarcoma with compartmentalizing fibrous bands. *B,* High-power micrograph of undifferentiated small cell proliferation in Ewing's sarcoma.

nucleoli. The cytoplasm characteristically stains with the periodic acid–Schiff stain, indicating the presence of glycogen. Although glycogen staining by this technique is helpful in diagnosis, some otherwise histologically acceptable cases of Ewing's sarcoma have yielded negative results. In addition, other tumors that mimic Ewing's sarcoma may contain glycogen.

Differential Diagnosis. Microscopically, Ewing's sarcoma is sufficiently undifferentiated or anaplastic that its appearance is readily simulated by other so-called small round cell tumors common to childhood and adolescence. This differential diagnosis includes lymphoma/leukemia, metastatic neuroblastoma, mesenchymal chondrosarcoma, small cell osteosarcoma, and, although rare for this age group, metastatic carcinoma. Routine light microscopy can often be used to discriminate between these similar-appearing neoplasms, but electron microscopy or immunohistochemistry must often be used to reach a conclusive diagnosis. By electron microscopy, the cells of Ewing's sarcoma are characterized by pools of cytoplasmic glycogen, sparse organelles, and rare primitive intercellular junctions. By immunohistochemistry, all Ewing's sarcomas contain abundant vimentin intermediate filaments. The presence of other classes of intermediate filaments has been demonstrated in frozen tissue specimens. The heterogeneity of antigenic expression in these primitive neoplasms suggests that Ewing's sarcoma is a true blastoma, derived from primitive totipotential cells that may differentiate along numerous lines. In contrast to the PNET spectrum of tumors, Ewing's sarcomas lack morphologic evidence of neural morphologic differentiation but share a high level of expression of the CD99 antigen (MIC-2 gene product) detected by antibodies 12 E7, HBA 71, or O13.

Treatment and Prognosis. The highly malignant nature of this sarcoma is reflected in its propensity for metastasis, especially to lungs, other bones, and lymph nodes. Multiple-method treatment protocols, involving surgery or radiation for local control and chemotherapy for systemic micrometastases, have dramatically improved the formerly dismal 10% 5-year survival. With these newer intensive therapies, 79% 2-year disease-free survival and 60% 5-year actuarial survival rates have been reported. Clinical features associated with poor prognosis include presentation before age 10 years, the presence of metastatic disease, systemic symptoms, a high erythrocyte sedimentation rate, elevated serum lactate dehydrogenase value, and thrombocytosis. In addition, the site of involvement appears to be of prognostic significance in Ewing's sarcomas—patients with man-

dibular tumors are noted to have a more favorable overall survival than those with any other bone site of origin.

BURKITT'S LYMPHOMA

Burkitt's lymphoma is a high-grade non-Hodgkin's lymphoma that is endemic in Africa and occurs only sporadically in North America. It was first recognized by Dennis Burkitt in Uganda in 1958 as a jaw sarcoma occurring with high frequency in African children. By 1961, further reports demonstrated the distinctive clinical and pathologic features of this tumor, by then confirmed to be a malignant lymphoma. Subsequently, nonendemic forms of Burkitt's lymphoma were recognized in the United States. The African and American forms of Burkitt's lymphoma are histologically and immunophenotypically identical. Clinical differences exist, however, between the African and American forms.

Both American and African forms of Burkitt's lymphoma are characterized by a translocation of the distal part of chromosome 8 to chromosome 14. The former is the site of the *c-myc* oncogene, and the latter, the immunoglobulin heavy-chain locus. This translocation may be directly involved in the enhanced tumor cell proliferation of Burkitt's lymphoma, which has been shown to have the highest proliferation rate of any neoplasm in humans, with a potential doubling time of 24 hours and a growth fraction of nearly 100%.

Clinical Features. In Africa, malignant lymphoma accounts for 50% of all childhood malignancies, but it composes only 6 to 10% of childhood malignancies in the United States and Europe. Whereas the African form of Burkitt's lymphoma has a peak incidence between 3 and 8 years of age and a 2-to-1 male predominance, the American form affects a slightly older age group, with a mean age of 11 years, and has no gender predilection. The overwhelming majority (77%) of cases of American Burkitt's lymphoma occur in whites.

African Burkitt's lymphoma typically involves the mandible, maxilla, and abdomen, with extranodal involvement of retroperitoneum, kidneys, liver, ovaries, and endocrine glands. The incidence of jaw tumors in African Burkitt's lymphoma is related to the age of the patient, with 88% of those younger than 3 years and only 25% of those older than 15 years showing jaw involvement. Involvement of the jaws is relatively uncommon in the American form of this disease, with a 16% incidence at presentation. The American Burkitt's lymphoma presents most often as an abdominal mass involving the mesenteric lymph nodes or ileocecal region, often with an intestinal obstruction. Involvement of the retroperitoneum, gonads, and other viscera occurs less frequently. Although predominantly an extranodal disease, involvement of cervical lymph nodes or bone marrow has also been noted. A notable difference between the endemic (African) and nonendemic (American) forms of Burkitt's lymphoma is that the Epstein-Barr virus genome can be detected in 90% of the African cases but in only 10% of the American cases.

When the mandible and maxilla are involved, the initial focus is usually in the posterior region, more commonly in the maxilla than the mandible (Fig. 14–19). The tumors in the American population appear more localized, whereas in the African form, they more commonly involve all four quadrants. The usual signs associated with jaw lesions are an expanding intraoral mass and mobility of teeth. Pain and paresthesia are occasionally present. In addition to a facial mass, in the American population, toothache is a common complaint as well as paresthesia of the lip. Burkitt's lymphoma has also been noted to invade the dental pulp, especially in developing teeth. Radiographically, a moth-eaten, poorly marginated destruction of bone is observed. The cortex may be expanded, eroded, or perforated, with soft tissue involvement.

Histopathology. Burkitt's lymphoma is a neoplastic B cell proliferation that contains cell-surface B-lineage differentiation antigens and monoclonal surface immunoglobulin. Although the lymphoma may be nodular, most often it is a diffuse proliferation of small transformed or noncleaved follicular center cell lymphocytes that are considered undifferentiated in the Rappaport classification. The proliferation is extremely monomorphic, composed of intermediate-sized lymphocytes with round nucleoli and three to five small basophilic nuclei. Throughout the lymphoid proliferation are numerous scattered macrophages containing pyknotic debris, contributing to the so-called starry-sky appearance (Fig. 14–20). The narrow rim of cytoplasm is pyroninophilic with the methyl green–pyronine stain. In touch imprints, cytoplasmic vacuoles containing lipid can be demonstrated.

The histologic differential diagnosis includes other subtypes of non-Hodgkin's lymphoma, undifferentiated carcinoma and sarcoma, metastatic neuroblastoma, and acute leukemia.

Treatment and Prognosis. Burkitt's lymphoma was at one time invariably fatal within 4 to 6 months of diagnosis. However, because of its high proliferation rate, Burkitt's lymphoma has proved to be extremely sensitive to combination chemotherapy and, therefore, potentially curable. The African and American forms of Burkitt's lymphoma show similar complete response rates to chemotherapy, with similar rates of relapse and survival. With combination chemotherapy, the

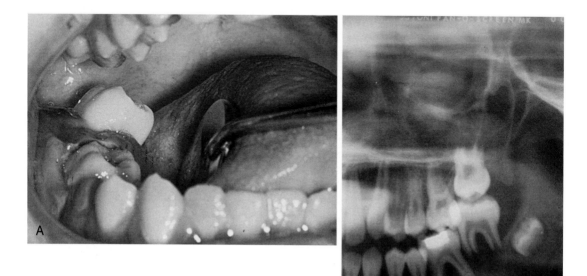

Figure 14–19. *A,* Burkitt's lymphoma of the mandible resulting in extrusion of the second molar. *B,* Radiograph showing an ill-defined diffuse lucency in the molar area. (*A* and *B,* Courtesy of Dr. R. Robert.)

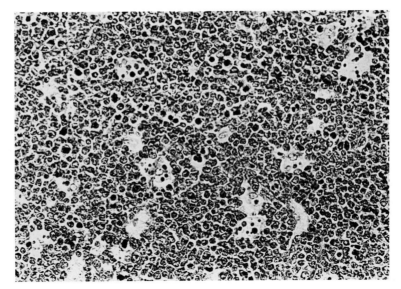

Figure 14–20. Burkitt's lymphoma showing a monotonous proliferation of small noncleaved lymphocytes with interspersed macrophages containing engulfed pyknotic debris lending a starry-sky appearance.

overall 2-year survival is 54%, with a range of 80% for low-stage disease and 41% for advanced-stage disease.

PLASMA CELL NEOPLASMS

Multiple Myeloma

Plasma cell neoplasms are derived from bone marrow stem cells of B lymphocyte lineage, and they are functionally differentiated in their ability to produce and secrete immunoglobulin. Because these tumors are derived from a single neoplastic clone, they are associated with the production of monoclonal immunoglobulin components, with the immunoglobulin light chain restricted to either the kappa or the lambda type. These tumors may present in soft tissue as extramedullary plasmacytoma, in bone as a solitary lytic lesion known as a plasmacytoma of bone, or most commonly, as part of the multifocal disseminated disease multiple myeloma. Eighty percent of the extramedullary plasmacytomas involve the head and neck region, with a predilection for the nasopharynx, nasal cavity, paranasal sinuses, and tonsils. The tumors have also been reported in gingiva, palate, floor of the mouth, and tongue. Solitary plasmacytoma of bone is rare in the jaws; it more commonly appears in the ileum, femur, humerus, thoracic vertebrae, and skull. Multiple myeloma is a disease of the hematopoietic marrow–bearing bone of the skeleton, but 70 to 95% of affected individuals have also had radiographic involvement of the bones of the maxilla or mandible.

Clinical Features. Rarely encountered before the fifth decade of life, multiple myeloma appears at a mean age of 63 years. It has a slight male predominance. Involvement of the jaws may be asymptomatic or may produce pain, swelling, expansion, numbness, mobility of teeth, or pathologic fracture. Rarely is there an associated soft tissue mass. Some patients may exhibit weakness, weight loss, anemia, and hyperviscosity syndromes. Approximately 10% of patients with multiple myeloma develop systemic amyloidosis. Eighty-five percent of patients with multiple myeloma have abnormal results of a skeletal radiographic survey. Although the remaining patients have an apparently normal radiographic series, they demonstrate plasmacytosis on marrow aspirate or biopsy.

The most common peripheral blood abnormality is anemia, with rouleau formation and, rarely, circulating plasma cells. The production of monoclonal immunoglobulin components by the neoplastic plasma cells results in an excess of abnormal protein that circulates in serum and can often be detected in urine. On serum protein electrophoresis, most patients with myeloma are found to have a decreased quantity of normal immunoglobulin and an abnormal monoclonal immunoglobulin protein peak known as an *M spike*. The immunoglobulin is usually of the IgG or IgA class, with a monoclonal light-chain component. Some plasma cell neoplasms may secrete only a monoclonal light chain. These monoclonal immunoglobulin components can be demonstrated by immunoelectrophoresis of both serum and urine in 91 to 97% of patients with myeloma. Urinary monoclonal light chains, so-called Bence Jones proteinuria, may be detected by a less sensitive

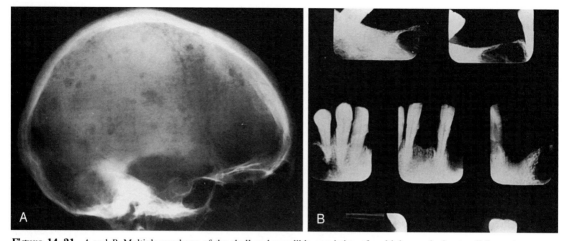

Figure 14–21. *A* and *B*, Multiple myeloma of the skull and mandible consisting of multiple punched-out radiolucencies.

heat test in approximately half of the patients with myeloma. Two percent of myeloma cases are nonsecretory, although monoclonal immunoglobulin may be demonstrated within plasma cell cytoplasm by the immunoperoxidase method.

The radiographic appearance of myeloma can vary. Typically seen are multiple sharply punched-out but noncorticated radiolucent areas of bone destruction in the jaws and in many of the hematopoietic marrow–containing bones of the skeleton (Fig. 14–21). Plasma cell tumors in the jaws may be expansile and on rare occasions may be osteosclerotic. The finding of a solitary plasma cell tumor in the jaws is more often a manifestation of systemic disease than of a solitary plasmacytoma of bone.

Histopathology. Histologically, all clinical manifestations of plasma cell tumors are similar.

Tumors are composed of a monotonous proliferation of pure plasma cells. The neoplastic plasma cells may display a wide range of differentiation, from mature-appearing plasma cells (Fig. 14–22) to less differentiated forms resembling immunoblastic large cell lymphomas. The abundant plasma cells within bone marrow can be distinguished from plasma cells of a chronic osteomyelitis or periapical granuloma by the associated proliferation of small vessels and fibroblasts with admixed neutrophils and macrophages in the reactive lesions. In addition, with the immunoperoxidase technique, a monoclonal intracytoplasmic immunoglobulin light chain can be demonstrated in nearly all plasma cell neoplasms, whereas reactive plasma cell infiltrates are uniformly polyclonal.

Differential Diagnosis. Although the punched-out lytic appearance is characteristic, the radio-

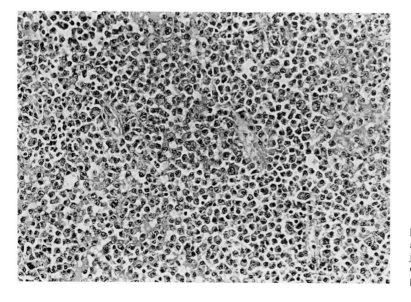

Figure 14–22. This well-differentiated plasma cell myeloma in the jaw is a monotonous proliferation of readily recognizable neoplastic plasma cells.

graphic differential diagnosis of these jaw lesions includes other malignant neoplasms of the jaws, such as metastatic carcinoma, lymphoma, and idiopathic histiocytosis. Therefore, diagnosis must be confirmed by tissue biopsy or aspirate. Histologically, very poorly differentiated plasma cell neoplasms may simulate other relatively undifferentiated malignant neoplasms, such as lymphoma, leukemia, undifferentiated carcinoma, metastatic malignant melanoma, and neuroblastoma. These entities can be distinguished by immunoperoxidase detection of the leukocyte common antigen in lymphomas/leukemias, cytokeratin in carcinomas, S-100 protein and melanoma-associated antigens in melanoma, and neuron-specific enolase in neuroblastoma. Plasma cell tumors do not express these antigens.

Treatment and Prognosis. Most patients with myeloma die of infection and, less commonly, of renal failure, disseminated myeloma, cardiac complications, and hematologic complications of hemorrhage or thrombosis. Multiple myeloma is treated with chemotherapeutic alkylating agents and steroids, with local radiation directed to painful bone lesions. Newer therapeutic regimens (none curative) have included combination chemotherapy, bone marrow transplantation, and the biologic response modifier interferon-alpha as maintenance therapy. The overall median survival is related to stage of disease and ranges from more than 60 months in patients with low stage I disease to 23 months in those presenting in high-stage III disease. Indicators of prognosis correlate with myeloma cell burden and include hemoglobin level, serum calcium level, serum and urine M-component, degree of bone involvement, and creatinine levels indicative of renal failure.

Solitary Plasmacytoma of Bone

Like multiple myeloma, solitary plasmacytoma of bone is a disease of adulthood, with a mean age of 50 years at presentation and a predominance in males. Solitary plasmacytomas rarely occur in the jaws, but when they do, they are often located in the angle of the mandible. For a diagnosis of solitary plasmacytoma to be established a radiologic bone survey and random bone marrow aspirate and biopsy should reveal no evidence of plasmacytosis in other areas of the body. However, 32 to 75% of cases of solitary plasmacytoma of bone eventually progress to multiple myeloma. It is not possible to predict which patients will develop disseminated disease and which will not. As with

multiple myeloma, the clinical symptoms include pain, swelling, and pathologic fracture.

Radiographically, solitary plasmacytoma is a well-defined lytic lesion that may be multilocular, resembling the appearance of central giant cell granuloma. Solitary plasmacytomas may destroy the cortical bone and spread into adjacent soft tissue. Unlike those with multiple myeloma, patients with solitary plasmacytoma of bone have a normal peripheral blood picture and a normal differential and clinical chemistry profile. In 17 to 25% of cases of solitary plasmacytoma of bone, a monoclonal immunoglobulin can be demonstrated in serum or urine. Biopsy material of solitary plasmacytoma of bone reveals a histologic appearance identical to that of multiple myeloma, with a monotonous proliferation of neoplastic plasma cells producing monoclonal immunoglobulin components.

Solitary plasmacytoma of bone is treated primarily by local radiotherapy. Accessible lesions may be surgically excised, followed by radiation therapy. Ten to 15% of patients have local recurrence of the solitary plasmacytoma, and small numbers of patients may develop an additional solitary plasmacytoma of bone. Although a significant proportion of cases progress to multiple myeloma, the overall survival of patients with solitary plasmacytoma is 10 years, in contrast to the 20-month mean survival of patients initially diagnosed with multiple myeloma. This appears to indicate that many solitary plasmacytomas are biologically low-grade but slowly progressive forms of multiple myeloma.

METASTATIC CARCINOMA

The most common malignancy affecting skeletal bones is metastatic carcinoma. However, metastatic disease to the mandible and maxilla is unusual; it is estimated that 1% of malignant neoplasms metastasize to these sites. Approximately 80% of these metastases are to the mandible, 14% to the maxilla, and 5% to both jaws. In adults, metastases to the jaws most commonly originate from primary carcinomas of the breast in women and of the lung in men. Other common primary sites in decreasing order of frequency are the kidney, colon and rectum, prostate, and thyroid gland. In children, neuroblastoma (adrenal gland) is the most common primary site in the first decade of life and bone malignancies in the second decade of life. Jawbone metastasis may be the first sign of malignancy in as many as 30% of cases.

Clinical Features. Individuals likely to be affected by metastatic carcinoma to the jaws are in

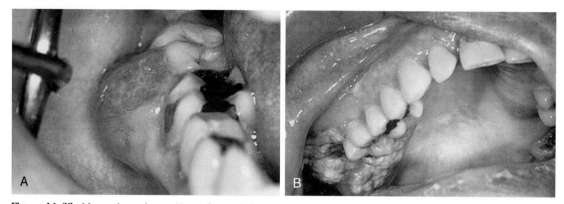

Figure 14–23. Metastatic carcinoma (*A,* esophagus; *B,* lung) to the mandible and presenting as gingival masses.

the older age groups, most in the fifth to seventh decades of life, with an average age of 45 years reflecting the greater prevalence of malignancy in this population. The mechanism of spread to the jaws is usually hematogenous from the primary visceral neoplasm or from lung metastases. Within the jaw, the premolar-molar region, the angle, and the body of the mandible are more commonly involved by metastatic disease. Bone pain, loosening of teeth, lip paresthesia, bone swelling, gingival mass (Fig. 14–23), and pathologic fracture may be clinically evident.

The radiographic appearance of most jaw metastases is poorly marginated, radiolucent, irregular, moth-eaten, expansile defects (Fig. 14–24). Some metastatic carcinomas, notably prostate and thyroid, are often characterized by an osteoblastic process. Although the appearance of osteomyelitis is also a moth-eaten radiolucency, it rarely expands the cortical bone.

Histopathology. The histologic appearance of metastatic carcinoma can be extremely variable, reflecting tumor type and grade of tumor differentiation. A prominent desmoplastic stromal response is often present. The diagnosis of metastatic carcinoma in difficult cases can be verified with an immunoperoxidase stain for cytokeratin, which is present in all carcinoma cells. In addition, immunoperoxidase staining to identify tissue-specific markers such as prostate-specific antigen, prostatic alkaline phosphatase, thyroglobulin, and calcitonin can indicate a primary origin in the prostate or thyroid gland. Antibodies to tumor type–specific antigens that are reactive in formalin-fixed, paraffin-embedded material and capable of pointing to primary sites in lung, breast, colon, or kidney are not yet available. It is anticipated that with advances in monoclonal antibody development, this technique will be very useful in identifying carcinomas of unknown metastatic origin.

Differential Diagnosis. The differential diagnosis of poorly differentiated carcinoma includes anaplastic sarcoma, lymphoma, and amelanotic melanoma. The very rare primary intraosseous

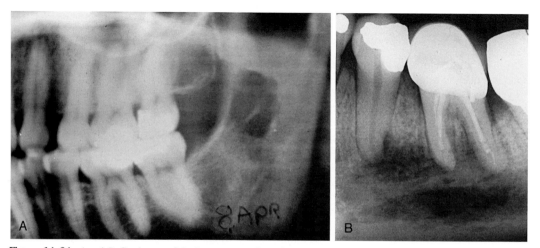

Figure 14–24. *A* and *B,* Carcinoma of the breast metastatic to the mandible.

carcinoma of probable odontogenic origin was considered in Chapter 11. The presence of cytokeratin within the tumor cells is diagnostic of carcinoma. Immunoperoxidase stains for the leukocyte common antigen verify a diagnosis of lymphoma/leukemia, whereas immunoreactivity with melanoma-associated antigens and S-100 protein indicates a diagnosis of melanoma. Although many of these sophisticated diagnostic techniques can be used to identify the nature of an anaplastic neoplasm, there is no substitute for an accurate medical history and physical examination, especially in the diagnosis of metastatic carcinoma.

Treatment and Prognosis. Metastatic carcinoma of the jaws requires further work-up to identify the primary site and to stage the degree of metastatic involvement. This is useful in identifying whether the jaw metastasis represents a solitary focus or, as is often the case, is merely the clinical sign of disseminated skeletal disease. A single focus may be treated by surgical excision or chemoradiotherapy. Generalized skeletal metastases are usually an ominous event and are treated palliatively. The prognosis for patients with metastatic carcinoma of the jaws is grave, with a dismal 10% 5-year survival and more than two thirds dead within a year.

Bibliography

Osteosarcoma

Ahuja S, Villacin A, Smith J, et al. Juxtacortical (parosteal) osteogenic sarcoma. Histologic grading and prognosis. J Bone Joint Surg 59A:632–647, 1977.

Banerjee S. Juxtacortical osteosarcoma of mandible: review of literature and report of case. J Oral Surg 39:535–538, 1981.

Bertone F, Unni KK, McLeod RA, Dahlin DC. Osteosarcoma resembling osteoblastoma. Cancer 55:416–426, 1985.

Bras J, Donner R, van der Kwast W, et al. Juxtacortical osteogenic sarcoma of the jaws. Review of the literature and report of a case. Oral Surg 50:535–544, 1980.

Caron A, Hajdu S, Strong E. Osteogenic sarcoma of the facial and cranial bones. A review of 43 cases. Am J Surg 122:719–725, 1971.

Chambers R, Mahoney W. Osteogenic sarcoma of the mandible. Current management. Am Surg 36:463–471, 1970.

Clark J, Krishnan K, Unni M, et al. Osteosarcoma of the jaw. Cancer 51:2311–2316, 1983.

Dahlin D. Bone Tumors. General Aspects and Data on 6,221 Cases, 3rd ed. Springfield, IL, Charles C Thomas, 1978, pp 226–273.

DeSantos L, Murray J, Finklestein J, et al. The radiographic spectrum of periosteal osteosarcoma. Radiology 127:123–129, 1978.

Gardner D, Mills D. The widened periodontal ligament of osteosarcoma of the jaws. Oral Surg 41:652–656, 1976.

Garrington G, Scofield H, Cornyn J, et al. Osteosarcoma of the jaws. Analysis of 56 cases. Cancer 20:377–391, 1967.

Kerpel S, Freedman P, Troyer S. Expansile mass of the body of the mandible. J Oral Maxillofac Surg 50:627–632, 1992.

Kurt A-M, Unni KK, McLeod RA, Pritchard DJ. Low-grade intraosseous osteosarcoma. Cancer 65:1418–1428, 1990.

Okada K, Frassica FJ, Sim FH, et al. Parosteal osteosarcoma: a clinicopathological study. J Bone Joint Surg 76A:366–378, 1994.

Raymond AK. Surface osteosarcoma. Clin Orthop Rel Res 270:140–148, 1991.

Regezi J, Zarbo R, McClatchey K, et al. Osteosarcomas and chondrosarcomas of the jaws: immunohistochemical correlations. Oral Surg Oral Med Oral Pathol 64:302–307, 1987.

Schajowicz F. Juxtacortical chondrosarcoma. J Bone Joint Surg 59B:473–480, 1977.

Scranton P, DeCicco F, Totten R, et al. Prognostic factors in osteosarcoma. A review of 20 years' experience at the University of Pittsburgh Health Center Hospitals. Cancer 36:2179–2191, 1975.

Unni K, Dahlin D, Beabout J, et al. Periosteal osteogenic sarcoma. Cancer 37:2476–2485, 1976.

Unni K, Dahlin D, Beabout J, et al. Parosteal osteogenic sarcoma. Cancer 37:2466–2475, 1976.

Zarbo R, Regezi J, Baker S. Periosteal osteogenic sarcoma of the mandible. Oral Surg 57:643–647, 1984.

Chondrosarcoma

Arlen M, Tollefsen H, Huvos A, et al. Chondrosarcoma of the head and neck. Am J Surg 120:456–460, 1970.

Evans H, Ayala A, Romsdahl M. Prognostic factors in chondrosarcoma of bone: a clinicopathologic analysis with emphasis on histologic grading. Cancer 40:818–831, 1977.

Fu Y, Perzin K. Non-epithelial tumors of the nasal cavity, paranasal sinuses, and nasopharynx: a clinicopathologic study. 3. Cartilaginous tumors (chondroma, chondrosarcoma). Cancer 34:453–463, 1974.

Hackney F, Aragon S, Aufdemorte T, et al. Chondrosarcoma of the jaws: clinical findings, histopathology and treatment. Oral Surg Oral Med Oral Pathol 71:139–143, 1991.

Salvador A, Beabout J, Dahlin D. Mesenchymal chondrosarcoma: observations on 30 new cases. Cancer 28:605–615, 1971.

Sato K, Nukaga H, Horikoshi T. Chondrosarcoma of the jaws and facial skeleton: a review of the Japanese literature. J Oral Surg 35:892–897, 1977.

Saito K, Unni KK, Wollan PC, Lund BA. Chondrosarcoma of the jaw and facial bones. Cancer 76:1550–1558, 1995.

Ewing's Sarcoma

Delattre O, Zucman J, Melot T, et al. The Ewing family of tumors—a subgroup of small-round-cell tumors defined by specific chimeric transcripts. N Engl J Med 331:294–299, 1994.

Graham-Poole J. Ewing's sarcoma: treatment with high dose radiation and adjuvant chemotherapy. Med Pediatr Oncol 7:1–8, 1979.

Kretschmar CS. Ewing's sarcoma and the "peanut" tumors (editorial). N Engl J Med 331:325–327, 1994.

Moll R, Inchul L, Gould V, et al. Immunocytochemical analysis of Ewing's tumors. Patterns of expression of intermediate filaments and desmosomal proteins indicate cell type heterogeneity and pluripotential differentiation. Am J Pathol 127:288–304, 1987.

Pomeroy T, Johnson R. Prognostic factors for survival in Ewing's sarcoma. Am J Roentgenol Radium Ther Nucl Med 123:598–606, 1975.

Pritchard D, Dahlin D, Dauphine R, et al. Ewing's sarcoma. A clinicopathological and statistical analysis of patients surviving five years or longer. J Bone Joint Surg 57A:10–16, 1975.

Rosen G, Caparros B, Nirenberg A, et al. Ewing's sarcoma: ten-year experience with adjuvant chemotherapy. Cancer 47:2204–2213, 1981.

Siegal G, Oliver W, Reinus W, et al. Primary Ewing's sarcoma involving the bones of the head and neck. Cancer 60:2829–2840, 1987.

Som P, Krespi Y, Hermann G, et al. Ewing's sarcoma of the mandible. Ann Otol Rhinol Laryngol 89:20–23, 1981.

Telles N, Rabson A, Pomeroy T. Ewing's sarcoma: an autopsy study. Cancer 41:2321–2329, 1978.

Burkitt's Lymphoma

Adatia A. Radiology of dental changes in Burkitt's lymphoma. *In* Proceedings of the Third International Congress of Maxillofacial Radiologists, Tokyo. Toyko, Japan Science Press, 1974, pp 405–414.

Berard C, Greene M, Jaffe E, et al. A multidisciplinary approach to non-Hodgkin's lymphomas. Ann Intern Med 94:218–235, 1981.

Grogan T, Warnke R, Kaplan H. A comparative study of Burkitt's and non-Burkitt's "undifferentiated" malignant lymphoma: immunologic, cytochemical, ultrastructural, cytologic, histopathologic, clinical, and cell culture features. Cancer 49:1817–1828, 1982.

Levine P, Kamaraju L, Connelly R, et al. The American Burkitt's lymphoma registry. Eight years' experience. Cancer 49:1016–1022, 1982.

Sariban E, Donahue A, MaGrath I. Jaw involvement in American Burkitt's lymphoma. Cancer 53:1777–1782, 1984.

Ziegler J. Burkitt's lymphoma. N Engl J Med 305:735–745, 1981.

Ziegler J. Treatment results of 54 American patients with Burkitt's lymphoma are similar to the African experience. N Engl J Med 297:75–80, 1977.

Plasma Cell Neoplasms

Alexanian R, Balcerzak S, Bonnet J, et al. Prognostic factors in multiple myeloma. Cancer 36:1192–1201, 1975.

Bataille R, Sany J. Solitary myeloma: clinical and prognostic features of a review of 114 cases. Cancer 48:845–851, 1981.

Corwin J, Lindberg R. Solitary plasmacytoma of bone vs extramedullary plasmacytoma and their relationship to multiple myeloma. Cancer 43:1007–1013, 1979.

Kapadia S. Multiple myeloma. A clinicopathologic study of 62 consecutively autopsied cases. Medicine (Baltimore) 59:380–392, 1980.

Kyle R. Multiple myeloma. Review of 869 cases. Mayo Clin Proc 50:29–40, 1975.

Meyer J, Schulz M. "Solitary" myeloma of bone. A review of 12 cases. Cancer 34:438–440, 1974.

Oken MM. Multiple myeloma: prognosis and standard treatment. Cancer Invest 15:57–64, 1997.

Regezi J, Zarbo R, Keren D. Plasma cell lesions of the head and neck: immunofluorescent determination of clonality from formalin-fixed paraffin-embedded tissue. Oral Surg 56:616–621, 1983.

Woodruff R, Malpas J, White F. Solitary plasmacytoma. 2. Solitary plasmacytoma of bone. Cancer 43:2344–2347, 1979.

Metastatic Carcinoma

Batsakis J. Tumors of the Head and Neck. Clinical and Pathological Considerations, 2nd ed. Baltimore, Williams & Wilkins, 1979, p 241.

Hirshberg A, Leibovich P, Buchner A: Metastatic tumors to the jawbones: analysis of 390 cases. J Oral Pathol Med 23:337–341, 1994.

15

Metabolic and Genetic Jaw Diseases

METABOLIC CONDITIONS

Paget's Disease

Etiology and Pathogenesis. Paget's disease, or osteitis deformans, is a chronic, slowly progressive condition of unknown cause. Numerous theories of origin have been postulated since the early concept of a chronic inflammatory process. These included autoimmunity, an endocrine abnormality related to hyperthyroid disease, an inborn error of connective tissue metabolism, an autonomic nervous system–mediated vascular disorder, a paramyxovirus infection, and a slow virus–type infection, although no causative link has been established between infective agents and Paget's disease.

The disease may be thought of as consisting of three stages. The initial phase is the bone resorptive phase. The second or vascular phase appears with concomitant haphazard osteoblastic repair. In this phase, symptoms become evident and often cause patients to seek treatment. The final phase is an appositional or sclerosing phase in which mineralization of previously deposited bony matrix occurs, with diminution of the overall cellularity and vascularity of the lesions.

Paget's disease is generally encountered in patients older than 50 years, although it can occur in younger patients. It is relatively common and has been reported to occur in 3 to 4% of the middle-aged and as many as 10 to 15% of the elderly. In approximately 14% of cases, a positive family history can be elicited. Paget's disease has a 3-to-2 male predilection, and it seems to occur more frequently in patients of European descent.

The most frequent sites of involvement include the spine, femora, cranium, pelvis, and sternum.

Clinical Features. The maxilla and mandible are involved in approximately 17% of cases, usually bilateral and symmetric. The maxilla is affected approximately twice as often as the mandible. Enlargement of the jaws as well as the skull is common. At initial presentation, symptoms often relate to deformity or pain in the affected bones; however, monostotic involvement can occur. Bone pain is described as deep and aching. Perception of skin temperature alteration is often stated. Neurologic complaints—including headache, auditory or visual disturbances, facial paralysis, vertigo, and weakness—may be related, in large part, to narrowing of skull foramina, resulting in compression of vascular and neural elements. Approximately 10 to 20% of patients are asymptomatic, however, and are incidentally diagnosed after radiographic or laboratory studies are performed for unrelated problems.

Classically, dental patients who wear complete dentures may complain of newly acquired poor prosthetic adaptation and function as the maxilla progressively enlarges. The alveolar ridge ultimately widens, with a relative flattening of the palatal vault (Fig. 15–1). When teeth are present,

417

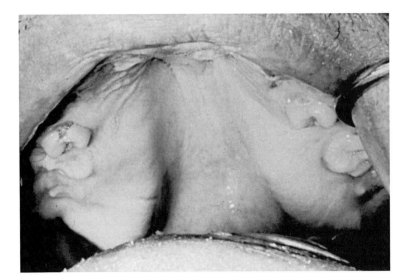

Figure 15–1. Paget's disease of the maxilla. Note bilateral enlargement of the ridges.

increased spacing as well as loosening is noted (Fig. 15–2). In severe cases, continued enlargement of the maxilla or mandible can make closure of the lips difficult or impossible.

The classic radiographic findings in later stages of Paget's disease relate to a haphazard arrangement of newly formed bone providing a patchy radiopaque pattern termed *cotton wool* by many (Fig. 15–3). In the jaws, this pattern of bone change may be associated with hypercementosis of tooth roots, loss of lamina dura, obliteration of the periodontal ligament space, and resorption of roots (Fig. 15–4).

Histopathology. Histologically, in the initial resorptive phase, random osteoclastic bone resorption is evident. The osteoclasts contain large numbers of nuclei. Resorbed bone is replaced by dense, vascularized connective tissue, which is often seen in direct apposition to eroded bony spicules. The second phase represents a dynamic composite of osteolysis and osteogenesis (Fig. 15–5). Broad osteoid bands or seams that are in the process of mineralization are evident. A characteristic histologic pattern develops; it is known as a *mosaic* because of irregular bone formation with numerous cemental or reversal lines. In the final, sclerotic phase, a decrease in osteoclastic activity and an increase in osteoblastic function are seen (Fig. 15–6).

The laboratory can provide important information about the diagnosis of Paget's disease. Serum calcium and serum phosphate levels are normal in the presence of sometimes markedly elevated alkaline phosphatase levels. The intense osteoblas-

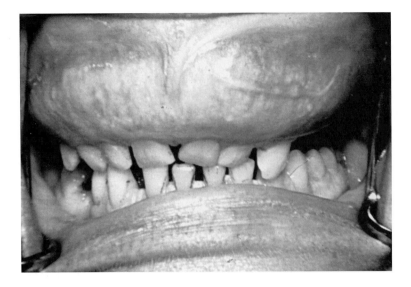

Figure 15–2. Paget's disease causing increased spacing of teeth.

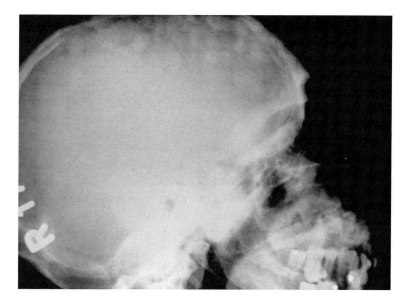

Figure 15–3. Patchy opaque pattern (cotton wool) noted in Paget's disease of the skull.

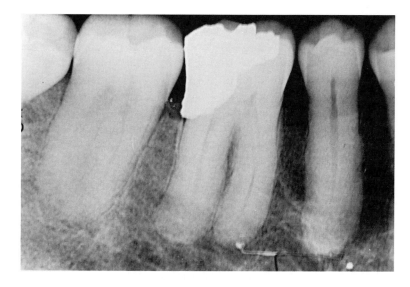

Figure 15–4. Hypercementosis of Paget's disease.

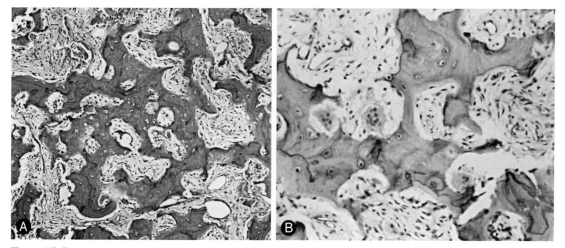

Figure 15–5. *A* and *B,* Intense osteoblastic and osteoclastic activity occurring in Paget's disease. Note the reversal lines.

419

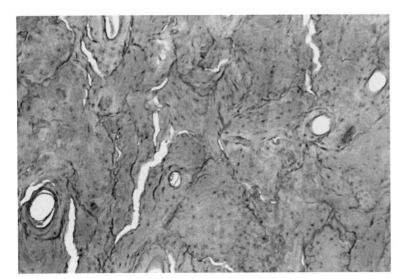

Figure 15–6. Dense sclerotic bone as seen in the late stage of Paget's disease.

tic activity in this metabolically active bone is believed to be responsible for the elevated alkaline phosphatase levels. The amount of bone resorption may be correlated to increases in urinary calcium and hydroxyproline levels. The differential diagnosis in Paget's disease may include acromegaly, florid osseous dysplasia, sclerosing osteomyelitis, osteosarcoma, and possibly the adult or acquired form of osteopetrosis. The primary indicator for therapeutic intervention is patient discomfort. Elevation of alkaline phosphatase levels to twice normal levels also warrants treatment.

Treatment. Therapy is essentially symptomatic, with analgesics used for pain control. Use of calcitonin or bisphosphonate as parathormone antagonists has been effective. Both suppress bone resorption and deposition, as reflected in reduction in the biochemical indexes, including alkaline phosphatase and urinary hydroxyproline levels. A 50% reduction in either index constitutes a good therapeutic response.

Unfortunately, Paget's disease is a slowly progressive disorder. It is seldom fatal. Relief of symptoms, in particular bone pain, with orally administered bisphosphonates has been dramatic and may persist for years after cessation of treatment. Complications relate to skeletal deformity, weakened bones, neurologic deficits, and pathologic fracture. In a small percentage of cases, malignant transformation into osteosarcoma may occur. Depending on the series reported, this has ranged from 1 to 15%.

Hyperparathyroidism

Hyperparathyroidism may be considered as represented by three forms: primary, secondary, and a hereditary type. Rarely, cases of hyperparathyroidism may be associated with a Noonan-like syndrome. The hereditary form has been shown to be an autosomal dominant condition mapped to chromosome 1q21-q31, the location of the HRPT2 endocrine tumor gene.

Primary hyperparathyroidism is characterized by hypersecretion of parathyroid hormone from hyperplastic parathyroid glands, a parathyroid adenoma, or less commonly an adenocarcinoma. In the hyperplastic state, there is usually an increase in the total amount of parathyroid tissue represented by an increase in both size and number of cells. The most consistent abnormal findings are elevated parathormone levels and hypercalcemia, the hypersecreting parathyroid glands being less sensitive to the negative feedback effects of increased serum calcium levels. Serum hypercalcemia results from parathormone stimulation of osteoclastic mediated bone resorption and from decreasing calcium excretion in the kidneys.

The finding of elevated or normal serum parathyroid hormone levels in the presence of elevated serum calcium values confirms the diagnosis of hyperparathyroidism. The primary form occurs from intrinsic disease within the gland, and the secondary form occurs as a compensatory response to hypocalcemia, as may be found in renal failure and in patients undergoing renal dialysis.

Etiology. In most instances, the cause of primary hyperparathyroidism is unknown. It has been suggested that prior irradiation may be a possible cause. Because the disease is more common in postmenopausal women, the possibility that diminished levels of estrogen may be partially responsible for this disease has also been suggested. In a small percentage of cases, the disease may be hereditary, occurring in patients with one of the multiple endocrine neoplasia syndromes.

Clinical Features. The disease spectrum of primary hyperparathyroidism ranges from asymptomatic cases (diagnosed by routine serum calcium determinations) to severe cases manifesting as lethargy and occasionally coma. Early symptoms include fatigue, weakness, nausea, anorexia, polyuria, thirst, depression, and constipation. Bone pain and headaches are frequently reported.

Several clinical features are associated with the primary form of this disease, classically described as "stones, bones, groans, and moans." Lesions of the kidneys, skeletal system, gastrointestinal tract, and nervous system are responsible for this syndrome complex. The renal component includes the presence of renal calculi or, more rarely, nephrocalcinosis.

Severe osseous changes (called, in the past, *osteitis fibrosa cystica*) result from significant bone demineralization, with fibrous replacement producing radiographic changes that appear cyst-like. The latter are of chief importance as far as the maxilla and especially the mandible are concerned. The most characteristic radiographic sign of the disease is subperiosteal resorption, occurring typically in locations such as the radial aspect of the second and third phalanges and the distal portions of the clavicles. Long bones may fracture and the vertebrae may collapse. Skeletal deformity is not uncommon (Fig. 15–7).

Gastrointestinal manifestations include peptic ulcer, secondary to increase in gastric acid, pepsin, and serum gastrin levels. Rarely, pancreatitis may develop, secondary to obstruction of the smaller pancreatic ducts by calcium deposits.

Finally, the neurologic manifestations may become evident when serum calcium levels are very high, exceeding 16 to 17 mg/dl. In such instances, coma or parathyroid crisis may occur. Loss of memory and depression are common, and rarely, true psychosis may appear. Some of the neurologic findings may be attributed to calcium deposits in the brain. Metastatic calcifications of the oral mucosa may rarely be seen in hyperparathyroidism. This is to be distinguished from dystrophic calcification, which occurs at sites of previous tissue injury in the presence of normal levels of serum calcium and phosphorus.

The chief oral finding is the appearance of well-defined cystic radiolucencies of the jaw, which may be monolocular or multilocular (Fig. 15–8). Less obvious radiographic pathology may include an osteoporotic appearance of the mandible and maxilla, reflecting a more generalized condition. Loosening of the teeth may also occur, as well as corresponding obfuscation of trabecular detail and overall cortical thinning. Partial loss of lamina dura is seen in a minority of patients with hyperparathyroidism (Fig. 15–9). Pulpal obliteration, with complete calcification of the pulp chamber and canals, has been reported in association with secondary hyperparathyroidism; therefore, this must be included within the differential diagnosis of pulpal obliteration. Other conditions to be included in the latter are dentinogenesis imperfecta and dentinal dysplasia.

Histopathology. The bone lesions of hyperparathyroidism, although not specific, are important in establishing the diagnosis. The bony trabeculae exhibit osteoclastic resorption as well as formation of osteoid trabeculae by large num-

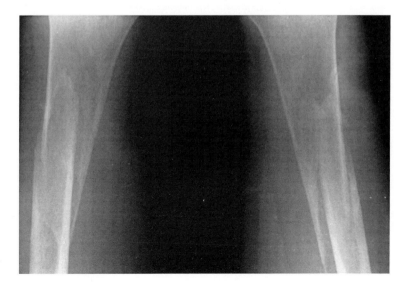

Figure 15–7. Bilateral fractures in primary hyperparathyroidism.

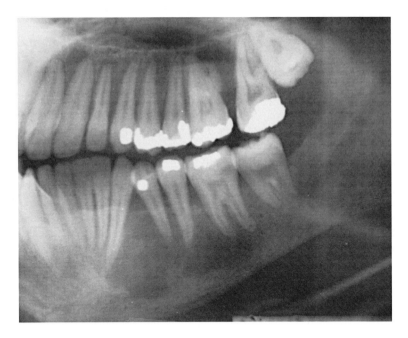

Figure 15–8. Radiolucencies of hyperparathyroidism.

bers of osteoblasts (Fig. 15–10). In these areas, large numbers of capillaries and endothelium-lined spaces are seen, with multinucleated giant cells scattered within a delicate fibrocellular stroma. Accumulations of hemosiderin and extravasated red blood cells also are noted. As a result, the tissues may appear reddish brown, accounting for the term *brown tumor.* The lesions are microscopically identical to central giant cell granulomas.

Treatment. Management of primary hyperparathyroidism is aimed at eliminating the parathyroid pathology and monitoring the fall in C-terminal parathyroid hormone concentration. Surgery is the treatment of choice in most instances because it offers the best opportunity for long-term cure. It has been observed that long-term hypercalcemia can be associated with increased morbidity, usually as a result of compromised renal function. Owing to the extensive use of routine multichannel serum autoanalyzers with early identification of asymptomatic hypercalcemia, complicating features of primary hyperparathyroidism are less commonly encountered today.

Treatment of secondary hyperparathyroidism

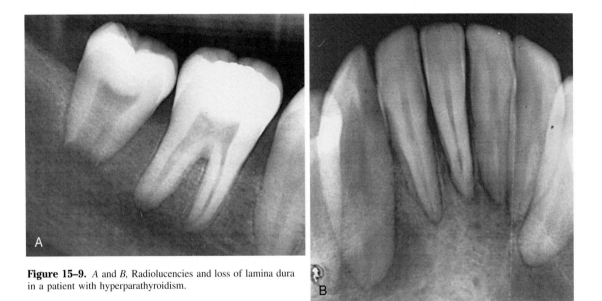

Figure 15–9. *A* and *B,* Radiolucencies and loss of lamina dura in a patient with hyperparathyroidism.

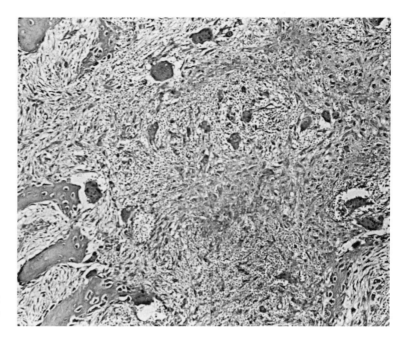

Figure 15–10. Bone replacement by fibrous tissue and giant cells in a patient with hyperparathyroidism.

due to increased parathyroid function resulting from chronic renal failure is aimed at management of kidney disease. The dental and oral considerations in this form of hyperparathyroidism are similar to those in the primary form of the disease.

Hyperthyroidism

Hyperfunction of the thyroid gland, or hyperthyroidism, is characterized by excessive amounts of thyroid hormones T_3 (triiodothyronine) and T_4 (thyroxine) or by increased levels of thyroid-stimulating hormones (TSH). In adults, hyperthyroidism occurs with an incidence of 3 cases per 10,000 per year, with a distinct female preponderance of approximately 5 to 1. This disease is rare in children, most cases occurring between 10 and 14 years of age.

The most common disorder leading to clinical hyperthyroidism is Graves' disease, accounting for 70 to 85% of all cases. The exact cause of this particular process is obscure but appears to be related to production of abnormal thyroid stimulator (long-acting thyroid stimulator, LATS), which differs chemically and functionally from TSH. LATS acts similarly to TSH but over a longer period of time. The LATS substance is an IgG produced by B lymphocytes, which is capable of inducing thyroid hyperplasia and increasing iodine uptake by the thyroid, free of any pituitary gland influence. Thyrotoxicosis may also result from excess stimulation of the thyroid gland via the hypothalamic pituitary axis or by secretion of thy-

roid hormone from ectopic, endogenous, or exogenous sources.

Heat intolerance and hyperhidrosis are common findings. Fine motor tremor and muscle weakness, palpitations, diarrhea, anxiety, weight loss, and menstrual dysfunction are commonly encountered. Patients complain of altered complexion, which is often ruddy. Thinning and brittle hair is a frequent finding. Palmar erythema is also common. Ocular changes include upper lid retraction and so-called lid lag on normal blinking. The bright-eyed stare that often results from upper lid retraction may be further accentuated by exophthalmos. Pretibial myxedema and acropachy may be found in patients with Graves' disease.

Cardiac manifestations are among the earliest and most consistent features of this disease. The increased metabolic activity places greater demand on the cardiovascular system; accordingly, increases in stroke volume, pulse rate, and cardiac output are usually observed.

Although the oral manifestations of this condition are not specific, they are consistent. In children, premature or accelerated exfoliation of deciduous teeth and concomitant rapid eruption of permanent teeth are often noted. In adults, osteoporosis of the mandible and maxilla may be found. On occasion, patients may complain of a burning tongue as well as other nonspecific symptoms. Of interest is a reported threefold increase in the incidence of dental erosion in comparison with euthyroid control subjects.

Treatment consists of thyroid-suppressive drug therapy or radioactive iodine administration, which essentially inactivates the hyperfunctional thyroid tissue. Thyroid-suppressive drugs include thiocarbamides such as propylthiouracil and methimazole. These drugs inhibit iodine oxidation and iodination of tyrosyl residues, two steps in the synthesis of thyroid hormones. Surgical therapy remains an option, although the potential for parathyroid gland removal and subsequent hypoparathyroidism is a risk.

Of clinical importance is the need to reduce stress to minimize the risk of precipitating a thyroid crisis in patients with this disease. Use of certain drugs such as epinephrine and atropine is contraindicated because they may precipitate a thyroid storm, which is a life-threatening state of thyroid hormone–induced hypermetabolism.

Hypophosphatasia

Hypophosphatasia represents a deficiency of alkaline phosphatase. This hereditary disorder is transmitted in an autosomal recessive manner. Of chief importance is that this unusual genetic metabolic disease is one of the main causes of premature loss of the primary dentition. (Other conditions in which premature tooth exfoliation may be seen include cyclic neutropenia, idiopathic histiocytosis, juvenile periodontitis, acrodynia, rickets, and Papillon-Lefèvre syndrome.) Although the primary dentition is nearly exclusively involved, adolescent and adult patients with this condition may also experience dental abnormalities including reduced marginal alveolar bone, abnormal root cementum, focal areas of dentin resorption, altered mineralization of coronal dentin, and large coronal pulp chambers of the molar dentition.

The chief clinical features of hypophosphatasia include enlarged pulp chambers of the primary teeth, alveolar bone loss with a predisposition for the anterior portion of the mandible and maxilla, and hypoplasia or aplasia of cementum over the root surface. Root development may be deficient, especially toward the apex. The crowns of the involved teeth demonstrate rickets-like changes, chiefly characterized by hypoplastic enamel defects. Enamel hypoplasia, increased pulp spaces, and premature tooth exfoliation are present in the permanent and primary dentitions. The dental abnormalities are a result of inadequate formation of both dentin and cementin.

In addition, long bones show inadequate levels of mineralization. Abnormally wide osteoid seams have been noted. Serum chemistry studies indicate a reduction in alkaline phosphatase levels, with concomitant urinary findings of detectable phos-

phoethanolamine. Tissue levels of alkaline phosphatase are likewise decreased in this disorder.

Four clinical types of hypophosphatasia have been recognized: (1) A congenital type has a 75% rate of neonatal mortality. (2) An early infantile type appears within the first 6 months of life, with a mortality rate of 50%. Renal calcinosis may accompany this disease, as well as a risk of cranial synostosis, delayed motor development, and premature loss of teeth. (3) A late infantile or childhood type begins between 6 and 24 months of age. Skeletal findings tend to be less pronounced, but abnormalities of long bone structures, including irregular ossifications at the metaphysis, may be observed, along with rickets-type changes at the costochondral junctions. Of importance in this form of the disease is premature loss of the anterior primary teeth, often the first sign of the illness. (4) The adult type, although distinctly uncommon, is characterized by bone pain, pathologic fractures, and a childhood history of rickets.

No successful treatment is known, apart from controlling the hypercalcemia resulting from the hypophosphatasia. Large doses of vitamin D have occasionally produced partial improvement, although hypercalcemia and soft tissue calcinosis may result from such an approach. Genetic counseling of the family as well as early diagnosis is of great value.

Infantile Cortical Hyperostosis

Infantile cortical hyperostosis, or Caffey's disease, is a self-limited, short-lived proliferative bone disease characterized by cortical thickening of various bones. The mandible is frequently involved, and less commonly the clavicles, long bones, maxilla, ribs, and scapulae. In addition to the osseous changes, swelling of the overlying soft tissues usually occurs.

There are no gender, racial, or geographic predilections. The characteristic age of onset is usually by the seventh month of life, with the average age of onset being 9 weeks.

Many believe that genetic factors are involved in the origin of this disease process, and most of the reported cases have been familial. An autosomal dominant mode of inheritance with incomplete penetrance and variable expressivity has been cited. Congenital abnormality of blood vessels supplying the periosteum of the involved bones is a suggested cause of the familial form. More recently, a possible infectious cause has been proposed, with a long latency period reminiscent of that suggested for Paget's disease. Sporadic cases also occur, suggesting etiologic possibilities that have included an infectious agent, immunologic disorder, nutritional aberrations, allergy, trauma, hormonal disturbances, and disorders of collagen metabolism.

Clinically, the involvement of the mandible, maxilla, or other bones is characterized by firm, tender swelling with rather deep-seated edema. Pain, fever, and hyperirritability may precede or develop concurrently with the swelling. From 75 to 90% of cases demonstrate mandibular involvement, typically over the angle and ascending ramus symmetrically. Sporadic cases of infantile cortical hyperostosis almost always show mandibular involvement, with familial cases demonstrating such involvement approximately 60% of the time.

Radiographically, an expansile hyperostotic process is visible over the cortical surface, with rounding or blunting of the mandibular coronoid process. Initially, the hyperostotic element is separated from the underlying bone by a thin radiolucent line.

Diagnosis may be facilitated by the use of technetium (^{99m}Tc) scans, which are often positive before routine radiographic detection is made. Laboratory findings that are also helpful in establishing the diagnosis include an elevated erythrocyte sedimentation rate, increased phosphatase levels, anemia, leukocytosis, and occasionally thrombocytopenia or thrombocytosis.

Infantile cortical hyperostosis is usually a self-limiting process, with treatment generally directed at supportive care. Systemic corticosteroids and nonsteroidal anti-inflammatory drugs have been used with some success. This disease has a tendency to follow an uneven though predictable course, with relapses and remissions possible. During such recurrences or relapses, the use of naproxen has been recommended to control symptoms and arrest progression of the disease, suggesting that prostaglandins may have a role in the etiology. The resolution phase ranges from 6 weeks to 23 months, with an average of 9 months. Radiographic and histologic resolution may take up to several years, with a generally excellent prognosis despite the possibility of recurrences and occasional residual effects, such as severe malocclusion and mandibular asymmetry.

Phantom Bone Disease

Phantom bone disease, also known as massive osteolysis or vanishing bone disease, is an unusual process characterized by posttraumatic or spontaneous slow, progressive, localized destruction of bone. It is a nonneoplastic condition featured by a proliferative vascular and connective tissue response. The fibrovascular tissue may completely replace the involved bone, but the mechanism of bone destruction and resorption is unknown. This is a rare entity, with fewer than 150 cases reported since its initial description in 1838. The process has been described in virtually every bone in the body, with 15 cases reported in the maxillofacial region.

No ethnic or gender predilection has been noted. There appears to be no genetic basis for transmission. Various studies, including metabolic, endocrine, and neurologic tests, have not been helpful in determining the cause of phantom bone disease.

In most patients, the disease develops before the fourth decade of life, although it has been described in patients ranging from 18 months to 72 years of age. The onset of the disease is insidious; pain is usually not a feature unless there is concomitant pathologic fracture of the involved bone. Progressive atrophy of the affected bone resulting in significant deformity constitutes a useful diagnostic sign of massive osteolysis. Although most cases involve a single bone, the disease may also be polyostotic, affecting usually contiguous bones. This disease is progressive but variable—over time, the bone may completely disappear, or it may spontaneously stabilize. Significant regeneration has not been reported.

The earliest radiographic sign of the disease has been reported to be one or more intermedullary subcortical radiolucencies of variable size, usually with indistinct margins and thin radiopaque borders. In time, these foci enlarge and coalesce, eventually involving the cortex (Fig. 15–11). A characteristic tapering ultimately occurs when long bones are affected.

Laboratory studies fail to show biochemical abnormalities. Microscopically, replacement of bone by connective tissue with many dilated capillaries and anastomosing vascular channels is noted (Fig. 15–12). As the disease progresses, dissolution of both medullary and cortical bone is seen. A fibrotic band, thought to represent residual periosteum, persists.

There is no effective treatment for phantom bone disease, although moderate doses of radiation therapy (40 to 45 Gy in 2-Gy fractions) have resulted in good outcome with few long-term complications. Limited success has been obtained with bone grafts and implants.

Acromegaly

Acromegaly is a rare condition with a prevalence of approximately 50 to 70 cases per million

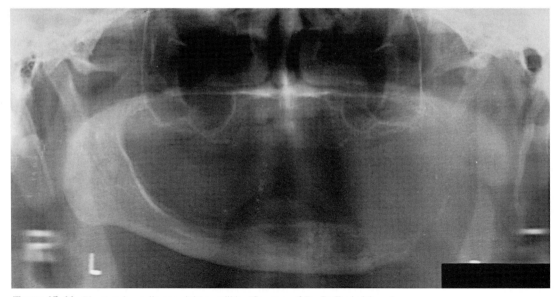

Figure 15–11. Phantom bone disease, right mandible. (Courtesy of Dr. D. Frederickson.)

population and an incidence of 3 cases per million per year. This disease is characterized by bony and soft tissue overgrowth and metabolic disturbances. These changes occur secondary to chronic hypersecretion of growth hormone subsequent to the closure of the epiphyseal plates. If hypersecretion occurs before epiphyseal closure, gigantism results.

Etiology. The cause in more than 90% of cases is hypersecretion of growth hormone from a benign pituitary adenoma, or so-called somatotropinoma. The pituitary tumor may occasionally produce prolactin along with growth hormone (somatomedin C) or other hormones, including TSH or adrenal corticotropic hormone (ACTH). Such adenomas, although most common in the pituitary gland itself, may also arise in ectopic locations along the migration path of Rathke's pouch. In general, growth hormone levels correlate proportionally to the size of the adenoma as well as the overall severity of the disease.

Clinical Features. Acromegaly presents most frequently in the fourth decade, with an even gender distribution and no racial or geographic predominance. This disorder is of insidious onset, with diagnosis often delayed for many years.

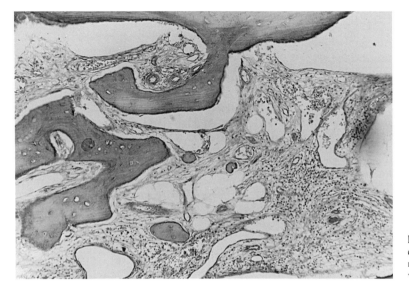

Figure 15–12. Phantom bone disease. Fibrous replacement of bone is noted in conjunction with increased vascularity.

Younger patients have more aggressive tumors and develop clinically recognizable acromegaly more rapidly.

Clinical signs and symptoms result from the local effects of the expanding pituitary mass and the effects of excess growth hormone secretion. Affected individuals present with hyperhidrosis; muscle weakness; paresthesia, especially carpal tunnel syndrome; dysmenorrhea; and decreased libido. Sleep apnea, hypertension, and heart disease are also encountered. Skin tag formation is common and may be a marker for colonic polyps. In the facial bones and the jawbones, new periosteal bone formation may be seen as well as cartilaginous hyperplasia and ossification. The resultant orofacial changes include frontal bossing, nasal bone hypertrophy, and relative mandibular prognathism or prominence. Enlargement of the paranasal sinuses as well as secondary laryngeal hypertrophy produces a rather deep, resonant voice, which is typical of acromegaly. Overall coarsening of facial features is noted, secondary to connective tissue hyperplasia (Fig. 15–13).

Oral manifestations include enlargement of the mandible and maxilla, with secondary separation of teeth due to alveolar overgrowth. Condylar hyperplasia with concomitant bone formation at the anterior portion of the mandible and a distinct increase in the bony angle produces a rather typical dental malocclusion and prognathism. Complete posterior crossbite is a common finding in such a circumstance. Thickened oral mucosa, increased salivary gland tissue, macroglossia, and prominent lips are also noted in most instances. It has been reported that with the concomitant changes in mandibular structure, marked alterations in the diameter of the inferior alveolar canal, myofascial pain dysfunction syndrome, and

speech abnormalities may result. Diagnostic is the demonstration of growth hormone levels that are nonsuppressible by glucose loading. Computed tomography or magnetic resonance imaging of the sella turcica may help confirm the diagnosis of acromegaly-associated tumor. Radioimmunoassay studies of somatomedin C may be used as a routine screening test.

Treatment. Treatment relates to a normalization of growth hormone levels, with concomitant preservation of normal pituitary function. Associated causes of death include hypertension, diabetes, pulmonary infections, and cancer. The most frequently used treatment is transsphenoidal surgery; a rapid therapeutic response is usually noted. Conventional radiotherapy to this area during a 4- to 6-week period carries a 70% rate of normalization of pituitary function, although hypopituitarism may be an unfavorable sequela. Current medical therapy uses bromocriptine, a dopamine agonist, or octreotide as adjunctive agents but not as primary modalities.

Successful management may be reflected in reversal of soft tissue abnormalities, although many of the facial deformities may persist. In such instances, corrective oral and maxillofacial surgery may be indicated, including mandibular osteotomy and partial glossectomy.

GENETIC ABNORMALITIES

Cherubism

Cherubism is a benign hereditary condition of the maxilla and mandible, usually found in children by 5 years of age. The term *cherubism* was chosen by Jones in 1933 to describe three siblings

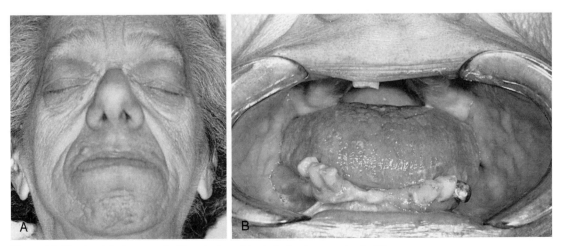

Figure 15–13. *A* and *B,* Acromegaly. Note tipping of the teeth due to macroglossia *(B).*

presenting with marked fullness of the jaws and cheeks and upwardly gazing eyes. The characteristically round and symmetrically full face is suggestive of a cherub's (Fig. 15–14).

Etiology and Pathogenesis. Cherubism usually occurs as an autosomal dominant disorder, with 100% penetrance in males and 50 to 75% penetrance in females, with a 2-to-1 male predominance. Sporadic cases have also been reported.

Mesenchymal alteration during the development of the jaw bones as a result of reduced oxygenation secondary to perivascular fibrosis has been suggested as a possible cause. It is usually a self-limiting disease, with rapid progression during childhood, often beginning by 2 years of age, through puberty. At this time, the bony lesions begin to regress, often to the degree that only a minor residual deformity may be present by age 30 years.

Clinical Features. The mandibular angle, ascending ramus, retromolar region, and posterior maxilla are most often affected. The coronoid process can also be involved, but the condyles are always spared. The vast majority of cases occur only in the mandible. The bony expansion is most

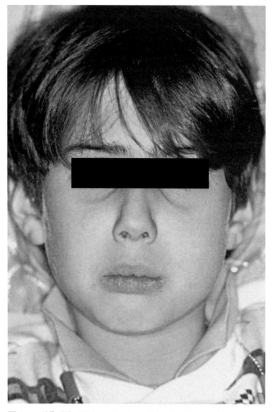

Figure 15–14. This patient exhibits the bilateral symmetric facial expansion often seen in cherubism.

frequently bilateral, although unilateral involvement has been reported.

Patients typically present with a painless symmetric enlargement of the posterior region of the mandible, with expansion of the alveolar process and ascending ramus. The clinical appearance may vary from a barely discernible posterior swelling of a single jaw to marked anterior and posterior expansion of both jaws, resulting in masticatory, speech, and swallowing difficulties. Intraorally, a hard, nontender swelling can be palpated in the affected area.

With maxillary disease, involvement of the orbital floor and anterior wall of the antrum occurs. Superior pressure on the orbit results in an increasing prominence of the sclera and the appearance of upturned eyes. The palatal vault may be reduced or obliterated. Maxillary involvement usually results in the greatest deformity. All four quadrants of the jaws may be simultaneously involved with this painless process of bony expansion. Premature exfoliation of the primary dentition may occur as early as 3 years of age. Displacement of developing tooth follicles results in poor development of selective permanent teeth and ectopic eruption. Permanent teeth may be missing or malformed, with the mandibular second and third molars most often affected. Significant malocclusions can be anticipated even with unifocal involvement.

Submandibular and upper cervical lymphadenopathy are common, although reactive regional lymphadenopathy, particularly of submandibular lymph nodes, usually subsides after 5 years of age. Intelligence is unaffected. Serum calcium and phosphorus levels are within normal limits, but alkaline phosphatase levels may be elevated.

Radiographic surveys may provide the only signs of disease. The radiographic lesions characteristically appear as numerous well-defined multilocular radiolucencies of the jaws (Fig. 15–15). The borders are distinct and divided by bony trabeculae. Seen in the mandible are expansion and thinning of the cortical plate, with occasional perforation; displacement of the inferior alveolar canal may be noted. An occlusal radiograph of the maxilla may give a soap bubble–like picture with maxillary antrum obliteration. Unerupted teeth are often displaced and appear to be floating in the cyst-like spaces.

Histopathology. Histologically, the lesions bear a close resemblance to those seen in central giant cell granulomas (Fig. 15–16). A highly vascularized fibrous stroma is noted, often arranged in a whorled pattern. Numerous fibroblasts and multinucleated giant cells with prominent nuclei and nucleoli are noted. Mature lesions exhibit a

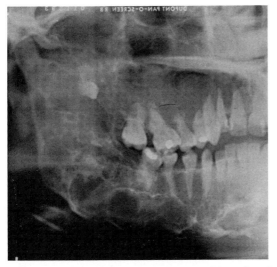

Figure 15–15. Well-defined multilocular radiolucencies of the mandible and maxilla characteristic of cherubism.

large amount of fibrous tissue and fewer giant cells. A distinctive feature is eosinophilic perivascular cuffing of collagen surrounding small capillaries throughout the lesion. Although this is not always present, perivascular collagen cuffing is regarded as pathognomonic for cherubism.

Differential Diagnosis. Diagnosis is supported by the radiographic features, clinical presentation, and family history. Clinical differential diagnosis of bilateral jaw swelling should include hyperparathyroidism, infantile cortical hyperostosis, and multiple odontogenic keratocysts. Unilateral swelling in children requires inclusion of fibrous dysplasia, central giant cell granuloma, histiocytosis, and odontogenic tumors.

Treatment and Prognosis. The prognosis is relatively good, particularly if the disease is limited to only one jaw—especially the mandible. After a rapid pace of bone expansion, the disease is usually self-limiting and regressive. Radiographic evidence of the condition tends to persist. Lesions of the maxilla act in a more aggressive manner and occasionally pose serious anatomic considerations. Although it is generally accepted that spontaneous regression begins at puberty, with relatively good resolution by age 30, no long-term follow-up of spontaneous resolution has been documented. Surgical intervention must be based on the need to improve function, prevent debility, and satisfy aesthetic considerations. If necessary, conservative curettage of the lesion with bone recontouring may be performed.

Osteopetrosis

Osteopetrosis is an uncommon hereditary bone condition characterized by a generalized symmetric increase in skeletal density and abnormalities of bone resorption remodeling. In 1904, the first case of generalized sclerosis of the skeleton was reported by Albers-Schönberg.

Osteopetrosis may be divided into three clinical groups. The infantile-malignant form is autosomal recessive in nature and is fatal within the first 2 to 3 years of life in the absence of treatment. An intermediate autosomal recessive type is nonfatal or "malignant," with onset usually within the first decade. An autosomal dominant form is the least severe form, with full life expectancy but with considerable morbidity secondary to orthopedic alterations.

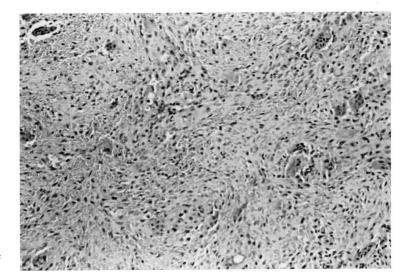

Figure 15–16. Cherubism. Note the giant cells in a fibrous stroma.

Etiology and Pathogenesis. The characteristic feature of osteopetrosis is an absence of physiologic bone resorption due to reduced osteoclastic activity. Animal studies have shown that osteoclasts do not respond appropriately to the presence of parathyroid hormone or to physiologic stimuli that normally promote bone resorption. The osteoclasts fail to undergo membrane elaboration to form the so-called ruffled border and allow release of lysosomal enzymes at the bone cell interface. The lack of bone resorption results in accumulation of bone mass and manifests itself in skeletal disturbances, including bone cavity occlusion, decreased hematopoietic activity, and growth retardation.

Recent progress toward further understanding of the mechanism of this disease has occurred at the molecular level and by way of gene mutation identification. The osteoclast defect may be intrinsic via osteoclast lineage or to the supportive environment of mesenchymal cell precursors of the osteoclast. Experimental studies have identified alternations of colony-stimulating factor (CSF-1), which serves as a growth factor for mononuclear phagocytes and osteoclasts. Experimental genetic manipulation by way of disruption of the *c-ser* proto-oncogene has led to osteopetrosis with formation of functional osteoclasts. A second oncogene, the *c-fos* proto-oncogene, when disrupted results in osteopetrosis by a complete absence of osteoclasts. The fundamental defect in the severe experimental forms of this condition concerns itself with the inability of hematopoietic precursors either to enter or to progress beyond the earliest stages of osteoclast development or differentiation. Carbonic anhydrase II deficiency in humans with the autosomal recessive form of this disease has been identified.

Clinical Features. Bone pain is the most frequent symptom. Cranial nerve compression may result in blindness, deafness, anosmia, ageusia, and sometimes facial paralysis. Normal cortical and cancellous bone is replaced by a dense, poorly structured bone that is fragile and has a propensity for pathologic fracture.

Delayed dental eruption is due to bony ankylosis, absence of alveolar bone resorption, and formation of pseudo-odontomas during apicogenesis. Premature exfoliation may be due to a defect in the periodontal ligament.

Infantile osteopetrosis is the most severe form of the disease. It is usually present at birth and is diagnosed within the first few months of life (Fig. 15–17). Patients with this condition rarely survive adolescence, and death is usually the result of infection or anemia. Hematologic manifestations result from a decrease in the marrow compartment, causing anemia, thrombocytopenia, and pancytopenia. Hepatosplenomegaly, secondary to compensatory extramedullary hematopoiesis, is often a feature.

The clinically benign adult form develops later in life and may not be diagnosed until the third or fourth decade. Bone involvement is similar to that

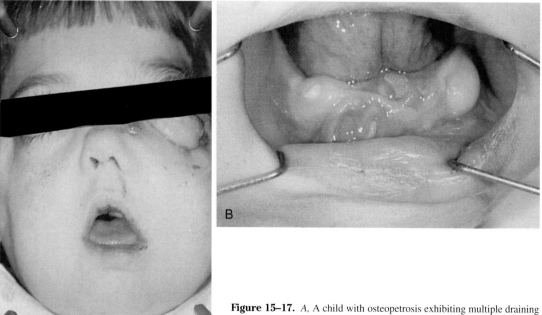

Figure 15–17. *A,* A child with osteopetrosis exhibiting multiple draining sinuses in the left infraorbital region. *B,* Malformed teeth with enamel hypoplasia and dental caries in this patient with osteopetrosis.

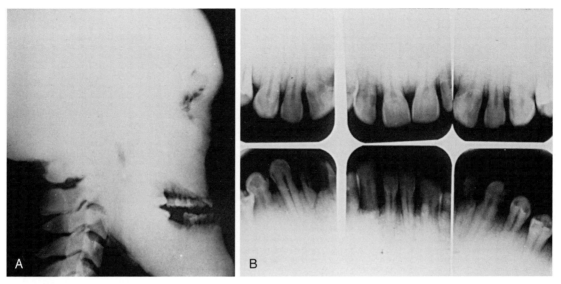

Figure 15–18. *A* and *B,* Radiographs obtained in the late stage of osteopetrosis.

in the malignant recessive type. Optic and facial nerve impairment is frequently present owing to narrowing of cranial foramina and resultant pressure on the nerves. The first sign of the disease often is pathologic fracture.

Dental findings include delayed eruption, congenitally absent teeth, unerupted and malformed teeth, and enamel hypoplasia. Decreased alveolar bone production, defective and abnormally thickened periodontal ligament, and marked mandibular prognathism have been reported. An elevated caries index may be secondary to enamel hypoplasia. This has serious implications owing to the propensity for development of osteomyelitis resulting from inadequate host response because of the diminished vascular component of osteopetrotic bone. Osteomyelitis is a serious complication of the disease; it occurs most frequently in the mandible and occasionally in the maxilla, scapula, and extremities.

Radiographic findings are characteristic of this disease. The classic bone-within-bone radiographic presentation is due to a defect in metaphyseal bone remodeling resulting in greatly thickened cortices and medullary space obliteration. The skeletal density generally is greatly increased owing to a uniform diffuse sclerosing of all bones (Fig. 15–18). The mandible is less frequently involved than are other bones. Loss of the distinct interface between the cortex and medulla appears, along with clubbing of the long bones with transverse peripheral banding.

Histopathology. Osteopetrosis is histologically characterized by normal production of bone with absence of physiologic bone resorption (Fig. 15–

19). The pattern of endochondral bone formation is disrupted, with a decrease in osteoclastic function and a compensatory increase in numbers of osteoclasts. This results in failure to develop normal lamellar structure in the bone and an absence of definable marrow cavities. Biopsy specimens of endochondral bone exhibit a core of calcified cartilage surrounded by bone matrix.

Endosteal bone has been described as exhibiting three distinct patterns: a pattern with a tortuous arrangement of lamellar trabeculae, an amorphous pattern, and an osteophilic pattern. An abundance of multinucleated osteoclasts and aggregated bony lacunae void of cellular components is often noted.

Unerupted teeth demonstrate areas of ankylosis at the cementum-bone interface in a jigsaw-puzzle pattern. The continuity of the periodontal membrane in ankylosed teeth is disrupted. The periodontal ligament is often composed of fibrous connective tissue, running parallel to the two surfaces, and an associated inflammatory infiltrate. In regions where osteomyelitis develops, marrow spaces appear fibrotic and contain chronic inflammatory cells.

Treatment and Prognosis. The prognosis for infantile osteopetrosis is poor, with patiens rarely surviving adolescence. Recent medical advances designed to increase osteoclast differentiation and activity using high-dose calcitrol have proved helpful. Bone marrow transplantation in the severe childhood or malignant forms of this disease have been performed in an effort to provide monocyte osteoclast precursors and the resultant production of cytokines with osteoclastotropic properties pro-

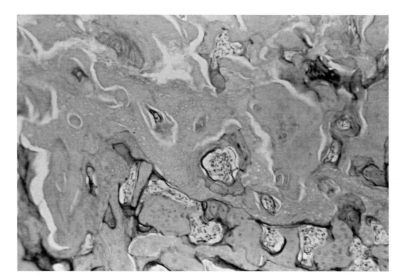

Figure 15–19. Photomicrograph of dense sclerotic bone of osteopetrosis.

duced within the microenvironment of bone remodeling packets.

Death results from secondary infection or anemia. The adult variety is more variable and insidious. Bone involvement is similar to the infantile recessive type but is usually less severe. The diagnosis often is not made until a pathologic fracture occurs. The differential diagnosis should include osteomalacia, Paget's disease, hyperparathyroidism, acromegaly, and malignant bone disease.

Management should be directed at recognition and treatment of complications, with frequent testing of visual fields and sight acuity and periodic radiographic examination of the optic foramina. Transfusion may be required for anemia, and splenectomy may be useful in some patients. Therapy is often directed at controlling the hematologic component of the disorder with systemic steroids.

Owing to the high risk of developing osteomyelitis, initiation of dental preventive regimens, similar to those for patients at risk for osteoradionecrosis, should be considered. This includes the implementation of frequent dental evaluations, use of topical and systemic fluorides, and fastidious home care programs.

Osteogenesis Imperfecta

Osteogenesis imperfecta represents a genetically heterogeneous group of heritable defects of connective tissue. Classically, this condition or syndrome may include fragile bones, blue sclerae, ligamentous laxity, hearing loss, and dentinogenesis imperfecta. Some affected patients exhibit extreme bone fragility with numerous fractures and die during the perinatal period; others suffer

only mild bone fragility and live a normal life span. Clinical presentation and severity are extremely variable. Patients with osteogenesis imperfecta are classified according to their clinical and radiographic manifestations, as well as by inheritance pattern. Four distinct types have been identified: two inherited as autosomal dominant traits, one inherited as an autosomal recessive trait, and one inherited as both an autosomal dominant and autosomal recessive trait. The presence of numerous long bone fractures early in life with dentinogenesis imperfecta, blue sclerae, or both is sufficient to establish the diagnosis. Early hearing loss in a patient or a member of a family with a history of fragile bones is highly suggestive of the disorder.

Etiology and Pathogenesis. Osteogenesis imperfecta is probably the most common inherited bone disease. It is estimated that approximately 30,000 individuals in the United States have osteogenesis imperfecta, and owing to its variable clinical expression, many mildly affected patients remain undiagnosed. Osteogenesis imperfecta type I is the most common variety; it has an incidence of about 1 in 30,000 live births. It is a mild to moderately severe disorder with an autosomal dominant mode of inheritance. Considerable variability in the inheritance is noted. Type II is the most severe form; it has a reported incidence of 1 in 100,000 deliveries. It has an autosomal recessive transmission, although spontaneous cases are reported. Type III, which has both an autosomal dominant and an autosomal recessive mode of inheritance, and type IV, which is transmitted autosomal dominantly, are intermediate in severity.

Biochemical findings suggest that osteogenesis imperfecta syndromes are a result of inborn errors of collagen metabolism. Most forms of the disease are believed to be caused by mutations in the structural genes for the collagen protein. The primary biochemical defect in most cases appears to involve the biosynthesis of type I collagen. The heterogeneity of these defects is at least in part explained by the more than 400 mutations in 6 of the 19 identified forms of collagen. More specifically, genetic mutations have been identified for both pro-alpha chains of type 1 procollagen in this disease.

Clinical Features. Osteogenesis imperfecta has also been termed *brittle bone disease* because of the principal clinical manifestation of bony fragility. Patients may exhibit joint hypermobility, excessive diaphoresis, and a tendency to bruise easily. Respiratory compromise and pulmonary infection are secondary to thoracic deformities. Mitral valve clicks are frequently auscultated. Hearing loss is common, and deafness may be conductive, sensorineural, or mixed in origin. Osteogenesis imperfecta type I is characterized by osteoporosis, bone fragility, blue sclerae, and conductive hearing loss in adolescents and adults. The sclera coloring is distinctive and is described as deep blue-black. Fractures may be present at birth in 10% of patients or may commence during infancy or childhood. There is considerable variability in the age of onset, frequency of fractures, and degree of skeletal deformity. Generally, birth weight and height are normal. Mild short stature is postnatal in onset and relates to the degree of involvement of the limbs and spine. Long bone deformities tend to be mild, with bowing of the limbs and angulation deformities occurring at previous fracture sites. Progressive kyphoscoliosis is seen in 20% of adults and may be severe. Hyperlaxity of ligaments of the hands, feet, and knees is common in children. Hearing impairment, which usually begins in the second decade of life, is present in 35% of adults. Dentinogenesis imperfecta is present in some patients with type I.

Type II osteogenesis imperfecta is a lethal syndrome, with half of all patients stillborn. It has an autosomal recessive mode of transmission, although spontaneous cases are reported. It is characterized in infancy by low birth weight, short stature, and broad thighs extending at right angles to the trunk. The limbs are short, curved, and grossly deformed. The skin is thin and frail and may be torn during delivery. Cranial vault ossification is lacking, and the facies is notable for hypotelorism, a small beaked nose, and a triangular shape. Defects in skeletal ossification lead to extreme bone fragility and frequent fractures, even during delivery. Dental abnormalities have been found, including atubular dentin with a lacework

of argyrophilic fiber structures, an absence of predentin, and an abundance of argyrophilic fibers in the coronal pulp.

Type III osteogenesis imperfecta is a rare disorder characterized in neonates by severe bone fragility, multiple fractures, and progressive skeletal deformity. The sclerae are blue at birth, but the color diminishes with age; adolescents and adults exhibit normal sclera coloration. Childhood mortality is high owing to cardiopulmonary complications, and prognosis is poor because of severe kyphoscoliosis. Individuals with type III exhibit the shortest stature of all patients with osteogenesis imperfecta. Dentinogenesis imperfecta is found in some patients with type III osteogenesis imperfecta. Hearing impairment has not been reported in these children.

Osteogenesis imperfecta type IV is a dominantly inherited osteopenia leading to bone fragility, without the other classic features associated with the osteogenesis imperfecta syndromes. The sclerae are bluish at birth only. Onset of fractures ranges from birth to adulthood, and the skeletal deformities are extremely variable. Bowing of the lower limbs at birth may be the only feature of this syndrome, and progressive deformities of the long bones and vertebral column may occur without fractures. Spontaneous improvement often occurs with puberty. Dentinogenesis imperfecta is seen in some patients with type IV. The frequency of hearing impairment in adults is low.

Dentinogenesis imperfecta associated with osteogenesis imperfecta is described as a blue, brown, or amber opalescent discoloration of teeth. The primary teeth are more severely affected than the permanent dentition (Fig. 15–20). Considerable variation is observed in expression of the discoloration, ranging from all teeth being affected to only a few. Teeth that are discolored are more prone to enamel wear and fracture. The crowns are described as shortened and bellshaped, with a cervical constriction. The roots are narrow and short, and partial or complete pulpal obliteration occurs. A high frequency of class II malocclusions and a high incidence of impacted first and second molars have been reported.

Differential Diagnosis. In children, osteogenesis imperfecta must be differentiated from other conditions resulting in multiple bony fractures. Fractures in children with normal skeletal mass may occur in battered baby and congenital indifference to pain syndromes. Idiopathic juvenile osteoporosis and Cushing's disease may cause a generalized osteopenia resulting in pathologic fractures.

Treatment and Prognosis. There is no specific treatment for this condition. Management of frac-

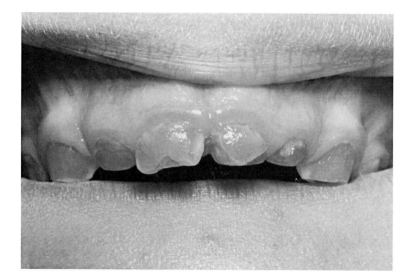

Figure 15–20. Primary teeth of a child with osteogenesis imperfecta. The classic opalescent discoloration is notable.

tures may be a significant orthopedic challenge. Rehabilitation and physical therapy for recurrent fractures, limb deformities, and kyphoscoliosis are suggested. Middle ear surgery may correct hearing loss. With the onset of puberty, the severity of this problem frequently lessens. When dentinogenesis imperfecta is a concern, management is focused around the preservation of the teeth. Generally, the primary dentition is more problematic. To prevent wear and improve aesthetic appearance, full crown coverage may be necessary.

Because of the wide variation in clinical expression, prognosis ranges from very good (dominant form) to very poor (recessive form). Genetic counseling is essential, and patient support groups may provide needed emotional support to affected individuals and their families.

Cleidocranial Dysplasia

Cleidocranial dysplasia is notable for aplasia or hypoplasia of the clavicles, characteristic craniofacial malformations, and the presence of numerous supernumerary and unerupted teeth.

Etiology and Pathogenesis. Cleidocranial dysplasia is transmitted by an autosomal dominant mode of inheritance with high penetrance and variable expressivity. A recessive form has been reported in two families. About one third of cases are sporadic and appear to represent new mutations. It occurs with equal frequency among males and females; there is no racial predilection. Most patients with the disease are of normal intelligence. Studies involving a large kindred of more than 1000 people in South Africa have isolated the origin of this disorder to the short arm of

chromosome 6 (a microdeletion defect). Studies have identified transcription factor (CBFA1) as causative in production of this disorder.

Intramembranous and endochondral bones in the skull are affected, resulting in a sagittally diminished cranial base, transverse enlargement of the calvarium, and delayed closure of the fontanelles and sutures. Hydrocephalic pressure on unossified regions of the skull, especially the fontanelles, causes biparietal and frontal bossing and extension of the cranial vault. The deficiency of the clavicles is responsible for the long appearance of the neck and the narrow shoulders. The combined abnormalities of the middle third of the face and the dental alveolar complex result in the characteristic facial appearance.

Delayed or failed eruption of the teeth has been associated with lack of cellular cementum. It is postulated that failure of cementum formation may be due to mechanical resistance to eruption by the dense alveolar bone overlying the unerupted teeth. Formation of supernumerary teeth is due to incomplete or severely delayed resorption of the dental lamina, which is reactivated at the time of crown completion of the normal permanent dentition.

Clinical Features. The clinical appearance of cleidocranial dysplasia is so distinct that it is pathognomonic. The stature is mildly to moderately shortened, with the neck appearing long and narrow and the shoulders markedly drooped. Complete or partial absence of clavicular calcification, with associated muscle defects, results in hypermobility of the shoulders, allowing for variable levels of approximation in an anterior plane (Fig. 15–21A).

The head is large and brachycephalic. Patients

have pronounced frontal, parietal, and occipital bossing. The facial bones and paranasal sinuses are hypoplastic, giving the face a small and short appearance. The nose is broad based, with a depressed nasal bridge. Ocular hypertelorism is frequently present. The entire skeleton may be affected, with defects of the pelvis, long bones, and fingers. Hemivertebrae and posterior wedging of the thoracic vertebrae may contribute to the development of kyphoscoliosis and pulmonary complications.

Maxillary hypoplasia gives the mandible a relatively prognathic appearance, although some patients may show variable mandibular prognathism due to increased length of the mandible in conjunction with a short cranial base. The palate is narrow and highly arched, and there is an increased incidence of submucosal clefts and complete or partial clefts of the palate involving the hard and soft tissues. Non-union of the symphysis of the mandible is seen.

The formation, maturation, and eruption of the deciduous dentition are usually normal. Extreme delay in physiologic root resorption occurs, however, and the result is prolonged exfoliation of primary teeth. The permanent dentition is severely delayed, and many teeth fail to erupt. Unerupted supernumerary teeth are frequently present in all regions (Fig. 15–21*B*). They develop on completion of normal crown formation in the permanent dentition lingual and occlusal to the normal unerupted crown. Only one supernumerary per normal tooth is generally noted. The over-retention of deciduous teeth, failure of eruption of permanent teeth, numerous supernumerary teeth, and maxillary hypoplasia result in severe malocclusion.

Radiographic findings of clinical significance pertain to the abnormalities of the craniofacial region, dentition, clavicles, and pelvis. Radiographs of the skull classically exhibit patent fontanelles and wormian bones, broad and anomalous cranial sutures, and underdeveloped paranasal sinuses. The clavicles may be aplastic unilaterally or bilaterally, or they may be hypoplastic, appearing as small fragments attached to the sternum or acromial process. The mandible and maxilla contain many unerupted and supernumerary teeth, which are often malpositioned.

Treatment. There is no specific treatment for patients with cleidocranial dysplasia. Genetic counseling is most important. Protective headgear may be recommended while fontanelles remain patent. The current mode of therapy for the dental anomalies combines early surgical intervention with orthodontic therapy. Extraction of supernumerary teeth and over-retained primary teeth, when the root formation of succedaneous teeth is greater than 50%, is followed by surgical exposure of unerupted teeth and orthodontic treatment. Early surgical exposure of unerupted teeth has resulted in stimulation of cementum formation and eruption of the dentition with normal root formation. Orthognathic surgery for correction of the

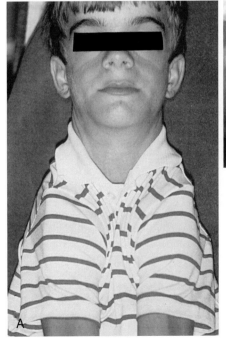
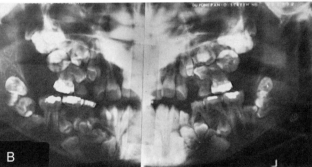

Figure 15–21. *A*, This patient with cleidocranial dysplasia is able to approximate his shoulders in this classic pose owing to hypoplasia of the clavicles. *B*, Multiple unerupted and malpositioned teeth are evident. The premolar regions are remarkable for numerous supernumerary teeth.

dental-facial deformity, postsurgical orthodontics, and prosthetics can be anticipated.

Crouzon's Syndrome (Craniofacial Dysostosis)

Crouzon's syndrome is characterized by variable cranial deformity, maxillary hypoplasia, and shallow orbits with exophthalmos and divergent strabismus. The character of the cranial deformity depends on the sutures affected, the degree of involvement, and the sequence of sutural fusion. Increased interpupillary distance and exophthalmos are constant features of Crouzon's syndrome and develop in early childhood owing to premature synostosis of the coronal suture. Systemic complications include mental retardation, hearing loss, speech and visual impairment, and convulsions.

Etiology and Pathogenesis. Craniofacial dysostosis is inherited in an autosomal dominant mode, with complete penetrance and variable expressivity. About one third of the cases reported arise spontaneously. The severity of expression of the disease increases in successive siblings, with the youngest child most severely affected.

Craniosynostosis results when premature fusion of the cranial sutures occurs. The cause is not known, but premature closure of these sutures can initiate changes in the brain, secondary to increased intracranial pressure.

The deformities of the cranial bones and orbital cavities are the result of the fusion of sutures and increased intracranial pressure. Underdevelopment of the supraorbital ridges and overgrowth of the sphenoid wing results in small and shallow orbits. Exophthalmos and reduced orbital volume are the result. Hypertelorism is accentuated by a downward and forward displacement of the ethmoid plate. Abnormalities of the bony orbit account for several functional ocular abnormalities. Severe distortion of the cranial base leads to reduced maxillary growth and nasopharyngeal hypoplasia with potential upper airway restriction.

Clinical Features. Patients with Crouzon's syndrome have a characteristic facies often described as frog-like. Midface hypoplasia and exophthalmos are striking (Fig. 15–22). Patients have relative mandibular prognathism, with the nose resembling a parrot's beak. The upper lip and philtrum are usually short, and the lower lip often droops. The cranial deformity is dependent on which sutures are involved. Proptosis with strabismus and orbital hypertelorism is common. Optic nerve damage occurs in 80% of cases.

Oral findings include severe maxillary hypopla-

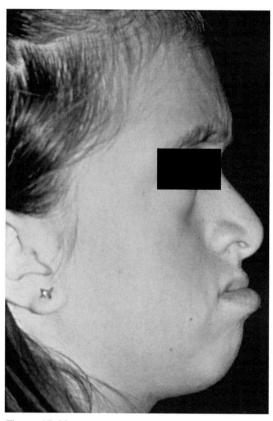

Figure 15–22. Severe maxillary hypoplasia, proptosis, and a short philtrum are noted in this patient with Crouzon's syndrome. (Courtesy of Dr. A. Shanske.)

sia, resulting in a narrowing of the maxillary arch and a compressed, high-arched palate. Bilateral posterior lingual crossbites are common. Premature posterior occlusion as a result of the inferiorly positioned maxilla results in an anterior open bite.

Radiographs of the skull reveal obliterated suture lines with obvious bony continuity. A hammered-silver appearance is often seen in regions of the skull where compensatory deformity cannot occur. Lordosis of the cranial base is apparent on lateral skull projections, and angular deformities with vertical sloping of the anterior cranial fossa can be visualized. A large calvarium with hypoplasia of the maxilla, shallow orbits, and a relatively large mandible is common.

The differential diagnosis of Crouzon's syndrome should include simple craniosynostosis, as well as the Apert, Pfeiffer, and Saethre-Chotzen syndromes.

Treatment and Prognosis. The age of onset and the degree of craniosynostosis influence the severity of the complications, which range from craniofacial dystrophy to hearing loss, speech and visual impairment, and mental retardation. With a high degree of suspicion, the condition is often identifiable at birth. Ultrasonic prenatal diagnosis of exophthalmos has been reported. Early recognition is essential to guide growth and development of the face and cranium. Surgical intervention may be necessary if exophthalmos is progressive, optic nerve damage or visual acuity is impaired, evidence of developing mental deficiency is noted, or intracranial pressure continues to rise. Treatment includes the surgical placement of artificial sutures to allow growth of the brain while minimizing intracranial pressure and secondary calvarial deformities. Orthodontic treatment with subsequent orthognathic surgical intervention has been successful in managing the concomitant dentofacial deformity.

Treacher Collins Syndrome (Mandibulofacial Dysostosis)

Treacher Collins syndrome primarily affects structures developing from the first branchial arch, but it also involves the second branchial arch to a minor degree. Individuals have a convex facial profile with a prominent nose and retrusive chin. It is generally a bilateral anomaly with a characteristic facies including downward sloping of the palpebral fissures, colobomas of the lower eyelid, mandibular and midface hypoplasia, and deformed pinnas.

Etiology and Pathogenesis. Treacher Collins syndrome is transmitted by an autosomal dominant mode of inheritance, although about half the cases are due to spontaneous mutation. The gene has a high degree of penetrance, but variable expressivity is common. Affected siblings are remarkably similar, and the syndrome becomes progressively more severe in succeeding generations. This disorder is relatively rare, with an incidence between 0.5 and 10.6 cases per 10,000 births.

It is believed that the embryologic and morphologic defects that result in the phenotypic expression of this syndrome begin as early as the sixth to seventh embryonic week. A defect in the stapedial artery during embryogenesis may be responsible for the anatomic deficits seen. Stapedial artery dysfunction gives rise to defects of the stapes and incus and the first arch vessels supplying the maxilla. Failure of the inferior alveolar artery to develop an ancillary vascular supply gives rise to mandibular abnormalities. Improper orientation and hypoplasia of the mandibular elevator muscles, resulting from an aplastic or hypoplastic zygomatic arch, may also be contributory.

Mandibular retrognathia and midface vertical excess may be accentuated by the pull of abnormally oriented mandibular elevator muscles, causing a backward rotation in mandibular growth pattern. The syndrome seems to be limited to defects of the bones and soft tissue of the face. Vascularization of the posterior portion of the second visceral arch by the stapedial artery seems unimpaired.

Clinical Findings. Treacher Collins syndrome is a manifestation of combined developmental anomalies of the second and, mainly, first branchial arches. It includes various degrees of hypoplasia of the mandible, maxilla, zygomatic process of the temporal bone, and external and middle ear. Abnormalities of the medial pterygoid plates and hypoplasia of the lateral pterygoid muscles are common. Right-to-left asymmetry of the deformities is generally seen. In the fully expressed syndrome, the facial appearance is characteristic and is often described as bird-like or fish-like (Fig. 15–23).

Notched or linear colobomas of the outer third of the lower eyelids are found in 75% of patients. The lower eyelashes are absent medial to the colobomas in about 50% of patients. Antimongoloid obliquity or downward slanting of the palpebral fissures is striking.

Congenital atresia of the external auditory canal and microtia are often present. The ears are low set, with deformed, crumpled, or absent pinnae. Middle ear defects include fibrous bands of the long process of the incus, malformed and fixed stapes and malleus, and accompanying conductive hearing loss. Ear tags and blind fistulas are often located between the pinna and the commissures of the mouth.

Atypical hair growth in the shape of a tongue-like process extends from the hairline toward the cheeks. Other associated anomalies such as skeletal deformities and facial clefts may be concomitant.

Oral findings include cleft palate in about 30% of patients and macrostomia in 15% of patients. High-arched palate and dental malocclusion consisting of apertognathia and widely separated and displaced teeth are common. Severe mandibular hypoplasia is most characteristic. The underdeveloped zygomaticomaxillary complex leads to a clinically severe midface deficiency.

Treacher Collins syndrome is notable for characteristic radiographic findings including downward sloping floors of the orbits, peaked bony nasal contour, aplastic or hypoplastic zygomatic process of the temporal bone, and obtuse mandibular angle. Lateral cephalograms demonstrate antigonial notching and broad curvature of the mandible. The peculiar broad and concave nature of the

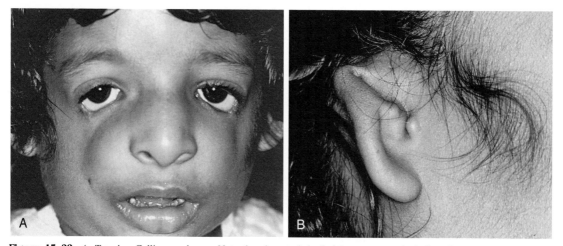

Figure 15–23. *A,* Treacher Collins syndrome. Note the characteristic facial appearance, including downward sloping of the palpebral fissures and colobomas of the lower eyelids. *B,* Microtia, or underdeveloped ear, and a narrow extension of hair over the preauricular region, known as a "hair lick," are common in patients with Treacher Collins syndrome.

inferior border of the mandible is characteristic and helps distinguish this condition from other syndromes involving the mandible. The condyle and coronoid processes are frequently flattened or aplastic.

Treatment and Prognosis. Treatment is directed at correction or reconstruction of the existing deformities. Neutralization of conductive hearing loss through surgery and hearing aids is helpful. Ophthalmologic surgery to correct eye deformities by orbital reconstruction is often performed. Extensive orthodontic treatment before orthognathic surgical reconstruction of the mandible and maxilla can be anticipated.

Pierre Robin Syndrome

The clinical presentation of micrognathia, glossoptosis, and high-arched or cleft palate in neonates has been termed the *Pierre Robin syndrome.* This malformation complex can occur as an isolated finding or as a component of various syndromes or developmental anomalies. The mandibular retrognathia and hypoplasia is considered the primary malformation. Respiratory and feeding problems are prevalent and may result in episodic airway obstruction, infant hypoxia, malnutrition, and failure to thrive.

Etiology and Pathogenesis. The incidence of Pierre Robin syndrome is 5.3 to 22.7 per 100,000 births, with 39% of the infants exhibiting no additional abnormalities. Of the remaining infants, 25% have known syndromes, and 36% have one or more anomalies that are not part of a known syndrome.

Fetal malposition and interposition of the tongue between the palatal shelves have long been considered the etiologic catalysts for palatal deformity and micrognathia. Arrest of mandibular development may prevent descent of the tongue and failure of palatal shelf elevation and fusion. Evidence suggests that the primary defect may be due to genetically influenced metabolic growth disturbances of the maxilla and mandible rather than to mechanical obstruction by the tongue during embryogenesis. Organogenetic differences lead to the variable presentation of micrognathia and cleft palate.

Clinical Features. Infants present with severe micrognathia and mandibular hypoplasia (Fig. 15–24). A U-shaped cleft palate is a common but not

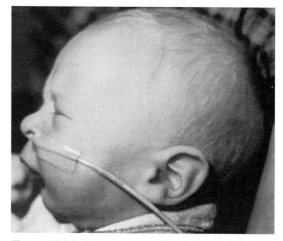

Figure 15–24. Severe micrognathia of the mandible in an infant with Pierre Robin syndrome. (Courtesy of Dr. A. Shanske.)

constant feature, and in some instances, the palate is highly arched. Glossoptosis is the result of the retropositional attachment of the genioglossus muscle because of the retrognathic mandible. The geniohyoid muscle is foreshortened, so that support to the hyoid bone and strap muscles of the larynx is also compromised.

Treatment and Prognosis. Respiratory and feeding problems are frequent in the immediate postnatal and neonatal periods. Constant medical supervision may be necessary to prevent airway obstruction and hypoxia, cor pulmonale, gastroesophageal reflux, bronchopneumonia, and exhaustion. In most cases, conservative repositioning of the infant and frequent prone posture are sufficient to prevent upper airway obstruction, by making optimal use of the effects of gravity during resting and feeding. Continuous pulse oximetry and apnea monitoring are prudent during the neonatal period. In severe cases with chronic upper airway obstruction and failure to thrive, intraoral or nasal pharyngeal airway placement, some surgical form of tongue and lip adhesion, and even tracheostomy as a last resort may be considered. Feeding infants with mandibular hypoplasia requires expertise and patience. Nasogastric feeding tubes may be required. After the first few months of life, mandibular growth and improved control of tongue musculature result in significant abatement of symptoms.

The growth of the mandible is remarkable during the first 4 years of life, and a normal profile is often achieved between 4 and 6 years of age. Some patients have a residual mild mandibular retrognathia requiring treatment later in life.

Marfan's Syndrome

Marfan's syndrome is a heritable disorder of connective tissue, characterized by abnormalities of the skeletal, cardiovascular, and ocular systems. It is currently estimated that 23,000 Americans have Marfan's syndrome. Diagnosis is problematic because of the extreme variability of clinical expression. The disorder is notable for a number of sudden catastrophic deaths that have occurred in affected (undiagnosed) athletes.

Etiology and Pathogenesis. Marfan's syndrome is an autosomal dominant–inherited disorder that affects 1 in 10,000 individuals. There are no ethnic, racial, or gender predilections. The condition exhibits complete but extremely variable penetrance, with the offspring of an affected individual having a 50% chance of acquiring the disorder. Approximately 15 to 35% of cases arise spontaneously, as a result of gamete gene mutation

in the ovum or sperm; a greater number occur with increasing paternal age. The Marfan gene is believed to produce a change in one of the proteins that provides strength to a component of connective tissue, probably collagen. The gene has been located on chromosome 15 and will provide for diagnostic testing in pairs at risk. Recent studies involving factors responsible for assisting in microfibril formation have identified the gene for fibrillin (FBN1) as the disease-causing gene in this disorder. Diagnosis is currently based on characteristic abnormalities of the musculoskeletal, ocular, and cardiovascular systems and a positive family history. Because most features progress with age, the diagnosis is often more obvious in older persons.

Clinical Features. Patients characteristically possess a tall, slender stature with relatively long legs and arms, large hands with long fingers, and loose joints. The arms, legs, and digits are disproportionately long compared with the patient's trunk. Chest deformities include a protrusion or indentation of the breast bone (pectus carinatum, pectus excavatum). The normal thoracic kyphosis is often absent, leading to a straight back. Various degrees of scoliosis are present. Oral findings include a narrow, high-arched palate and dental crowding. The face appears long and narrow.

The cardiovascular system is affected in nearly all persons. Mitral valve prolapse occurs in 75 to 85% of affected patients, and a small percentage develop mitral regurgitation. Ascending aortic dilatation may result in aortic regurgitation and heart failure. Progressive dissection of the aorta may lead to aneurysms, placing patients at great risk for a catastrophic episode.

Ocular findings include dislocation of the lens (ectopia lentis), which occurs in half these patients. The most common eye anomaly, however, is myopia (nearsightedness). Retinal detachment occurs infrequently, but it is more prevalent after lens removal.

Treatment and Prognosis. Morbidity and mortality are directly related to the degree of connective tissue abnormality in the involved organ systems. The cardiovascular abnormalities of ascending aorta dilatation and mitral valve prolapse, subluxation of the lens of the eye, chest cavity deformities and scoliosis, and potential for pneumothorax are serious prognostic indicators.

Treatment of patients with Marfan's syndrome consists of annual medical examinations with a cardiovascular emphasis, frequent ophthalmologic examination, scoliosis screening, and echocardiography. Physical activity often is restricted and redirected in an attempt to protect the aorta.

Antibiotic prophylaxis has been recommended

for infective endocarditis, regardless of the clinical evidence of valvular disease. Beta-blockers such as propranolol are often used to reduce aortic stress and have been shown to significantly reduce both the rate of aortic dilatation and the risk of serious complications. Mortality has been drastically reduced with the use of composite grafts to replace the aortic valve and the region containing the aortic aneurysm. The prognosis for untreated ascending aorta aneurysm is extremely poor.

Ehlers-Danlos Syndrome

The Ehlers-Danlos syndrome is an uncommon inherited disorder of connective tissue, clinically characterized by joint hypermobility, skin hyperextensibility, and fragility. The clinical manifestations of the disease are due to inherited defects in collagen metabolism. In addition to the skin and joint anomalies, severe cardiovascular and gastrointestinal complications may occur and coexist.

The condition has been classified into eight variants. The periodontal form (Ehlers-Danlos syndrome type VIII) is characterized by rapidly progressing periodontal disease resulting in complete tooth loss by the second or third decade of life.

Etiology and Pathogenesis. Various subtypes of Ehlers-Danlos syndrome are inherited as autosomal dominant, autosomal recessive, and X-linked traits. The clinical presentations of the recessively inherited forms are more severe.

At least 10 subtypes of Ehlers-Danlos syndrome have been classified, on the basis of genetic, biochemical, and clinical characteristics. For instance, in the potentially lethal type 4 variant, mutations in the gene for type III procollagen have been identified. Mutations in the lysyl hydrolase gene are associated with the type 6 variant, whereas types 7a and 7b are related to type I collagen gene mutations.

From a clinical standpoint, defects in type III collagen formation are associated with spontaneous mixture of the aorta or intestines, tissues rich in type III collagen. Deficiencies in collagen hydroxylysine are secondary to depressed levels of lysyl hydroxylase. Others may have a defect in collagen metabolism, preventing the conversion of procollagen to collagen. Also, a disorder of copper metabolism has been noted in some patients.

Clinical Features. Classic clinical features include marked hyperelasticity of the skin and extreme laxity of the joints (Fig. 15–25). The skin may be stretched for several centimeters, but when released, it resumes its former contours. Skin manifestations include a velvety appearance with a high degree of fragility and a tendency toward bruising. Minor trauma may produce ecchymoses, bleeding, and large gaping wounds with poor healing tendencies and cigarette-paper scar formation, especially evident on the forehead and lower legs and over pressure points. Other cutaneous findings include molluscoid pseudotumors, redundant skin on the palms and soles, and subcutaneous lipid-containing cysts, which may calcify.

Articular hypermobility is variable. It may be of sufficient severity to cause spontaneous dislocation of the joints. Extreme joint laxity leads to genu recurvatum (back knee), flat feet, habitual joint dislocation, kyphoscoliosis, and other skeletal deformities.

Patients may have severe cardiovascular, gastrointestinal, and pulmonary manifestations. Cardio-

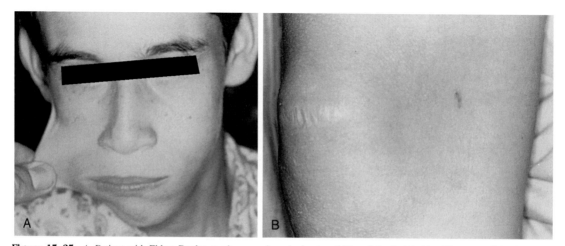

Figure 15–25. *A,* Patient with Ehlers-Danlos syndrome and marked extensibility of the facial skin. (Courtesy of Dr. H. Diner.) *B,* Minor trauma may produce cigarette-paper scar formation, as seen on the knee of this patient with Ehlers-Danlos syndrome.

vascular anomalies include dissecting aortic aneurysm, mitral valve prolapse, and rupture of major blood vessels. The majority of patients have a bleeding diathesis that may consist of a tendency to bruise, or may be severe, with hematoma formation and bleeding from the nose, gut, lungs, and urogenital tract.

Rupture of the bowel and bladder may occur. Pulmonary problems include spontaneous pneumothorax and respiratory impairment, secondary to chest wall deformities. Hernias, gastrointestinal diverticula, and ocular defects may be encountered.

Orofacial features include a narrow maxilla, flattened midface, and wide nasal bridge. Other facial findings include hypertelorism, epicanthal folds, a hollowed appearance of the eyes, and scarring of the forehead and chin. Fragility of gingival and mucosal tissues may be problematic. The incidence of temporomandibular joint dysfunction is increased as a result of profound laxity of the joint, contributing to hypermobility and dislocation. Marked extensibility of the tongue, enabling contact with the tip of the nose, has been described.

Dental findings include deep anatomic grooves and excessive cuspal height of the molars and premolars. Stunted or dilacerated roots and the presence of free-floating coronal pulp stones secondary to alteration and calcification of intrapulpal vascular structures have been noted. Irregular composition of dentinal tubules, denticles, and enamel hypoplasia is often seen.

Treatment and Prognosis. Prognosis is dependent on the severity of the systemic manifestations. The cardiovascular status of all patients should be evaluated and closely monitored. Sudden death in youth or early adult life may occur owing to dissecting aneurysms and ruptured arteries.

Surgical intervention must be tempered in light of connective tissue fragility. Joint ligament repair is often unsuccessful owing to suture failure. Wound healing is usually delayed, and prolonged bleeding may occur after injury. Osteoarthritis is a common complication in patients with repeated dislocations.

Down Syndrome (Trisomy 21)

Down syndrome is a common and easily recognizable chromosomal aberration. The incidence is reported to be 1 in 600 to 1 in 700 live births; however, more than half of the affected fetuses spontaneously abort during early pregnancy. Approximately 10 to 15% of all institutionalized patients have Down syndrome.

Most cases of trisomy 21 (94%) are caused by nondisjunction, resulting in an extra chromosome. The remaining patients with Down syndrome have various chromosomal abnormalities. The translocation type occurs in 3%, mosaicism occurs in 2%, and rare chromosomal aberrations make up the remaining 1% of cases. The incidence of this condition rises with increasing maternal age.

Etiology and Pathogenesis. Possible etiologies for Down syndrome include undetected mosaicism in a parent, repeated exposure to the same environmental insult, genetic predisposition to nondisjunction, an ovum with an extra 21 chromosome, or a preferential survival in utero of trisomy 21 embryos and fetuses with increasing maternal age. Parents of any age who have had one child with trisomy 21 have a significant risk (about 1%) of having a similarly affected child, a risk of recurrence equivalent to that affecting births to a mother older than 45 years. No racial, social, economic, or gender predilections have been identified.

Clinical Features. Patients with Down syndrome present with numerous characteristic clinical findings and various common systemic manifestations. A number of common phenotypic findings in children with Down syndrome have been identified; these can assist in establishing a diagnosis.

Various degrees of mental retardation exist in all patients with Down syndrome. Most mildly affected individuals are highly functioning and are able to perform well in a workshop environment. Dementia affects about 30% of patients with Down syndrome, and early aging is common. After age 35, nearly all individuals develop the neuropathologic changes analogous to those found in Alzheimer's disease, although 70% exhibit no clinically detectable behavioral changes. These two disorders have many neuropathologic and neurochemical similarities, and an increased risk for Down syndrome has been found in families with a predilection for Alzheimer's disease.

In Down syndrome, the skull is brachycephalic, with a flat occiput and prominent forehead (Fig. 15–26). A third or fourth fontanelle is present, and all the fontanelles are large and have extended patency. Sagittal suture separation greater than 5 mm is present in 98% of affected individuals. Frontal and sphenoid sinuses are absent, and the maxillary sinus is hypoplastic in more than 90% of patients. Midface skeletal deficiency is quite marked, with ocular hypotelorism, flattened nasal bridge, and relative mandibular prognathism.

The eyes are almond shaped, with upward-slant-

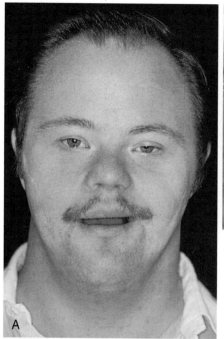

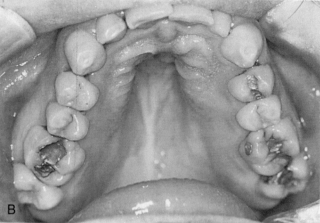

Figure 15–26. *A,* Typical facies of a patient with Down syndrome. Note the oblique palpebral fissures, prominent forehead, flat nasal bridge, and open mouth posture. *B,* The palate is highly vaulted, with decreased width and length.

ing palpebral fissures, epicanthic folds, and Brushfield spots of the iris frequently noted. Other ocular anomalies include convergent strabismus, nystagmus, refractive errors, keratoconus, and congenital cataracts.

Congenital heart disease is present in 30 to 45% of all patients with Down syndrome. Anomalies include complete atrioventricular canal, partial endocardial cushion abnormalities, and ventricular septal defects. A study revealed a 50% prevalence of mitral valve prolapse; one third of these patients had negative auscultatory findings. Tetralogy of Fallot, patent ductus arteriosus, and secundum atrial septal defects are seen less frequently.

It appears that T cell and probably B cell function is aberrant, with some affected children being more susceptible to infectious diseases. Respiratory tract infections are extremely common. Thyroid dysfunction occurs in upward of 50% of all patients. There is also an increased incidence of acute lymphocytic leukemia and hepatitis B antigen carrier status.

Skeletal problems include hypoplasia of the maxilla and sphenoid bones, rib and pelvic abnormalities, hip dislocation, and patella subluxation. Of particular concern is the presence of atlantoaxial instability in 12 to 20% of persons with Down syndrome, owing to the increased laxity of the transverse ligaments between the atlas and the odontoid process. Delay in recognizing this condition may result in irreversible spinal cord damage, which might occur during manipulation of the neck in patients undergoing dental therapy or general anesthesia.

Oral manifestations of Down syndrome are common. The tongue is often fissured, and macroglossia is usually relative to the small oral cavity, although true macroglossia is possible. Open-mouth posture is common, because a narrow nasopharynx and hypertrophied tonsils and adenoids cause upper airway compromise. A protruding tongue and frequent mouth breathing result in drying and cracking of the lips. Palatal width and length are significantly decreased, and bifid uvula and cleft lip and palate are occasionally observed. Elevated concentrations of sodium, calcium, and bicarbonate ion have been demonstrated in parotid saliva.

The dentition exhibits a number of characteristic anomalies, and periodontal disease is prevalent. The incidence of dental caries, however, appears to be no greater than in normal individuals. Considering the existence of poor oral hygiene, this may reflect the greater buffering capacity of the saliva or the ability to control dietary intake in institutional and home settings. The defective immune system directly contributes to rampant and precocious periodontal disease.

Eruption of both the primary and the permanent dentitions is delayed in 75% of cases. Abnormalities in eruption sequence occur frequently. Hypodontia occurs in both dentitions, and microdontia is often seen. Developmental tooth anomalies, including crown and root malformations, are often present. Almost 50% of patients with Down syndrome exhibit three or more dental anomalies. Enamel hypocalcification occurs in about 20% of patients.

Occlusal disharmonies consisting of mesioclusion owing to a relative prognathism, posterior crossbites, apertognathia, and severe crowding of the anterior teeth are common. Posterior crossbites are of maxillary basal bone origin, whereas anterior open bites are due to dental-alveolar discrepancies.

Treatment and Prognosis. Infants with Down syndrome that includes significant congenital heart disease have a poor prognosis. Causes of death frequently include cardiopulmonary complications, gastrointestinal malformations, and acute lymphoblastic leukemia.

Recent technologic advances in cardiovascular diagnosis have brought about a marked improvement in prognosis. Newborns require chest x-rays, electrocardiograms, echocardiograms, and subsequent pediatric cardiac consultation if cardiovascular anomalies are detected.

Regular ophthalmologic and audiologic follow-ups are extremely important. They can intercept early visual and hearing problems that may affect learning and development. Detection of atlantoaxial instability may prevent a catastrophic spinal injury.

Dental therapy is directed at prevention of dental caries and periodontal disease. Frequent follow-up and institution of stringent home care regimens are critical. Highly functioning children may be candidates for orthodontic intervention and subsequent maxillofacial surgery, if required. Guidelines established by the American Heart Association for antibiotic prophylaxis should be followed for those patients with congenital heart disease.

Hemifacial Atrophy

Hemifacial atrophy is a rare disorder that represents a progressive unilateral atrophy of the face. It may occasionally affect other regions on the same side of the body. The cause of this condition is totally unknown, although trauma, dysfunction of the peripheral nervous system, infection, and genetic abnormalities have been suggested.

Hemifacial atrophy typically appears during young adulthood. The most common early sign is a painless cleft or furrow near the midline of the face. The condition involves both soft tissue and bone of the affected side. Orally, the tongue, lips, and salivary glands may show hemiatrophy. Developing teeth may show incomplete root develop-

ment and delayed eruption. Unilateral involvement of the brain, ears, larynx, esophagus, diaphragm, and kidneys has been reported. Various associated ophthalmologic conditions are often encountered.

Progressive hemifacial atrophy associated with contralateral jacksonian epilepsy, trigeminal neuralgia, and changes in the eyes and hair is known as *Romberg's syndrome.* Unilateral atrophy of the upper lip with visible exposure of the maxillary teeth on the affected side is characteristic in moderately and severely involved cases.

The differential diagnosis should include facial hypoplasia, scleroderma, fat necrosis, and oculoauriculovertebral-related disorders. The distinction between Romberg's syndrome and localized scleroderma is often difficult and depends on the absence or presence of skin pigmentation and other inflammatory changes.

Hemifacial Hypertrophy

Congenital hemihypertrophy is a rare disorder characterized by gross body asymmetry. It may be simple, limited to a single digit; segmental, involving a specific region of the body; or complex, encompassing half the body. The enlargement is usually unilateral, although limited bilateral crossover does occur. All tissues in the region of abnormal growth may be involved, but a selective number of tissues are occasionally affected. Histologically, it has been determined that there is an actual increase in the number of cells present rather than an increase in cell size. It classically presents as a unilateral, localized overgrowth of the facial soft tissues, bones, and teeth.

Etiology and Pathogenesis. Gross asymmetry has been found in 1 in 86,000 patients, with a 3-to-2 female preponderance. In males, involvement of the right side is more common. Almost all cases appear to be sporadic. There are equal numbers of segmental and complex forms, with neither side of the body exhibiting a greater incidence of involvement. Wilms' tumor is the most common neoplasm reported in association with hemihypertrophy.

Multiple etiologic factors have been implicated in the development of hemihypertrophy, including anatomic and functional vascular or lymphatic abnormalities, endocrine dysfunction, altered intrauterine environment, central nervous system disturbances, chromosomal abnormalities, and asymmetric cell division. Etiologic heterogeneity may be responsible for the varied clinical presentation, affecting single or multiple systems, and the degree of tissue involvement.

Clinical Features. The varieties and complexities of hemihypertrophy have resulted in a wide range of reported dentofacial findings. In some patients, the face is involved solely, but unilateral facial enlargement is often associated with hypertrophy of a portion of the body. The tissues involved frequently are not affected uniformly, accentuating the variable clinical presentation.

Craniofacial findings include asymmetry of the frontal bone, maxilla, palate, mandible, alveolar process, condyles, and associated overlying soft tissue (Fig. 15–27). The skin may be thickened, with excessive secretions by sebaceous and sweat glands and hypertrichosis. The pinnae are often remarkably enlarged. Unilateral enlargement of one of the cerebral hemispheres may be responsible for mental retardation in 15 to 20% of patients and for the occurrence of seizure disorders.

The oral findings are quite striking, affecting the dentition and tongue to a significant degree. The tongue is unilaterally hyperplastic and often distorted in appearance, with a distinct midline demarcation. The fungiform papillae are usually enlarged and resemble soft polypoid excrescences. Dysgeusia has been reported. Intraoral soft tissues are thickened and anatomically enlarged, often being described as overabundant and lying in soft velvety folds.

Dental findings include abnormalities in crown

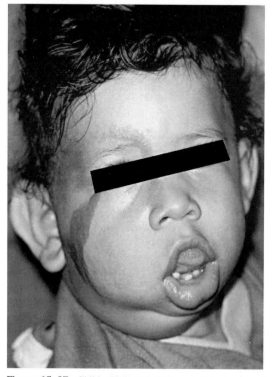

Figure 15–27. Child with hemifacial hypertrophy (as part of epidermal nevus syndrome).

size and root size and shape as well as precocious development and eruption. The permanent canines, premolars, and first molars are most frequently enlarged. When the primary dentition is affected, abnormalities are limited to the second molars and, less frequently, the canines. Unilateral macrodontia approaches but does not exceed a 50% increase in crown dimension in mesiodistal and buccolingual diameters. Root size and shape are proportionately enlarged or uncommonly shortened, and premature apical development is usual. The primary teeth on the affected side calcify, erupt, and exfoliate sooner than the contralateral teeth. Eruption of the affected permanent teeth by age 4 or 5 years has been reported.

Dental malocclusions are common owing to asymmetric growth of the maxilla, mandible, and alveolar process and abnormalities of tooth morphology and eruption patterns. Midline deviations, severely canted occlusal planes, and open bites are common.

Lateral and posterior anterior cephalograms demonstrate pronounced bony asymmetry and facial bone hypertrophy as well as evidence of hypertrophied soft tissues, such as tonsillar enlargement. Root anomalies, crown enlargement, and evidence of premature eruption are easily identifiable by panoramic or periapical radiography.

Differential Diagnosis. The diagnosis of true congenital hemifacial hypertrophy rests on the presence of unilateral hypertrophy of the craniofacial structures and associated soft tissue, including the dentition. Perception of contralateral dissimilarity may be difficult and often subjective, resulting in delayed diagnosis of congenital hemifacial hypertrophy in the infant. Angio-osteohypertrophy (Klippel-Trenaunay-Weber syndrome) can be ruled out by the absence of an overlying cutaneous nevus flammeus. Neurofibromatosis may cause gross enlargement of the soft tissue and skeleton of half the face, but it does not affect tooth size and eruption sequence. Lymphangioma and hemangioma are characterized by soft tissue enlargement; they do not affect tooth morphology. Acromegaly produces symmetric bilateral jaw enlargement. Fibrous dysplasia, craniofacial dysostosis, and chronic inflammatory diseases should also be ruled out.

Congenital hemifacial hypertrophy has been reported concomitantly with conductive hearing loss, seizure disorders, and Wilms' tumor. Other syndromes and conditions that produce soft and hard tissue hypertrophy and asymmetry include Russell's, or Silver's, syndrome, Beckwith-Wiedemann syndrome, congenital lymphedema, arteriovenous aneurysms, multiple exostoses, and facial tumors of childhood.

Treatment and Prognosis. During infancy and childhood, patients should be examined frequently to facilitate early identification of potential neoplasms involving the liver, adrenal glands, and kidneys. Growth and development should be observed closely for evidence of mental impairment or abnormalities of sexual development.

Abnormalities during the mixed dentition phase relate to tooth size–arch size discrepancies and abnormalities in eruption sequence. Asymmetric growth of the craniofacial complex and dental alveolus require early orthodontic intervention, including space maintenance, minor tooth movement, and functional appliances. Surgical reconstruction of hard and soft tissue anomalies to improve function and aesthetics must be anticipated.

The frequent association of congenital hemihypertrophy with vascular anomalies, embryonal neoplasms, and mental retardation requires a multidisciplinary team of dental and medical specialists.

Clefts of the Lip and Palate

Clefts of the lip and palate are frequently encountered congenital anomalies that often result in severe functional deficits of speech, mastication, and deglutition. The prevalence of associated congenital malformations as well as learning disabilities secondary to hearing deficits is frequently increased.

Generally, clefts of the lip and palate are classified into four major types: (1) cleft lip, (2) cleft palate, (3) unilateral cleft lip and palate, and (4) bilateral cleft lip and palate. Other clefts of the lip and mouth include lip pits, linear lip indentations, submucosal clefts of the palate, bifid uvula and tongue, and numerous facial clefts extending through the nose, lips, and oral cavity. Clefting deformities are extremely variable in character; they may range from furrows in the skin and mucosa to extensive cleavages involving muscle and bone. A combination of cleft lip and palate is the most common clefting deformity seen.

Etiology and Pathogenesis. Cleft lip and palate account for approximately 50% of all cases, whereas isolated cleft lip and isolated cleft palate each occur in about 25% of cases. The incidence of cleft lip and cleft palate has been reported to be 1 in 700 to 1000 births, with variable racial predilection. Isolated cleft palate is less common, with an incidence of 1 in 1500 to 3000 births. Cleft lip with or without cleft palate is more frequent in males, and cleft palate alone is more common in females.

The majority of cases of cleft lip or cleft palate or both can be explained by the multifactorial threshold hypothesis. The multifactorial inheritance theory implies that many contributory risk genes interact with one another and the environment and collectively determine whether a threshold of abnormality is breached, resulting in a defect in the developing fetus. Multifactorial or polygenic inheritance explains the transmission of isolated cleft lip or palate, and it is extremely useful in predicting occurrence risks of this anomaly among family members of an affected individual.

Disruption of normal patterns of facial growth, including deficiencies of any of the facial processes, may lead to maldevelopment of the lips and palate. Cleft lip generally occurs at about the sixth to seventh week *in utero*; it is a result of failure of the epithelial groove between the medial and the lateral nasal processes to be penetrated by mesodermal cells.

Cleft palate is a result of epithelial breakdown at about the eighth week of embryonic development, with ingrowth failure of mesodermal tissue and lack of lateral palatal segment fusion. Most embryologists believe that true tissue deficiencies exist in all clefting deformities and that actual anatomic structures are absent. Various degrees of cleft lip and palate may occur, ranging from mild notching of the vermilion border or bifid uvula to severe bilateral complete clefts of the lip, alveolus, and entire palate.

Clinical Features. The Veau system of classification for cleft lip and palate is widely used by clinicians; it helps to describe the variety of lip and palatal clefts seen. The system classifies cleft lip and cleft palate separately into four major categories, with emphasis on the degree of clefting present.

Cleft lip may vary from a pit or small notch in the vermilion border to a complete cleft extending into the floor of the nose (Fig. 15–28). Using the Veau classification, a class I cleft of the lip is a unilateral notching of the vermilion border that does not extend into the lip. If the unilateral notching of the vermilion extends into the lip but does not involve the floor of the nose, it is designated as a class II cleft. Class III lip clefts are unilateral clefts of the vermilion border extending through the lip into the floor of the nose. Any bilateral cleft of the lip, exhibiting incomplete notching or a complete cleft, is classified as a class IV cleft.

Clefting deformities of the palate can also be divided into four clinical types using the Veau system (Fig. 15–29). A cleft limited to the soft palate is a class I palatal cleft. Class II clefts are

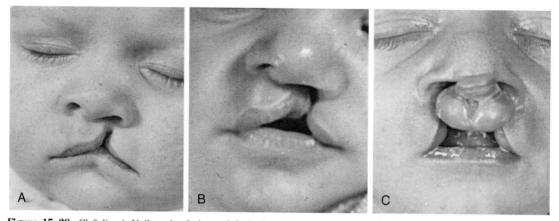

Figure 15–28. Cleft lip. *A,* Unilateral soft tissue cleft. *B,* Complete unilateral cleft extending through the alveolus and into the floor of the nose. *C,* Complete bilateral cleft lip.

defects of the hard and soft palate; they extend no farther than the incisive foramen and, therefore, are limited to the secondary palate only. Clefts of the secondary palate may be complete or incomplete. A complete cleft includes the soft and hard palate to the incisive foramen. An incomplete cleft involves the velum and a portion of the hard palate, not extending to the incisive foramen. Complete unilateral clefts extending from the uvula to the incisive foramen in the midline and the alveolar process unilaterally are designated as class III palatal clefts. Class IV clefts are complete bilateral clefts involving the soft and hard palate and the alveolar process on both sides of the premaxilla, leaving it free and often mobile.

Submucosal clefts are not included in this system of classification, but they can be identified clinically by the presence of a bifid uvula, palpable notching of the posterior portion of the hard and soft palate, and the presence of a zona pellucida or a thin translucent membrane covering the defect.

Clefts of the soft palate, including submucosal clefts, are often associated with velopharyngeal incompetence or eustachian tube dysfunction. Recurrent otitis media and hearing deficits are common complications. Palatal pharyngeal incompetence results from failure of the soft palate and pharyngeal wall to make contact during swallowing and speech, thus preventing the necessary muscular seal between the nasal and the oral pharynx. Speech is often characterized by air emission from the nose and has a hypernasal quality.

The prevalence of dental anomalies associated with cleft lip and palate is remarkable (Fig. 15–30). Abnormalities of tooth number, size, morphology, calcification, and eruption have been well described. Both deciduous and permanent denti-

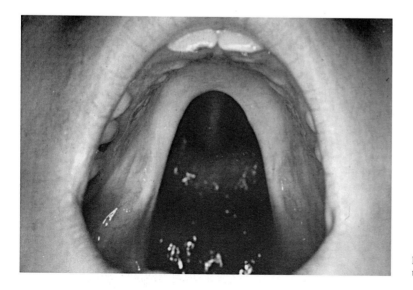

Figure 15–29. Complete cleft of the palate.

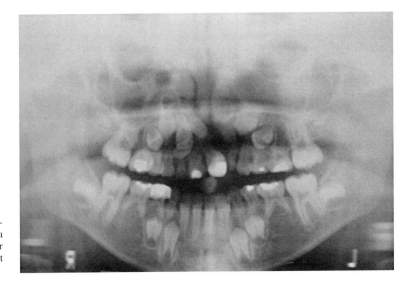

Figure 15–30. Panographic radiograph (Panorex) of a patient with a unilateral maxillary dental alveolar cleft. Note the alveolar bone defect and malpositioned teeth.

tions may be affected. The lateral incisor in the vicinity of the cleft is often involved, but teeth outside the cleft area exhibit developmental defects to a greater degree than is seen in unaffected patients.

The incidence of congenitally missing teeth is high, especially among deciduous and permanent maxillary lateral incisors adjacent to the alveolar cleft. The prevalence of hypodontia increases directly with the severity of the cleft. Complete unilateral and bilateral alveolar clefts are often associated with supernumerary teeth as well, usually the maxillary lateral incisors. Tooth formation is often delayed, and enamel hypoplasia, microdontia or macrodontia, and fused teeth are seen frequently.

Treatment and Prognosis. Prognosis is dependent on the severity of the clefting disorder. Aesthetic considerations and hearing and speech deficits often result in significant developmental problems.

Treatment is chronologically sequenced and often requires a multidisciplinary team concept, owing to the extensive nature of the problem and its impact on the child and the immediate family. Craniofacial or cleft palate teams are made up of dental, medical, and surgical specialists, with the assistance of allied health professionals in social services, child development, and hearing and speech therapy.

Generally, cleft lip repair is accomplished during early infancy when the child is stable, weighs at least 10 pounds, and has hemoglobin levels of 10 mg/dl. Cheiloplasty is often required later in life. Orthodontic or surgically placed orthopedic devices are being used in infants to guide the dentoalveolar segments into normal anatomic rela-

tionships and facilitate plastic closure. Closure of soft palate defects with sliding or pharyngeal flaps is often recommended by 1 year of age to promote normal speech development. Palatal obturators are often fabricated for infants who have cleft palate disorders and who are having difficulty feeding or are regurgitating food or liquids through the nasal cavity. Early audiologic and speech evaluation is highly recommended, and hearing aids are often indicated to prevent associated learning problems in children who have cleft palate and frequent episodes of otitis media. Chronic otitis media and associated low-frequency hearing loss are results of improper orientation of the eustachian tubes and inserting muscles resulting in middle ear fluid stasis and retrograde infection.

Preventive dental services are extremely important, because an intact dentition is the foundation for future orthodontic therapy. Treatment is often required to correct developmental dental defects. Orthodontic treatment is sometimes initiated during the primary dentition to correct unilateral and bilateral posterior maxillary crossbites and to retract an anterior displaced premaxillary segment.

Once into the mixed dentition phase of development, conventional orthodontic therapy is initiated to establish a normal maxillary arch form (Fig. 15–31). This is often done in preparation for an autogenous bone graft (commonly iliac crest) to the alveolar cleft to reestablish maxillary arch continuity. It is recommended that the grafting procedure be performed when root formation of the unerupted permanent tooth associated with the alveolar defect (usually the maxillary canine) has reached one-quarter to one-half completion. These teeth have been shown to successfully erupt passively or mechanically through the graft site, con-

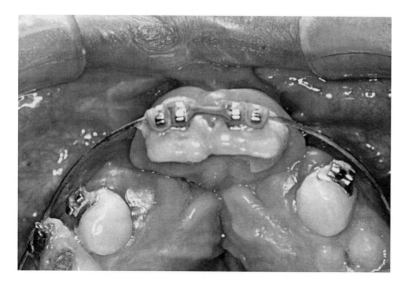

Figure 15–31. Patient with bilateral dental alveolar cleft and cleft of the palate undergoing early orthodontic treatment.

solidating the arch, preserving the graft, and reestablishing alveolar competence.

Further orthodontic treatment, followed by orthognathic surgery, is often required for those patients with significant dentofacial deformities. Frequent plastic surgical procedures to correct the aesthetics and function of the vermilion border, lip, philtrum, and nose can be anticipated.

Fragile X Syndrome

It has long been recognized in the general population that more males than females are mentally deficient. The large percentage of mentally disabled males and historical documentation of families with affected male and unaffected female children are highly suggestive of an X-linked inheritance pattern. Since the report in 1943 of a family with 11 severely retarded males delivered to an apparently unaffected mother, multiple case reports have identified a syndrome (fragile X syndrome) characterized by X-linked mental retardation, macro-orchidism, and a characteristic phenotypic presentation.

Etiology and Pathogenesis. The fragile X syndrome, believed to account for 30 to 50% of all families with X-linked mental retardation, takes its name from an identifiable fragile site on the X chromosome that is a reliable diagnostic marker. It is now recognized that X-linked mental retardation may be as common as Down syndrome in males; it accounts for approximately 25% of all mentally disabled males, with an incidence of 0.3 to 1 affected child per 1000 male births. The finding of 20 to 30% of female carriers with various degrees of mental retardation may be explained by lyonization or random inactivation of one of the X chromosomes.

The family history remains the primary tool for recognition of patients with X-linked mental retardation. In the fragile X syndrome, specific cytogenetic studies can aid in the diagnosis. In affected males, only 4 to 50% of cells exhibit the chromosomal changes, an abnormal secondary constriction near the terminal end of the long arm

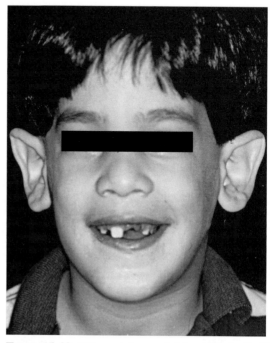

Figure 15–32. This mentally retarded boy with fragile X syndrome demonstrates the typical clinical features, including a long, narrow face and large ears.

(q) of the X chromosome. This segment is often broken and has been termed the *fragile site.* In 50% of female carriers, the fragile X chromosome cannot be detected at all. Abnormalities of speech have also been noted in the fragile X syndrome, and it has been theorized that major genes related to verbal function are located on the X chromosome and are disrupted at the fragile site. Recent genetic and biochemical studies have isolated a specific nucleotide alteration. This involves an expanded CGG repeat at one end (5′) of the FMR1 gene, which in turn is related to a methylation step in the production of FMR protein formation. Degrees of altered methylation by way of FMR gene product may help explain the range of clinical findings.

Clinical Features. The classic clinical presentation is that of a mentally retarded male with postpubescent macro-orchidism, large ears, prognathism, and a long narrow face with a high forehead and prominent supraorbital ridges (Fig. 15–32). Other findings include hyperextensible joints, mitral valve prolapse, cleft palate, and an association with Pierre Robin syndrome. Patients have a characteristic repetitive jocular speech and may exhibit hyperactive behavior or autism. The characteristic speech pattern has been termed *cluttering* or is hurried and presents as repetitive sentences that come out in a rush. The hands are often large and fleshy, and the iris may be pale. Hand biting has been reported. Oral findings include a high-arched palate, prominent lateral palatine ridges, anterior and posterior dental crossbites, and increased occlusal attrition. A high-normal birth weight is common, and increased head circumference during infancy and childhood is noted.

The degree of mental retardation is variable, even among affected siblings. Results of testicular biopsies and endocrine function tests are found to be within normal limits.

Treatment and Prognosis. The significance of identification of X-linked retardation in families cannot be overemphasized. Because the syndrome is inherited as an X-linked trait and the fragile X site can be identified in 30 to 50% of families with X-linked mental retardation, early diagnosis and genetic counseling are imperative.

Fragile X syndrome screening of the mentally retarded population has proved to be cost effective. Genetic counseling of families with positive histories may help to advise potential or proven carriers of the risks of bearing an affected child. The only reliable means of prenatal diagnosis currently is by examination of fetal chromosomes. There is no method of excluding carrier status in females who do not express the fragile X chromosome.

Mitral valve prolapse has been reported to occur in as many as 80% of males affected with this syndrome, supporting the need for definitive cardiac evaluation before dental therapy.

Bibliography

Metabolic Conditions

Basle MF, Rebel A, Fournier JG, et al. On the trail of paramyxoviruses in Paget's disease of bone. Clin Orthop 217:9–14, 1987.

Bernstein RM, Zaleske DJ. Familial aspects of Caffey's disease. Am J Orthop 24:777–781, 1995.

Broadus AE, Rasmussen H. Clinical evaluation of parathyroid function. Am J Med 70:475–478, 1981.

Carrillo R, Morales A, Rodriguez-Peralto JL, et al. Benign fibro-osseous lesions in Paget's disease of the jaws. Oral Surg Oral Med Oral Pathol 71:588–592, 1991.

Dickson GR, Hamilton A, Hayes D, et al. An investigation of vanishing bone disease. Bone 11:205–210, 1990.

Dunbar SF, Rosenberg A, Mankin H, et al. Gorham's massive osteolysis: the role of radiation therapy and a review of the literature. Int J Radiol Oncol Biol Phys 26:491–497, 1993.

Ellis G, Connole P. Diffuse mandibular enlargement caused by osteitis deformans. Ear Nose Throat J 64:466–477, 1985.

Ezzat S, Forster MJ, Berchtold P, et al. Acromegaly. Clinical and biochemical features in 500 patients. Medicine (Baltimore) 73:233–240, 1994.

Frederiksen NL, Wesley RK, Sciubba JJ, et al. Massive osteolysis of the maxillofacial skeleton. A clinical, radiographic, histologic, and ultrastructural study. Oral Surg 55:470–480, 1983.

Freedy RM, Bell KA. Massive osteolysis (Gorham's disease) of the temporomandibular joint. Ann Otol Rhinol Laryngol 101:1018–1020, 1992.

Goepferd SJ. Advanced alveolar bone loss in the primary dentition. J Periodontol 52:753–757, 1981.

Hampton RE. Acromegaly and resulting myofascial pain and temporomandibular joint dysfunction. J Am Dent Assoc 114:625–631, 1987.

Heyman E, Laver J, Beer S. Prostaglandin synthetase inhibitor in Caffey's disease. J Pediatr 101:314, 1982.

Houston MS, Hay ID. Practical management of hyperthyroidism. Am Fam Physician 41:909–916, 1990.

Jadresic A, Banks LM, Child DF, et al. The acromegaly syndrome: relation between clinical features, growth hormone values, and radiological characteristics of the pituitary tumors. Q J Med 51:189–204, 1982.

Kanzler A, Farmand M, DiGiacomi B, et al. Pathologic changes in the face and skull in acromegaly. Swiss Dent 13:35–44, 1992.

Kjellman M, Oldfelt V, Nordenram A, et al. Five cases of hypophosphatasia with dental findings. Int J Oral Surg 2:152–158, 1973.

Lederman DA. Oral radiographic manifestations of systemic disease: bone disorders. Clin Prev Dent 5:22–26, 1983.

Macfarlane JD, Swart JGN. Dental aspects of hypophosphatasia: a case report, family study, and literature review. Oral Med 67:521–526, 1989.

Maclachlan AK, Gerrard JW, Houston CS, et al. Familial infantile cortical hyperostosis in a large Canadian family. Can Med Assoc J 130:1172–1174, 1984.

Melmed S. Acromegaly. N Engl J Med 322:966–977, 1990.

Melmed S, Fagin JA. Acromegaly update—etiology, diagnosis, and management. West J Med 146:328–333, 1987.

Merkow RL, Lane JM. Paget's disease of bone. Orthop Clin North Am 21:171–189, 1990.

Murphy JB, Doker HC, Carter BC. Massive osteolysis: phantom bone disease. J Oral Surg 36:318–322, 1978.

Olsson A, Matsson L, Blomquist HK, et al. Hypophosphatasia affecting the permanent dentition. J Oral Pathol Med 25:343–347, 1996.

Parisien M, Silverberg SJ, Shane E, et al. Bone disease in primary hyperparathyroidism. Endocrinol Metab Clin North Am 19:19–34, 1990.

Petti GH Jr. Hyperparathyroidism. Otolaryngol Clin North Am 23:339–355, 1990.

Piatelli A. Symmetrical pulpal obliteration in mandibular first molars. J Endod 18:515–516, 1992.

Reginster JY, Lecont MP. Efficacy and safety of drugs for Paget's disease of bone. Bone 17(Suppl 5):485S–488S, 1995.

Roth RN, McAuliffe MJ. Hyperthyroidism and thyroid storm. Emerg Med Clin North Am 7:873–883, 1989.

Saul RA, Lee WH, Stevenson RE, et al. Caffey's disease revisited: further evidence of autosomal dominant inheritance with incomplete penetrance. Am J Dis Child 136:56–60, 1982.

Shear M, Copelyn M. Metastatic calcification of the oral mucosa in renal hyperparathyroidism. Br J Oral Surg 42:81–87, 1966.

Stafne EC, Austin LT. A study of dental roentgenograms in cases of Paget's disease (osteitis deformans), osteitis fibrosa cystica, and osteoma. J Am Dent Assoc 25:1202–1214, 1938.

Szabo J, Heath B, Hill VM, et al. Hereditary hyperparathyroidism–jaw tumor syndrome: the endocrine gene HRPT2 maps to chromosome 1q21-q31. Am J Hum Genet 56:944–950, 1995.

Thometz JG, DiRaimiondi CA. A case of recurrent Caffey's disease treated with naproxen. Clin Orthop 323:304–309, 1996.

Thomas DW, Tate RJ, Shepherd JP. Paget's disease of bone: current concepts in pathogenesis and treatment. J Oral Pathol Med 23:12–16, 1994.

van Damme PA, Mooren RE. Differentiation of multiple giant cell lesions, Noonan-like syndrome and (occult) hyperparathyroidism. Int J Oral Maxillofac Surg 23:32–36, 1994.

Xhonga FA, Herle AV. The influence of hyperthyroidism on dental erosion. Oral Surg 36:349–357, 1973.

Zachariades N, Skordalaki A, Papanicolaou S, et al. Infantile cortical hyperostosis: report of two cases. J Oral Maxillofac Surg 44:644–648, 1986.

Genetic Abnormalities

Augarten A, Sagy M, Yahav J, et al. Management of upper airway obstruction in Pierre Robin syndrome. Br J Oral Maxillofac Surg 28:105–108, 1990.

Barnett ML, Friedman D, Kastner T. The prevalence of mitral valve prolapse in patients with Down's syndrome: implications for dental management. Oral Surg Oral Med Oral Pathol 66:445–447, 1988.

Beighton AP, Lord J, Dickson E. Variants of the Ehlers-Danlos syndrome: clinical, biochemical, hematological, and chromosomal features of 100 patients. Ann Rheum Dis 28:228–244, 1969.

Bell RA, McTigue DJ. Complex congenital hemihypertrophy: a case report and literature review. J Pedod 8:300–313, 1984.

Bhatia R, Deka RC. Treacher-Collins syndrome with deviated nasal septum. Indian J Pediatr 51:739–741, 1984.

Bjorvtan K, Gilhuus-Moe O. Oral aspects of osteopetrosis. Scand J Dent Res 87:245–252, 1979.

Bollerslev J. Osteopetrosis. Clin Genet 31:86–90, 1987.

Braun TW, Sotereanos GC. Alveolar reconstruction in adolescent patients with cleft palates. J Oral Surg 39:510–517, 1981.

Braun TW, Sotereanos GC. Orthognathic surgical reconstruction of cleft palate deformities in adolescents. J Oral Surg 39:255–263, 1981.

Bull MJ, Givan DC, Sadove AM, et al. Improved outcome in Pierre Robin syndrome: effect of multidisciplinary evaluation and management. Pediatrics 86:294–301, 1990.

Byers PH, Bonadio JF, Steinmann B. Invited editorial comment: osteogenesis imperfecta: update and perspective. Genetics 17:429–435, 1984.

Caputo PJ, Walter JH Jr. Osteogenesis imperfecta. J Am Podiatr Med Assoc 73:456–460, 1983.

Carpenter NJ, Leichtman LG, Say B. Fragile X-linked mental retardation. Am J Dis Child 136:392–398, 1982.

Christian J, Gorlin RJ, Anderson VE. The syndrome of pits of the lower lip and cleft lip and/or palate, genetic considerations. Clin Genet 2:95–103, 1971.

Cohen MM Sr, Cohen M Jr. The oral manifestations of trisomy 21 (Down's syndrome). Birth Defects 7:241–251, 1971.

Cutter NR, Heston LL, Davies P, et al. Alzheimer's disease and Down's syndrome: new insights. Ann Intern Med 103:566–578, 1985.

Dean DH, Hiramoto RN. Osteogenesis imperfecta congenita: dental features of a rare disease. J Oral Med 39:119–121, 1984.

de Vries BB, Jansen CC, Duits AA, et al. Variable FMR1 gene methylation of large expansions leads to variable phenotype in three males from one fragile X family. J Med Genet 33:1007–1010, 1996.

Dicks JL, Dennis ES. Down's syndrome and hepatitis: an evaluation of carrier status. J Am Dent Assoc 114:637–639, 1987.

El Deeb M, Messer LB, Lehnert MW, et al. Canine eruption into grafted bone in maxillary alveolar cleft defects. Cleft Palate J 19:9–16, 1982.

Edwards JRG, Newall DR. The Pierre Robin syndrome reassessed in the light of recent research. Br J Plast Surg 38:339–342, 1985.

Felix R, Hofstetter W, Cecchini MG. Recent developments in the understanding of osteopetrosis. Eur J Endocrinol 134:143–156, 1996.

Fraser FC. The genetics of cleft lip and cleft palate. Am J Hum Genet 22:336–352, 1970.

Fridrich KL, Fridrich HH, Kempf KK, et al. Dental implications in Ehlers-Danlos syndrome. Oral Surg Oral Med Oral Pathol 69:431–435, 1990.

Friedman E, Eisenbud L. Surgical and pathological considerations in cherubism. Int J Oral Surg 10(Suppl 1):52–57, 1981.

Geormaneanu M, Iagaru N, Popescu-Miclosanu SP, et al. Congenital hemihypertrophy. Tendency to association with other abnormalities and/or tumors. Morphol Embryol (Bucur) 29:39–45, 1983.

Gluckman E. Bone marrow transplantation in children with hereditary disorders. Curr Opin Pediatr 8:42–44, 1996.

Gorlin RJ, Cohen MM, Levin LS. Syndromes of the Head and Neck, 3rd ed. Oxford University Press, New York, 1990.

Gott VL, Pyeritz RE, Macgovern GJ Jr, et al. Surgical treatment of aneurysms of the ascending aorta in the Marfan syndrome. N Engl J Med 314:1070–1074, 1986.

Grayson BH, Bookstein FL, McCarthy JG. The mandible in mandibulofacial dysostosis: a cephalometric study. Am J Orthodont 5:393–398, 1986.

Hatziioannou N. Presurgical oral orthopedic appliances for infants with cleft lip and palate. J Pedod 14:18–26, 1989.

Helms JA, Speidel TM, Denis KL. Effect of timing on long-term clinical success of alveolar cleft bone grafts. Am J Orthod Dentofacial Orthop 92:232–240, 1987.

Henessy WT, Cromie WJ, Duckett JW. Congenital hemihypertrophy and associated abdominal lesions. Urology 18:576–579, 1981.

Horton WA, Schimke RN, Iyama T. Osteopetrosis: further heterogeneity. J Pediatr 97:580–585, 1980.

Hume WJ. Hemifacial hypertrophy associated with endocrine disharmony. Br Dent J 139:16–20, 1975.

Ireland AJ, Eveson JW. Cherubism: A report of a case with an unusual post-extraction complication. Br Dent J 164:116–117, 1988.

Jacenko O. c-fos and bone loss. A proto-oncogeal regulater osteoclast lineage determination. Bioassays 17:277–281, 1995.

Jahrsdoerfer RA, Yeakley JW, Aguilar EA, et al. Treacher Collins syndrome: an otologic challenge. Ann Otol Rhinol Laryngol 98:807–812, 1989.

Jensen BL, Kreiborg S. Development of the dentition in cleidocranial dysplasia. J Oral Pathol Med 19:89–93, 1990.

Jones JE, Friend GW. Cleft orthotics and obturation. Oral Maxillofac Surg Clin North Am 3:517–529, 1991.

Kahler SG, Burns JA, Aylsworth AS. A mild autosomal recessive form of osteopetrosis. Am J Med Genet 17:451–464, 1984.

Kainulainen K, Pulkkinen L, Savolainen A, et al. Location on chromosome 15 of the gene defect causing Marfan syndrome. N Engl J Med 323:935–939, 1990.

Kerr BD. Cleidocranial dysplasia. J Rheumatol 15:359–361, 1988.

Khalifa MC, Ibrahim RA. Cherubism. J Laryngol Otol 102:568–570, 1988.

Kivirikko KI. Collagens and their abnormalities in a wide spectrum of diseases. Ann Med 25:113–126, 1993.

Koch PE, Hammer WB. Case reports: cleidocranial dysostosis: review of literature and report of case. J Oral Surg 36:39–42, 1978.

Kwon HJ, Waite DE, Stickel FR, et al. The management of alveolar cleft defects. J Am Dent Assoc 102:848–853, 1981.

Lawoyin JO, Daramola JO, Lawoyn DO. Congenital hemifacial hypertrophy. Oral Surg Oral Med Oral Pathol 68:27–30, 1989.

Levin LS, Salinas CF, Jorgenson RJ. Classification of osteogenesis imperfecta by dental characteristics. Lancet 1(8059):332–333, 1978.

Levin S. The immune system and susceptibility to infections in Down's syndrome. In McCoy EE, Epstein CJ (eds). Oncology and Immunology of Down Syndrome. New York, AR Liss, 1987, pp 143–162.

Loesch DZ, Hay DA, Mulley J. Transmitting males and carrier females in fragile X—revisited. Am J Med Genet 51:392–399, 1994.

Loh HS. Congenital hemifacial hypertrophy. Br Dent J 153:111–112, 1982.

Losken HW, Morris WMM, Uys PB, et al. Crouzon's disease. Part I. One-stage correction by combined face and forehead advancement. S Afr Med J 75:274–279, 1989.

Marsh JL, Celin SE, Vannier MW, et al. The skeletal anatomy of mandibulofacial dysostosis (Treacher Collins syndrome). Plast Reconstr Surg 78:460–468, 1986.

McIntee RA, Moore IJ, Yonkers AJ. A general review of maxillofacial cleft deformities with emphasis on dental anomalies. Ear Nose Throat J 65:286–290, 1986.

Menashe Y, Ben Baruch G, Rabinovitch O, et al. Exophthalmus—prenatal ultrasonic features for diagnosis of Crouzon syndrome. Prenat Diagn 9:805–808, 1989.

Mixon JC, Dev VG. Understanding the fragile X syndrome. Ala J Med Sci 21:284–286, 1984.

Miyamato RT, House WF. Neurologic manifestations of the osteopetroses. Arch Otolaryngol 106:210–214, 1980.

Monasky GE, Winkler S, Icenhower JB, et al. Cleidocranial

dysostosis—two case reports. NY State Dent J 49:236–238, 1983.

Muchnick RS, Aston SJ, Rees TD. Ocular manifestations and treatment of hemifacial atrophy. Am J Ophthalmol 85:889–897, 1979.

Mundlos S, Otto F, Mulliken JB, et al. Mutations involving the transcription factor CBFA1 cause cleidocranial dysplasia. Cell 89:773–779, 1997.

Mundy GR. Cytokines and local factors which affect osteoclast function. Int J Cell Cloning 10:215–222, 1992.

Nunn JH, Durning P. Fragile X (Martin Bell) syndrome and dental care. Br Dental J 168:160, 1990.

Pasyayan HM, Lewis M. Clinical experience with the Robin sequence. Cleft Palate J 21:270–276, 1984.

Prockop DJ, Kivirikko KI. Collagens: molecular biology, diseases, and potentials for therapy. Annu Rev Biochem 64:403–434, 1995.

Prockop DJ, Kuivaniemi H, Tromp G. Molecular basis of osteogenesis imperfecta and related disorders of bone. Clin Plast Surg 21:407–413, 1994.

Pyertitz RE. The Marfan syndrome. Am Fam Physician 34:83–94, 1986.

Pyeritz RE, McKusick V. Basic defects in the Marfan syndrome. N Engl J Med 305:1011–1012, 1981.

Ramesar RS, Greenberg J, Martin R, et al. Mapping of the gene for cleidocranial dysplasia in historical Cape Town (Arnold) kindred and evidence for locus homogeneity. J Med Genet 33:511–514, 1996.

Ramon Y, Engelberg IS. An unusually extensive case of cherubism. Oral Maxillofac Surg 44:325–328, 1986.

Ranalli DN, Guzman R, Schmutz JA. Craniofacial and intraoral manifestations of congenital hemifacial hyperplasia: report of case. ASDC J Dent Child 57:203–208, 1990.

Ranta R. Incomplete median cleft of the lower lip associated with cleft palate, the Pierre Robin anomaly or hypodontia. Int J Oral Surg 13:555–558, 1984.

Reade P, McKellar G, Radden B. Unilateral mandibular cherubism: brief review and case report. J Maxillofac Surg 22:189–194, 1984.

Reinhardt DP, Chalberg SC, Sakai LY. The structure and function of fibrillin. Ciba Found Symp 192:128–143, 1995.

Richardson A, Deussen FF. Facial and dental anomalies in cleidocranial dysplasia: a study of 17 cases. Int J Pediatr Dent 4:225–231, 1994.

Rintala A, Ranta R, Stegars T. On the pathogenesis of cleft palate in the Pierre Robin syndrome. Scand J Plast Reconstr Surg 18:237–240, 1984.

Rosen HM, Witaker LA. Cranial base dynamics in craniofacial dysostosis. J Maxillofac Surg 12:56–61, 1984.

Rousseau F, Heitz D, Biancalana V, et al. Direct diagnosis by DNA analysis of the fragile X syndrome of mental retardation. N Engl J Med 325:1673–1681, 1991.

Sandham A. Classification of clefting deformity. Early Hum Dev 12:81–85, 1985.

Scarbrough PR, Cosper P, Finley SC, et al. Fragile X syndrome—an overview. Ala J Med Sci 21:68–72, 1984.

Sculerati N, Jacobs JB. Congenital facial hemihypertrophy: report of a case with airway compromise. Head Neck Surg 8:124–128, 1985.

Shapiro F. Osteopetrosis. Current clinical considerations. Clin Orthop 294:34–44, 1993.

Shellhart WC, Casamassimo PS, Hagerman RJ, et al. Oral findings in fragile X syndrome. Am J Med Genet 23:179–187, 1986.

Shprintzen RJ, Siegel-Sadewitz VL, Amato J, et al. Anomalies associated with cleft lip, cleft palate, or both. Am J Med Genet 20:585–595, 1985.

Spengler DE. Staging in cleft lip and palate habilitation. Oral Maxillofac Surg Clin North Am 3:489–499, 1991.

Steiner M, Gould AR, Means WR. Osteomyelitis of the mandible associated with osteopetrosis. J Oral Maxillofac Surg 41:395–405, 1983.

Stewart RE, Barber TK, Troutman KC, et al (eds). Pediatric Dentistry: Scientific Foundations and Clinical Practice. St Louis, CV Mosby, 1982.

Sulik KK, Johnston MC, Smiley SJ, et al. Mandibulofacial dysostosis (Treacher Collins syndrome): a new proposal for its pathogenesis. Am J Med Genet 27:359–372, 1987.

Sunderland EP, Smith CJ. The teeth in osteogenesis and dentinogenesis imperfecta. Br Dent J 149:287–289, 1980.

Svoboda PJ, Mendieta C, Reeve CM. Albers-Schönberg disease complicated with periodontal disease. J Periodontol 54:592–597, 1983.

Tiegs RD. Heritable metabolic and dysplastic bone diseases. Endocrinol Metab Clin North Am 19:133–173, 1990.

Trimble LD, West RA, McNeil RW. Cleidocranial dysplasia: comprehensive treatment of the dentofacial abnormalities. J Am Dent Assoc 105:661–666, 1982.

Trusler S, Beatty-DeSana J. Fragile X syndrome: a public health concern. Am J Public Health 75:771–772, 1985.

Turvey TA, Vig K, Moriarty J, et al. Delayed bone grafting in the cleft maxilla and palate: a retrospective multidisciplinary analysis. Am J Orthod 86:244–256, 1984.

Ulseth JO, Hestnes A, Stovner LJ, Storhaug L. Dental caries and periodontitis in persons with Down syndrome. Special Care Dent 11:71–74, 1991.

Vig KW, Turvey TA. Orthodontic-surgical interaction in the management of cleft lip and palate. Clin Plast Surg 12:735–749, 1985.

Welbury RR. Ehlers-Danlos syndrome: historical review, report of two cases in one family and treatment needs. ASDC J Dent Child 56:220–224, 1989.

Whyte M, Murphy W, Fallon M, et al. Osteopetrosis, renal tubular acidosis and basal ganglia calcification in three sisters. Am J Med 69:64–74, 1980.

Winship IM. Ehlers-Danlos syndrome in the Western Cape. S Afr Med J 67:509–511, 1985.

Winter RM. Fragile X mental retardation. Arch Dis Child 64:1223–1224, 1989.

Yeswell HN, Pinnell SR. The Ehlers-Danlos syndromes. Semin Dermatol 12:229–240, 1993.

Younai F, Eisenbud L, Sciubba JJ. Osteopetrosis: a case report including gross and microscopic findings in the mandible at autopsy. Oral Surg Oral Med Oral Pathol 65:214–221, 1988.

Zachariades N, Papanicolaou S, Xypolyta A, et al. Cherubism. Int J Oral Surg 14:138–145, 1985.

16

Abnormalities of Teeth

ALTERATIONS IN SIZE

Microdontia

In generalized microdontia, all teeth in the dentition appear smaller than normal. Teeth may actually be measurably smaller than normal, as in pituitary dwarfism, or they may be relatively small in comparison with a large mandible and maxilla.

In focal or localized microdontia, a single tooth is smaller than normal (Fig. 16–1). The shape of these microdonts is also often altered with the reduced size. This phenomenon is most commonly seen with maxillary lateral incisors in which the tooth crown appears cone or peg shaped, prompting the designation *peg lateral* (Fig. 16–2). An autosomal dominant inheritance pattern has been associated with this condition. Peg laterals are of no significance, other than cosmetic appearance. The second most commonly seen microdont is the maxillary third molar, followed by supernumerary teeth.

Macrodontia

Generalized macrodontia is characterized by the appearance of enlarged teeth throughout the dentition. This may be absolute, as seen in pituitary gigantism, or it may be relative owing to a disproportionately small maxilla and mandible. The latter results in crowding of teeth and possibly an abnormal eruption pattern because of insufficient arch space.

Focal or localized macrodontia is characterized by an abnormally large tooth or group of teeth (Fig. 16–3). This relatively uncommon condition is usually seen with mandibular third molars. In the rare condition known as *hemifacial hypertrophy*, teeth on the affected side are abnormally large compared with the unaffected side.

ALTERATIONS IN SHAPE

Gemination

Gemination is the fusion of two teeth from a single enamel organ (Fig. 16–4). The typical result is partial cleavage, with the appearance of two crowns that share the same root canal. Complete cleavage or twinning occasionally occurs, resulting in two teeth from one tooth germ. Although trauma has been suggested as a possible cause, the cause of gemination is unknown. These teeth may be cosmetically unacceptable and may cause crowding.

Fusion

Fusion is the joining of two developing tooth germs, resulting in a single large tooth structure

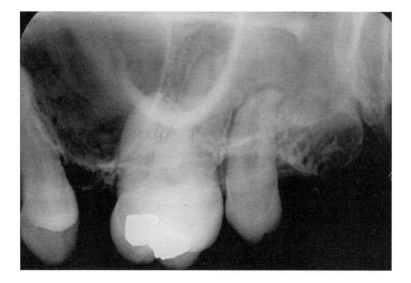

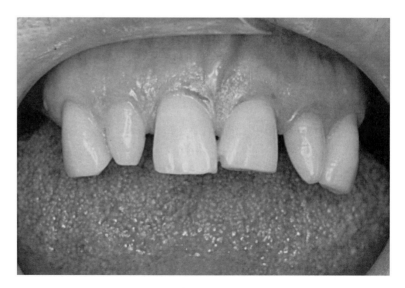

Figure 16–1. Microdont in the third molar position.

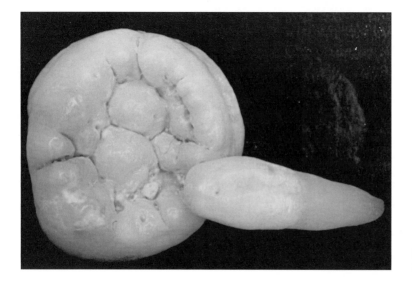

Figure 16–2. Peg laterals.

Figure 16–3. Occlusal view of a macrodont (molar) and a peg lateral.

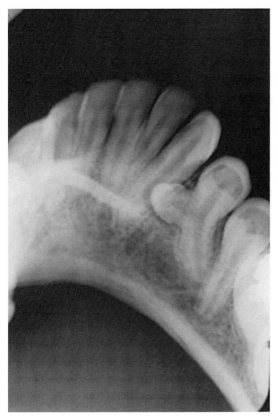

Figure 16–4. Gemination of a mandibular first premolar. (Courtesy of Dr. R. Courtney.)

(Fig. 16–5). The fusion process may involve the entire length of the teeth, or it may involve the roots only, in which case cementum and dentin are shared. Root canals may also be separate or shared. It may be impossible to differentiate fusion of normal and supernumerary teeth from gemination. The cause of this condition is unknown, although trauma has been suggested.

Concrescence

Concrescence is a form of fusion in which the adjacent already formed teeth are joined by cementum (Fig. 16–6). This may take place before or after eruption of teeth and is believed to be related to trauma or overcrowding. Concrescence is most commonly seen in association with the maxillary second and third molars. This condition is of no significance, unless one of the teeth involved requires extraction. Surgical sectioning may be required to save the other tooth.

Dilaceration

Dilaceration is an extraordinary curving or angulation of tooth roots (Fig. 16–7). The cause of this condition has been related to trauma during root development. Movement of the crown or of the crown and part of the root from the remaining developing root may result in sharp angulation after the tooth completes development. Hereditary factors are believed to be involved in a small number of cases. Eruption generally continues without problems. However, extraction may be difficult. Obviously, if root canal fillings are required in these teeth, the procedure is challenging.

Dens Invaginatus

Also known as *dens in dente* or *tooth within a tooth*, dens invaginatus is an uncommon tooth

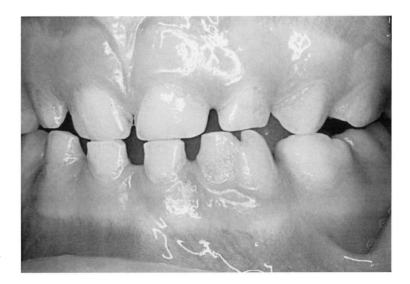

Figure 16–5. Fusion of a primary incisor and cuspid.

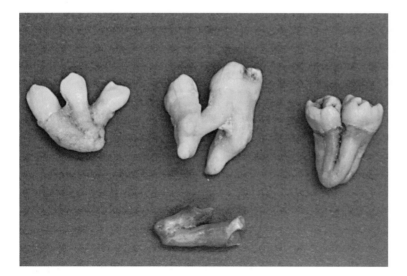

Figure 16–6. Concrescence.

anomaly that represents an exaggeration or accentuation of the lingual pit (Fig. 16–8). This defect ranges in severity from superficial, in which only the crown is affected, to deep, in which both the crown and the root are involved. The permanent maxillary lateral incisors are most commonly involved, although any anterior tooth may be affected. Bilateral involvement is frequently seen. The cause of this developmental condition is unknown. Genetic factors are believed to be involved in only a small percentage of cases.

Because the defect cannot be kept free of plaque and bacteria, dens invaginatus predisposes the tooth to early decay and subsequent pulpitis. Prophylactic filling of the pit is recommended to avoid this complication. Because the defect may often be identified on radiographic examination before tooth eruption, the patient can be prepared

in advance of the procedure. In cases in which pulpitis has led to nonvitality, endodontic procedures may salvage the affected tooth.

Dens Evaginatus

This is a relatively common developmental condition affecting predominantly premolar teeth. It has been reported almost exclusively in Asians, Eskimos, and Native Americans (Fig. 16–9). The defect, frequently bilateral, is an anomalous tubercle or cusp located in the center of the occlusal surface. Because of occlusal abrasion, the tubercle wears relatively quickly, causing early exposure of an accessory pulp horn that extends into the tubercle. This may result in periapical pathology in young caries-free teeth, often before completion

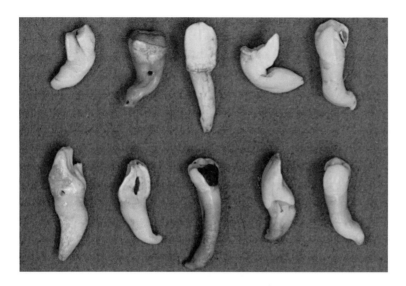

Figure 16–7. Dilaceration.

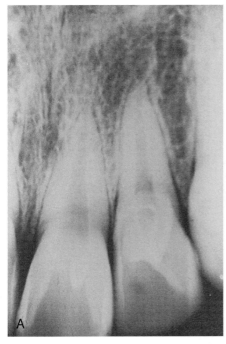

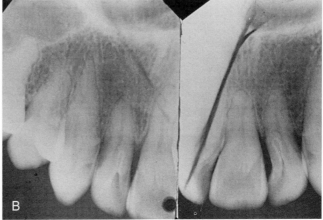

Figure 16–8. *A* and *B*, Dens invaginatus of the maxillary lateral incisors.

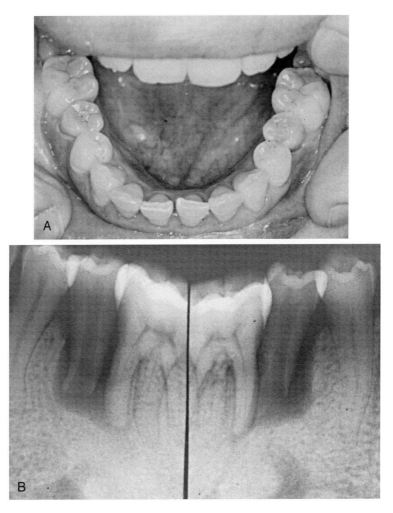

Figure 16–9. *A* and *B*, Dens evaginatus of second premolars. Note the apical lucencies resulting from pulp exposures. (*A* and *B*, Courtesy of E. S. Senia.)

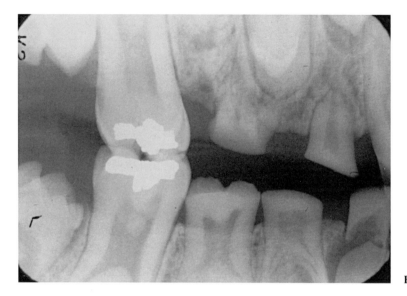

Figure 16–10. Taurodontism.

of root development and apical closure, making root canal fillings more difficult. Judicious grinding of the opposing tooth or the accessory tubercle to stimulate secondary dentin formation may prevent the periapical sequelae associated with this defect.

Taurodontism

Taurodontism is a variation in tooth form in which teeth have elongated crowns or apically displaced furcations, resulting in pulp chambers that have increased apical-occlusal height (Fig. 16–10). Because this abnormality resembles teeth in bulls and other ungulates, the term *taurodontism* was coined. Various degrees of severity may be seen, but subclassifications that have been developed to describe them appear to be of academic interest only. Taurodontism may be seen as an isolated incident, in families, in association with syndromes such as Down and Klinefelter's, and in past primitive populations such as Neanderthals. Although taurodontism is generally an uncommon finding, it has been reported to have a relatively high prevalence in Eskimos, and it has been reported to be as high as 11% in a Middle Eastern population. Other than a possible relationship to other genetically determined abnormalities, taurodontism is of little clinical significance. No treatment is required.

Supernumerary Roots

Accessory roots are most commonly seen in mandibular canines, premolars, and molars (espe-

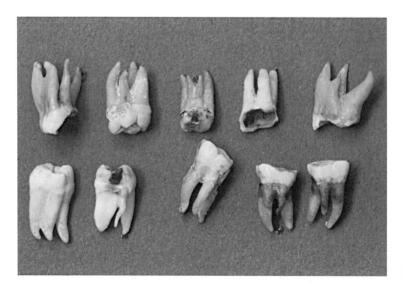

Figure 16–11. Supernumerary roots.

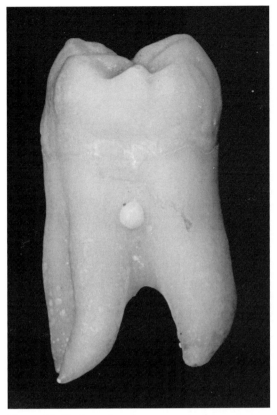

Figure 16–12. Enamel pearl.

cially third molars). They are rarely found in upper anterior teeth and mandibular incisors (Fig. 16–11). Radiographic recognition of an extraordinary number of roots becomes important when extractions or root canal fillings are necessary.

Enamel Pearls

Droplets of ectopic enamel or so-called enamel pearls may occasionally be found on the roots of teeth (Fig. 16–12). They occur most commonly in the bifurcation or trifurcation of teeth but may appear on single-rooted premolar teeth as well. Maxillary molars are more frequently affected than are mandibular molars. These deposits are occasionally supported by dentin and rarely have a pulp horn extending into them. This developmental disturbance of enamel formation may be detected on radiographic examination. It is generally of little significance, except when located in an area of periodontal disease. In such cases, it may contribute to the extension of a periodontal pocket, because periodontal ligament attachment would not be expected, and hygiene would be more difficult.

Attrition, Abrasion, Erosion

Attrition is the physiologic wearing of teeth resulting from mastication. It is an age-related process and varies from one individual to another. Factors such as diet quality, dentition, jaw musculature, and chewing habits can significantly influence the pattern and extent of attrition.

Abrasion is the pathologic wearing of teeth as a result of an abnormal habit or abnormal use of abrasive substances orally. Pipe smoking, tobacco chewing, aggressive tooth brushing, and use of abrasive dentifrices are among the more common causes (Figs. 16–13 and 16–14). The location and pattern of abrasion are directly dependent on the

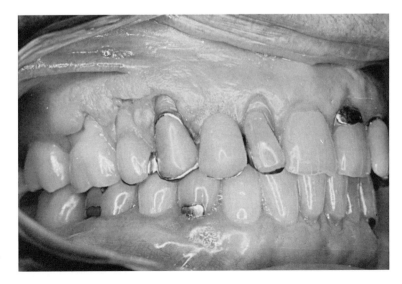

Figure 16–13. Toothbrush abrasion of the cervical zone of the maxillary teeth.

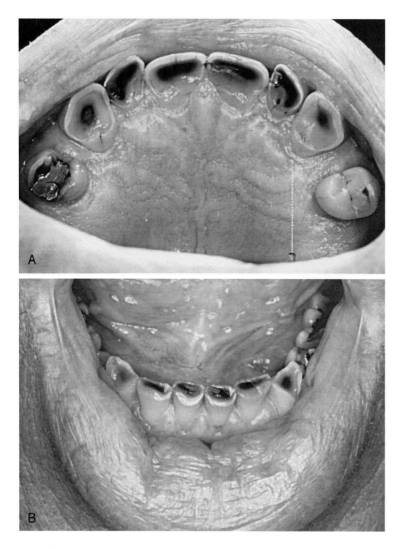

Figure 16–14. *A* and *B*, Tooth abrasion from cigar chewing.

cause, with so-called toothbrush abrasion along the cementoenamel junction an easily recognized pattern.

Erosion is the loss of tooth structure from a nonbacterial chemical process (Fig. 16–15). Most commonly, acids are involved in the dissolution process from either an external or an internal source. Externally, the acid may be found in the work environment (e.g., battery manufacturing) or in the diet (e.g., citrus fruits and acid-containing soft drinks). The internal source of acid is most probably from regurgitation of gastric contents. This may be seen in any disorder in which chronic vomiting is a part. Self-induced vomiting as a component of anorexia nervosa or bulimia syndrome has become an increasingly important cause of dental erosion and other oral abnormalities. The pattern of erosion associated with vomiting is usually generalized tooth loss on lingual surfaces of maxillary teeth. However, all surfaces may be affected, especially in individuals who compensate for fluid loss by excessive intake of fruit juices. In many cases of tooth erosion, no cause is found.

ALTERATIONS IN NUMBER

Anodontia

Absence of teeth is known as *anodontia*. It is further qualified as complete anodontia, when all teeth are missing; as partial anodontia, when one or several teeth are missing; as pseudoanodontia, when teeth are absent clinically because of impaction or delayed eruption; and as false anodontia, when teeth have been exfoliated or extracted. Partial anodontia is relatively common. Congenitally missing teeth are usually third molars, followed by second premolars and maxillary lateral

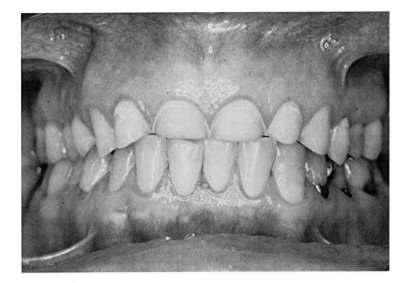

Figure 16–15. Erosion of the maxillary anterior teeth.

incisors (Fig. 16–16). The cause of partial anodontia is unknown, although hereditary factors are frequently involved. Complete anodontia is rare but is often associated with a syndrome known as *hereditary ectodermal dysplasia*, which is usually transmitted as an X-linked recessive disorder. Partial anodontia is more typical of this syndrome, however (Fig. 16–17). The few teeth that are present are usually conical.

IMPACTION

Impaction of teeth (pseudoanodontia) is a common event that most frequently affects the mandibular third molars and maxillary cuspids (Fig. 16–18). Less commonly, premolars, mandibular cuspids, and second molars are involved. It is rare to see impactions of incisors and first molars. Impaction occurs because of obstruction from crowding or from some other physical barrier. It may occasionally be due to an abnormal eruption path, presumably because of unusual orientation of the tooth germ. *Ankylosis*, the fusion of a tooth to surrounding bone, is another cause of impaction. This usually occurs in association with erupted primary molars (Fig. 16–19). It may result in impaction of a subjacent permanent tooth. The reason for ankylosis is unknown, but it is believed to be related to periapical inflammation and subsequent bone repair. With the focal loss of the periodontal ligament, bone and cementum become inextricably mixed, causing fusion of the tooth to alveolar bone.

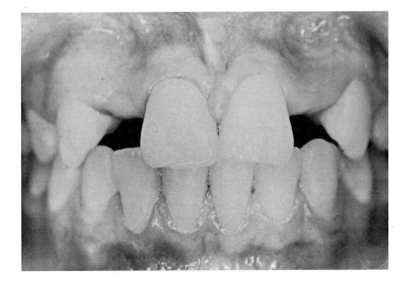

Figure 16–16. Congenitally missing maxillary lateral incisors.

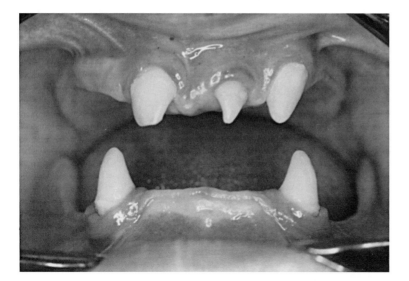

Figure 16–17. Partial anodontia in a patient with hereditary ectodermal dysplasia.

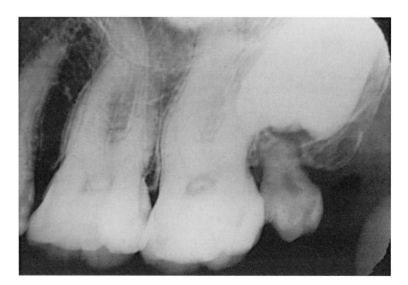

Figure 16–18. Impaction of a maxillary third molar. Note the supernumerary microdont and pulp stones.

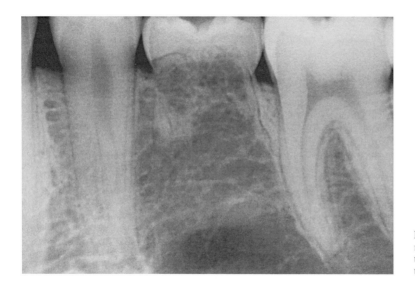

Figure 16–19. Ankylosis of primary molar tooth. Note the congenitally missing subjacent permanent tooth.

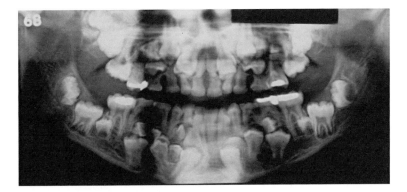

Figure 16–20. Supernumerary and impacted teeth in a patient with cleidocranial dysplasia.

Supernumerary Teeth

Extra or supernumerary teeth in the dentition most probably result from continued proliferation of the permanent or primary dental lamina to form a third tooth germ. The resulting teeth may have a normal morphology or may be rudimentary and miniature. Most are isolated events, although some may be familial and others may be syndrome associated (Gardner syndrome and cleidocranial dysplasia [Fig. 16–20]). Supernumerary teeth are found more often in the permanent than in the primary dentition and are much more frequently seen in the maxilla than in the mandible (10:1) (Fig. 16–21). The anterior midline of the maxilla is the most common site, in which case the supernumerary tooth is known as a *mesiodens* (Fig. 16–22). The maxillary molar area (fourth molar or paramolar) is the second most common site. The significance of supernumerary teeth is that they occupy space. When they are impacted, they may block the eruption of other teeth, or they may cause delayed eruption or maleruption of adjacent teeth. If supernumerary teeth erupt, they may cause malalignment of the dentition, and they may be cosmetically objectionable.

Supernumerary teeth appearing at the time of birth, known as *natal teeth*, are believed to be a rare event (Fig. 16–23). More commonly seen are prematurely erupted deciduous teeth, usually mandibular central incisors. Not to be confused with both these phenomena is the appearance of the common gingival or dental lamina cysts of the newborn.

Supernumerary teeth appearing after the loss of the permanent teeth are known as *postpermanent dentition*. This is generally regarded as a rare event. Most teeth appearing after extraction of the permanent teeth are believed to arise from eventual eruption of previously impacted teeth.

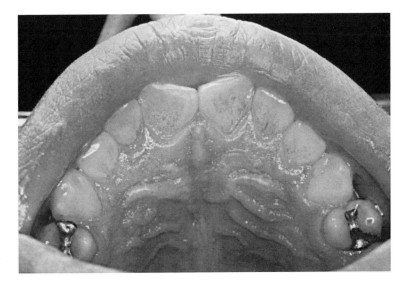

Figure 16–21. Supernumerary incisor teeth.

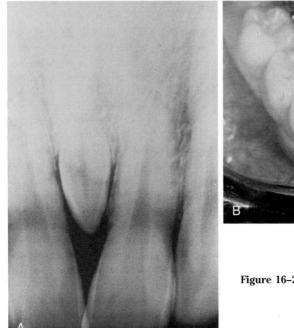

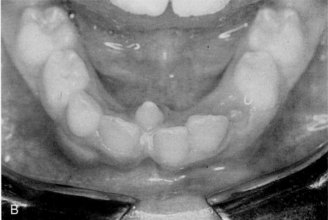

Figure 16–22. *A* and *B*, Mesiodens.

DEFECTS OF ENAMEL

Environmental Defects of Enamel

During enamel formation, ameloblasts are susceptible to various external factors that may be reflected in erupted teeth. Metabolic injury, if severe enough and long enough, can cause defects in quantity and shape of enamel or in the quality and color of enamel. Quantitatively defective enamel, when of normal hardness, is known as *enamel hypoplasia*. Qualitatively defective enamel, in which normal amounts of enamel are produced but are hypomineralized, is known as *enamel hypocalcification*. In this defect, the enamel is softer than normal. The extent of the enamel defect is dependent on three conditions: (1) the intensity of the etiologic factor, (2) the duration of the factor's presence, and (3) the time at which the factor occurs during crown develop-

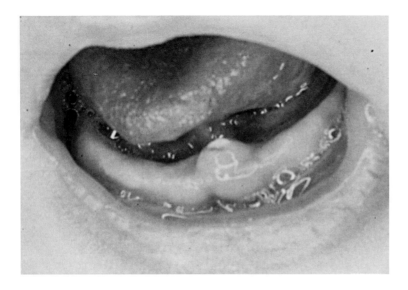

Figure 16–23. Natal tooth.

ment. The factors that lead to ameloblast damage are highly varied, although the clinical signs of defective enamel are the same.

Etiologic factors may occur locally, affecting only a single tooth, or they may act systemically, affecting all teeth in which enamel is being formed. Local trauma or abscess formation can adversely affect the ameloblasts overlying a developing crown, resulting in enamel hypocalcification or hypoplasia. Affected teeth may have areas of coronal discoloration, or they may have actual pits and irregularities. This is most commonly seen in permanent teeth in which the overlying deciduous tooth becomes abscessed or is physically forced into the enamel organ of the permanent tooth. The resulting hypoplastic or hypocalcified permanent tooth is sometimes known as *Turner's tooth* (Fig. 16–24).

For systemic factors to have an effect on developing permanent teeth, they must generally occur after birth and before the age of 6 years. During this time, the crowns of all permanent teeth (with the exception of the third molars) develop. Because most enamel defects affect anterior teeth and first molars, systemic factors will have occurred predominantly during the first year and a half of life (Fig. 16–25). Primary teeth and possibly the tips of first permanent molars and permanent central incisors may reflect ameloblast dysfunction occurring *in utero*, as these are the teeth undergoing enamel calcification during this period. The specific causes of systemically induced enamel defects are often obscure but are usually attributed to childhood infectious diseases. This, however, has not been well substantiated with research data. Other cited causes of enamel hypo-

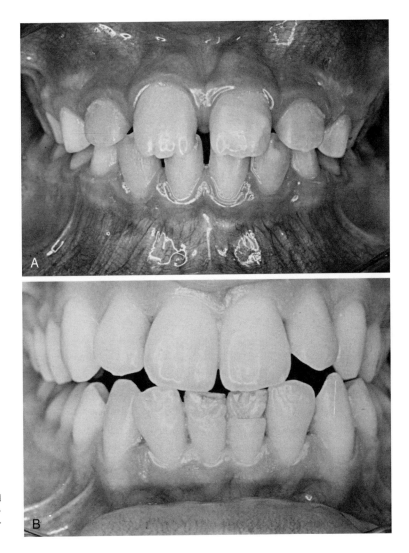

Figure 16–24. *A,* Hypocalcified maxillary left-central incisor (Turner's tooth). *B,* Hypoplastic mandibular central incisors.

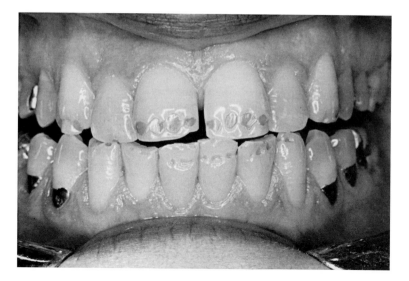

Figure 16–25. Environmental hypoplasia of the anterior teeth.

plasia or hypocalcification include nutritional defects such as rickets (Fig. 16–26), congenital syphilis, birth trauma (neonatal line in primary teeth), fluoride, and idiopathic factors. The enamel hypoplasia that may be seen with congenital syphilis is rather characteristic. The *in utero* infection by *Treponema pallidum* affects the developing permanent incisors and first molars (Fig. 16–27). Affected incisors, also known as *Hutchinson's incisors*, are tapered incisally and are notched centrally on the incisal edge. Affected molars, also known as *mulberry molars*, show a lobulated or crenated occlusal surface.

Ingestion of drinking water containing fluoride at levels greater than 1 part per million during the time crowns are being formed may result in enamel hypoplasia or hypocalcification, also known as *fluorosis* (Fig. 16–28). Endemic fluorosis is known to occur in areas where the drinking water contains excessive naturally occurring fluoride. As with other causative agents, the extent of damage is dependent on duration, timing, and intensity or concentration. Mild to moderate fluorosis ranges clinically from white enamel spots to mottled brown and white discolorations. Severe fluorosis appears as pitted, irregular, and discolored enamel. Although fluoride-induced enamel hypoplasia or hypocalcification is caries resistant, it may be cosmetically objectionable, making aesthetic dental restorations desirable.

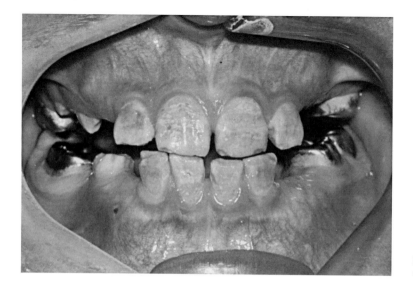

Figure 16–26. Enamel hypoplasia due to rickets.

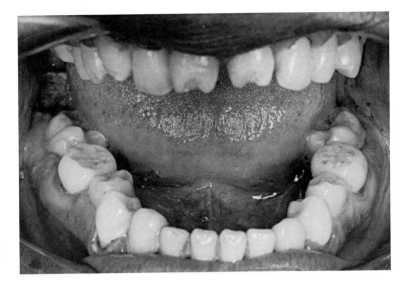

Figure 16–27. Notched incisors and mulberry molars resulting from congenital syphilis.

Amelogenesis Imperfecta

Amelogenesis imperfecta is a group of similar-appearing hereditary disorders of enamel formation in both dentitions. Most cases fall into one of two major types, hypoplastic or hypocalcified. A third type, known as *hypomaturation*, has been added to the list. Numerous subtypes of the three major groups are also recognized; these are based on different inheritance patterns and clinical appearances. The hereditary patterns range from autosomal dominant or recessive to X-linked dominant or recessive.

In the hypoplastic type, teeth erupt with insufficient amounts of enamel (Fig. 16–29), ranging from pits and grooves in one patient to complete absence (aplasia) in another. Because of reduced enamel thickness in some cases, abnormal contour and absent interproximal contact points may be evident. In the hypocalcified type, the quantity of enamel is normal, but it is soft and friable, so that it fractures and wears readily (Fig. 16–30). The color of the teeth varies from tooth to tooth and patient to patient—from white opaque to yellow to brown. Teeth also tend to darken with age, owing to exogenous staining. Radiographically, enamel appears reduced in bulk, often showing a thin layer over occlusal and interproximal surfaces. Dentin and pulp chambers appear normal. Other than cosmetic restoration, no treatment is

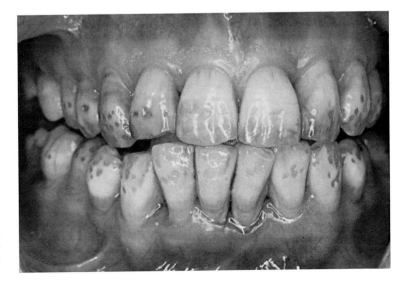

Figure 16–28. Enamel hypoplasia (fluorosis) resulting from excessive levels of fluoride in the drinking water.

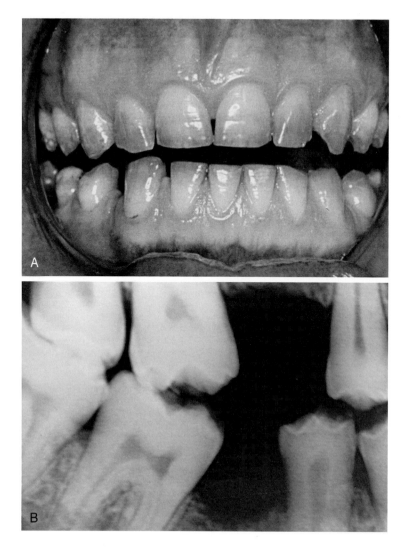

Figure 16–29. *A* and *B,* Amelogenesis imperfecta, hypoplastic type.

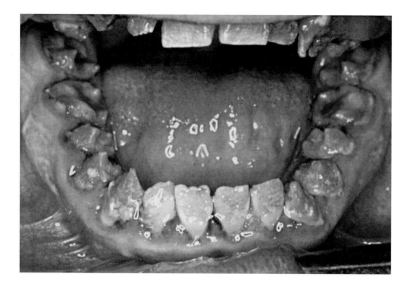

Figure 16–30. Amelogenesis imperfecta, hypocalcified type.

necessary. Although the enamel is soft and irregular, teeth are not caries prone.

DEFECTS OF DENTIN

Dentinogenesis Imperfecta

Dentinogenesis imperfecta is an autosomal dominant trait with variable expressivity. It affects dentin of both the primary and the permanent dentition. Because of the clinical discoloration of teeth, this condition has also been known as (hereditary) *opalescent dentin.*

Dentinogenesis imperfecta has been divided into three types: type I, in which the dentin abnormality occurs in patients with concurrent osteogenesis imperfecta. In this form, primary teeth are more severely affected than permanent teeth. In type II, patients have only dentin abnormalities

and no bone disease (Figs. 16–31 and 16–32). In type III, or Brandywine type (discovered in the triracial Brandywine isolate in Maryland), only dental defects occur, similar to type II but with some clinical and radiographic variations (Fig. 16–33). Features of type III that are not seen in types I and II include multiple pulp exposures, periapical radiolucencies, and a variable radiographic appearance.

Clinically, all three types share numerous features. In both dentitions, teeth exhibit an unusual translucent, opalescent appearance with color variation from yellow-brown to gray. The entire crown appears discolored owing to the abnormal underlying dentin. Although the enamel is structurally and chemically normal, it fractures easily, resulting in rapid wear. The enamel fracturing is believed to be due to the poor support provided by the abnormal dentin and possibly in part to the absence of the microscopic scalloping normally seen between

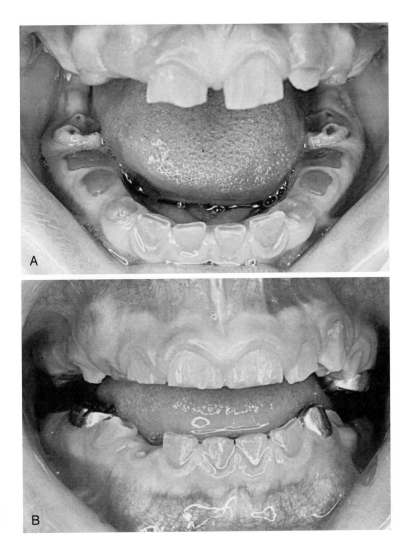

Figure 16–31. *A* and *B,* Dentinogenesis imperfecta in two brothers. Note the severe wear and abnormal color.

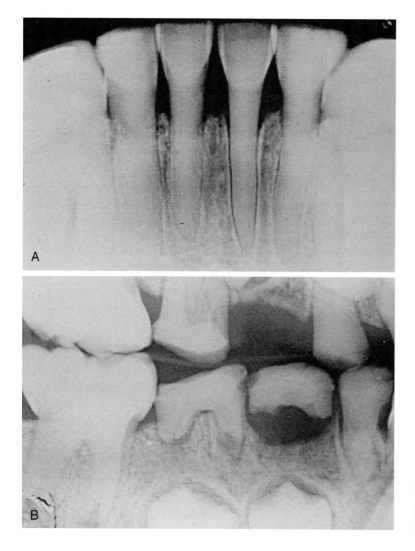

Figure 16–32. *A* and *B,* Dentinogenesis imperfecta. Note the obliterated pulps, bell-shaped crowns, and short roots.

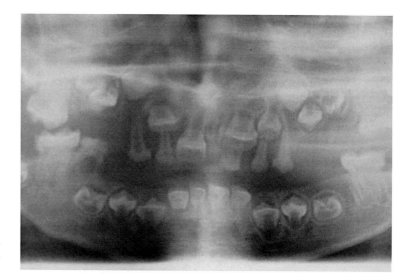

Figure 16–33. Dentinogenesis imperfecta, type III (Brandywine type), in a child in his mixed dentition.

dentin and enamel that is believed to help mechanically lock the two hard tissues together. Overall tooth morphology is unusual for its excessive constriction at the cementoenamel junction, giving the crowns a tulip or bell shape. Roots are shortened and blunted. The teeth do not exhibit any greater susceptibility to caries, and they may in fact show some resistance because of the rapid wear and absence of interdental contacts.

Radiographically, types I and II exhibit identical changes. Opacification of dental pulps occurs owing to continued deposition of abnormal dentin. The short roots and the bell-shaped crowns are also obvious on radiographic examination. In type III, the dentin appears thin and the pulp chambers and root canals extremely large, giving the appearance of thin dentin shells—hence, the previous designation of *shell teeth.*

Microscopically, the dentin of teeth in dentinogenesis imperfecta contains fewer but larger and irregular dentinal tubules. The pulpal space is nearly completely replaced over time by the irregular dentin. Enamel appears normal, but the dentinoenamel junction is smooth instead of scalloped.

Treatment is directed toward protecting tooth tissue from wear and toward improving the aesthetic appearance of the teeth. Generally, fitting with full crowns at an early age is the treatment of choice. Despite the qualitatively poor dentin, support for the crowns is adequate. These teeth should not be used as abutments, because the roots are prone to fracture under stress.

Dentin Dysplasia

Dentin dysplasia is another autosomal dominant trait that affects dentin. This is a rare condition that has been subdivided into type I or radicular type (Figs. 16–34 and 16–35) and a more rare type II or coronal type that varies slightly in its clinical presentation. In type II dentin dysplasia, the color of the primary dentition is opalescent, and the permanent dentition is normal; in type I, both dentitions are of normal color. The coronal pulps in type II are usually large ("thistle tube") and are filled with globules of abnormal dentin. Also, periapical lesions are not a regular feature of type II as they are in type I.

Clinically, the crowns in dentin dysplasia type I appear to be normal in color and shape. Premature tooth loss may occur because of short roots or periapical inflammatory lesions. Teeth show greater resistance to caries than do normal teeth.

Radiographically, in type I dentin dysplasia, roots appear extremely short and pulps are almost completely obliterated. Residual fragments of pulp tissue appear typically as horizontal lucencies (chevrons). Periapical lucencies are typically seen; they represent chronic abscesses, granulomas, or cysts. In type II dentin dysplasia, deciduous teeth are similar in radiographic appearance to type I, but permanent teeth exhibit enlarged pulp chambers that have been described as "thistle tube" in appearance.

Microscopically, the enamel and the immediately subjacent dentin appear normal. Deeper layers of dentin show atypical tubular patterns, with amorphous, atubular areas and irregular organization. On the pulpal side of the normal-appearing mantle of dentin, globular or nodular masses of abnormal dentin are seen.

Treatment is directed toward retention of teeth for as long as possible. However, because of the short roots and periapical lesions, the prognosis for prolonged retention is poor. This dental condition has not been associated with any systemic connective tissue problems.

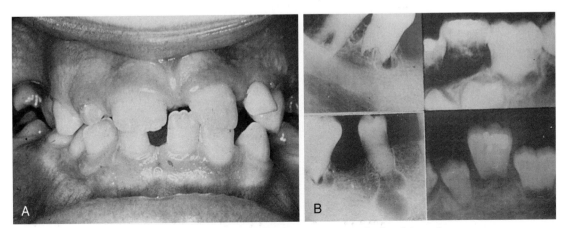

Figure 16–34. *A* and *B,* Dentin dysplasia, type I (radicular type). Note the normal color of the teeth.

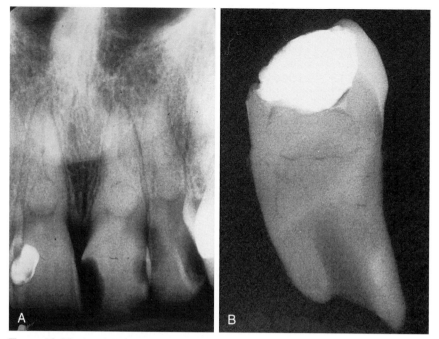

Figure 16–35. *A* and *B,* Dentin dysplasia, type I, with intrapulpal calcification and short roots. Note the thin zone of pulp tissue in the coronal areas.

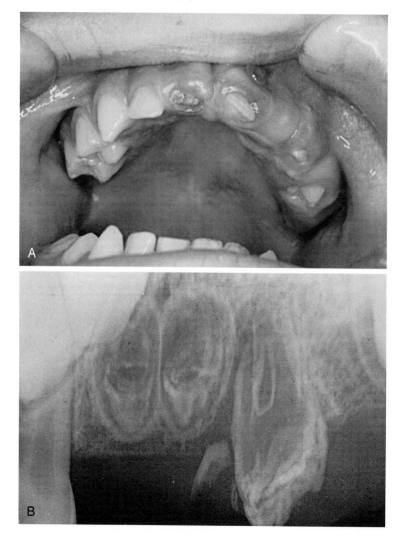

Figure 16–36. *A* and *B,* Regional odontodysplasia of the maxilla.

DEFECTS OF ENAMEL AND DENTIN

Regional Odontodysplasia

Regional odontodysplasia is a dental abnormality that involves the hard tissues that are derived from both epithelial (enamel) and mesenchymal (dentin and cementum) components of the tooth-forming apparatus. The teeth in a region or quadrant of the maxilla or mandible are affected to the extent that they exhibit short roots, open apical foramina, and enlarged pulp chambers (Fig. 16–36). The thinness and poor mineralization quality of the enamel and dentin layers have given rise to the term *ghost teeth*. The permanent teeth are affected more than the primary teeth, and the maxillary anterior teeth are affected more than other teeth. Eruption of the affected teeth is delayed or does not occur.

The cause of this rare dental abnormality is unknown, although numerous etiologic factors have been suggested, including trauma, nutritional deficiencies, infections, metabolic abnormalities, systemic diseases, and genetic influences.

Because of the poor quality of the affected teeth, their removal is usually indicated. The resulting edentulous zone can then be restored with a prosthesis.

ABNORMALITIES OF DENTAL PULP

Pulp Calcification

This is a rather common phenomenon that occurs with increasing age for no apparent reason. There appears to be no relation to inflammation, trauma, or systemic disease. Pulp calcification may be of microscopic size or may be large enough to be detected radiographically (Fig. 16–37). Calcifications may be either diffuse (linear) or nodular (pulp stones). The diffuse or linear deposits are typically found in the root canals and generally are parallel to the blood vessels. Pulp stones are usually found in the pulp chamber. When they are composed predominantly of dentin, they are referred to as *true denticles*; when they represent foci of dystrophic calcification, they are referred to as *false denticles*. Pulp stones are occasionally subdivided into attached and free types, depending on whether they are incorporated into the dentin wall or are surrounded by pulpal tissue.

Pulp stones appear to have no clinical significance. They are not believed to be a source of

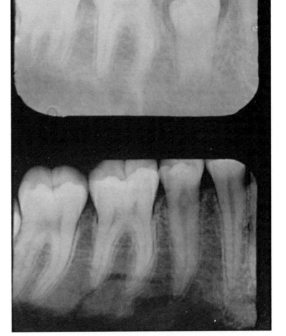

Figure 16–37. Pulp stone in an erupting second premolar (top) and an erupted tooth in the same patient.

pain and are not associated with any forms of pulpitis. They may, however, be problematic during endodontic therapy of nonvital teeth.

Internal Resorption

Resorption of the dentin of the pulpal walls may be seen as part of an inflammatory response to pulpal injury, or it may be seen in cases in which no apparent trigger can be identified (Fig. 16–38). The resorption occurs as a result of the activation of osteoclasts or dentinoclasts on internal surfaces of the root or crown. Resorption lacunae are seen, containing these cells and chronic inflammatory cells. Reversal lines may also be found in the adjacent hard tissue, indicating attempts at repair. In time, the root or crown is perforated by the process, making the tooth useless.

Any tooth may be involved, and usually only a single tooth is affected, although cases in which more than one tooth is involved have been described. In advanced cases, teeth may appear pink owing to the proximity of pulp tissue to the tooth

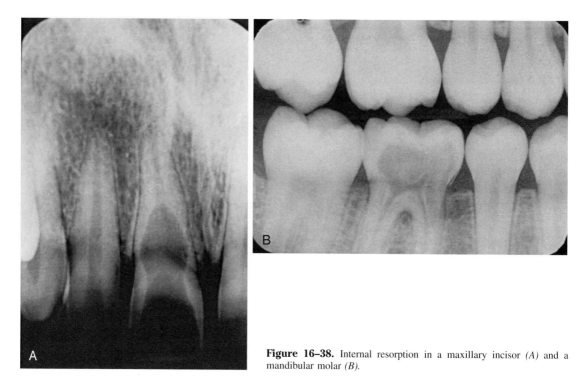

Figure 16–38. Internal resorption in a maxillary incisor *(A)* and a mandibular molar *(B)*.

surface. Until root fracture or communication with a periodontal pocket occurs, patients generally have no symptoms.

The treatment of choice is root canal therapy before perforation. Once there is communication between pulp and periodontal ligament, the prognosis for saving the tooth is very poor. The process occasionally may spontaneously arrest for no apparent reason.

External Resorption

Resorption of teeth from external surfaces may have one of several causes. This change may be the result of an adjacent pathologic process, such as (1) chronic inflammatory lesions, (2) cysts, (3) benign tumors, and (4) malignant neoplasms. The pathogenesis of external resorption from these causes has been related to release of chemical mediators, increased vascularity, and pressure. External resorption of teeth may also be seen in association with (1) trauma, (2) reimplantation or transplantation of teeth, and (3) impactions (Fig. 16–39). Trauma that causes injury to or necrosis of the periodontal ligament may initiate resorption of tooth roots. This trauma may be from a single event, from malocclusion, or from excessive orthodontic forces. Because reimplanted and transplanted teeth are nonvital and have no surrounding viable periodontal ligament, they are eventually

resorbed and replaced by bone. This is basically a natural physiologic process in which the calcified collagen matrix of the tooth serves as a framework for the deposition of new viable bone. Impacted teeth, when they impinge or exert pressure on adjacent teeth, may cause root resorption of the otherwise normally erupted tooth. Impacted teeth themselves may occasionally undergo resorption. The cause of this phenomenon is unknown, although it is believed to be related to a partial loss of the protective effect of the periodontal ligament or reduced enamel epithelium.

Finally, external resorption of erupted teeth may be idiopathic. This may occur in one or more teeth. Any tooth may be involved, although molars are least likely to be affected. One of two patterns may be seen. In one, resorption occurs immediately apical to the cementoenamel junction, mimicking a pattern of caries associated with xerostomia (Fig. 16–40). In external resorption, however, the lesions occur on root surfaces below the gingival epithelial attachment. In the other pattern of external resorption, the process starts at the tooth apex and progresses occlusally (Fig. 16–41).

External resorption is a particularly frustrating type of dental abnormality for both patients and practitioners, because there is no plausible or evident explanation for the condition and no effective treatment. Over an extended clinical course, resorption eventually causes loss of the affected tooth.

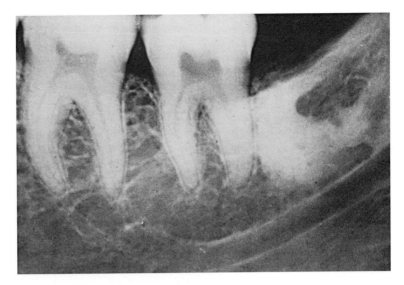

Figure 16–39. External resorption of an impacted third molar.

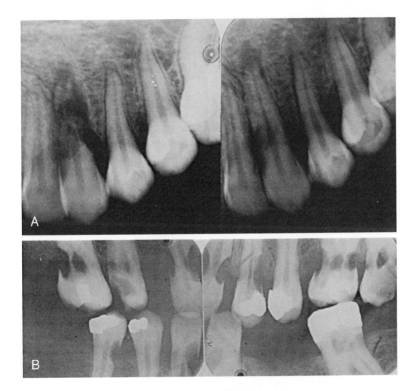

A

B

Figure 16–40. *A* and *B*, External resorption in the cervical areas of permanent teeth.

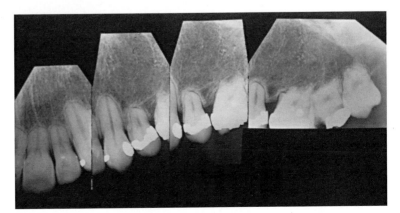

Figure 16–41. External resorption beginning at the apices of permanent teeth.

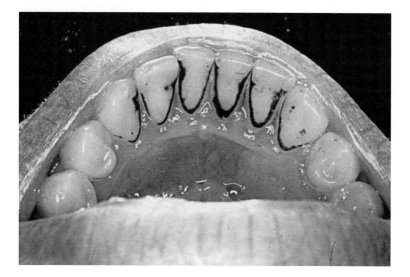

Figure 16–42. Black stain.

ALTERATIONS IN COLOR

Exogenous Stains

Stains on the surface of teeth that can be removed with abrasives are known as *exogenous* or *extrinsic stains*. The color change may be caused by pigments in dietary substances (e.g., coffee, betel nut, tobacco) or by the colored byproducts of chromogenic bacteria in dental plaque. Chromogenic bacteria are believed to be responsible for brown, black, green, and orange stains observed predominantly in children. Brown and black stains are typically seen in the cervical zone of teeth, either as a thin line along the gingival margin or as a wide band (Fig. 16–42). This type of stain is also often found on teeth adjacent to salivary duct orifices. Green stain is tenacious and is usually found as a band on the labial surfaces of the maxillary anterior teeth (Fig. 16–43). Blood pigments are thought to contribute to the green color. Orange or yellow-orange stains appear on the gingival third of teeth in a small percentage of children. These are generally easily removed.

Endogenous Stains

Discoloration of teeth resulting from deposits of systemically circulating substances during tooth development is defined as *endogenous* or *intrinsic staining*.

Systemic ingestion of *tetracycline* during tooth development is a well-known cause of endogenous staining of teeth. Tetracycline has an affinity for teeth and bones and is deposited in these sites

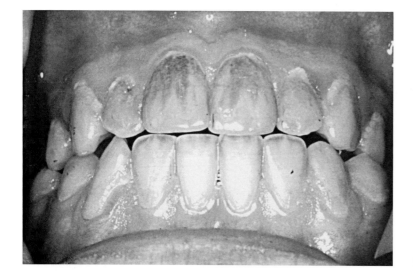

Figure 16–43. Green stain.

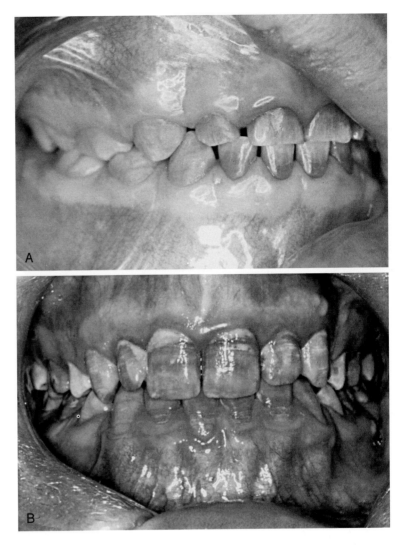

Figure 16–44. *A* and *B,* Tetracycline stain. Note the dark (gray) staining of the anterior teeth due to oxidization of tetracycline.

during metabolic activity. The drug's bright yellow color is reflected in the subsequently erupted teeth (Fig. 16–44). The fluorescent property of tetracycline can be demonstrated with an ultraviolet light in clinically erupted teeth. With time, the tetracycline oxidizes, resulting in a color change from yellow to gray or brown with the loss of its fluorescent quality. Because tetracycline can cross the placenta, it may stain primary teeth if taken during pregnancy. If it is administered between birth and age 6 or 7 years, permanent teeth may be affected. Only a small minority of children given tetracycline for various bacterial diseases, however, exhibit clinical evidence of discoloration. Staining is directly proportional to the age at which the drug is administered and the dose and duration of drug usage.

The significance of tetracycline staining lies in its cosmetically objectionable appearance. Because other equally effective antibiotics are available, tetracycline should not be prescribed for children younger than 7 years, except in unusual circumstances.

It should be noted that minocycline, a semisynthetic derivative of tetracycline, can stain the roots of adult teeth. It also may stain skin and mucosa in a diffuse or patchy pattern (see Chapter 5).

Rh incompatibility (erythroblastosis fetalis) has been cited as a cause of endogenous staining in primary teeth. Because of red blood cell hemolysis resulting from maternal antibody destruction of fetal red blood cells, blood breakdown products (bilirubin) are deposited in developing primary teeth. The teeth appear green to brown. Treatment is not required, because only primary teeth are affected.

Congenital porphyria, one of several inborn errors of porphyrin metabolism, is also a potential cause of endogenous pigmentation (Fig. 16–45). This autosomal recessive trait is also associated

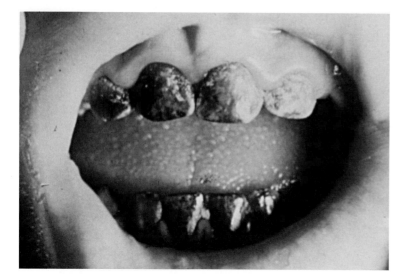

Figure 16–45. Porphyrin stain.

with photosensitivity, vesiculo-bullous skin eruptions, red urine, and splenomegaly. Teeth may appear red to brown because of deposition of porphyrin in the developing teeth. Affected teeth fluoresce red with ultraviolet light.

Liver disease, *biliary atresia* and *neonatal hepatitis*, may produce discoloration of the primary dentition. In biliary atresia, the teeth may assume a green discoloration; a yellowish-brown color is noted in cases of neonatal hepatitis. This is secondary to the deposition or incorporation of bilirubin in developing enamel and dentin.

Bibliography

Ahlquist M, Grondahl H. Prevalence of impacted teeth and associated pathology in middle-aged and older Swedish women. Community Dent Oral Epidemiol 19:116–119, 1991.

Brady W. The anorexia nervosa syndrome. Oral Surg Oral Med Oral Pathol 50:509–516, 1980.

Congleton J, Burkes E. Amelogenesis imperfecta with taurodontism. Oral Surg Oral Med Oral Pathol 48:540–544, 1979.

Escobar V, Goldblatt L, Bixler D. A clinical, genetic, and ultrastructural study of snowcapped teeth: amelogenesis imperfecta, hypomaturation type. Oral Surg Oral Med Oral Pathol 52:607–614, 1981.

Ferguson F, Friedman S, Frazzetto V. Successful apexification technique in an immature tooth with dens in dente. Oral Surg Oral Med Oral Pathol 49:356–359, 1980.

Gorlin R, Goldman H. Toma's Oral Pathology, 6th ed. St Louis, CV Mosby, 1970, Chaps 3 and 4.

Grover P, Carpenter W, Allen G. Panographic survey of United States' Army recruits: analysis of dental health status. Milit Med 147:1059–1061, 1982.

Grover P, Lorton L. Gemination and twinning in the permanent dentition. Oral Surg Oral Med Oral Pathol 59:313–318, 1985.

Grover P, Lorton L. The incidence of unerupted permanent teeth and related clinical cases. Oral Surg Oral Med Oral Pathol 59:420–425, 1985.

Heimler A, Sciubba J, Lieber E, et al. An unusual presentation of opalescent dentin and Brandywine isolate hereditary opalescent dentin in an Ashkenazic Jewish family. Oral Surg Oral Med Oral Pathol 59:608–615, 1985.

Jaspers M. Taurodontism in the Down syndrome. Oral Surg Oral Med Oral Pathol 51:632–636, 1981.

Jaspers M, Witkop C. Taurodontism, an isolated trait associated with syndromes and X-chromosomal aneuploidy. Am J Hum Genet 32:396–413, 1980.

Levin L, Leaf S, Jelmini R, et al. Dentinogenesis imperfecta in the Brandywine isolate (DI type III): clinical, radiologic, and scanning electron microscopic studies of the dentition. Oral Surg Oral Med Oral Pathol 56:267–274, 1983.

Lin L, Chance K, Skribner J, et al. Dens evaginatus: a case report. Oral Surg Oral Med Oral Pathol 63:86–89, 1987.

Rotstein I, Stabholz A, Friedman S. Endodontic therapy for dens invaginatus in a maxillary second premolar. Oral Surg Oral Med Oral Pathol 63:237–240, 1987.

Rubin M, Nevins A, Berg M, et al. A comparison of identical twins in relation to three dental anomalies: multiple supernumerary teeth, juvenile periodontosis, and zero caries incidence. Oral Surg Oral Med Oral Pathol 52:391–394, 1981.

Ruprecht A, Batniji S, El-Neweihi E. The incidence of taurodontism in dental patients. Oral Surg Oral Med Oral Pathol 63:743–747, 1987.

Sclare R. Hereditary opalescent dentin (dentinogenesis imperfecta). Br Dent J 84:164–166, 1984.

Spyropoulos N, Patsakas A, Angelopoulos A. Simultaneous presence of partial anodontia and supernumerary teeth. Oral Surg Oral Med Oral Pathol 48:53–56, 1979.

Witkop C. Hereditary defects of dentin. Dent Clin North Am 19:25–45, 1975.

Witkop C, Jaspers M. Teeth with short, thin, dilacerated roots in patients with short stature: a dominantly inherited trait. Oral Surg Oral Med Oral Pathol 54:553–559, 1982.

Wright J, Robinson C, Shoe R. Characterization of the enamel ultrastructure and mineral content in hypoplastic amelogenesis imperfecta. Oral Surg Oral Med Oral Pathol 72:594–601, 1991.

17

Common Skin Lesions

Ginat W. Mirowski and Todd W. Rozycki

MACULES AND PATCHES
Hypopigmented (White or Pink)
  Vitiligo
Hyperpigmented (Brown)
  Ephelides
  Café au Lait Macules (Café au Lait
    Spots)
  Solar Lentigo (Liver Spot)
  Melasma (Mask of Pregnancy)
Erythematous (Red)
  Erysipelas
  Telangiectasia
  Petechiae
  Purpura
  Ecchymoses
  Splinter Hemorrhages
PAPULES AND PLAQUES
Flesh-Colored/Yellow/Hypopigmented
  Acrochordon (Skin Tag)
  Fibrous Papule
  Adenoma Sebaceum (Angiofibroma)
  Neurofibroma
  Syringoma
  Molluscum Contagiosum
  Sebaceous Hyperplasia
  Xanthelasma
  Milia
  Favre-Racouchot Syndrome
Hyperpigmented (Brown)
  Nevus
  Melanoma
  Seborrheic Keratosis
Erythematous (Red)
  Acne
  Perioral Dermatitis
  Folliculitis
  Furuncle
  Miliaria
  Granuloma Faciale
  Cherry Hemangioma
  Strawberry Hemangioma
  Spitz Nevus
  Acute Febrile Neutrophilic Dermatosis
    (Sweet's Syndrome)
  Morbilliform Drug Eruptions
Violaceous (Blue or Purple)

  Lichen Planus
  Venous Lake
  Blue Nevus
  Angiosarcoma
NODULES
  Basal Cell Carcinoma
  Keratoacanthoma
  Squamous Cell Carcinoma
WHEALS
  Urticaria (Hives)
  Angioedema
PAPULOSQUAMOUS DERMATOSES
  Actinic Keratoses (Solar Keratoses)
  Seborrheic Dermatitis
  Psoriasis
  Atopic Dermatitis
  Keratosis Pilaris
  Pityriasis Rosea
  Verruca Vulgaris (Warts)
  Flat Wart (Verruca Plana)
VESICLES/BULLAE/PUSTULES
  Herpes Simplex Infection
  Varicella-Zoster Infection
  Contact Dermatitis
  Impetigo
  Rosacea
  Erythema Multiforme
  Pemphigus Vulgaris/Foliaceus/
    Erythematosus
EROSIONS/FISSURES/ULCERS/SCARS
  Perlèche
  Pyoderma Gangrenosum
  Burns
  Keloid
  Radiodermatitis
CONNECTIVE TISSUE DISEASES
  Dermatomyositis
  Lupus Erythematosus
  Scleroderma
  Temporal Arteritis

MACULES AND PATCHES

A macule is defined as a well-circumscribed, flat, discolored area approximately 0.5 cm in diameter. It may be brown, red, blue, white, yellow, or pink. A larger, flat, discolored area is a patch.

Hypopigmented (White or Pink)

VITILIGO

Vitiligo is an autoimmune condition characterized by loss of melanocytes and pigment from affected tissues. Vitiligo occurs at any age and in both men and women. The clinical course is unpredictable. Spontaneous repigmentation may occur but is rare. Toxic destruction of melanocytes after chemical exposure has occasionally been noted.

Clinical Features. Depigmented macules and patches have relatively distinct and possibly hyperpigmented margins. Perioral and periocular tissues are preferentially affected, as are the nape of the neck and areas of repeated trauma, such as the knees, elbows, and hands (Fig. 17–1).

Treatment. Treatment is difficult and may center on the use of cosmetic products such as tanning creams and cosmetic cover-ups of affected areas or depigmentation of normal adjacent skin. Sunscreens with a sun protection factor of 15 or greater should be used to prevent both sunburns and future skin cancers. Patients only rarely respond to topical steroids. Topical or systemic PUVA (psoralens and ultraviolet light) therapy may be effective but requires months of treatment. Autologous mini-grafts may accelerate repigmentation.

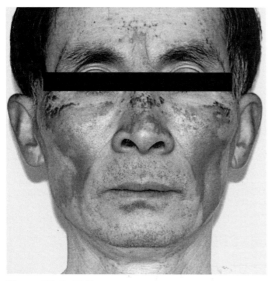

Figure 17–1. Vitiligo.

Hyperpigmented (Brown)

EPHELIDES

Ephelides, or freckles, are small (less than 0.5 cm) tan to brown discrete macules on sun-exposed skin (Fig. 17–2).

Clinical Features. Ephelides are found on the nose, cheeks, dorsal surface of the arms, and upper trunk of fair individuals with red-blond hair.

Histopathology. In ephelides, melanocytes are approximately one-third less abundant than in normal skin; however, they contain a greater number of melanosomes that also tend to be large, elongated, or rodshaped.

Treatment. No treatment is indicated. Trichloroacetic acid is occasionally used to peel off a few at a time; results are variable.

CAFÉ AU LAIT MACULES (CAFÉ AU LAIT SPOTS)

Café au lait macules (CALM) are discrete, pale brown macules or patches that vary in size from 0.2 to 2 cm and have irregular or serrated margins (Fig. 17–3). CALM are noted at birth or soon thereafter. As many as three CALM may be seen in normal children, but the presence of numerous or larger macules is usually associated with either neurofibromatosis (NF) or Bloom's syndrome. Ultraviolet (UV) light frequently darkens CALM; however, in contrast to ephelides, they do not disappear with shading from light. Neurofibromatosis (von Recklinghausen's disease) is an autosomal dominant neurocutaneous syndrome characterized by numerous neurofibromas (discussed later) of the skin, nerves, and central nervous system. The presence of five or more CALM greater than 0.5 cm in diameter in children younger than 5 years or the presence of six or more CALM greater than 1.5 cm in diameter in adults strongly suggests the diagnosis of NF. Axillary freckling accompanied by the presence of six or more CALM is pathognomonic for NF. Patients with NF may also develop generalized hyperpigmentation and, rarely, hypopigmented macules.

Two forms of NF are recognized on the basis of their clinical manifestations and according to the genetic defect. Patients with NF1 have a mutation of the tumor-suppressor gene for neurofibromin, which is located on chromosome 17. Patients with NF2 have a mutation in the tumor-suppressor gene for schwannomin, and the defect is localized to chromosome 22. Patients with NF1 present with multiple cutaneous tumors, CALM,

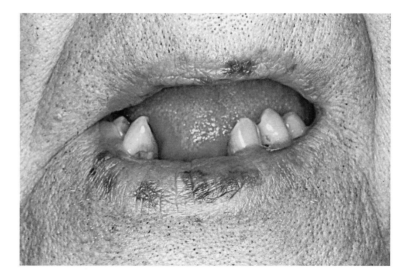

Figure 17–2. Ephelides (freckles).

and central nervous system tumors. On the other hand, patients with NF2 have bilateral acoustic neuromas and fewer cutaneous lesions, one or more plexiform neurofibromas, and two or more Lisch nodules on slit-lamp examination.

Albright's syndrome (polyostotic fibrous dysplasia), a sporadic disorder, is considered to be strongly associated with somatic mutation of the Gs, alpha gene. It most often includes pseudocysts of long bones, endocrine dysfunction, CALM, and precocious puberty in girls; however, possible variants have been associated with primary biliary cirrhosis and alopecia. The CALM of Albright's tend to be large and unilateral and to have very irregular borders.

Histopathology. Microscopically, CALM of NF have an increased number of morphologically normal melanocytes that may contain macromela-

nosomes in melanocytes and/or keratinocytes. CALM of Albright's lack these macromelanosomes. Although macromelanosomes are frequently found in CALM of NF, their absence does not exclude NF as the diagnosis.

Treatment. CALM do not require treatment; evaluation for an underlying genetic disease may be required.

SOLAR LENTIGO (LIVER SPOT)

Solar lentigo is a benign, irregularly shaped, hyperpigmented macule. Solar lentigines tend to be larger and darker than ephelides (Figs. 17–4 and 17–5).

Clinical Features. These discrete macules occur in skin that has been chronically exposed to

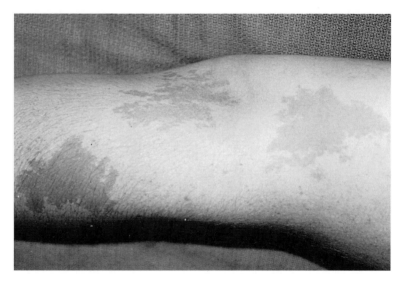

Figure 17–3. Café au lait macules.

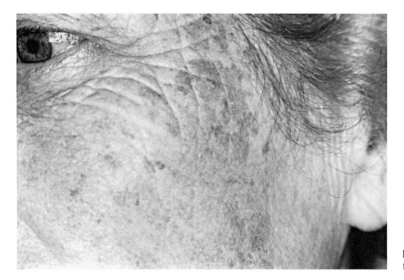

Figure 17–4. Solar lentigines of the face.

the sun; however, unlike freckles, which tend to fade when protected from solar exposure, solar lentigines remain. Lentigines are associated with other signs of chronic sun exposure, such as depigmented macules, actinic purpura, and actinic keratoses. Although lentigines are benign, any lentigo that enlarges or develops increased pigmentation, localized thickening, or a highly irregular border should be evaluated for melanoma. Perioral lentigines are associated with Addison's disease, Peutz-Jegher's syndrome, and Laugier-Hunziker syndrome.

Histopathology. Lentigines contain a marked increase in melanocyte density, increased pigmentation of the basal cell layer and adjacent keratinocytes, and elongation of rete ridges. Melanophages may be present in the upper dermis (Fig. 17–6).

Treatment. Most normal-appearing solar lentigines do not require treatment. If any underlying

pathologic change is suspected, a biopsy is required, with possible excision pending final diagnosis. Cosmetic ablation may be performed with cryotherapy (liquid nitrogen), laser vaporization, or topical tretinoin.

MELASMA (MASK OF PREGNANCY)

Melasma is an acquired hypermelanosis, commonly noted in pregnancy and in women taking birth control pills; 10% of cases are seen in males. Melasma occurring during pregnancy usually disappears several months after delivery; however, discontinuing oral contraceptives rarely eliminates melasma even 5 years after discontinued use. The

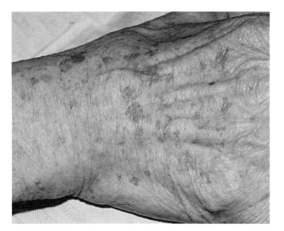

Figure 17–5. Solar lentigines of the hand.

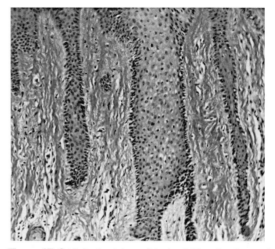

Figure 17–6. Solar lentigines of the hand. Note the elongated and hyperpigmented rete ridges.

infrequency of melasma in postmenopausal women on estrogen replacement indicates that estrogen alone is not the etiologic agent. Sunlight seems to have an important role in the development and darkening of melasma.

Clinical Features. Melasma is an acquired hypermelanosis characterized by well-demarcated and often symmetric brown to grayish patches on the face. It has a predilection for the cheeks, forehead, and upper lip; however, concurrent involvement of the nipples and genital region is occasionally seen.

Histopathology. Three types of melasma are seen histologically: (1) epidermal type, (2) dermal type, and (3) mixed type. All types show an increase in the number and activity of melanocytes, as well as increased transfer of melanosomes. In epidermal melasma, melanin is also increased in the basal and suprabasal layers. In dermal melasma, melanin-laden macrophages are found in the mid and upper dermis.

Treatment. Wood's lamp evaluation of epidermal melasma (positive) versus dermal melasma (negative) is an aid in treatment considerations. Epidermal melasma may be treated with bleaching agents such as 2 to 4% hydroquinone and concomitant use of strong sunscreens and topical tretinoin cream at night. Dermal melasma does not respond to treatment.

Erythematous (Red)

Erythema is reddening of the skin caused by vasodilatation of superficial blood vessels. Erythema is nonspecific and may occur in many skin conditions.

ERYSIPELAS

Erysipelas is an acute superficial cellulitis characterized by marked lymphatic vessel involvement. It is due to group A streptococci in children or group B streptococci in neonates. Rarely, *Staphylococcus aureus* may be responsible.

Clinical features. Erysipelas occurs in infants, young children, and the elderly. A small break in the skin with subsequent contamination with streptococci is the typical precedent. A recent history of an upper respiratory tract infection with streptococci is often elicited. Erysipelas presents as bright to dusky red, warm, shiny skin that is often indurated and edematous. The sharply demarcated, advancing raised border may be painful. The bridge of the nose and one or both cheeks are often affected; the process usually stops at the

beard or hairline. Patients present with a high fever, general malaise, and a leukocytosis of 15,000 or greater. Complications such as abscess formation, spreading necrosis of the soft tissues, and septicemia are rare but may occur after inadequate therapy or in immunocompromised patients.

Histopathology. The epidermis is usually unaffected. Marked edema and lymphatic dilatation are noted in the dermis, with a diffuse, mostly neutrophilic infiltrate extending throughout the dermis and occasionally into the subcutaneous fat. Gram stain reveals streptococci in the tissue and lymphatics.

Treatment. Uncomplicated erysipelas is often a self-limited process, remaining confined to the lymphatics and subcutaneous tissues and subsiding over 7 to 10 days. Antibiotic therapy shortens this process; however, more than a week may be required for more complete resolution. Recurrences are frequent.

TELANGIECTASIA

Telangiectasias are permanently dilated dermal blood vessels that appear as red or violaceous threads in different patterns. They occur in many cutaneous and systemic conditions. Some of these include actinic-damaged skin, basal cell carcinoma, CREST syndrome (calcinosis, Raynaud's, esophageal constriction, sclerodactyly, and telangiectasias), systemic lupus erythematosus (SLE), rosacea, cirrhosis, and pregnancy. They are only cosmetic problems, and bleeding occurs very rarely.

Treatment. Spider angiomas, one type of telangiectatic pattern, are often treated either by electrodesiccation of the central arteriole or by laser ablation. In general, telangiectasias are not treated.

PETECHIAE

Petechiae are tiny, well-circumscribed macules. These nonspecific findings represent punctate hemorrhages in the dermis. Conditions in which petechiae may occur include gonococcemia, meningococcemia, amyloidosis, and various leukocytoclastic vasculitides. Petechiae disappear after the underlying disease process has ceased.

PURPURA

Purpura are circumscribed intradermal deposits of hemorrhage that measure more than 0.1 to 5.0 cm in diameter. Purpura are nonspecific findings that may accompany platelet abnormalities, Rocky Mountain spotted fever, scurvy, or trauma.

ECCHYMOSES

Ecchymoses, or bruises, are large dermal hemorrhages that occur most often after blunt trauma but may be due to platelet dysfunction or amyloidosis. They may be purple-red initially, but in time, they become lighter and may be rust colored, yellow, or greenish.

SPLINTER HEMORRHAGES

Splinter hemorrhages are longitudinal linear hemorrhages in the nail bed (Fig. 17–7). Their presence, along with supportive clinical history, is highly suggestive of bacterial endocarditis. Along with Osler's nodes (painful nodules of digital tufts) and Janeway lesions (nontender papules on palms/plantar surfaces), splinter hemorrhages are the cutaneous manifestations of bacterial endocarditis. In as many as 20% of patients, splinter hemorrhages are nonspecific. Some other causes include trauma, vasculitis, scurvy, and trichinosis. Diagnosis and treatment of the underlying cause is required.

PAPULES AND PLAQUES

A papule is a raised bump that measures up to 0.5 cm in diameter. A plaque is an elevated, plateau-like area that measures greater than 0.5 cm and may be formed by the confluence of multiple papules.

Flesh-Colored/Yellow/ Hypopigmented

ACROCHORDON (SKIN TAG)

An acrochordon is a soft, flesh-colored, often pedunculated benign tumor of the skin. Acrochordons may have irregular or smooth surfaces. They occur around the eyelids, neck, and axillae and remain asymptomatic unless the pedicle twists, resulting in infarction.

Histopathology. Acanthosis, hyperkeratosis, and papillomatosis of the epithelium are noted. The stalk is composed of loose collagen fibers and dilated capillaries.

Treatment. Skin tags may be removed by snipping with curved iris scissors, or they may be destroyed using electrocautery or cryotherapy.

FIBROUS PAPULE

Clinical Features. Fibrous papules are dome-shaped, firm, flesh-colored papules measuring less than 0.5 cm and having a broad base (Fig. 17–8); they occasionally are pedunculated. These occur in middle age and affect both genders equally.

Histopathology. The epidermal changes observed include hyperkeratosis with a slight degree of hypergranulosis and flattened epithelial ridges. The primary alterations are within the dermis and consist of hyperplastic collagen and spindle-

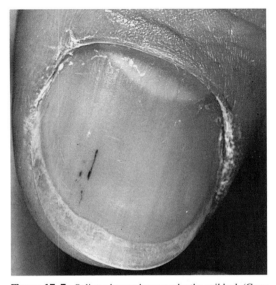

Figure 17–7. Splinter hemorrhages under the nail bed. (Courtesy of Dr. C.W. Lewis.)

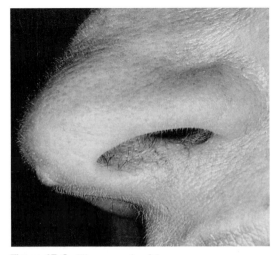

Figure 17–8. Fibrous papule of the nose.

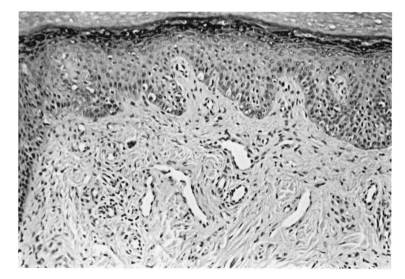

Figure 17–9. Fibrous papule showing prominent vessels and spindle cells in a collagenous stroma.

shaped to stellate cells that are often multinucleated (Fig. 17–9). Collagen bundles are coarse and are often arranged vertically toward the superficial aspects of the dermis. Blood vessels are usually increased in number and dilated.

Treatment. Treatment is surgical in nature. Curettage followed by cautery of the surgical bed generally prevents recurrence.

ADENOMA SEBACEUM (ANGIOFIBROMA)

Angiofibromas occur as solitary papules or as part of the triad (mental deficiency, epilepsy, and multiple angiofibromas of the face) of tuberous sclerosis, an autosomal dominant syndrome.

Clinical Features. Angiofibromas appear as small (0.1 to 0.3 cm), flesh-colored, brown or reddish, smooth, shiny papules on both sides of the nose, on the medial cheeks, and extending slightly down the nasolabial folds.

Histopathology. Angiofibromas are indistinguishable histologically from the solitary fibrous papule of the face. The epidermis is normal in architecture, the papillary dermis is absent, there is considerable dermal fibrosis, with collagen fibers running perpendicular to the epidermis, and capillaries are dilated. In the papillary dermis, stellate, glia-like cells and occasional multinucleated giant cells are present. The sebaceous glands are generally atrophic.

Treatment. Shave excision is often curative; however, when many lesions are present, as in tuberous sclerosis, dermabrasion or laser treatment may be helpful. Recurrence is common.

NEUROFIBROMA

Neurofibromas are benign nerve sheath tumors that may be solitary or multiple. Multiple neurofibromas are noted in NF (discussed earlier).

Clinical Features. Dermal neurofibromas are soft, flesh-colored papules or nodules that may be pedunculated or sessile. They often invaginate when depressed (Fig. 17–10). Subcutaneous neurofibromas tend to be larger and firmer than dermal neurofibromas. These tumors may be found anywhere but favor the trunk.

Histopathology. Well-circumscribed unencapsulated tumors are seen to infiltrate the surrounding dermis. Large tumors may extend into the fat. Typical neurofibromas are composed of thin, wavy, slightly eosinophilic collagen fibers that extend in various directions. A sizable number of uniform, spindle-shaped nuclei are present within these strands. A large number of mast cells are often found, but elastic fibers are absent.

Treatment. Solitary neurofibromas may be excised. However, if an identified nerve is involved, the nerve may have to be sacrificed. Excision is not practical in patients with NF but can be reserved for especially painful or unsightly lesions.

SYRINGOMA

The syringoma is a benign tumor that represents an adenoma of intraepidermal eccrine ducts.

Clinical Features. Clinically, numerous firm, flesh-colored to yellowish papules, 0.2 to 0.4 cm in diameter, are found under the eyelids and on the cheeks, axillae, pubic area, and abdomen. Hormonal influences have been postulated because

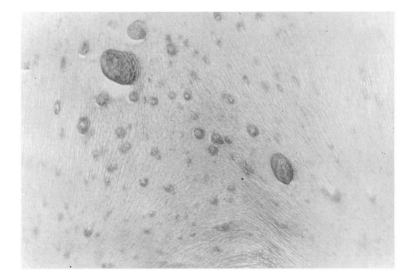

Figure 17–10. Neurofibromas of von Recklinghausen's disease.

they proliferate at puberty and women are more commonly affected. Syringomas proliferate and increase is size during pregnancy and premenstrually (Fig. 17–11).

Histopathology. The epidermis may show keratin-filled ductal lumina with occasional keratohyalin-containing cells. In the papillary dermis are many small, cystic ducts and solid epithelial strands embedded in a fibrous stroma. Some of the ducts may have small comma-like excrescences that may give them the appearance of tadpoles.

Treatment. These tumors have no malignant potential but are disfiguring and may be removed for purely cosmetic reasons by electrodesiccation, curettage, or excision.

MOLLUSCUM CONTAGIOSUM

Molluscum contagiosum is a common viral skin disease that presents as discrete white/skin-colored, umbilicated papules on the skin and rarely the vermilion. The etiologic agent is a large DNA poxvirus. The clinical presentation and treatments depend on the age and immune status of the host. Molluscum contagiosum is transmitted by direct contact and ultimately involutes spontaneously, with an associated mild inflammatory reaction and tenderness. In immunosuppressed individuals, *Cryptococcus neoformans* may present as umbilicated papules that clinically resemble molluscum contagiosum.

Clinical Features. In children, 1 to 50 or more

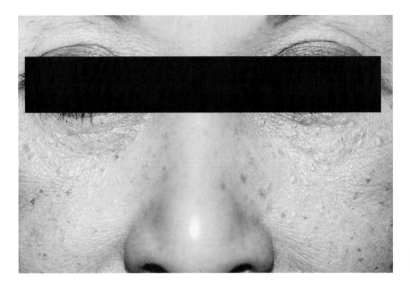

Figure 17–11. Multiple syringomas under the eyes.

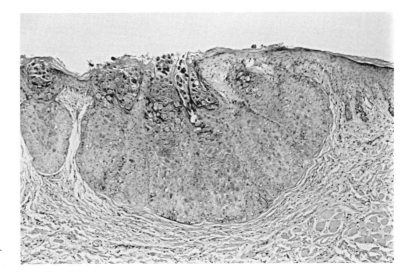

Figure 17–12. Molluscum contagiosum papule.

papules may be noted on the skin. These develop 2 to 3 months after the initial inoculation and are typically asymptomatic. The lesions have a predilection for the neck, trunk, eyelids, and anogenital area. Dozens or even hundreds of such lesions can be seen in immunosuppressed individuals, in whom spontaneous involution does not occur.

Histopathology. A striking characteristic of the epidermis in molluscum lesions is the appearance of a widened epithelial ridge as great as six times normal. Intracytoplasmic inclusions, called *molluscum bodies* or *Henderson-Patterson bodies*, are noted in infected cells and extend toward the surface, eventually completely obliterating the epithelium (Figs. 17–12 and 17–13). These inclusions are pathognomonic.

Treatment. Molluscum contagiosum often re-solves spontaneously. Treatment may shorten the duration as well as reduce the chance for autoinoculation and transmission to others. Curettage followed by minimal electrocautery or cryotherapy with liquid nitrogen or dry ice may be effective at decreasing the size and number of lesions. In immunocompromised individuals, the lesions are particularly recalcitrant to all treatments.

SEBACEOUS HYPERPLASIA

Clinical Features. Sebaceous hyperplasia presents with small (0.1 to 0.3 cm), soft, yellow, slightly umbilicating papules on the face or forehead of middle-aged or older people.

Histopathology. Usually noted is a single enlarged sebaceous gland composed of many lobules

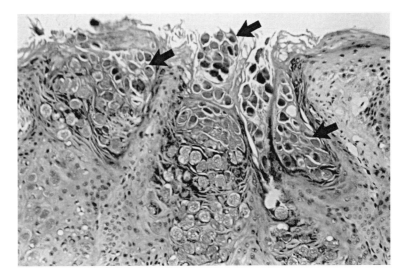

Figure 17–13. Molluscum contagiosum papule. Note the molluscum bodies in the upper epidermis *(arrows).*

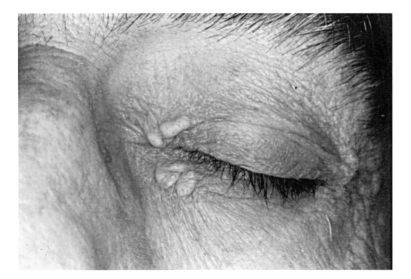

Figure 17–14. Xanthelasma palpebarum.

grouped around a central dilated duct. The sebaceous glands usually are fully mature, but there may be more than one peripheral row of undifferentiated cells that possess very little lipid.

Treatment. Treatment is removal of the elevated portion of the papule by shave biopsy, curettage, electrodesiccation, or treatment with trichloroacetic acid. Oral isotretinoin is dramatically effective, but side effects limit its usefulness.

XANTHELASMA

Xanthelasma presents as yellow papules and plaques or macules that may or may not be associated with hyperlipidemia. The upper eyelids are the predominant sites, and the lesions are not associated with hyperlipoproteinemia (Fig. 17–14).

Histopathology. Histologically, foam or xanthoma cells, which are macrophages that have ingested lipid material (Fig. 17–15), are present within the superficial dermis and are surrounded by fibrous connective tissue.

Treatment. No treatment is indicated; however, excision or the sequential application of trichloracetic acid may be used for cosmetic purposes. Xanthelasma may recur.

MILIA

Milia are small (0.1 to 0.2 cm) white superficial cysts of the upper segment of the hair follicle

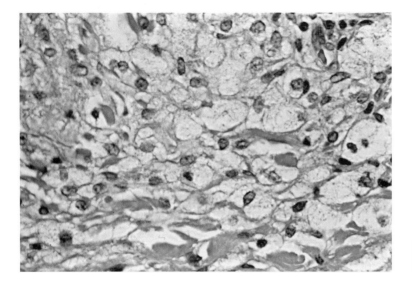

Figure 17–15. Xanthelasma palpebarum. Foamy macrophages are found in the dermis.

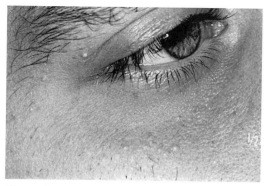

Figure 17–16. Milia.

(Fig. 17–16). No treatment is necessary. Milia may be removed for cosmetic considerations by incising the overlying epidermis and gently extracting the cyst contents.

FAVRE-RACOUCHOT SYNDROME

Favre-Racouchot syndrome is a condition of the elderly in which facial skin (especially lateral to the eyes) exhibits extensive sun damage. Clinically, numerous open, dilated, and cystic comedones are evident.

Histopathology. The surrounding epidermis appears normal, but the dermis may have variable solar elastosis. Characteristically seen are dilated pilosebaceous openings with distended, horn-filled hair follicles. Sebaceous gland atrophy with rare inflammation occurs because the comedones are open.

Treatment. Treatment is limited because of severe underlying solar damage.

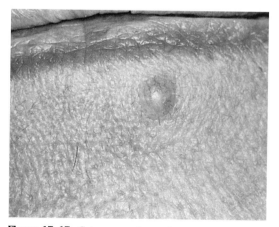

Figure 17–17. Cutaneous melanocytic nevus.

Hyperpigmented (Brown)

NEVUS

A nevus is commonly known as a mole. Nevi are flat or slightly raised light brown to brown-black papules measuring 0.1 to 0.6 cm (Figs. 17–17 and 17–18). Dysplastic nevi are asymmetric moles with irregular borders and characteristic histologic features. Individuals with numerous large dysplastic nevi are at a higher risk for melanoma.

Clinical Features. Nevi are rare at birth and usually appear after the age of 2 years. After childhood, some flat nevi change into compound nevi (elevate). Degeneration into melanoma is exceedingly rare. Epidemiologic studies have found that many nonfreckling, lighter-skinned individuals and light-skinned blacks may have nevi.

Histopathology. Clusters of melanocytes are found at the dermal-epidermal junction, in the dermis, or both in the dermis and at the junction of the dermis and epidermis.

Treatment. Clearly, removing all cutaneous moles is an impossible and inappropriate task. However, if a particular mole exhibits transformation or is irritated, removal with pathologic evaluation is indicated.

MELANOMA

The incidence of melanomas of the skin has been increasing during the past several years. Mel-

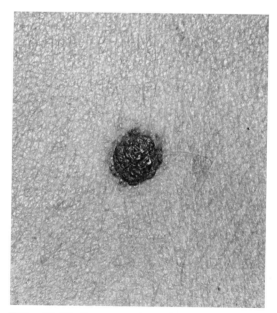

Figure 17–18. Cutaneous melanocytic nevus.

Table 17–1. Melanoma Thickness and Prognosis

THICKNESS (mm)	SURVIVAL RATE (%)
<0.75	Nearly 100
0.75–1.5	90
1.5–3.5	40

Breslow A. Thickness, cross-sectional areas and depth of invasion in the prognosis of cutaneous melanoma. Ann Surg 172:902–908, 1970.

anoma now represent approximately 2% of all cancers (excluding basal cell and squamous cell carcinomas of the skin). Predisposing risk factors include a positive family history, light natural pigmentation, and acute intermittent exposure to sunlight, especially in childhood. Most melanomas arise *de novo*, although some arise from preexisting pigmented lesions. The best indicator of prognosis is the microscopic depth of invasion of the tumor. This may be measured with a relatively subjective assessment using Clark's levels (1 to 5) or with an objective determination known as *Breslow's measurement* (Table 17–1). With Breslow's technique, the thickness of the primary lesion is measured with a microscope ocular micrometer, from the top of the granular layer to the deepest tumor cell. Obviously, the thinner the neoplasm, the better is the prognosis. Generally, the larger the lesion and the greater the spread, the poorer is the prognosis.

Clinical Features. Approximately 20% of all melanomas occur on the head and neck. Melanomas are characterized by two growth phases—a horizontal and a vertical phase. Melanomas are classified into three predominant types according to their clinical features. *Superficial spreading melanomas* account for approximately 60% of all melanomas. Nodular melanomas account for 30%, and lentigo maligna melanomas account for 10% of melanomas. A *superficial spreading melanoma* advances across the skin, producing an irregular patch of various colors (Fig. 17–19). Neoplastic cells are found in nests at the epidermal-dermal junction and extend laterally from the center of the lesion. While in this prolonged horizontal or *radial growth phase*, the lesion may be designated microscopically as melanoma *in situ*. Treatment during the radial or *in situ* growth phase yields excellent results.

A vertical growth phase is signaled by the appearance of clusters of neoplastic cells within the underlying dermis. The lesion develops metastatic potential that significantly affects prognosis. A *nodular melanoma* has only a vertical growth phase and thus exhibits a poorer prognosis. These present as darkly pigmented papules or nodules (Fig. 17–20) that may ulcerate or may exhibit rapid growth. Neoplastic melanocytes are found in both the dermis and epidermis.

Lentigo maligna melanoma occurs predominantly on sun-exposed skin of the elderly. Its radial growth phase may last as long as 25 or 30 years. Clinically, lentigo maligna melanoma appears as a flat, irregularly pigmented patch with ill-defined margins. Prognosis is generally considered excellent until the lesion enters a vertical phase.

Treatment. Surgical excision remains the treatment of choice for all types of melanomas. Generally, 1-cm margins are recommended for thin lesions and 2- to 3-cm margins are recommended for thicker lesions. Elective dissection of regional

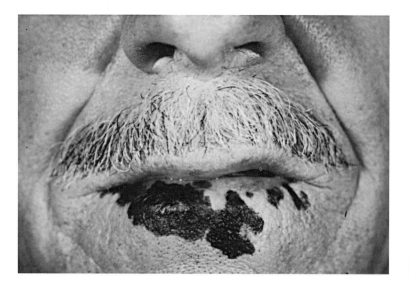

Figure 17–19. Superficial spreading melanoma.

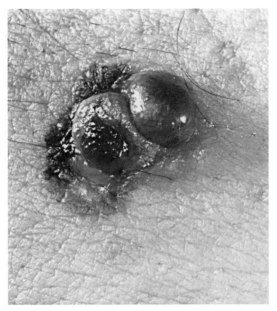

Figure 17–20. Cutaneous nodular melanoma. (Courtesy of Dr. W. G. Sprague.)

lymph nodes is a controversial issue but is more likely to be performed with excision of thicker neoplasms. Chemotherapy, immunotherapy, and radiation therapy may be added to the treatment regimen.

SEBORRHEIC KERATOSIS

Seborrheic keratosis is a benign epidermal proliferation with increasing frequency from middle age to the later years. The cause is unknown.

Clinical Features. Seborrheic keratosis may present as a solitary lesion, but several lesions are frequently found. Plaques range from light brown to black, with sharp, delineated margins. Clinically, seborrheic keratosis has a greasy-feeling keratotic crust that is loosely attached (Figs. 17–21 and 17–22). A stuck-on quality is typical. The surface may be rough or warty because of tightly aggregated fine fissures or clefts. During the early phases of development, seborrheic keratoses may be flat, with a dull or matte surface quality similar in appearance to solar or simple lentigines. Larger pigmented lesions may be mistaken for pigmented basal cell carcinoma or nodular melanoma.

Histopathology. Seborrheic keratoses show a wide range of histologic variation. Many microscopic subtypes may be seen in the same lesion. Common features of all lesions include hyperkeratosis, acanthosis, and papillomatosis (Fig. 17–23). They are characterized by a biphasic hyperplasia of both the epidermis and supporting papillary dermis. Small keratotic pseudocysts or horn cysts appear as a result of invagination of the stratum corneum. Commonly, a mild chronic inflammatory cell infiltrate can be found in the dermis, occasionally producing a lichenoid pattern. If the lesion is irritated, small whorls of prematurely keratinizing cells known as *squamous eddies* can be seen.

Treatment. If lesions become cosmetically objectionable, removal is advised. Curettage with superficial electrocautery of the base, cryotherapy, or electrosurgery may be used.

Erythematous (Red)

ACNE

Acne is a chronic skin disease that originates in the pilosebaceous apparatus of the neck and trunk.

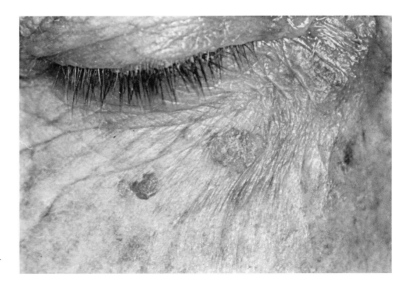

Figure 17–21. Elevated and pigmented seborrheic keratoses.

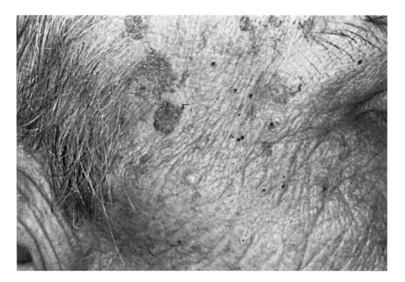

Figure 17–22. Elevated and pigmented seborrheic keratoses. Note the black comedones and white milia.

Acne may range in severity from trivial to disfiguring (conglobata form) and may have a profound impact on the psychologic outlook of affected individuals. The cause appears to be multifactorial, and treatment regimens are directed toward these various factors.

At least three major, interrelated contributing events appear to initiate acne: (1) follicular hyperkeratosis, (2) follicular bacterial proliferation, and (3) increased sebum production. Hyperkeratosis of the follicular epithelium leads to follicular plugging, which in turn produces the primary lesion, a *comedone*. A noninflamed collection of keratin, sebum, and bacteria that does not communicate with the surface is a *closed comedone* (whitehead), whereas an *open comedone* (blackhead) communicates with the skin surface. Oxidation of pigment causes the lesion to appear black.

Propionibacterium acnes, a diphtheroid, is a gram-negative resident of the pilosebaceous unit. *P. acnes* proliferates, especially with follicular plugging, and produces lipases that act on triglycerides, a major component of sebum, resulting in the formation of free fatty acids that diffuse into the perifollicular tissues, where they act as irritants and inflammatory stimuli. *P. acnes* also produces enzymes and chemical mediators that promote follicular and perifollicular inflammation. Increased production of sebum appears to have a major role in the cause of acne because sebum acts as a substrate for *P. acnes*. Increased sebum production occurs predominantly through the stimulation of sebaceous glands by androgens and, in part, by progestins. Chronic mechanical trauma, stress, and drugs such as birth control pills, corticosteroids, lithium, cyclosporine, phenytoin, and barbiturates

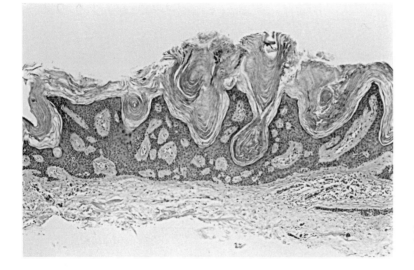

Figure 17–23. Seborrheic keratosis with characteristic histologic features.

may exacerbate acne. Cosmetics may promote comedogenesis. Genetic influences also have been noted.

Clinical Features. The face, back, and trunk are commonly affected by acne. Comedones may become inflamed, resulting in pustules. Healing of larger, deeper nodules or cysts may result in pitted or depressed scars, hypertrophic scars, or keloids. Hypopigmentation or hyperpigmentation may also be seen.

Treatment. Topical measures are recommended for mild to moderate disease: systemic medications (with or without topical agents) are recommended for severe or recalcitrant acne. Therapeutic measures are generally targeted at the major etiologic components. Topical treatments include the use of benzoyl peroxide preparations, antibiotics, or both. The antikeratinizing agent retinoic acid (tretinoin) may be effective when used alone or in combination with other topical agents. Systemic antibiotics such as erythromycin, clindamycin, tetracycline, and trimethoprim-sulfamethoxazole are effective in reducing bacterial numbers and inflammation. Oral 13-*cis*-retinoic acid (isotretinoin) can be particularly effective in controlling nodulocystic acne. However, isotretinoin is associated with significant side effects that include cheilitis, dry skin, elevation of serum triglyceride and cholesterol levels, elevation of liver enzymes, pseudotumor cerebri, and, most important, high teratogenicity. Patient education, to keep expectations realistic and compliance high, must be part of the patient treatment package.

PERIORAL DERMATITIS

Perioral dermatitis is an inflammatory eruption characterized by periorificial papules and pustules.

Use of topical steroids predisposes to this acneiform eruption, although tartar control dentifrices have also been implicated. Women between the ages of 15 and 45 years are predominantly affected, although it is occasionally seen in children and in men.

Clinical Features. Perioral dermatitis usually presents as a symmetric eruption consisting of tiny papules, microvesicles, or small pustules around the nasal alae and the mouth and on the chin (Fig. 17–24). The eruption may also be seen in the glabellar and eyelid regions. These changes are superimposed on a diffuse or patchy erythematous base associated with variable degrees of scaling. A highly characteristic feature is the appearance of a narrow margin of normal skin between the vermilion and the eruption.

Histopathology. Epidermal changes tend to be relatively mild and include slight acanthosis, spongiosis, and parakeratosis. Scattered throughout the dermis is a mild inflammatory cell infiltrate of lymphocytes, plasma cells, and macrophages.

Treatment. If sensitizing agents are identified, withdrawal of these should be curative. To prevent rebound due to discontinuation of topical steroids, application of 1% hydrocortisone for a short time has proved beneficial in some cases. A short course of systemic antibiotics (1 to 2 months) may be necessary for acute control, but topical antibiotics (metronidazole) are the mainstay of treatment.

FOLLICULITIS

Folliculitis, or inflammation of the hair follicle, may be due to various factors. Infection with *Staphylococcus* and *Candida* is a frequent cause.

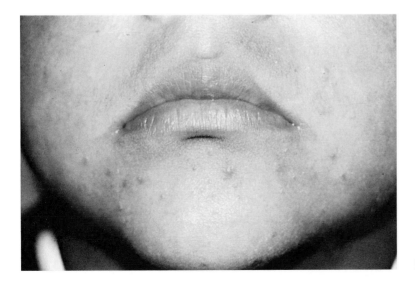

Figure 17–24. Perioral dermatitis.

Pseudofolliculitis barbae, or razor bumps, is a foreign-body reaction to ingrown hairs and is more prevalent in African-Americans. Dermatophyte infection of the hair follicles may produce a similar picture and should be considered in the differential diagnosis. Candidal infection most often involves perioral hairs and is accompanied by flaking of the skin. Bacterial infection may occur after injury, abrasion, or occlusive steroid treatment and is usually due to *Staphylococcus*. However, follicular infection with dermatophytes can occur, usually limited to the beard and mustache areas. Bacterial cultures, Gram staining, or potassium hydroxide preparations may be helpful in diagnosis.

Clinical Features. Folliculitis is manifested as a painless or slightly tender pustule with surrounding erythema.

Histopathology. Pustules show considerable perifollicular infiltrate of neutrophils or lymphocytes, with occasional necrosis of the hair follicle and perifollicular epidermis. Follicular pus collections are noted. Pseudofolliculitis barbae usually demonstrates hair growth back into the epidermis, with resulting neutrophilic infiltrate.

Treatment. The cause dictates the treatment. If razor irritation is suspected, postponement of shaving, later use of hydrating lubricants, and use of new razors is recommended. Warm, wet compresses or oral antibiotics may be useful. Fungal infection with *Candida* or dermatophytes should be treated with appropriate systemic antifungals.

FURUNCLE

The furuncle, or boil, is a deep, painful, fluctuant inflammatory nodule that is preceded by staphylococcal folliculitis. Furuncles occur in areas of heavy perspiration or friction such as the face, neck, axillae, and buttocks.

Clinical Features. A furuncle is a firm, tender, erythematous nodule. Rupture may occur spontaneously, with extrusion of pus and sometimes a necrotic core.

Histopathology. Perifollicular necrosis with many neutrophils and fibrinoid material is identified, and a large abscess is located in the subcutaneous tissue. A Gram stain reveals gram-positive cocci, and the cultures are positive for *S. aureus*.

Treatment. Moist heat application may decrease pain and promote drainage. Incisional drainage may be required, as well as oral antibiotics if the lesions are accompanied by fever, are difficult to eradicate, or are complicated by cellulitis. Rarely, furuncles may result in bacteremia. Squeezing furuncles located around the lips and nose may seed the cavernous sinus via the facial and angular emissary veins.

MILIARIA

Miliaria, or heat rash, is a dermatologic condition that occurs in predisposed individuals after exercise or heat exposure. It is due to obstruction of the intraepidermal eccrine ducts, with subsequent leakage of sweat into the surrounding tissue and an inflammatory response. Three distinct types are noted, depending on the histologic level of leakage: miliaria crystallina, miliaria rubra, and miliaria profunda.

Clinical Features. Miliaria crystallina is characterized by small, asymptomatic, superficial papules or vesicles (dewdrops) that often occur after an insult to the horny layer such as in a sunburn. Miliaria rubra, or prickly heat, develops when the eccrine duct is obstructed deeper in the epidermis after excessive sweating, especially in skin covered by clothing. These are pruritic or prickly papulovesicles surrounded by erythema. Anhidrosis and heat intolerance can occur. Miliaria profunda most often develops in people in tropical climates, particularly after several episodes of miliaria rubra. In this case, the occlusion occurs at the dermal-epidermal junction. The lesions are white to flesh-colored papules and are not pruritic. Anhidrosis can be severe.

Histopathology. Miliaria crystallina is characterized by intracorneal or subcorneal vesicles in continuity with the underlying eccrine ducts, with a neutrophilic infiltrate at the periphery of the vesicle. The surrounding epidermis is spongiotic, and the papillary dermis is edematous. In miliaria rubra, spongiotic vesicles in the spiny layer are continuous with sweat ducts. Spongiosis and a lymphocytic infiltrate of the periductal area are usually noted. Miliaria profunda is similar to miliaria rubra but involves the lower epidermis and the upper dermis.

Treatment. Treatment is supportive and includes allowing air to circulate, control of fever, and application of a camphor-menthol–containing lotion to relieve the itching.

GRANULOMA FACIALE

Granuloma faciale is a cutaneous lesion of unknown cause; however, some immunofluorescence data have suggested that it is immune complex mediated. No systemic involvement is noted.

Clinical Features. The lesions of granuloma faciale classically are asymptomatic soft, brown-red papules, plaques, or nodules. They range in size from a few millimeters to several centimeters. They occasionally become annular and are sometimes made worse or darkened after exposure to sunlight. These granulomas are seen primarily in middle life and are more common in men and in Caucasians. Granuloma faciale does not ulcerate, but telangiectasias may occur on its surface.

Histopathology. The epidermis is unaffected. A dense, mostly neutrophilic infiltrate is found in the dermis and occasionally extending into the subcutaneous tissue. A grenz zone (unaffected border) separates the infiltrate from the epidermis. Immunofluorescence studies have shown deposition of IgG, IgM, complement, and fibrin around vessels and at the dermal-epidermal junction.

Treatment. Granuloma faciale is notoriously resistant to treatment and has a high rate of recurrence. Radiation, cryotherapy, cauterization, and systemic corticosteroids all provide unpredictable control of these lesions. Surgical removal and dermabrasion have shown better results, but recurrence is still likely.

CHERRY HEMANGIOMA

The cherry hemangioma is a small, raised, bright red to purple papule that varies in size from a barely visible point to several millimeters in diameter (Fig. 17–25). These benign papules are typically seen on the trunk and upper extremities of middle-aged to elderly patients.

Histopathology. Many newly formed capillaries with narrow lumina and with prominent endothelial cells are arranged in lobules. In time, the capillaries dilate and the intercapillary stroma becomes edematous. The epidermis is often thinned to the point of forming a collarette around the hemangioma.

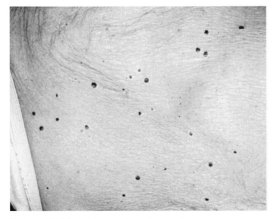

Figure 17–25. Multiple cherry hemangiomas.

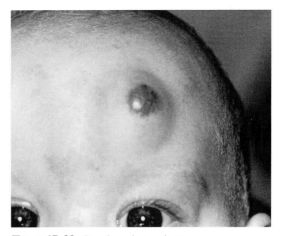

Figure 17–26. Strawberry hemangioma.

Treatment. Hemangiomas tend to persist indefinitely, and treatment is necessary only for cosmetic purposes. If elected, electrodesiccation or laser therapy is effective.

STRAWBERRY HEMANGIOMA

Strawberry hemangioma, a vascular tumor of infancy, usually appears during the third to fifth week of life, grows rapidly, and spontaneously regresses. It occurs in 1 to 3% of all infants and has a predominance in girls. These hemangiomas consist of one or more bright red, well-demarcated, soft nodules on the head, but they may occur anywhere (Fig. 17–26). Initially, the lesion may simply be an ill-defined vascular macule that grows rapidly for weeks to months, to a maximum size of several centimeters. Compression of vital structures or obstruction of vision may result in amblyopia or blindness, and rapidly growing hemangiomas may ulcerate, resulting in bacterial invasion. The strawberry hemangioma begins to involute by 3 years of age; complete resolution occurs by 7 years of age in 70% of patients.

Histopathology. Lobular architecture is a constant feature, but other features may differ as the tumor evolves. Initially noted is extensive endothelial cell proliferation with large and mitotically active cells. More mature lesions show flattening of the endothelium and enlarging lumina, with eventual fibrosis.

Treatment. Uncomplicated strawberry hemangiomas should be allowed to involute spontaneously. Those that remain after 7 years of age will probably not involute and will require intervention (usually surgical). Rapidly growing lesions that compromise vital structures are treated aggressively with systemic or intralesional corticosteroids or surgery until partial remission occurs.

SPITZ NEVUS

The Spitz nevus (benign juvenile melanoma) is a worrisome-appearing benign tumor of children and young adults. Its clinical and histologic appearance is similar to that of melanoma.

Clinical Features. Spitz nevi appear as hairless, red to reddish-brown, dome-shaped papules or nodules with a verrucous or smooth surface. Most Spitz nevi measure less than 0.6 cm. They are usually solitary but occasionally are numerous, appearing suddenly on the face and lower extremities.

Histopathology. Differentiation between Spitz nevus and melanoma may be difficult. Architecturally, Spitz nevi are symmetric and resemble nevi with compound, junctional, or intradermal patterns. The epidermis is often hyperplastic and has elongated rete ridges; permeation of the epidermis by nevus cells is usually slight. Cytologically, large spindle and epithelioid cells differentiate the Spitz nevus from nevi and most melanomas. Maturation of the cells with increasing depth and uniformity of cells from one side to the other is also an important differentiating feature. Mitoses are found in approximately one half of Spitz nevi; however, atypical mitoses are not frequent.

Treatment. Spitz nevi should be removed for histologic examination because they cannot be differentiated from melanoma on a purely clinical basis, especially at or beyond puberty.

ACUTE FEBRILE NEUTROPHILIC DERMATOSIS (SWEET'S SYNDROME)

Acute febrile neutrophilic dermatosis is an uncommon, recurrent cutaneous disease first described by Sweet in 1964. The disease occurs typically in middle-aged women after nonspecific illnesses of the gastrointestinal or respiratory tract. An underlying malignancy may occur in as many as 20% of cases. The acute onset of fever, leukocytosis, and erythematous papules and plaques infiltrated with neutrophils is characteristic. Some series have shown that fever and leukocytosis are not consistently observed. Therefore, the two major diagnostic criteria for Sweet's syndrome are abrupt onset of tender, erythematous plaques and a predominantly neutrophilic infiltrate in the dermis without leukocytoclastic vasculitis.

Histopathology. The perivascular dermis has a dense infiltrate composed mostly of neutrophils along with prominent dermal edema. Extensive vascular damage does not occur. Subepidermal blister formation occasionally occurs.

Treatment. High-dose oral steroids are very effective, but oral potassium iodide and colchicine have also proved useful. Recurrences have been noted.

MORBILLIFORM DRUG ERUPTIONS

Morbilliform, or maculopapular, eruptions are the most common of the drug-induced reactions. Although any drug may be implicated, antibiotics are the most likely class of medications to cause morbilliform eruptions. The history of use of a new medication is highly suggestive.

Clinical Features. The eruption presents as symmetric erythematous, blanching macules and papules that may become confluent. The eruption appears on the trunk or on areas of physical trauma, at any time from less than a week after starting treatment until several weeks after discontinuing the drug. Patients may experience involvement of mucous membranes, mild fever, or pruritus. The major differential diagnosis is that of viral exanthems; laboratory findings are nonspecific and generally unrewarding. However, if fever and eosinophilia are associated with the eruption, the drug should be discontinued and the patient evaluated for evidence of liver toxicity, as is encountered in the Dilantin hypersensitivity syndrome.

Histopathology. Some vacuolation of the dermal-epidermal junction may be observed. A variable, mainly perivascular infiltrate of lymphocytes and sometimes eosinophils is characteristic. Occasionally noted are papillary edema and fibrinoid deposition.

Treatment. The eruption often disappears or decreases in severity despite ongoing use of the causative agent. Discontinuation of the offending agent is curative; however, the eruption may not disappear for several weeks. Further support measures include topical steroids and antihistamines.

Violaceous (Blue or Purple)

LICHEN PLANUS

Lichen planus (LP) is characterized by a papulosquamous or erosive, severely pruritic eruption of the skin and mucous membranes. LP tends to occur in middle-aged persons, without a racial or sexual predilection. LP-like eruptions can also occur with use of certain drugs such as gold compounds, penicillamine, and methyldopa. Although the cause of LP is not known, current evidence suggests that it is a reflection of a cell-mediated immune response and probably is not due to an infectious agent.

Clinical Features. The classic cutaneous lesions of LP are flat, pruritic, polygonal purple papules that range from 0.2 to 1.0 cm. Often observed is a flat, fine semitransparent scale or a network of fine white lines called *Wickham's striae*. LP can occur anywhere on the body, but most lesions are found on the flexor surfaces of the limbs, the shins, lower back, genitalia, and oral cavity. Koebner's phenomenon (an isomorphic response in which lesions appear at the site of trauma) is a frequent finding in the acute phase of LP. In healing lesions, hyperpigmentation and, rarely, hypopigmentation may occur.

Histopathology. Distinct variants of LP exist, but typical findings include orthokeratosis, wedge-shaped hypergranulosis, irregular acanthosis, damage to the basal cells, and a band-like lymphocytic infiltrate in the upper dermis. Plasma cells may be present. The majority of the lymphocytes are T lymphocytes, with T-suppressor cells predominating in later lesions.

Treatment. Topical corticosteroids are effective in treating localized LP of the skin and mucous membranes, but short-term systemic steroids may be beneficial if lesions are extensive. Long-term systemic steroid treatment is rarely warranted in LP.

VENOUS LAKE

Clinical Features. Venous lakes are soft, slightly raised dark blue papules occurring most commonly on the face, lips, and ears of elderly people. They usually measure 0.2 to 1 cm in diameter and are composed of dilated, blood-filled venous channels. As a diagnostic maneuver, venous lakes may be partially blanched (emptied of the majority of their blood) simply using sustained tactile pressure.

Histopathology. In the upper dermis, either one large, dilated space or many interconnected dilatations lined by a single layer of endothelium and filled with erythrocytes are seen.

Treatment. The lesions can be removed by excision or electrodesiccation or can be vaporized with laser treatment.

BLUE NEVUS

Blue nevi are aggregates of melanin-producing cells in the dermis. They appear blue because melanin deep in the dermis absorbs long-wavelength light, and blue is reflected to the observer (Tyndall effect). Blue nevi have no malignant potential.

Clinical Features. Blue nevi appear as small (less than 1.0 cm), well-circumscribed, dome-shaped blue to black papules on the hands, feet, and head. They may be congenital but are most commonly acquired by late childhood.

Histopathology. The epidermis is normal. The dermis contains elongated, wavy, dendritic melanin-containing cells whose processes extend in bundles parallel to the epidermis. The cells may extend to the subcutaneous fat or approach the epidermis.

Treatment. Small, unchanging blue nevi in adults require no therapy. If a blue lesion suddenly appears, enlarges, or exceeds 1.0 cm, histologic examination is required to rule out melanoma.

ANGIOSARCOMA

Angiosarcoma is a malignant tumor of endothelial cell origin. One of the most frequent presentations is insidious progressive erythema on the scalp or face of an elderly patient. Extension of tumor, not metastasis, is frequently the cause of death. It occurs most often in males, with an ethnic predilection for white and Asian persons.

Clinical Features. These lesions arise as erythematous or dusky patches or plaques with later development of nodules or ulceration. The scalp and middle or upper face are the most frequently involved sites (Fig. 17–27).

Histopathology. This tumor is characterized by anastomosing vascular channels lined by a layer of enlarged, atypical endothelial cells that frequently infiltrate and surround individual collagen bun-

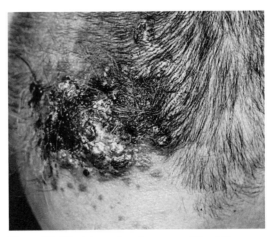

Figure 17–27. Advanced angiosarcoma of the scalp.

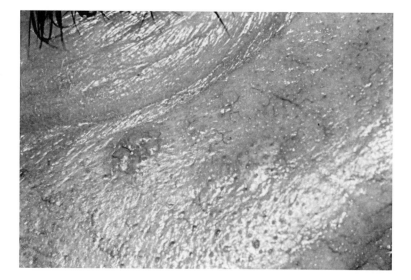

Figure 17–28. Early basal cell carcinoma.

dles. In highly malignant tumors, the endothelial cells may grow as sheets without lumen formation.

Treatment. The prognosis is poor, because most cases are diagnosed very late. Early surgical excision or Mohs' microsurgical technique may lead to a better prognosis. Radiotherapy may be palliative.

NODULES

A nodule is an elevated, circumscribed, solid lesion that measures more than 0.5 cm.

Basal Cell Carcinoma

Basal cell carcinoma is the most prevalent cancer of the skin, and it is also the most prevalent cancer of the head and neck. The midface is the area in which most basal cell carcinomas are found. The lesion is most frequently encountered in older patients. Men are more commonly affected than women, presumably because of greater cumulative sun exposure. This malignancy arises from basal cells of the skin. The vast majority of basal cell carcinomas occur on sun-exposed skin. Except in very rare instances, basal cell carcinoma does not occur on mucous membranes.

Individuals at increased risk for the development of basal cell carcinoma are those with lighter natural skin pigmentation, those with a long history of chronic sun exposure, and those with one of several predisposing hereditary syndromes. Among the latter is nevoid basal cell carcinoma syndrome, in which individuals have numerous

odontogenic keratocysts, skeletal abnormalities, and multiple basal cell carcinomas.

Clinical Features. Basal cell carcinoma presents as an indurated pearly papule or nodule with telangiectatic vessels coursing over its surface (Figs. 17–28 and 17–29). With time, the center of the tumor becomes ulcerated and crusted. If untreated, the tumor exhibits a slow but relentless locally destructive nature (Figs. 17–30 and 17–31). Other clinical forms may on occasion be seen. The pigmented form of basal cell carcinoma presents in a manner similar to the noduloulcerative type, with the addition of melanin pigmentation within or at the periphery. The superficial form presents as a scaly erythematous lesion flush with the skin surface, occasionally appearing as

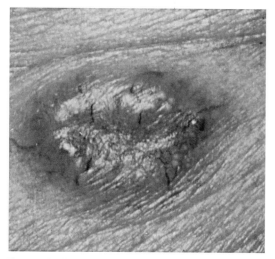

Figure 17–29. Basal cell carcinoma of lower eyelid. (Courtesy of Dr. S. K. Young.)

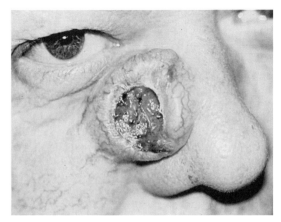

Figure 17–30. Large ulcerating basal cell carcinoma.

Mohs' microscopically guided surgery) and irradiation can be used to treat basal cell carcinoma. The type of treatment depends on the size and location of the neoplasm as well as the experience and training of the clinician.

Keratoacanthoma

Solitary keratoacanthoma is an epidermal tumor that is classified as a type of squamous cell carcinoma. Keratoacanthomas characteristically occur in elderly and immunocompromised patients; multiple keratoacanthomas may be associated with the Muir-Torre syndrome (multiple sebaceous neoplasms).

Clinical Features. Keratoacanthoma is characterized by a firm, smooth, dome-shaped nodule that is flesh colored to erythematous. It commonly reaches its full size (1.0 to 2.5 cm) within 6 to 8 weeks. Keratoacanthoma usually develops a central horny crust (Fig. 17–34). Common sites are the hands, arms, trunk and face, but any hairy skin surface may be involved. Considerable controversy exists about their malignant potential. These tumors may involute spontaneously within 6 months, but healing often results in a depressed scar. The smooth surface maintained throughout the evolution of the lesion aids in differentiation from squamous cell carcinoma.

Histopathology. In early lesions, the epidermis appears to invaginate into the dermis. Keratin fills this invagination, and the epithelium exhibits nuclear atypia and many mitotic figures. A pronounced inflammatory infiltrate is found in the dermis. Mature lesions have a central, keratin-

an atrophic scar-like process. The fibrosing form of basal cell carcinoma presents as an indurated yellowish plaque that may be slightly depressed or flat, resembling a slow or insidiously enlarging scar in the absence of trauma. Because basal cell carcinomas are generally slow growing and rarely metastatic, the prognosis is very good.

Histopathology. In basal cell carcinomas, nests and cords of cuboidal cells arise from the region of the epidermal basal cells. The neoplastic cells around the periphery of the invading nests and strands are usually palisaded and often columnar (Fig. 17–32). In some infiltrative basal cell carcinomas, tiny infiltrative nests are found in a fibroblastic stroma (Fig. 17–33). This has been described as an aggressive growth pattern and may portend a more aggressive clinical course.

Treatment. Various surgical procedures (standard scalpel surgery, cryosurgery, electrosurgery,

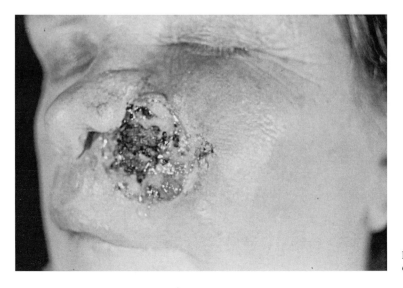

Figure 17–31. Advanced basal cell carcinoma.

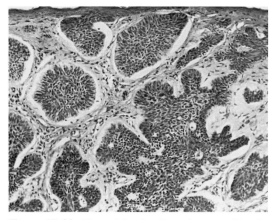

Figure 17–32. Nests of basal cell carcinoma proliferative from the epidermis. Note the retraction spaces around the tumor islands.

filled crater, multiple epidermal proliferations, and keratin pearls.

Treatment. Many keratoacanthomas heal spontaneously with scarring, and some do metastasize. Therefore, delay in treating is not advisable. Keratoacanthomas may be treated by electrodesiccation or excision or with medical therapies including 5-fluorouracil (topical or intralesional), podophyllum, or oral isotretinoin.

Squamous Cell Carcinoma

In the vast majority of cases, squamous cell carcinoma of the face and lower lip arises from epidermal keratinocytes that have been damaged by sunlight. Unlike basal cell carcinoma, this neoplasm has significant potential to metastasize to regional lymph nodes and beyond. As with basal cell carcinoma, several factors contribute to the etiology of squamous cell carcinoma; however, the chief factor remains repeated and chronic damage due to sunlight. The highest incidence is noted in fair-skinned individuals after long-term exposure to sunlight. In addition, carcinogens such as tars, oils, and arsenicals; exposure to x-rays, and the presence of skin diseases that cause scarring, such as severe burns and discoid lupus erythematosus (DLE), also predispose to malignant transformation of the epithelium.

Clinical Features. The clinical course is insidious, evolving over months to years. A central ulcer with slightly raised indurated margins and surrounding erythema eventually forms. Lesions may occasionally appear as verrucous growths, papules, or plaques. Areas of the face most commonly affected include the lower lip, tip of the ear, forehead, and infraorbital/nasal bridge region. Lesions are firm and indurated, reflecting tumor infiltration of adjacent tissues.

It is important to appreciate that lesions arising within solar keratoses are less aggressive than those arising *de novo* or in some sun-protected locations. Squamous cell carcinomas arising in sites of irradiation, burns, or chronic degenerative skin disorders are more aggressive than their sun-exposure counterparts. A squamous cell carcinoma arising in solar cheilitis tends to invade and metastasize at an earlier point than its counterpart in sun-damaged skin.

Histopathology. This tumor consists of atypical keratinocytes that invade the dermis and beyond. As with intraoral squamous cell carcinoma, cytologic features include increased nuclear-cytoplasmic ratio, nuclear hyperchromatism, individ-

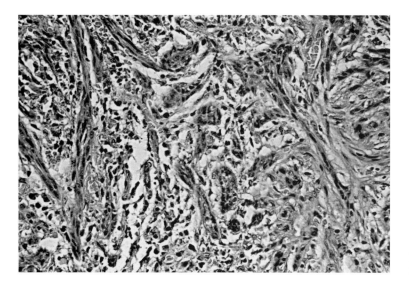

Figure 17–33. Basal cell carcinomas. Aggressive growth pattern.

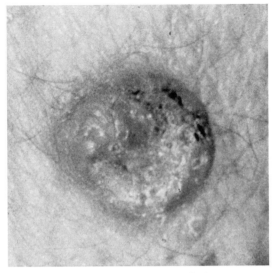

Figure 17–34. Keratoacanthoma on the cheek.

ual cell keratinization, tumor giant cells, atypical mitotic figures, and increased mitotic rate.

Treatment. The mainstay of therapy remains excision. The mode of excision, however, depends on the size and location of the lesion. Larger carcinomas may be treated with wide excision, often with reconstructive grafts, or irradiation therapy. Microscopically directed surgery, Mohs' surgery, may be used because of its advantage in tissue conservation. The overall 5-year cure rate for squamous cell carcinoma of the skin is approximately 90%.

WHEALS

A wheal is a transient papule or plaque formed by serum exudation into the dermis. Wheals are produced by vasodilatation and fluid leakage secondary to histamine release from mast cells and basophils.

Urticaria (Hives)

Clinical Features. Urticaria, or wheals, may be erythematous or white, they may be of any size, and they usually are pruritic. Urticaria may be caused by a reaction to foods, insect venom, infections, drugs, systemic disease, and physical stimuli. Physical hives include dermographism and cholinergic, solar, and cold urticaria.

Histopathology. Histopathologic features include dermal edema, dilated venules, and swelling of endothelial cells, without many inflammatory cells. In chronic lesions, the edema may be accompanied by a mixed inflammatory cell infiltrate.

Treatment. Avoidance of the precipitating factor with use of antihistamines and possibly corticosteroids or epinephrine for severe or refractory cases is curative. Skin biopsy and further work-up for internal disease may occasionally be necessary.

Angioedema

Clinical Features. Angioedema is a wheal-like swelling that is caused by increased vascular permeability in the subcutaneous tissue. It is due to IgE-dependent hypersensitivity, as seen in urticaria. Skin and tissue of the gastrointestinal and respiratory tracts may be involved. The lips, extremities, trunk, and genitalia are most often involved, with accompanying burning and pain but not pruritus (see Chapter 2). Angioedema of the head and neck may compromise the airway acutely and require emergent care. Angioedema may be caused by allergies to drugs, food, or insect venom or by idiopathic or hereditary factors.

Histopathology. The epidermis is not involved. Dermal and subcutaneous edema with few inflammatory cells is observed.

Treatment. Removal of the inciting agent is the initial step if possible. Antihistamines are the mainstay of treatment. Epinephrine may be used emergently if laryngeal edema is compromising the airway.

PAPULOSQUAMOUS DERMATOSES

Actinic Keratoses (Solar Keratoses)

Actinic keratoses are epithelial changes noted typically in light-complexioned individuals who have had long-term exposure to sunlight. A small percentage of these lesions develop into squamous cell carcinoma. Outdoor workers and individuals participating in extensive outdoor recreation are particularly prone to the development of actinic keratoses.

Clinical Features. Oval plaques usually less than 1 cm in diameter are typically found on the forehead, cheeks, temples, lower lip, ears, and lateral portions of the neck. The color may vary from yellow-brown to red, and texture is usually rough and sandpaper-like (Figs. 17–35 and 17–36).

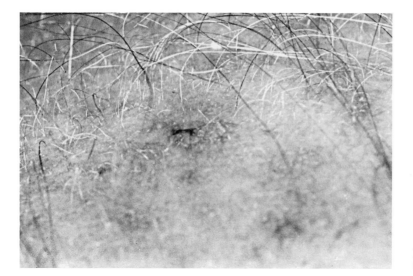

Figure 17–35. Actinic keratosis of the forehead.

Histopathology. Common to the many actinic keratosis microscopic subtypes are nuclear atypia, increased nuclear-cytoplasmic ratio, and atypical proliferation of basal cells. The dermis generally contains a lymphocytic inflammatory cell infiltrate. Elastotic or basophilic change of collagen and irregular clumps of altered elastic fibers and regenerated collagen are noted in these areas.

Treatment. Individual actinic keratoses may be treated with cryotherapy. However, in patients with confluent actinic keratoses, the therapeutic mainstay is topical application of 5-fluorouracil. Additional treatment modalities include curettage and surgical excision. For lesions that are indurated or nodular or that demonstrate marked inflammation, a biopsy to rule out invasive squamous cell carcinoma is necessary.

Seborrheic Dermatitis

Seborrheic dermatitis is a chronic waxing and waning papulosquamous eruption. Although the cause is unknown, it is more common in individuals of northern European or Celtic background. Seborrheic dermatitis can also be seen in individuals with zinc deficiency, those receiving hyperalimentation, and those with Parkinson's disease or in an immunosuppressed state.

Clinical Features. The onset of seborrheic dermatitis is gradual, usually with symptoms of pruritus, often increased with perspiration. Worsening during winter months is typical. Commonly affected is the scalp, followed by the eyelid margins, nasolabial folds, cheeks, forehead, and eyebrows

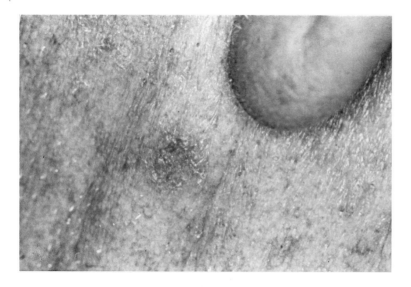

Figure 17–36. Actinic keratosis of the skin inferior to the ear.

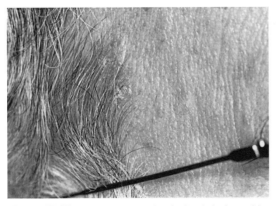

Figure 17–37. Erythematous scale of seborrheic dermatitis.

(Fig. 17–37). At times, otitis externa may be the presenting manifestation of this reaction.

Seborrheic dermatitis may present within the first few weeks of life but more commonly between 20 and 50 years. Males are more commonly affected. Affected areas may appear yellowish red to gray to white. Dry, scaling macules or papules of various sizes and with diffuse margins are often present. Lesions tend to assume nummular (coin-shaped) or polycyclic (clustered or coalesced circular arrays) patterns. In contrast, scalp psoriasis tends to be sharply circumscribed and raised, with a silvery scale that is more compact.

Histopathology. The early lesions of seborrheic dermatitis are characterized by widely dilated superficial blood vessels with corresponding edema within the papillary dermis and a sparse perivascular lymphocytic infiltrate. The epidermis exhibits a slight degree of focal spongiosis. On the surface, a scale or crust containing neutrophils is noted at the follicular ostia. Later, follicular plugging, crusts at the infundibular ostia, spongiosis, and superficial perivascular round cell infiltrates are noted. Chronic lesions tend to be psoriasiform.

Treatment. Conservative therapy is recommended, especially in mild cases. Recurrences and remissions are characteristic. The use of topical steroids or systemic or topical ketoconazole provides significant benefit.

Psoriasis

Psoriasis is a common skin disease (2% incidence). It is of unknown cause but is strongly linked to heredity. Triggering factors include systemic infections, stress, and drugs. Psoriasis appears to be an immunoregulatory disorder in which epidermal changes are related to a defect in the control of keratinocyte proliferation. The hyperproliferative state of the affected epidermis produces a turnover rate that is as much as eight times greater than normal.

Clinical Features. Psoriasis occurs at any age but most commonly appears during young adult life. It is a chronic disease that may persist throughout life, with periods of exacerbation and remission. Various triggers, such as trauma, infection, and stress, may precipitate new episodes. The development of psoriatic lesions after trauma of normal-appearing skin is known as *Koebner's reaction* or *phenomenon*.

The basic skin lesion of psoriasis is a well-defined erythematous macule or plaque covered by silvery scales (Fig. 17–38). When the scales are removed, small pinpoint bleeding is seen because of increased vascularity under focal areas of epidermal thinning. This feature of psoriasis is known as the *Auspitz sign.* Oral lesions of psoriasis are rare. Geographic tongue has also been listed as an oral manifestation of psoriasis, but this may simply be a coincidental finding.

In a small percentage of psoriatic patients, a seronegative polyarthritis may be identified. The temporomandibular joint may occasionally be one of the joints involved in this process. Pain and restricted motion are encountered with erosion of the condyle.

Histopathology. Because of the hyperproliferative nature of psoriasis, epithelial hyperplasia due to acanthosis and parakeratosis is seen (Figs. 17–39 and 17–40). Connective tissue papillae contain lymphocytes and prominent capillaries that are covered by thinned epithelium. Neutrophils are usually found in the epithelium, often in aggregates between epithelial cells, producing microabscesses that are called *Munro microabscesses.*

Treatment. A wide variety of drugs are available for the treatment of cutaneous psoriasis. The

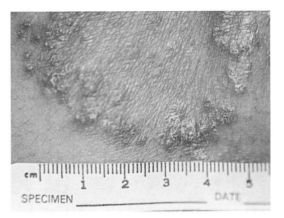

Figure 17–38. Plaques of psoriasis.

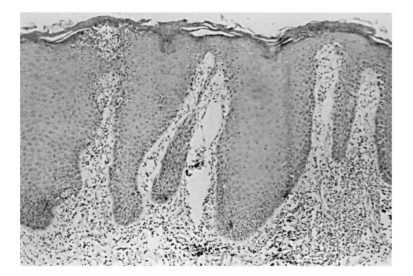

Figure 17–39. Psoriasis featuring epithelial hyperplasia with intermittent thinning and microabscesses of Munro.

drug or combination of drugs used depends on the clinician's training and experience and the patient's response. Topical preparations (tars, anthralin, and corticosteroids), systemic agents (methotrexate and retinoids), and photochemotherapy (PUVA) all have their advantages and proponents.

Atopic Dermatitis

Atopic dermatitis (AD) is a chronic relapsing inflammatory condition affecting all age groups, but infants, children, and adolescents are predominantly affected. Usually elicited is a family history of AD, eczema, asthma, hay fever, or sinusitis. AD has a female predominance and frequently an association with an elevated serum IgE level.

Many patients with AD have other atopic disorders such as asthma or allergic rhinitis.

Clinical Features. AD is characterized by periods of exacerbation and remission. AD presents as small follicular, erythematous papules associated with considerable pruritus. However, these may enlarge and become lichenified or may evolve into vesicles or bullae. In infants, AD predominates on the face. As afflicted children mature, AD tends to affect flexural skin. In older children and adults, AD involves the antecubital and popliteal fossae and the sides of the neck.

Histopathology. The epidermis exhibits mild spongiosis and parakeratosis in early phases of AD, with lymphocytes and histiocytes scattered around the superficial vascular plexus. AD of longer duration is marked by elongation of the

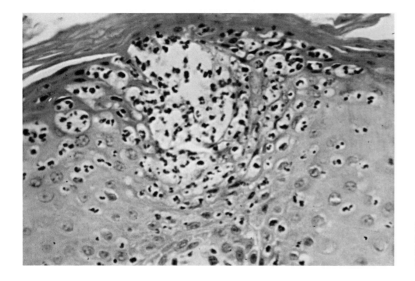

Figure 17–40. Psoriasis featuring epithelial hyperplasia with intermittent thinning and microabscesses of Munro.

rete ridges, hyperkeratosis, and wedge-shaped hypergranulosis with areas of developing parakeratosis. Spongiosis and cellular infiltrates are less prominent. Eosinophils are less common in AD than in allergic contact dermatitis.

Treatment. Treatment of AD is usually empirical, and decisions about treatment are based on the skin findings at a specific time. Follicular eczema can be improved by eliminating irritating factors and using topical steroids temporarily. When lichenified, AD does not resolve unless the chronic irritant or trauma is eliminated. Treating with hydration and water trapping with hydrophobic agents is helpful. Histamine receptor (types 1 and 2) blocking agents may also provide benefit in preventing and controlling the associated pruritus.

Keratosis Pilaris

Keratosis pilaris is a very common asymptomatic and persistent skin condition associated with atopic dermatitis. Areas typically affected include the lateral aspects of the arms, the thighs, buttocks, and face. Keratosis pilaris is more severe in the winter months.

Clinical Features. Discrete keratotic, follicular papules are surrounded by a rim of erythema.

Histopathology. The orifice and upper portion of the follicular infundibulum are blocked and dilated by an orthokeratotic plug of keratin. A twisted villous hair may be trapped within the plug. A mild mononuclear cell infiltrate is often present in the surrounding dermis.

Treatment. A lubricating cream may help to smooth the rough skin; keratolytic agents such as lactic acid lotions, salicylic acid, or retinoic acid may benefit in severe cases.

Pityriasis Rosea

Pityriasis rosea (PR) is an acute self-limited dermatitis that follows a distinctive course. PR affects women more often than men, occurs from late childhood to middle age, and is of unknown cause. Although PR has many similarities to viral exanthems, no infective agent has been isolated. PR-like rashes have also been described after initiating treatment with drugs such as barbiturates, bismuth, and angiotensin-converting enzyme inhibitors, but these rashes tend to show some atypia when compared with classic PR. PR is often preceded by a prodrome with symptoms of fever, malaise, loss of appetite, nausea, and joint pain.

Clinical Features. The primary plaque, or herald patch, is a round or oval salmon-colored, peripherally scaling plaque that is seen in the majority of cases. It is commonly located on the trunk. The secondary eruption appears simultaneously or up to several weeks later. It is characterized by either small plaques that resemble miniature versions of the primary plaque or small erythematous papules on the trunk, neck, or back. Both may occur at the same time. They appear in a Christmas tree pattern on the back because they lie in skin cleavage lines. The secondary eruption reaches its peak within 2 weeks, lasts for 2 to 10 weeks, and is variably pruritic.

Histopathology. In the secondary lesions, spongiosis due to intracellular edema, variable acanthosis, focal parakeratosis, and exocytosis of lymphocytes are noted in the epidermis. A dermal lymphoid infiltrate with eosinophils or macrophages and erythrocyte extravasation in the dermis is seen. The herald patch has similar but amplified findings.

Treatment. Because PR is self-limited, active therapy usually is not needed. Irritants should be minimized, with severe itching treated with zinc oxide, calamine lotion, or oral antihistamines. In more severe cases, topical corticosteroids or even a short course of oral corticosteroids may be useful.

Verruca Vulgaris (Warts)

Verruca vulgaris, the common wart, is caused by human papillomavirus (HPV). Many subtypes of HPV are responsible.

Clinical Features. Warts appear as firm, circumscribed, verrucous papules or nodules on the hands, face, or scalp. Any skin site may be affected, including the lips and oral mucosa.

Histopathology. Warts show hyperkeratosis, acanthosis, and papillomatosis. Also seen are foci of koilocytic cells (vacuolated cells) in the stratum malpighii, focal areas of parakeratosis, and clumped keratohyaline granules.

Treatment. Most warts regress spontaneously within 2 years. Treatment for warts is nonspecific destruction; various destructive methods include cryotherapy, salicylates, and excision. Cimetidine has been reported to be effective in children.

Flat Wart (Verruca Plana)

Clinical Features. Flat warts are flat, smooth papules that typically measure 0.2 to 0.4 cm. They are usually flesh colored or hyperpigmented and have minimal scale. The dorsal aspects of the hands and the face are frequently involved sites.

Like other warts, flat warts are caused by HPV, specifically subtypes 3 and 10. These subtypes have not been associated with malignant transformation.

Histology. The epidermis shows hyperkeratosis, acanthosis, and slight elongation of rete ridges but no papillomatosis or parakeratosis. The cells of the granular layer often have diffuse vacuolation with basophilic nuclei. The dermis appears normal.

Treatment. Treatment is often difficult and frustrating. Results often depend on the modality used. These include application of dry ice, liquid nitrogen, caustic agents, or retinoic acid.

VESICLES/BULLAE/PUSTULES

Vesicles, bullae, and pustules represent a circumscribed collection of fluid within or just beneath the epithelium. Vesicles measure up to 0.5 cm, whereas bullae measure greater than 0.5 cm in diameter. Pustules are circumscribed collections of pus (leukocytes and serum) that vary in size from 0.1 to 2 cm. Pustules may be primary or secondary lesions.

Herpes Simplex Infection

Herpes simplex virus (HSV) infections occur in mucosa, in skin, and on the vermilion of the lips. Infection occurs because of direct inoculation by HSV type I and occasionally HSV type II. Viral particles are shed from lesions until a crust forms, about 5 to 7 days after the earliest appearance of the disease. Shedding of virus during the latent or asymptomatic period has been documented.

Cutaneous lesions of primary and secondary herpes are initially vesicular in nature (Fig. 17–41), followed quickly by an ulcerative stage. The disease is self-limited and is currently best treated with antiviral agents (acyclovir, famciclovir, valacyclovir). Chronic mucocutaneous HSV infection is defined as unresolved HSV infection lasting longer than one month. Chronic mucocutaneous HSV may appear as large unhealing ulcers or as inflammatory tumors and is a diagnostic defining criterion for acquired immunodeficiency syndrome (see Chapter 1).

Varicella-Zoster Infection

Varicella-zoster virus (VZV) infections affect mucosa and skin in a similar fashion. Both primary (varicella) and secondary (zoster) infections begin as vesicles that ultimately ulcerate and crust (Figs. 17–42 and 17–43). The most commonly affected site is the trunk, followed by the head and neck and then the lumbosacral region. Pain is a frequent complication during and after clinical healing. Postzoster neuralgia is defined as pain lasting longer than 4 to 6 weeks. Zoster infections may signal the presence of a lymphoma or an immunocompromising condition.

Treatment. Acyclovir and its derivatives are not as effective against VZV as they are against HSV. However, with higher doses, acyclovir provides adequate control. Even though systemic corticosteroids are generally contraindicated in infectious disease, they have been used in VZV

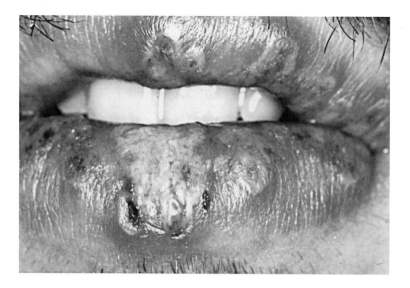

Figure 17–41. Herpes simplex labialis.

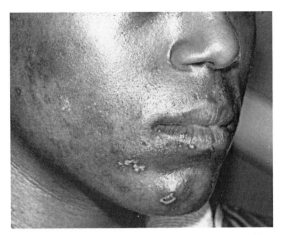

Figure 17–42. Unilateral vesiculo-ulcerative eruption of herpes zoster.

infections to help control postzoster neuralgia (see also Chapter 1).

Contact Dermatitis

Contact dermatitis (CD) is a spongiotic dermatitis (also referred to as *eczematous*) that is a reaction to environmental substances. CD may be classified as irritant or allergic CD. Irritant CD is a nonallergic inflammation of the skin caused by direct toxic effects of irritants. Toxic chemicals include alkalis, detergents, and organic solvents. Even repeated wetting and drying is very irritating. Allergic CD is a delayed-type hypersensitivity reaction that is precipitated by specific antigens that include *Rhus* (poison ivy, oak, and sumac), nickel, rubber, preservatives in cosmetics, and topical medications.

Clinical Features. Allergic and irritant CD are not always clinically distinguishable. However,

CD may present as simple dryness, cracking, or erythema but may be vesicular, necrotic, or ulcerative. The reaction depends on the type of chemical, concentration, mode of exposure, local barriers, and body site. Allergic CD may present 24 to 72 hours after exposure to the antigen as pruritic, erythematous vesicles and papules. Sharply demarcated reaction patterns are diagnostic of an allergic CD and represent the exact shape of the offending substance.

Histopathology. The histologic pattern of irritant CD ranges from the spongiotic changes of allergic CD to extensive ulceration. Necrosis, often into the dermis, neutrophilic infiltration, and acantholysis are much more frequent in irritant CD than in the allergic form. In early allergic CD, the epidermis is spongiotic, and vesicles, if present, may contain Langerhans cells. Eosinophils are often present in the dermal infiltrate and areas of spongiosis. Continued exposure to the antigen may eventually produce lichen simplex chronicus.

Treatment. Diagnosis and identification of the offending compound by history or by testing for delayed hypersensitivity reaction (patch testing) is the first step in managing suspected allergic contact dermatitis. In both allergic and irritant dermatitis, subsequent avoidance of the offending substance is required, and desensitization for the antigenic substances may be beneficial if it is identified.

Impetigo

Impetigo is an acute superficial bacterial infection of the skin. This superficial infection of the skin is due to group A streptococci, *S. aureus*, or a mixture of the two. Complications associated with impetigo are unusual. Nonetheless, glomeru-

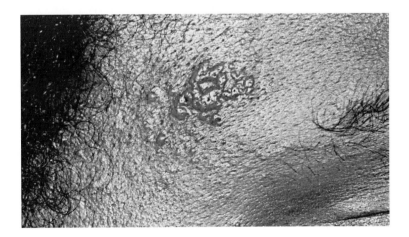

Figure 17–43. Unilateral vesiculo-ulcerative eruption of herpes zoster.

lonephritis can occur with some strains of streptococci. In the vast majority of cases, however, impetigo clears rapidly with proper therapy.

Clinical Features. This infection, common in children and adolescents, is highly contagious and spreads readily within the home, school, or institution. The initial lesion is a small vesicle on the face, extending periorally and along the base of the nose (Fig. 17–44). As vesicles rupture, crusts form and pus appears. Autoinoculation produces spread to other sites. Areas affected are pruritic and typically measure from 1 to 3 cm. Central healing is noted as the lesions progress centrifugally (polycyclic pattern). In the perioral region, impetigo may be confused with recurrent or secondary HSV infections.

Treatment. Antibiotics are required to treat impetigo. Penicillinase-stable antibiotics may be necessary if *Staphylococcus* is an etiologic agent. New generations of potent topical antibiotics such as mupirocin are also clinically effective.

Rosacea

Rosacea represents an inflammatory process that involves the infundibular portion of the hair follicles, with various levels of severity. The specific cause of rosacea is unknown, but several factors can influence the evolution of this condition. An underlying vasomotor instability that is worsened by intake of hot beverages, alcohol, and hot or spicy foods is believed to be involved. Environmental factors such as extreme temperatures and sunlight can also exacerbate this condition. Vasodilator drugs can produce flushing and worsen the condition. Rosacea may develop in association with use of topical corticosteroid medications, sometimes called *steroid rosacea*. Topically applied potent preparations initially produce vasoconstriction. On discontinuation of this therapy, however, rebound vasodilatation takes place and often worsens the underlying condition.

Clinical Features. Rosacea is characterized by facial erythema with or without an overlying papular/pustular eruption. Comedones of acne are absent. Distribution is over the central portion of the face, especially the cheeks, nose, and chin (Fig. 17–45). The condition usually begins in the fourth decade of life and may occur later in women in association with menopause. The eyes may also be involved, with attendant symptoms of conjunctivitis, blepharitis, and keratitis.

Severe and long-standing cases of rosacea may result in formation of bulbous, greasy, and hypertrophic lesions of the nose. This condition, known as *rhinophyma*, occurs particularly in men older than 40 years (Fig. 17–46). The nasal tip and alae are usually involved by persistent lymphedema and sebaceous gland hyperplasia, resulting in the clinical appearance of extremely dilated follicles containing large plugs of keratin and sebaceous material.

Histopathology. Rosacea is essentially a follicular inflammatory process that progresses to a suppurative folliculitis and ultimately to a granulomatous form with associated dermatitis. Epithelioid granulomas may form. In rhinophyma, massive sebaceous gland hyperplasia and associated infundibular cysts are seen. Cysts tend to rupture or leak into the surrounding dermis, causing a granulomatous response and suppuration.

Treatment. The mainstay of therapy remains systemic tetracycline and topical metronidazole.

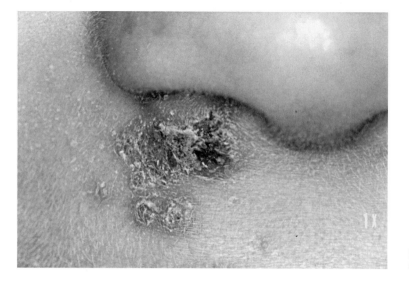

Figure 17–44. Impetigo above the upper lip.

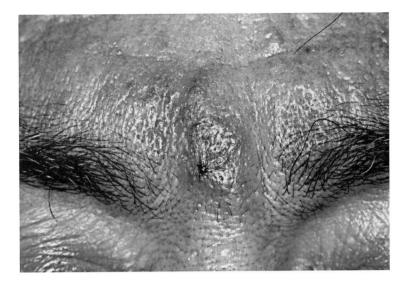

Figure 17–45. Rosacea of the forehead.

Patients are urged to avoid heat, cold, sunlight, alcohol, coffee, and spicy foods. Rhinophyma management is surgical.

Erythema Multiforme

Erythema multiforme (EM) is an acute inflammatory skin disease. The clinical spectrum of EM is variable and is generally classified by the degree of involvement of the skin or the number of mucous membranes affected. EM is associated with infectious agents (*Mycoplasma* or HSV), drugs, connective tissue disease, or internal malignancies. However, many cases are idiopathic. EM

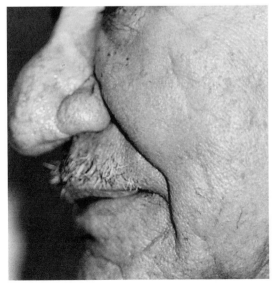

Figure 17–46. Rhinophyma.

major, or Stevens-Johnson syndrome, is an extremely severe mucocutaneous eruption that often has considerable systemic involvement (see Chapter 2).

Clinical Features. Erythema multiforme is associated with a mild prodrome (symptoms including malaise, fever, and itching or burning of the skin where the lesions will later appear). In EM minor, the cutaneous lesions are typically symmetric red macules, papules, or target-like papules less than 2 cm in diameter, located on the extremities and face. Lesions disappear in about 1 month. When the lips are involved, a hemorrhagic crust associated with superficial erosions is characteristically located on the lower lip and extends into the oral cavity.

In EM major (Stevens-Johnson), fever and upper respiratory tract symptoms precede the eruption by days to several weeks. Vesicles and bullae appear on the two or more mucosal sites with an associated maculopapular eruption. Pneumonitis occasionally accompanies the cutaneous findings. Mortality rates in patients with untreated Stevens-Johnson syndrome may be as great as 5 to 15%.

Histopathology. The hallmark of EM is death of individual keratinocytes in the stratum malpighii. Orthokeratosis, vacuolization of the basal cell layer, and a sparse perivascular lymphoid infiltrate are noted. Edema of the papillary dermis with considerable inflammation and spongiosis may also be observed. Bullous lesions demonstrate full-thickness epidermal necrosis. Immunofluorescence testing often shows deposits of IgM, C3, and fibrinogen in the walls of superficial dermal vasculature and along the dermal-epidermal junction.

Treatment. EM minor with a minimal number

of lesions is usually not treated. More extensive involvement may be treated with a short course of oral corticosteroids. The offending drug should be discontinued. If HSV is the cause, prophylaxis is appropriate. Recurrences are common. The use of corticosteroids to treat EM major remains a controversial but commonly used therapy. Symptomatic treatment and antibiotic therapy for secondary bacterial infection are appropriate.

Pemphigus Vulgaris/ Foliaceus/Erythematosus

Pemphigus vulgaris is an autoimmune bullous eruption characterized by intraepidermal separation of keratinocytes one from another. One third of patients present with oral erosions and ulcers. However, cutaneous flaccid bullae are characteristic (see Chapter 1). Two variants of pemphigus occur without oral involvement. Pemphigus foliaceus is a superficial, less severe form of pemphigus. It is also rarer than pemphigus vulgaris. The age of onset of pemphigus foliaceus is variable, but it usually develops in middle-aged persons. Pemphigus erythematosus resembles, occurs simultaneously with, and has immunologic markers identical to systemic lupus erythematosus (SLE).

Pemphigus foliaceus begins as localized areas of erythema with eventual evolution of scaling, crusting, and occasionally bullae that itch or burn on the scalp, face, upper trunk, and back. Oral lesions are present only rarely. Pemphigus erythematosus is characterized by a malar rash and bullous lesions with a seborrheic quality located elsewhere on the body.

Histopathology. Pemphigus foliaceus may have the following histologic patterns: (1) eosinophilic spongiosis, (2) subcorneal blistering with few acantholytic keratinocytes, and (3) subcorneal blistering with dyskeratotic granular cells. A variable inflammatory infiltrate is found. Immunofluorescence testing reveals deposition of IgG in the epidermal intercellular substance. Pemphigus erythematosus is histologically identical to pemphigus foliaceus. However, immunofluorescence testing reveals IgG deposition both in the epidermal intercellular substance and in the granular deposition of IgG, IgM, and C3 at the dermal-epidermal junction (positive lupus band test result).

Treatment. Pemphigus foliaceus tends to follow a fluctuating course. Severe flares respond to systemic corticosteroids. However, adjuvant therapy with drugs such as cyclophosphamide, azathioprine, or dapsone may be necessary. In the case of pemphigus erythematosus, a search for concom-

itant SLE should be undertaken because of overlap between the two entities.

EROSIONS/FISSURES/ ULCERS/SCARS

These secondary skin lesions all represent focal destruction of cutaneous tissue. Erosions are defined as loss of the epidermis only. Erosions heal without scar. Ulcers are defined as epidermal loss and dermal damage. Cutaneous ulcers heal with scar. Scars are permanent alterations in the appearance of skin and are due to damage and collageneous repair of the skin.

Perlèche

Perlèche, or angular cheilitis, is inflammation and atrophy of the skin folds at the angles of the mouth. This may be due to excessive lip licking, thumb sucking, or sagging of facial skin in edentulous or elderly persons. Prolonged contact with saliva results in maceration, with possible secondary infection by *Candida* or staphylococci.

Clinical Features. The skin at the angles of the mouth has erythematous fissures with frequent exudate and crust (Fig. 17–47). Further licking to moisten the inflamed area exacerbates the problem.

Treatment. Treatment consists of applying antimicrobial creams, followed by low-potency steroid creams until the symptoms resolve. Protective lip balm may help prevent recurrence.

Pyoderma Gangrenosum

Pyoderma gangrenosum (PG) is a rare inflammatory condition that may occur in association with systemic disease such as ulcerative colitis, Crohn's disease, rheumatoid arthritis, and chronic active hepatitis. PG is in the spectrum of neutrophilic dermatoses.

Clinical Features. PG starts out as a painful nodule or pustule that ulcerates. The ulcer is surrounded by a dusky to purplish undermined border with a purulent base. PG may occur anywhere, but lesions are found commonly on the lower legs, buttocks, head, and neck. PG may occur at any age. The course typically extends over weeks to months or even years.

Histopathology. The histology of PG is nonspecific; however, a neutrophilic and an undermined ulceration is suggestive. The infiltrate often extends into the deep dermis or subcutis.

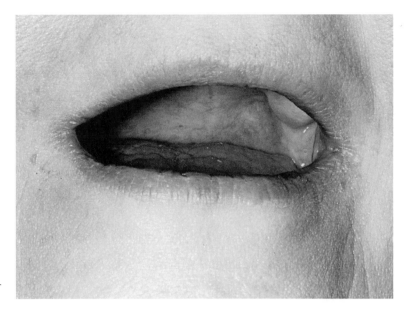

Figure 17–47. Perlèche, or angular cheilitis.

Treatment. Diagnosis and treatment of the underlying systemic disease are necessary as initial treatment. Individual ulcers respond variably to intralesional or systemic steroids. Dapsone and immunosuppressive drugs have also shown success. Local care with wet compresses is essential. Aggressive débridement is contraindicated.

Burns

The skin is burned on exposure to extremes of heat, with severity depending on temperature, skin thickness, and duration of exposure. Thermal damage to the skin causes coagulation necrosis, enzymatic inactivation, and capillary damage.

Clinical Features. Healing is slow, with considerable scarring. *First-degree* burns are superficial burns that appear soft and hyperemic without blister formation. Healing occurs without scarring. *Second-degree* burns may be superficial or deep and involve the dermis to some extent. *Third-degree* burns involve full-thickness destruction of the skin with extensive scar formation that almost always requires grafting.

Histopathology. *First-degree* burns show intraepidermal edema and occasionally superficial necrosis. In *second-degree* burns, variable epidermal necrosis, blister formation, and epidermal edema are noted. Superficial necrosis of dermal collagen may be observed. *Third-degree* burns are characterized by full-thickness necrosis of the epidermis and dermis. Scars show homogeneous collagen and loss of skin appendages.

Treatment. Treatment depends on the type of burn and exceeds the scope of this chapter.

Keloid

Clinical Features. Keloids are hyperplastic scars that persist or enlarge over the course of one to several years (Fig. 17–48). These lesions are often tender, painful, or hyperesthetic, especially early in development. They are commonly located on the shoulder, chest, or head but may occur anywhere, usually after injury. Keloids are more common in African-Americans.

Histopathology. The epidermis may be flattened, and adnexal structures or elastic fibers may be few. In the dermis, nodules of hypereosinophilic collagen are arranged in thick, compacted bands.

Treatment. Treatment includes surgical removal, steroid injections, cryotherapy, or silicone gel sheeting. Recurrences are very common.

Radiodermatitis

Clinical Features. Acute radiodermatitis, in contrast to sunburns, develops after large doses of high-energy radiation. Within about 1 week after exposure, erythema develops, with desquamation or blister formation. Ulcers may form after very large doses of radiation; lesions may scar or not heal at all. Long-term administration of smaller doses results in atrophy, telangiectasias, or pigment changes. Squamous cell carcinoma may develop in areas of severe radiation damage.

Histopathology. Early in the course of radiodermatitis, the epidermis has intracellular edema with pyknosis of nuclei. Adnexal structures show

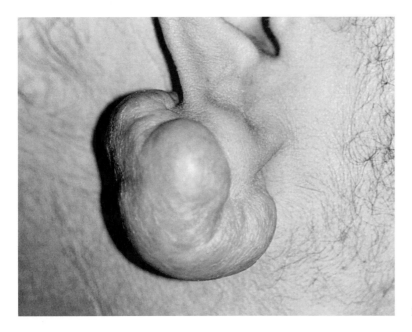

Figure 17–48. Keloid of the ear.

acute degenerative changes. Vasodilatation and an inflammatory infiltrate are noted throughout the dermis and into the epidermis. Late changes include concomitant atrophy and hyperplasia of the epidermis, swelling of irregularly staining collagen bundles, and the presence of large, irregular fibroblasts. Telangiectasias are present.

Treatment. Initial treatment includes avoiding UV exposure, applying cool compresses, washing with water only, and drying with powders. Antibacterial ointments may also be helpful to prevent secondary invasion of bacteria. After the initial exudative phase, oil and water emulsions are useful, but corticosteroids have little effect.

CONNECTIVE TISSUE DISEASES

Dermatomyositis

Dermatomyositis is one of the major systemic inflammatory diseases of connective tissue. It is manifested as an inflammatory myopathy with characteristic cutaneous findings. Dermatomyositis is an uncommon disease with characteristic dual peaks of occurrence, one in childhood and one in late middle age. Systemic manifestations of dermatomyositis include proximal symmetric muscle weakness, elevated levels of muscle enzymes, characteristic muscle biopsy findings, muscle pain, and eventually muscle atrophy. Dermatomyositis may be associated with malignancy, especially in adults.

Clinical Features. The main dermatologic findings in dermatomyositis are the heliotrope rash and Gottron's papules. The heliotrope rash is a distinctive violaceous, slightly edematous periorbital swelling. It is found most often on the upper eyelids (Fig. 17–49). Gottron's papules are discrete purple-red papules over bony prominences such as the knees, knuckles, and elbows (Fig. 17–50). Evolution of these papules into plaques with telangiectasis and pigmentary changes is known as *Gottron's sign*.

Histopathology. The histologic changes may be almost indistinguishable from those seen in SLE. The epidermis is thinned, the basement membrane is fragmented, a sparse lymphocytic infiltrate is found perivascularly, and interstitial mucin is deposited. Severe inflammatory changes may include subepidermal fibrin deposition. Unlike SLE, dermatomyositis is not characterized by immune complexes at the dermal-epidermal junction.

Treatment. Treatment of dermatomyositis is usually with prednisone and bed rest, with tapering initiated once muscle weakness has started to improve. Other modalities used for unresponsive cases include plasmapheresis, cytotoxic drugs, and total body irradiation. Improvement usually occurs with use of steroids; however, this is often a very chronic and debilitating disease. Treatment of the underlying malignancy, if present, resolves the symptoms.

Lupus Erythematosus (LE)

In its systemic form, LE affects major organs such as the kidneys, heart, lungs, and joints, and

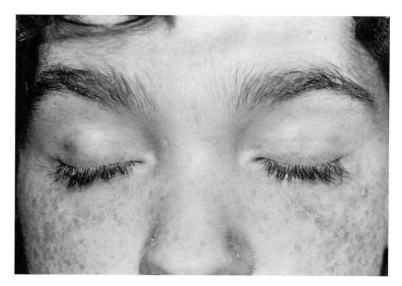

Figure 17–49. The heliotrope rash of dermatomyositis.

results of laboratory tests for autoantibodies are positive. The discoid/cutaneous form may result in cosmetically unacceptable lesions, whereas the systemic form may cause organ dysfunction and ultimately death. Discoid lupus erythematosus (DLE) is the most frequent form of cutaneous lupus erythematosus and usually involves only the skin above the neck. Cutaneous lesions typically appear as erythematous patches that may develop central scarring. Although related to SLE, DLE lacks the systemic manifestations except in infrequent cases of generalized DLE (when lesions are present both above and below the neck) (see Chapter 2).

Clinical Features. DLE presents as discrete erythematous, infiltrated plaques characterized by follicular plugging and thick, adherent scales (car-pet tacks). Older lesions often appear atrophic and may have pigmentary changes (Figs. 17–51 and 17–52). Some lesions may show verrucous hyper-keratosis at the periphery. The most commonly affected sites in DLE are the face (malar area), scalp, ears, oral mucosa, and vermilion of the lips. Oral mucosal involvement is seen in approximately 15% of cases of DLE, with either characteristic silvery-white striae on the vermilion border or sunburst-like plaques of the oral mucosa. SLE may develop in generalized DLE and DLE can be identified in patients with SLE. A thorough history and physical examination should help identify any systemic manifestations. Results of laboratory tests in DLE are generally negative. However, persistently high-titer-positive antinuclear antibody, hypergammaglobulinemia, and positive re-

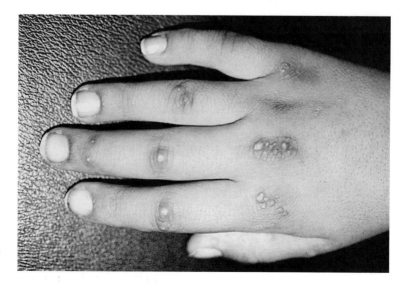

Figure 17–50. Gottron's papules of dermatomyositis.

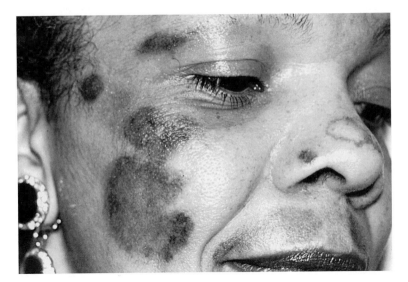

Figure 17–51. Discoid lupus erythematosus.

sults of a lupus band test usually indicate systemic disease.

Histopathology. Histopathologic findings of DLE include hyperkeratosis of the stratum corneum with follicular plugging, with dyskeratosis and flattening of the stratum malpighii and vacuolar degeneration of the basal layer. The basement membrane is often thickened and tortuous, with a junctional or appendageal lymphoid infiltrate that may extend subcutaneously. Edema and mucin deposition are noted in the dermis. Immunofluorescence studies of DLE lesions demonstrate a thick band of immunoglobulin at the dermal-epidermal junction.

Treatment. DLE can produce permanent scarring; therefore, the lesions should be treated aggressively with local measures. Topical or intralesional corticosteroids (care must be used on the face) are the mainstay of treatment. For lesions that do not respond to local measures, antimalarial agents (i.e., hydroxychloroquine or dapsone) are the next line of therapy; systemic corticosteroids are not indicated for solely cutaneous involvement. All patients with DLE must be meticulous about sun protection in order to limit their risk of developing skin cancers and activating their disease.

Scleroderma

Scleroderma is a chronic disease of unknown cause, although it is generally regarded as an immune dysfunction condition. Two basic forms are

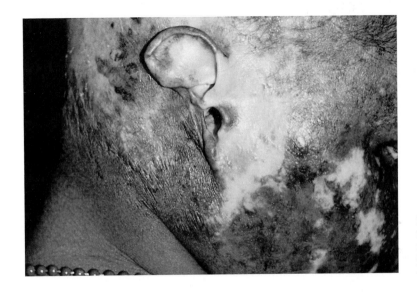

Figure 17–52. Discoid lupus erythematosus. Patient had ear resection for aggressive squamous cell carcinoma, which developed within a DLE lesion.

recognized: a relatively inconsequential but disfiguring localized cutaneous form known as *morphea* and a potentially life-threatening form known as *systemic scleroderma*. The remainder of this discussion focuses on the systemic type. It often occurs in conjunction with other autoimmune conditions such as rheumatoid arthritis, lupus erythematosus, dermatomyositis, and Sjögren's syndrome. Rheumatoid factor and antinuclear antibodies are typically demonstrable in patients with scleroderma. Hypergammaglobulinemia and an elevated sedimentation rate are also noted. Along with an increased rate of collagen synthesis is the appearance of vascular changes. Inflammatory and obstructive changes are seen microscopically in arterioles and capillaries, supporting the notion that vessel changes are important in the pathogenesis of scleroderma. Also, Raynaud's phenomenon, a peripheral vascular condition, frequently precedes the other manifestations of the disease. Systemic scleroderma appears usually during middle age (30 to 50 years) and predominantly in women (4:1). There is no racial predilection.

Clinical Features. The disease can affect any organ and may progress to affect many organ systems. The skin is typically affected first, although joint involvement may provide the initial sign. In time, as fibrosis of organs progresses, signs of organ failure begin to appear.

Cutaneous manifestations are typified by pitting edema early, followed by tightness and rigidity of the skin (Fig. 17–53). The skin eventually becomes indurated, smooth, and atrophic, with telangiectasias. The face becomes expressionless and seems mask-like. Fibrosis of the fingers leads to stiffness and atrophy of the skin over the digits.

Vascular compromise may result in ischemia and ulceration of the fingertips—a phenomenon seen in both scleroderma and Raynaud's phenomenon.

The rigidity of the perioral skin causes restriction of the oral orifice. Oral hygiene and routine dental care become difficult. Fibrosis of the salivary glands gives rise to xerostomia and potentially to cervical caries. Mandibular bone resorption and uniformly widened periodontal membranes (as seen in periapical films) are also characteristic oral manifestations of this disease.

Histopathology. The primary histologic feature of scleroderma is the deposition of vast amounts of relatively acellular collagen. Perivascular lymphocytic infiltrates are also typical. Minor salivary gland changes include pronounced interstitial fibrosis and acinar atrophy.

Treatment. Systemic disease stabilizes in most patients after a time. Patients with progressive disease are likely to succumb to renal, cardiac, or pulmonary failure. Other than supportive therapy, there is no satisfactory treatment for scleroderma. Corticosteroids may provide some benefit early but are not likely to give lasting control in progressive cases. Other drugs such as penicillamine and azathioprine have shown some promise.

Temporal Arteritis

Temporal arteritis, a variant of giant-cell arteritis, is encountered primarily in the elderly. Patients present with headache, scalp tenderness, claudication of the temporalis and masseter, visual disturbances (including blindness), and stroke. Results of laboratory tests are nonspecific, but an erythrocyte sedimentation rate greater than 50 mm/hr is

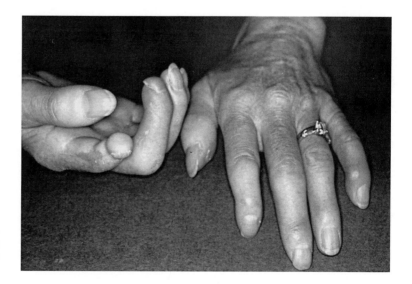

Figure 17–53. Scleroderma resulting in cutaneous atrophy. Note loss of the tip of the right index finger.

commonly found. Prompt referral and initiation of treatment with high-dose prednisone are necessary to prevent irreversible blindness.

Bibliography

Café au Lait Macule

Benedict PH, Szabo G, Fitzpatrick TB, Sinesi SJ. Melanotic macules in Albright's syndrome and in neurofibromatosis. JAMA 205:618–626, 1968.

Jimbow K, Szabo G, Fitzpatrick TB. Ultrastructure of giant pigment granules (macromelanosomes) in the cutaneous pigmented macules of neurofibromatosis. J Invest Dermatol 61:300–309, 1973.

Solar Lentigo

Montagna W, Hu F, Carlisle K. A reinvestigation of solar lentigines. Arch Dermatol 116:1151–1154, 1980.

Griffiths CE, Goldfarb MT, Finkel LJ, et al. Topical tretinoin (retinoic acid) treatment of hyperpigmented lesions associated with photoaging in Chinese and Japanese patients: a vehicle-controlled trial. J Am Acad Dermatol 30:76–84, 1994.

Melasma

Sanchez NP, Pathak MA, Sato S, et al. Melasma: a clinical, light microscopic, ultrastructural, and immunofluorescence study. J Am Acad Dermatol 4:698–710, 1981.

Erysipelas

Bisno AL, Stevens DL. Streptococcal infections of skin and soft tissues. N Engl J Med 334:1478, 1996.

Neurofibromatosis/Café au Lait Macules

Riccardi VM. Von Recklinghausen neurofibromatosis (review). N Engl J Med 305:1617–1627, 1981.

Sebaceous Hyperplasia

Rosian R, Goslen JB, Brodell RT. The treatment of benign sebaceous hyperplasia with the topical application of bichloracetic acid. J Dermatol Surg Oncol 17:876–879, 1991.

Syringoma

Friedman SJ, Butler DF. Syringoma presenting as milia. J Am Acad Dermatol 16:310–314, 1987.

Favre-Racouchot

Hassounah A, Pierard GE. Kerosis and comedos without prominent elastosis in Favre-Racouchot disease. Am J Dermatopathol 9:15–17, 1987.

Nevi

Rhodes AR, Silverman RA, Harrist TJ, Melski JW. A histologic comparison of congenital and acquired nevomelanocytic nevi. Arch Dermatol 121:1266–1273, 1985.

Folliculitis

Pravada DJ, Pugliese MM. Tinea faciei. Arch Dermatol 114:250–252, 1978.

Furuncle

Pinkus H. Furuncle. J Cutan Pathol 6:517–518, 1979.

Granuloma Faciale

Bergfeld WF, Scholes HT, Roenigk HH Jr. Granuloma faciale—treatment by dermabrasion. Report of a case. Cleve Clin Q 37:215–218, 1970.

Nieboer C, Kalsbeek GL. Immunofluorescence studies in granuloma eosinophilicum faciale. J Cutan Path 5:68–75, 1978.

Strawberry Hemangioma

Garden JM, Bakus AD. Clinical efficacy of the pulsed dye laser in the treatment of vascular lesions. J Dermatol Surg Oncol 19:321–326, 1993.

Illingworth RS. Thoughts on treatment of strawberry naevi (review). Arch Dis Child 51:138–140, 1976.

Reyes BA, Vazquez-Botet M, Capo H. Intralesional steroids in cutaneous hemangioma. J Dermatol Surg Oncol 15:828–832, 1989.

Spitz Nevus

Paniago-Pereira C, Maize JC, Ackerman AB. Nevus of large spindle and/or epithelioid cells (Spitz's nevus). Arch Dermatol 114:1811–1823, 1978.

Weedon D, Little JH. Spindle and epithelioid cell nevi in children and adults. A review of 211 cases of the Spitz nevus. Cancer 40:217–225, 1977.

Sweet's Syndrome

Von den Driesch P. Sweet's syndrome (acute febrile neutrophilic dermatosis). J Am Acad Dermatol 31:535–556, 1994.

Lichen Planus

Buechner SA. T cell subsets and macrophages in lichen planus. In situ identification using monoclonal antibodies and histochemical techniques. Dermatologica 169:325–329, 1984.

Ellis FA. Histopathology of lichen planus based on analysis of one hundred biopsy specimens. J Invest Dermatol 48:143–148, 1967.

Holmstrup P, Dabelsteen E. Changes in carbohydrate expression of lichen planus affected oral epithelial cell membranes. J Invest Dermatol 73:364–367, 1979.

Venous Lakes

Alcalay J, Sandbank M. The ultrastructure of cutaneous venous lakes. Int J Dermatol 26:645–646, 1987.

Angiosarcoma

Haustein UF. Angiosarcoma of the face and scalp. Int J Dermatol 30:851–856, 1991.

Holden CA, Spittle MF, Jones EW. Angiosarcoma of the face and scalp, prognosis and treatment. Cancer 59:1046–1057, 1987.

Rosai J, Summer HW, Kostianovsky M, Perez-Mesa C. Angiosarcoma of the skin. A clinicopathologic and fine structural study. Hum Pathol 7:83–109, 1976.

Wart/Flat Wart

Gross G, Pfister H, Hagedorn M, Gissmann L. Correlation between human papillomavirus (HPV) type and histology of warts. J Invest Dermatol 78:160–164, 1982.

Lutzner MA. The human papillomaviruses. A review. Arch Dermatol 119:631–635, 1983.

Keratoacanthoma

Muir EG, Bell AJ, Barlow KA. Multiple primary carcinomata of the colon, duodenum, and larynx associated with keratoacanthomata of the face. Br J Surg 54:191–195, 1967.

Wade TR, Ackerman AB. The many faces of keratoacanthomas. J Dermatol Surg Oncol 4:498–501, 1978.

Atopic Dermatitis

Cooper KD. Atopic dermatitis: recent trends in pathogenesis and therapy (review). J Invest Dermatol 102:128–137, 1994.

Leung DY, Bhan AK, Schneeberger EE, Geha RS. Characterization of the mononuclear cell infiltrate in atopic dermatitis using monoclonal antibodies. J Allergy Clinical Immunol 71:47–56, 1983.

Stone SP, Muller SA, Gleich GJ. IgE levels in atopic dermatitis. Arch Dermatol 108:806–811, 1973.

Pityriasis Rosea

Panizzon R, Bloch PH. Histopathology of pityriasis rosea Gibert. Qualitative and quantitative light-microscopic study of 62 biopsies of 40 patients. Dermatologica 165:551–558, 1982.

Erythema Multiforme

Bushkell LL, Mackel SE, Jordon RE. Erythema multiforme: direct immunofluorescence studies and detection of circulating immune complexes. J Invest Dermatol 74:372–374, 1980.

Detjen PF, Patterson R, Noskin GA, et al. Herpes simplex virus associated with recurrent Stevens-Johnson syndrome.

A management strategy. Arch Intern Med 152:1513–1516, 1992.

Howland WW, Golitz LE, Weston WL, Huff JC. Erythema multiforme: clinical, histopathologic, and immunologic study. J Am Acad Dermatol 10:438–446, 1984.

Levy M, Shear NH. *Mycoplasma pneumoniae* infections and Stevens-Johnson syndrome. Report of eight cases and review of the literature. Clin Pediatr 30:42–49, 1991.

Pemphigus

Amerian ML, Ahmed AR. Pemphigus erythematosus. Presentation of four cases and review of literature. J Am Acad Dermatol 10:215–222, 1984.

Pyoderma Gangrenosum

Hurwitz RM, Haseman JH. The evolution of pyoderma gangrenosum. A clinicopathologic correlation. Am J Dermatopathol 15:28–33, 1993.

Powell FC, Schroeter AL, Su WP, Perry HO. Pyoderma gangrenosum and monoclonal gammopathy. Arch Dermatol 119:468–472, 1983.

Dermatomyositis

Callen JP. Malignancy in polymyositis/dermatomyositis. Clin Dermatol 6:55–63, 1988.

Cronin ME, Plotz PH. Idiopathic inflammatory myopathies. Rheum Dis Clin North Am 16:655–665, 1990.

Janis JF, Winkelmann RK. Histopathology of the skin in dermatomyositis. A histopathologic study of 55 cases. Arch Dermatol 97:640–650, 1968.

Discoid Lupus Erythematosus

Coburn PR, Shuster S. Dapsone and discoid lupus erythematosus. Br J Dermatol 106:105–106, 1982.

Millard LG, Rowell NR. Abnormal laboratory test results and their relationship to prognosis in discoid lupus erythematosus. A long-term follow-up study of 92 patients. Arch Dermatol 115:1055–1058, 1979.

Prystowsky SD, Gilliam JN. Discoid lupus erythematosus as part of a larger disease spectrum. Correlation of clinical features with laboratory findings in lupus erythematosus. Arch Dermatol 111:1448–1452, 1975.

Weiss JS. Antimalarial medications in dermatology. A review. Dermatol Clin 9:377–385, 1991.

Index

Note: Page numbers in *italics* refer to illustrations; page numbers followed by t refer to tables. Page numbers preceded by "O-" refer to overview section.

519

ISBN 0-7216-7731-2

90038